Management of Rare Adult Tumours

Springer

Paris
Berlin
Heidelberg
New York
Hong Kong
Londres
Milan
Tokyo

Management of Rare Adult Tumours

Editors

Yazid Belkacémi
René-Olivier Mirimanoff
Mahmut Ozsahin

Springer

Yazid Belkacémi MD PhD

Professor in Radiation Oncology
Deputy Head of the Department of Radiation Oncology
Hôpital Henri-Mondor
51, avenue du Maréchal-de-Lattre-de-Tassigny
94000 Créteil Cedex
France

René-Olivier Mirimanoff MD

Professor in Radiation Oncology
Head of the Department of Radiation Oncology
Centre hospitalier universitaire Vaudois
Rue du Bugnon
CH-1011 Lausanne
Switzerland

Mahmut Ozsahin MD PhD

Associate Professor in Radiation Oncology
Department of Radiation Oncology
Centre hospitalier universitaire Vaudois
Rue du Bugnon
CH-1011 Lausanne
Switzerland

ISBN-13 : 978-2-287-92245-9 Springer Paris Berlin Heidelberg New York

Imprimé en France

Springer-Verlag France est membre du groupe Springer Science + Business Media

Maquette de couverture : Jean-François Montmarché

List of Contributors

Stefan Aebi, Pr., Dr.
Department of Medical Oncology
University Hospital/Inselspital
Freiburgstrasse
3000 Berne
Switzerland

Ingrid Alexandre
Université Pierre et Marie Curie
Department of Medical Oncology
Hôpital Tenon
APREC, Assistance Publique – Hôpitaux de Paris
4, rue de la Chine
75970 Paris Cedex 20
France

Yavuz Anacak, Dr.
Department of Radiation Oncology
Ege University Tip Fakültesi, Bornova
35100 Izmir
Turkey

Martine Antoine
Service d'Anatomie Pathologique
Faculté de Médecine Pierre et Marie Curie
Université Paris-VI
Hôpital Tenon
Assistance publique – Hôpitaux de Paris
4, rue de la Chine
75970 Paris
France

David Azria, MD
Département d'oncologie radiothérapie
CRLC Val d'Aurelle
208, rue des Apothicaires - Parc Euro-médecine
34298 Montpellier Cedex 5
France

Marie-Christine Baranzelli, Dr., MD
Centre de lutte contre le cancer Oscar-Lambret
3, rue Fréderic-Combemale
BP307
59020 Lille Cedex
France

Jean Bauer MER, Dr., Médecin Adjoint
Centre Pluridisciplinaire d'Oncologie
University Hospital (CHUV)
Rue du Bugnon
CH-1011 Lausanne
Switzerland

Karl Thomas Beer, MD, EMBA
Centre de Radio-oncologie Bienne-Seeland-Jura Bernois
38, Chemin des vignes
2503 Bienne
Switzerland

Yazid Belkacémi, MD, PhD
Professor in Radiation Oncology
Deputy Head of the Department of Radiation Oncology
Hôpital Henri-Mondor
51, avenue du Maréchal-de-Lattre-de-Tassigny
94000 Créteil Cedex
France

Jean-Yves Blay, Pr.
Université Claude Bernard
Cancer Center Léon-Bérard
28, rue Laënnec
69008 Lyon
France

Jacques Bonneterre
University Lille-II
Department of Radiation Oncology

Centre de lutte contre le cancer Oscar-Lambret
3, rue Fréderic-Combemale
BP307
59020 Lille Cedex
France

Augustin Bonnichon, Dr.
Department of Pneumology-Oncology
Hôpital d'Instruction des Armées Laveran
34, boulevard Laveran
13013 Marseille

Noureddine Bouaouina
Department of Radiotherapy
Farhat Hached University Hospital
Avenue Ibn-El-Jazzar
4000 Sousse
Tunisia

Guilhem Bousquet, Dr., MD
Department of Medical Oncology
Hôpital Saint-Louis
1, avenue Claude-Vellefaux
75010 Paris
France

Hamouda Boussen, Pr.
Department of Medical Oncology
Institut Salah Azaiz
Boulevard du 9-Avril
1006. Bab Saadoun
Tunis
Tunisia

Luc Bron
Otolaryngology Service
Department of Head and Neck Surgery
University Hospital (CHUV)
Rue du Bugnon
CH-1011 Lausanne
Switzerland

Jacques Cadranel
Faculté de Médecine Pierre et Marie Curie
Université Paris-VI
Service de Pneumologie et Réanimation
Hôpital Tenon
Assistance Publique – Hôpitaux de Paris
4, rue de la Chine
75970 Paris Cedex 20

Mònica Caro
Department of Radiation Oncology
H. Universitari Germans Trias
Institut Català d'Oncologia
08916 Badalona
Barcelona

David Christie, MBChB, FRANZCR, A/Pr.
Premion, John Flynn Private Hospital
42, Inland Drive
Tugun
Queensland 4224
Australia

Jean-François Cordier
Pilot Unit for the Management of Rare Intrathoracic Tumors
Department of Respiratory Medicine
Louis-Pradel Hospital
28, Avenue Doyen-Lépine
69500 Bron
France

Bruno Cutuli, Dr.
Radiothérapie-Oncologie
Polyclinique de Courlancy
38, rue de Courlancy
51100 Reims
France

Eric Dansin, Dr.
Department of General Oncology
Centre de lutte contre le cancer Oscar-Lambret
3, rue Fréderic-Combemale
BP307
59020 Lille Cedex
France

Jean-François Delaloye
Département de Gynécologie et d'Obstétrique
University Hospital (CHUV)
Rue du Bugnon
CH-1011 Lausanne
Switzerland

Nicolas Demartines
Department of Visceral Surgery
University Hospital (CHUV)
Rue du Bugnon
CH-1011 Lausanne
Switzerland

Sylvain Dewas, MD
Pôle de chirurgie thoracique
CHRU de Lille
Boulevard du Professeur-Leclerq
59037 Lille

Fazilet Öner Dinçbaş, Pr., MD
Cerrahpaşa Tıp Fakültesi
Radyasyon Onkolojisi Anabilim Dali
34098 Arakay
Istanbul
Turkey

Anne-Claire Dupont-Gossart
Gastroenterology Department
CHU Jean-Minjoz
2, boulevard Fleming
25030 Besançon Cedex
France

Catherine Durdux, Dr.
Université Paris-Descartes
Department of Oncology-Radiotherapy
Hôpital Européen Georges-Pompidou
20, rue Leblanc
75015 Paris
France

Pierre Duvillard
University Paris XI
Department of Pathology
Institut Gustave-Roussy
39, rue Camille-Desmoulins
94805 Villejuif
France

Charles Ferté
Centre de lutte contre le cancer Oscar-Lambret
3, rue Fréderic-Combemale
BP307
59020 Lille Cedex
France

Maryse Fiche
Institut Universitaire de Pathologie
University Hospital (CHUV)
Rue du Bugnon
CH-1011 Lausanne
Switzerland

Alain Fourquet
Service de Radiothérapie Oncologique
Institut Curie
26, Rue d'Ulm
75005 Paris
France

Nicolas Girard
Human Oncology and Pathogenesis Program
Memorial Sloan-Kettering Cancer Center
1275, York Avenue
New York 10065
USA

Pilot Unit for the Management of Rare Intrathoracic Tumors
Department of Respiratory Medicine
Louis-Pradel Hospital
28, Avenue Doyen-Lépine
69500 Bron
France

Joseph Gligorov, Dr.
University Paris VI
Department of Medical Oncology
Hôpital Tenon
Assistance Publique – Hôpitaux de Paris
4, rue de la Chine
75970 Paris Cedex 20

Günther Gruber, PD, Dr.
Institute of Radiotherapy
Klinik Hirslanden
Witellikerstrasse 60
CH-8032 Zuerich
Switzerland

Bernard Guillot, MD
Department of Dermatology
University of Montpellier I
Hôpital Saint-Eloi
80, avenue Augustin-Fliche
34295 Montpellier Cedex 5
France

Melis Gültekin MD
Department of Radiation Oncology
Hacettepe University Oncology Institute
06100 Ankara
Turkey

Christine Haie-Meder, Dr.
Head of the Brachytherapy Service
Institut Gustave-Roussy
39, rue Camille-Desmoulins
94800 Villejuif
France

Nermin Halkic
Department of Visceral Surgery
University Hospital (CHUV)
Rue du Bugnon
CH-1011 Lausanne
Switzerland

Elizabeth Horn
George Washington University
2121 I Street, N.W.
Washington, D.C. 20052
USA

A. Şefik Hoşal, MD, Pr.
Department of Otolaryngology-Head and Neck Surgery
Hacettepe University Medical Faculty
Sıhhiye
06100 Ankara
Turkey

Martin Hübner
Department of Visceral Surgery
University Hospital (CHUV)
Rue du Bugnon
CH-1011 Lausanne
Switzerland

Florence Huguet, MD
Faculté de Médecine Pierre et Marie Curie
University of Paris-VI
Service d'Oncologie-Radiothérapie
Hôpital Tenon
Assistance Publique – Hôpitaux de Paris
GHU-Est
4, rue de la Chine
75020 Paris
France

Christos Ikonomidis
Otolaryngology Service
Department of Head and Neck Surgery
University Hospital (CHUV)
Rue du Bugnon
CH-1011 Lausanne
Switzerland

Mehrdad Jafari
Gastrointestinal and Genitourinary Oncology Department
Centre de lutte contre le cancer Oscar-Lambret
3, rue Fréderic-Combemale
BP307
59020 Lille Cedex
France

Wendy Jeanneret Sozzi
Department of Radiation Oncology
University Hospital (CHUV)
Rue du Bugnon
CH-1011 Lausanne
Switzerland

Serra Kamer
Department of Radiation Oncology
Ege University Tip Fakültesi, Bornova
35100 Izmir
Turkey

Kaouthar Khanfir, MD
Department of Radiation Oncology
Hôpital de Sion-CHCVs-RSV
Grand-Champsec 81
1951 Sion
Switzerland

Youlia M. Kirova, MD
Service de Radiothérapie Oncologique
Institut Curie
26, Rue d'Ulm
75005 Paris
France

Marco Krengli, Pr., MD
Department of Radiotherapy
University of Piemonte Orientale
Hospital Maggiore della Carità
Corso Mazzini 18
28100 Novara (NO)
Italy

Abraham Kuten, Pr., MD
Department of Oncology
Rambam Health Care Campus
PO Box 9602
Haïfa 31096
Israel

Hannah Lamallem, MD
Centre de Radiotherapie Haute Energie Hartmann
1 bis, rue des Dames-Augustines
92200 Neuilly-sur-Seine
France

Axel Le Cesne
Department of Medicine
Institut Gustave-Roussy
39, rue Camille-Desmoulins
94805 Villejuif
France

Hervé Le Floch
Department of Pneumology
Hôpital d'instruction des Armées Percy
101, avenue Henri-Barbusse
92140 Clamart
France

Émilie Le Rhun
Département de sénologie
Centre de lutte contre le cancer Oscar-Lambret
3, rue Fréderic-Combemale
BP307
59020 Lille Cedex
France

Anne Lesoin, Dr., MD
Centre de lutte contre le cancer Oscar-Lambret
3, rue Fréderic-Combemale
BP307
59020 Lille Cedex
France

Catherine Lhommé
University Paris XI
Department of Medical Oncology
Institut Gustave-Roussy
39, rue Camille-Desmoulins
94805 Villejuif
France

Serge Leyvraz, Pr.
Cancer Center
University Hospital (CHUV)
Rue du Bugnon
CH-1011 Lausanne
Switzerland

Yexiong Li, Dr.
Department of Radiation Oncology
Cancer Hospital and Institute
Chinese Academy of Medical Sciences (CAMS)
and Peking Union Medical College (PUMC)
Beijing 100021
China

Jean-Pierre Lotz
University Paris VI
Department of Medical Oncology
Hôpital Tenon
Assistance Publique – Hôpitaux de Paris
4, rue de la Chine
75970 Paris Cedex 20
France

Philippe Maingon
Department of Radiation Oncology
Centre Georges-François Leclerc
1, rue Professeur-Marion
21079 Dijon
France

Jacques Margery
Department of Pneumology
Hôpital d'instruction des Armées Percy
101 avenue Henri-Barbusse
92140 Clamart

Laura Masini, Dr.
Department of Radiotherapy
University of Piemonte Orientale
Hospital Maggiore della Carità
Corso Mazzini 18
I-28100 Novara
Italy

Oscar Matzinger, Dr.
Department of Radiation Oncology
University Hospital (CHUV)
Rue du Bugnon
CH-1011 Lausanne
Switzerland

Renaud Mazeron
Department of Curitherapy
Institut Gustave-Roussy
39, rue Camille-Desmoulins
94800 Villejuif
France

Robert C. Miller, MD
Department of Radiation Oncology
Mayo Clinic
Charlton Bldg. Desk R
200 First Street SW
Rochester, MN 55905
USA

Olivier Mir, Dr.
Department of medical Oncology
Hôpital Cochin
27, rue du Faubourg Saint-Jacques
75014 Paris

René-Olivier Mirimanoff, MD
Professor in Radiation Oncology
Head of the Department of Radiation Oncology
Centre hospitalier universitaire Vaudois
Rue du Bugnon
CH-1011 Lausanne
Switzerland

Michael Montemurro, Dr.
Cancer Center
University Hospital (CHUV)
Rue du Bugnon
CH-1011 Lausanne
Switzerland

Virginie Monnard
Department of Radiation Oncology
University Hospital (CHUV)
Rue du Bugnon
CH-1011 Lausanne
Switzerland

Philippe Morice
University Paris XI
Department of Surgical Oncology
Institut Gustave-Roussy
39, rue Camille-Desmoulins
94800 Villejuif
France

Françoise Mornex, Pr., MD, PhD
Department of Radiotherapy
Centre Hospitalier Lyon-Sud
165, chemin du Grand-Revoyet
69495 Pierre-Bénite Cedex
France

Cristina Nay Fellay, Dr.
Department of Oncology Riviera-Chablais
Site de la Providence
Rue de la Prairie 5
1800 Vevey
Switzerland

Thanh Van France Nguyen, MD
Department of Radiation Oncology
CHU Jean-Minjoz
2, boulevard Fleming
25030 Besançon Cedex
France

Kjell Öberg, Pr., MD, PhD
Department of Endocrine Oncology
Uppsala University Hospital
Entrance 78D
SE-751 85 Uppsala
Sweden

Enis Özyar, MD
Department of Radiation Oncology
Acibadem University, Kozyatagi
34742 Istanbul
Turkey

Esat Mahmut Ozsahin, MD, PhD
Associate Professor in Radiation Oncology
Department of Radiation Oncology
Head of the Department of Radiation Oncology
Centre hospitalier universitaire Vaudois
Rue du Bugnon
CH-1011 Lausanne
Switzerland

Renato G. Panizzon, MD
Chairman Dept of Dermatology
Centre hospitalier universitaire Vaudois
Rue du Bugnon
CH-1011 Lausanne
Switzerland

David Pasquier, MD, PhD
Department of Radiation Oncology
Centre Galilée
Polyclinique de la Louvière
69, rue de la Louvière
59800 Lille
France

Patricia Pautier
University Paris XI
Department of Medical Oncology
Institut Gustave-Roussy
39, rue Camille-Desmoulins
94805 Villejuif
France

Avivit Peer, MD
Department of Oncology
Rambam Health Care Campus
PO Box 9602
Haïfa 31096
Israel

Karine Peignaux, Dr.
Department of Radiation Oncology
Centre Georges-François Leclerc
1, rue Professeur Marion
21079 Dijon
France

Nicolas Penel
Équipe d'accueil 2694 : Santé publique, épidémiologie et modélisation des modèles chroniques
Université Lille-II
Département de cancérologie générale
Centre de lutte contre le cancer Oscar-Lambret
3, rue Fréderic-Combemale
BP307
59020 Lille Cedex
France

Jean Yannis Perentes, Dr.
Department of Thoracic and Vascular Surgery
University Hospital (CHUV)
Rue du Bugnon
CH-1011 Lausanne
Switzerland

Francesco Pia, Pr.
Otolaryngology
University of Piemonte Orientale
Hospital Maggiore della Carità
Corso Mazzini 18
I-28100 Novara
Italy

Alessia Pica, MD
Department of Radiation Oncology
University Hospital (CHUV)
Rue du Bugnon
CH-1011 Lausanne
Switzerland

Philip M.P. Poortmans, MD, PhD
Department of Radiation Oncology
Dr. Bernard Verbeeten Instituut
PO Box 90120
5000 LA Tilburg
The Netherlands

Henri Porte, MD, PhD
Pôle de chirurgie thoracique
CHRU de Lille
Boulevard du Professeur-Leclerq
59037 Lille

Eric Pujade Lauraine
University Paris V
Department of Medical Oncology
Hôtel-Dieu
Assistance publique – Hôpitaux de Paris
1, place du Parvis-Notre-Dame
75181 Paris Cedex 4

Khaled Rahal
Departments of Surgical Oncology
Institut Salah Azaiz
Boulevard du 9-Avril
1006. Bab Saadoun
Tunis
Tunisia

Isabelle Ray-Coquard
Department of Medical Oncology
Centre Léon-Bérard
28, rue Laennec
69 373 Lyon

Nicolas Rezvoy, MD
Department of Radiation Oncology
University Lille-II
Centre de lutte contre le cancer Oscar-Lambret
3, rue Fréderic-Combemale
BP307
59020 Lille Cedex
France

Hans-Beat Ris, Dr.
Department of Thoracic and Vascular Surgery
University Hospital (CHUV)
Rue du Bugnon
CH-1011 Lausanne
Switzerland

Frédéric Rivière
Department of Pneumology
Hôpital d'instruction des Armées Percy
101 avenue Henri-Barbusse
92140 Clamart

Martine Roelandts
Department of Radiotherapy
Institut Bordet
Université Libre de Bruxelles
Boulevard de Waterloo 121
1000 Brussels
Belgium

Philippe Rouanet
Departement of Surgery
CRLC Val d'Aurelle
208, rue des Apothicaires - Parc Euromédecine
34298 Montpellier Cedex 5
France

Vanessa Samouëlian, Dr., MD, PhD
Centre de lutte contre le cancer Oscar-Lambret
3, rue Fréderic-Combemale
BP307
59020 Lille Cedex
France

Luciano Scandolaro, MD
Divisione di Radioterapia Oncologica
Ospedale Sant'Anna
Via Napoleona 60
22100 Como
Italy

Michel Schlienger
Université Paris-VI
Service d'Oncologie-Radiothérapie
Hôpital Tenon
Assistance Publique – Hôpitaux de Paris
GHU-Est
4, rue de la Chine
75020 Paris
France

Frederic Selle, Dr.
University Paris-VI
Department of Medical Oncology
Hôpital Tenon
APREC, Assistance Publique – Hôpitaux de Paris
4, rue de la Chine
75970 Paris Cedex 20
France

Michael Heinrich Seegenschmiedt, Pr. Dr. med.
Strahlenzentrum Hamburg
Langenhorner Chaussee 369
22419 Hamburg-Langenhorn
Germany

Mark Shilkrut, PhD, MD
Department of Oncology
Rambam Health Care Campus, and
Rappaport Faculty of Medicine
Technion - Israel Institute of Technology Haifa, P.O.Box 9602
31096 Israel

Marc Spielmann
Department of Medicine
Institut Gustave-Roussy
39, rue Camille-Desmoulins
94805 Villejuif
France

Moshe E. Stein, Dr.
Department of Oncology
Rambam Health Care Campus
POB 9602
Haifa 31096
Israel

Timothy Sullivan, MD
Department of Radiation Oncology
Massachusetts General Hospital
Harvard Medical School
100 Blossom Street
Boston, MA 02114
USA

Alphonse G. Taghian, MD, PhD
Chief of Breast Service
Department of Radiation Oncology
Massachusetts General Hospital
Associate Professor
Harvard Medical School
100 Blossom Street
Boston, MA 02114
USA

Alain Toledano
Centre de Radiotherapie Haute Energie Hartmann
1 bis, rue des Dames Augustines
92200 Neuilly-sur-Seine
France

Emmanuel Touboul, MD
Faculté de Médecine Pierre et Marie Curie
University of Paris-VI
Service d'Oncologie-Radiothérapie
Hôpital Tenon
Assistance Publique – Hôpitaux de Paris
GHU-Est
4, rue de la Chine
75020 Paris
France

Richard W. Tsang, MD, FRCPC
Department of Radiation Oncology
Princess Margaret Hospital
610 University Avenue
Toronto ON M5G 2M9, Ontario
Canada

Pelagia G. Tsoutsou
Medical School
Democritus University of Thrace
Dragana
68100 Alexandroupolis
Greece

Vic Tuset
Department of Radiation Oncology
H. Universitari Germans Trias
Institut Català d'Oncologia
08916 Badalona
Barcelona

Gamze Ugurluer
Department of Radiation Oncology
Yüzüncü Yil University Hospital
65200 Van
Turkey

Paul Van Houtte
Department of Radiotherapy
Institut Jules-Bordet
Université Libre de Bruxelles
Boulevard de Waterloo 121
1000 Brussels
Belgium

Fabien Vaylet
Department of Pneumology
Hôpital d'instruction des Armées Percy
101 avenue Henri-Barbusse
92140 Clamart
France

Sabine Vieillot
Département d'oncologie radiothérapie
CRLC Val d'Aurelle
208, rue des Apothicaires - Parc Euro-médecine
34298 Montpellier Cedex 5
France

Salvador Villà Freixa, MD
Department of Radiation Oncology
H. Universitari Germans Trias
Institut Català d'Oncologia
08916 Badalona
Barcelona

Damien C. Weber, PD Dr. med.
Vice-Chairman
Radiation Oncology Department
Geneva University Hospital
24, rue Micheli-du-Crest
CH-1211 Geneva 14
Switzerland

Marie Wislez
Faculté de Médecine Pierre et Marie Curie
Université Paris-VI
Hôpital Tenon
Assistance publique – Hôpitaux de Paris
4, rue de la Chine
75970 Paris
France

Laurent Zelek
Department of Oncology
Avicenne Hospital
Assistance Publique – Hôpitaux de Paris
125, rue de Stalingrad
93009 Bobigny Cedex
France

Abderrahim Zouhair, MD
Department of Radiation Oncology
University Hospital (CHUV)
Rue du Bugnon
CH-1011 Lausanne
Switzerland

Acknowledgements

We would like to thank Frances Godson for her generous efforts and expertise to review and finalize the manuscript.

Contents

SECTION 5. GYNECOLOGICAL TUMOURS

SECTION 6. BREAST TUMOURS

SECTION 7. LUNG AND INTRATHORACIC MALIGNANCIES

SECTION 8. MALIGNANCIES OF THE SKIN

SECTION 9. OTHER MALIGNANCIES

References in ***bold type*** *are key references.*

Preface

P.H. Levine

The importance of Studying Rare Malignancies

Rare cancers play an important role in the epidemiology of cancer in view of the clues they give us to cancer etiology in general. The most obvious example is the study of cancer clusters, which provide excellent opportunities to identify etiologic agents. The study of cancer clusters has many problems and is usually unproductive [8] because reported clusters often involve large numbers of common tumours with long latent periods, but the most dramatic successes involve rare malignancies. In such cases, alert clinicians play an important role as exemplified by Gottlieb in 1981 [3] who noticed the unusual new occurrence of Kaposi's sarcoma in gay San Francisco males which eventually led to the identification of Acquired Autoimmune Deficiency Syndrome (AIDS) as a potential public health problem and subsequent identification of Human Immunodeficiency Virus (HIV) as the etiologic agent. A non-infectious danger was recognized in Boston with the appearance of a rare cancer in young women, vaginal cancer, which was eventually traced to the administration of a hormone, diethylstilbestrol (DES) to the mothers to maintain a pregnancy [5]. DES proved to be unsuccessful in maintaining pregnancies but more important, the danger of this hormone being given to pregnant women was quickly identified.

Another important consideration in cancer epidemiology is the study of a rare tumour in one country that is not rare in other countries. The etiology or an etiologic component may or may not be known but it is important to understand the co-factors that increase or decrease the incidence of a specific malignancy after exposure to the suspected agent. Such studies these days involve the integration of laboratory studies into the development of epidemiologic protocols, and it now seems to be the exception rather than the rule that a large epidemiologic study does not include the collection of biospecimens for multiple laboratory investigations. Our experience in this area began with Burkitt's lymphoma (BL), a malignancy first described by Denis Burkitt in Sub-Saharan Africa geographically limited by climate and altitude to areas of holoendemic malaria. Because BL was unknown in England, where Burkitt had practiced as an experienced surgeon, he was fascinated by this rare tumour which led to extensive international collaborative studies involving clinicians, epidemiologists and laboratory investigators culminating in the discovery of the Epstein-Barr virus (EBV) [1, 4]. One of the epidemiologist-statisticians focusing on BL was Malcolm Pike who, noting the occasional clusters of the disease, proposed a "Factor X", an etiologic agent in addition to EBV and malaria, which could contribute to the etiology. He suggested that a comparison of the endemic African disease be compared with non-endemic cases where malaria was not a factor and thus the American Burkitt's Lymphoma Registry was initiated [6].

More than 143 cases of BL in the US were reported in eight years [7] and biospecimens, particularly paraffin blocks, revealed that at least two distinct forms of BL could be identified [2], the prototypical EBV-associated BL, the most common form in sub-Saharan Africa but rare in the US, and the non-EBV-associated form, the more common form in the U.S. with distinct chromosomal and clinical differences from African BL.

The identification of patients with rare tumours is now greatly facilitated by the internet, which is now being used to investigate a number of rare tumours, as demonstrated by the many interesting chapters in this book. The Rare Cancer Network (RCN) has been using the Internet to connect clinicians to improve the management of rare cancers, as described in these chapters. This is an important beginning, since much more needs to be done to understand the pathobiology and control of a variety of rare malignancies. As advances occur in the laboratory, more sophisticated studies are now feasible, such as the use of oral rinses to collect DNA for sophisticated analysis. The findings resulting in the study of rare tumours can be expected to have major implications for cancer etiology in general.

Paul Levine, MD
Research Professor in the Department of Epidemiology and Biostatistics
The George Washington University School of Public Health and Health Services
2300 Eye Street, NW
Washington DC 20037
USA

References

1. Burkitt DP, Charles S, Mott Award (2006) The discovery of Burkitt's Lymphoma. Cancer 10: 1772-86
2. Barriga F, Kiwanuka J, Alvarez-Mon M *et al.* (1988) Significance of chromosome 8 breakpoint location in Burkitt's lymphoma: correlation with geographical origin and association with Epstein-Barr virus. Curr Top Microbiol Immunol 141: 128-37
3. Centers for Disease Control and Prevention (CDC) (1981) Kaposi's sarcoma and *Pneumocystis* pneumonia among homosexual men–New York and Californa. MMWR Morb Mortal Wkly Rep 30: 305-8
4. Epstein MA, Achong BG, Barr YM (1969) Virus particles in cultured lymphoblasts from Burkitt's lymphoma. Lancet 1 702-3
5. Herbst AL, Ulfeder H, Poskanzer DC (1971) Adenocarcinoma of the vagina: Association with maternal stilbestrol therapy with tumor appearance in young women. N Eng J Med 284: 878-81
6. Levine PH. Wanted: Case reports of Burkitt's lymphoma in the U.S. (1971) Med Times 99 (2): 124-6
7. Levine PH, Kamaraju LS, Connelly RR *et al.* (1982) The American Burkitt's lymphoma registry: eight years' experience. Cancer 49 (5): 1016-22
8. Rothenberg RB, Steinberg KK, Thacker SB (eds) (1990) National Conference on Clustering of Health Events. Am J Epidemiol 132 (suppl) S1-S202

Foreword

R.C. Miller

This work addresses the problem of rare tumour management. By definition, these are uncommon malignancies whose diagnosis and treatment are made more complicated by a relative absence of information in the medical literature. A uniform definition of a "rare tumour" does not currently exist. In some instances, terminology even for individual disease entities remains indeterminate because of their infrequent occurrence. The National Institute of Health's Office of Rare Disease Research defines a "rare disease" as one effecting less than 200,000 individuals in the United States [2]. In contrast, the European Commission has more broadly defined rare diseases as those diseases which "are life-threatening or chronically debilitating diseases which are of such low prevalence that special combined efforts are needed to address them" or those that affect less than 5 per 10,000 persons. Although individually the incidence of any given rare disease is low, it is estimated that 6% to 8% of the population of the European Union has a disease classified as "rare" when all entities meeting this definition are considered in aggregate [3]. The unusual neoplastic processes presented in *Management of Rare Adult Tumours* range from the very rare, where the cases reported in the medical literature consist only of a few dozens of patients, such as Erdheim-Chester disease and primary spinal epidural lymphoma, to more common entities that clinicians may occasionally encounter, but where a low incidence has left their best management incompletely defined, such as thymoma and ductal carcinoma *in-situ* in very young women. The European Commission has identified rare diseases as a subject where cooperative action within the international community may be of benefit. On November 11th, 2008, the European Commission published proposed recommendations for European action in the field of rare diseases, calling for global action in concert given the rarity of these conditions and the often complex requirements of their diagnosis and management. *Management of Rare Adult Tumours* is a timely addition towards that effort.

In an era where evidence-based medicine (EBM) has become the focus of clinical research and medical practice, the treatment of rare diseases presents a unique challenge. EBM practice is founded on a hierarchy of evidence, with the greatest value being assigned to evidence derived from sources with robust statistical power, such as meta-analyses and randomized clinical trials. By definition, the study of rare tumours is problematic from the EBM perspective given that their infrequent occurrence prevents their study through prospective means. Despite the challenges of dealing with patient populations too small for testing research questions through randomized controlled trials, these problems are not insurmountable [1-4]. The internet has proved to be important in increasing communication and awareness of rare diseases, as well as providing a powerful tool for fostering cooperative investigations. International collaborations through such organizations as The Rare Cancer Network (www.rarecancer.net) permit a pooling of data and an increase in statistical power in the study of malignant entities in which no single institution can produce sufficient cases for definitive analysis.

Management of Rare Adult Tumours is meant to provide a concise summary of the state of the art of rare tumour management for clinicians and medical scientists interested in uncommon malignancies. Arranged on the basis of anatomic site of the primary tumours, the authors address the classification, diagnosis, and therapy of 61 rare tumours. The focus of their work is on providing a summary of the medical literature to date that can assist the clinician in decision making during the diagnosis and treatment of such tumours. The authors have been chosen because of their expertise in this difficult field of investigation. Their efforts are greatly appreciated and it is hoped that this book will serve as a valuable resource for those caring for adult patients with rare malignancies.

References

1. Behera M, Kumar A, Soares H *et al.* (2007) Evidence-based medicine for rare diseases: implications for data interpretation and clinical trial design. Cancer Control, 14(2), 160-6
2. National Institutes of Health Office of Rare Diseases Research, [homepage on the Internet]. Bethesda, MD (US) [cited 2009 Apr 20]. Available from: http://rare-diseases.info.nih.gov/RareDiseaseList.aspx
3. Proposal for a Council Recommendation in the Field of Rare Diseases (SEC(2008)2712-2713). Brussels (Belgium): Commission of the European Communities [cited 2009 Apr 20]. Available from: http://ec.europa.eu/health/ph_threats/non_com/rare_diseases_en.htm
4. Tan S, Dear K, Bruzzi P *et al.* (2003) Strategy for randomised clinical trials in rare cancers. BMJ, 327(7405), 47-9

Section 1
Central nervous system tumours

Germinal tumours of the central nervous system in adult patients

1

S. Villà Freixa, M. Caro and V. Tuset

Five Essential Points

1. *Germ cell tumours of the central nervous system are uncommon. Very few reports have been published on adult presentation and so therapeutic results from pediatric series have been extrapolated to the adult population.*
2. *Pre-therapeutic workup must include neuroaxis MRI, tumour marker analysis in serum and CSF, and cytology in CSF.*
3. *Histological subtypes are the most decisive prognostic factors.*
4. *In the absence of clinical phase III trials, for pure germinoma without dissemination at presentation, RT alone continues to be the standard of care. Controversies regarding volumes and total doses of RT have still not been definitively solved. However, taking into account long survival of these patients, it is logical to consider that the combination of CT and low doses and partial volumes of RT could become the standard, mainly in patients responding to CT. For non-germinomatous types, CT is needed and higher doses and volumes of RT remain necessary.*
5. *CT alone is not indicated due to high rates of relapse.*

Introduction

Germ cell tumours of the central nervous system (GCT-CNS) in the adult population are very uncommon. Furthermore, controversy remains concerning the treatment of intracranial GCTs, due largely to the complexity and rarity of these tumours, added to the lack of prospective randomized trials, involving this specific group of adult patients with this pathology, as in almost all rare cancers.

Although radiotherapy (RT) has long been the standard of care for GTC-CNS, agreement on the optimal management of these tumours with respect to treatment volume, total dose, and the use of neoadjuvant chemotherapy (CT) remains undefined. On the other hand, germinoma and nongerminomatous tumours have different prognoses [17] (see Table 1), and deserve different approaches. Until now, these approaches have been the same for both adults and children.

Table 1 – Different prognostic groups according histological subtypes for germ cell tumours of the central nervous system (adapted from Ogawa 2003).

Good prognosis group
Germinoma, pure
Mature teratoma
Intermediate prognosis group
Germinoma with syncytiotrophoblastic giant cells
Immature teratoma
Teratoma with malignant transformation
Mixed tumours (mainly composed by of germinoma and/or teratoma)
Poor prognosis group
Choriocarcinoma
Yolk sac tumour
Embryonal carcinoma
Mixed tumours (mainly composed of choriocarcinoma, yolk sac, or embryonal)

1

Incidence

Incidence varies depending on geography. These GCT are more frequent in the far-east of Asia. GCT-CNS accounts for 2-3% of primary brain tumours, and more in paediatric series (8-15%) [21]. In the West, it represents only 0.3-0.6% in the general population, and 3-4% in children. Incidence in the white population is higher than in the black [27]. The peak of incidence is between 10 and 14 years, and almost 90% of patients are under 25 years of age. Consequently, an elderly population with CNS-GCT is uncommon (1% of intracranial tumours). In adult age, congenital examples such as teratomas are more prevalent. Very few reports in the literature are dedicated only to adult patients (cut-off 16-18 years) [1, 8, 26]. Table 2 shows the main series of adult patients affected with GCT-CNS with a series where median age is 16 years or more, or where a significant number of patients are adults.

Table 2 – Series of adult patients affected with germ cell tumours of the central nervous system. It includes either pure adult series, adult median age (cut-off of 16-18 years), or significant proportion of adult patients.

Series	n	Median age	G	NG	Chemotherapy	CSI	Involved-field
Paris I [1]	19*	18	4	14	8 patients	-	16 patients (8 after chemotherapy and 8 as only treatment)
Barcelona [29]	16&	18	9	7	4 patients (mixed tumours)	27.3-29 Gy	52 Gy
London [14]	11	20	8	3	VCE 8 patients	35 Gy all patients	Boost 45-50 Gy
Japan I [18]	126	17	126	-	None	30.4 Gy in 56 patients	30 Gy WBI + boost 50 Gy 53 Gy in focal fields, only in 8 patients
Japan II [19]	103	16	103	-	EP/CE/ICE	13.5-25.2 Gy in 27 patients	50 Gy 46 Gy if previous chemotherapy
Milan [26]	20*	21	18	2	PVB	30 Gy (1 disseminated patient)	35 Gy
Gainesville-Atlanta [24]	31	18	31	-	-	20-25 Gy	Ventricular boost 9 Gy Tumour boost 19.5 Gy
Houston [16]	21	19	21	-	VP-16/CDDP/ Carbo / VCR in 12 patients previous focal RDT	24 Gy (in 12 patients)	Tumour boost 26 Gy (12 patients) Focal RT 30.6 Gy if previous chemotherapy
Paris II [8]	10*	27	10	-	EP in all patients	30-36 Gy	Boost 20-24 Gy

Abbreviations and notes: *: exclusive adult patient series; &: 14 out of 16 patients were adult; G: germinoma; NG: non-germinomatous tumours; CSI: craniospinal irradiation; CDDP: Cisplatin; VP-16: Etoposide; Carbo: Carboplatin; EP: Etoposide/Cisplatin; PVB: Cisplatin/Vinblastine/Bleomycine; VCR: vincristine; CE: Carboplatin/Etoposide; ICE: Ifosfamide/Cisplatin/Etoposide; VCE: Vincristine/Carboplatin/Etoposide.

Tumour location

GCT-CNS usually affects the midline of the brain [21]. The region of the pineal gland is the most common site, followed by the suprasellar area and cerebral hemisphere [14, 20]. Other less common locations such as the basal ganglia or thalamus have been described [28]. The proportion of cases with multifocal presentation in the brain is also quite significant [26]. The pineal region is more frequently affected in males [27], which is not the case in the suprasellar area [14].

Pathology

The WHO defines 7 different subtypes: pure germinoma, mature teratoma, immature teratoma, teratoma with malignant transformation, yolk sac tumour (so-called endodermal sinus tumour), embryonal carcinoma, and choriocarcinoma [21]. GCT of the CNS are morphological and immunophenotypic homologues of gonadal GCT [21]. The identification of subtypes of GCT-CNS is very important for treatment strategies and their prognosis [17]. They are often of mixed histology. In fact, only the germinoma and teratoma are likely to be pure tumour types.

Germinomas

These are the most common (2/3 of whole group) and are composed of large and undifferentiated cells. Nuclei are rounded, vesicular and centrally positioned with prominent nucleoli and relatively abundant cytoplasm with glycogen accumulation. Mitoses are usual but necrosis is rare. The fibrovascular septa, infiltrated by mainly T lymphocytes, is a usual feature. The identification of both mature lymphocytes and larger germinoma cells leads to diagnosis. Immunohistochemically, cell membrane labelling by c-kit and nuclear activity for OCT4 are the most characteristic of these tumours. On the other hand, typical germinomas may have syncytiotrophoblastic giant cells and cells that label for beta-HCG.

Nongerminomatous tumours

Teratoma

Teratomas are derived from ectodermal, endodermal and mesodermal lines [23].

Mature Teratoma

These are composed exclusively of pure adult type elements. Concerning ectodermal components, these are most frequently skin, nervous tissue or choroid plexus. More usual mesodermal components are cartilage, bone, fat and muscle while cyst lines of epithelial or respiratory or enteric type are more common endodermal components.

Immature teratoma

This variant is characterized by undifferentiated components resembling foetal tissue. This fact is sufficient to determine the immature type even when these features are minor. Cleft lines by melanotic neuroepithelium are often observed. Post treatment analysis of these immature neoplasms, frequently reveals only mature components due to effects of therapy. These residual tumours are known as *growing teratoma syndrome* [21]. Other teratomas with malignant epithelial or mesenchymal elements are considered to be teratomas with malignant transformation [23].

Yolk sac tumour

This tumour is composed of epithelial cells of primitive appearance, representing yolk sac endoderm, which contain compact sheets, ribbons, cords, or papillae. Schiller-Duval bodies are characteristic of GCT-CNS and confirm diagnosis [23]. Mitotic activity can vary considerably, but necrosis is rare. Immunoreactivity for AFP is characteristic, and is non-reactive for c-kit and OCT4.

Embryonal carcinoma

This other variant is defined as large cells that form abortive papillae or line irregular gland-like spaces. Nucleoli are enlarged with high mitotic index and zones of coagulative necrosis. Its diffuse cytoplasm is labelling for cytokeratins. They share PLAP and OCT4 immunoreactivity with most germinomas, but c-kit is not expressed in embryonal carcinoma.

Choriocarcinoma

The main characteristic of choriocarcioma is extra-embryonic differentiation along trophoblastic lines. The identification of cytotrophoblastic elements and syncytiotrophoblastic giant cells are needed for diagnosis. Vascular channels with blood lakes and hemorrhagic necrosis are also characteristic. Immunolabelling for beta-HCG and HPL are the rule.

Combinations of any of these above-mentioned tumour types are referred to as mixed germ cell tumours.

Clinical presentation

Clinical presentation and duration of symptoms vary with location and histological subtypes [14]. Germinomas are slower growing tumours than others and their clinical presentation is longer. If tumours are located at the pineal region, they often compress the cerebral aqueduct, resulting in hydrocephalus with increased cranial hypertension. Also, a tumour in this location invades the tectal plate producing a characteristic paralysis of upwards gaze and convergence, the so-called Parinaud's syndrome. Suprasellar and neurohypophyseal GCT typically affect the optic chiasm causing visual deficits [14] and also affect the hypothalamo-hypophyseal axis, leading to pituitary failure [14]. In the Boston series [12], the most common syndrome was endocrinopathies (diabetes insipidus, growth retardation or precocious puberty), followed by increased intracranial pressure or visual disturbance, including Parinaud's syndrome. This syndrome persisted after treatment [26]. On the other hand, in one fourth of patients, memory deficit and anorexia were detected [12]. Anecdotal reports suggest that solitary intradural focus could be seen [15].

Staging procedure

As with other brain tumours, a systematic work-up is necessary. Medical history and physical examination, MRI of the whole neuroaxis, spinal fluid cytology, complete blood cell count, chemistry panel, and tumour markers (alfa-fetoprotein and beta-human chorionic gonadotrophin) in serum and CSF are strongly recommended. Careful staging with modern imagery influenced survival in historical series [23]. Specifically, MRI is the first imaging carried out for staging GCT-CNS but the neuro-radiological profiles are non-specific. However, other than teratomas, GCT appears as a solid mass which is isodense or hyperdense in comparison with grey matter. Contrast enhancement is high. Germinomas located at the basal ganglia can be seen as hyperintensity in T2 sequences and with minimal contrast enhancement; some of them present as multiple midline lesions [12]. Teratoma, on the other hand, can exhibit intratumoral cysts and calcified or fatty regions. Intratumoral haemorrhage is more characteristic of choriocarcinomas. Neuroimaging studies are important to define hydrocephalus, invasion of other structures, as well as leptomeningeal dissemination in spinal cord. Ventricular endoscopy is especially sensitive in the localization of neoplasms and can watch nodules on the ependyma that are not detectable by MRI [30]. PET using 11C-methionine at diagnosis could be useful to avoid hazardous biopsies under some circumstances [14].

Cytology is considered mandatory to screen tumour cells from ventricular CSF or from lumbar puncture, if clinically possible. In the Boston series [12], 24% of pure germinoma cases had positive cytology. However, other authors found a lower incidence. Schild *et al.* [23] had just one positive case in a series of 57 patients (one case of mixed tumour).

Tumour markers

Alfa-fetoprotein and beta-human chorionic gonadotrophin can be detectable either in serum or in CSF. Alfa-fetoprotein elevation rules out the diagnosis of pure germinoma. However, a moderate increase of beta-human chorionic gonadotrophin is compatible with pure germinoma. In some series, almost 40% of patients presented abnormal levels in serum or CSF [12, 19]. Hence, definitive histology is not mandatory in nongerminomatous tumours [20]. Furthermore, monitoring of tumour markers will aid physicians in defining response [5].

Treatment

No high level clinical evidence to support treatment choice is found in the literature. There are two reasons for that:

1. low incidence of these tumours in children and, consequently, in an adult cohort;
2. lack of randomized trials due to the above.

As mentioned previously, two groups can be differentiated from a therapeutic point of view: germinoma and nongerminomatous histology, as in gonadal tumours.

Surgery

Surgical options depend on tumour location, multifocality, type of tumour and clinical presentation. Shunting procedure is indicated in patients presenting with ventricle obstruction. Biopsy only is more often indicated for lesions of the suprasellar area. Partial or complete resection has to be considered for tumours in the third ventricle/pineal region. Nowadays, in patients with negative tumour markers, histology is mandatory. Surgeons are more aggressive, in terms of amount of resection, for patients with nongerminomatous neoplasms [7, 17, 22]. Nevertheless, it has been shown that radical removal of germinoma offers no benefit over biopsy [12, 26].

For more than a decade, the use of the surgical microscope and stereotactic tools have increased precision and safety during tumour resection [23, 25].

Radiotherapy

Volumes and total doses of RT still remain controversial. Over the last two decades, there has been a tendency towards a lower total dose of RT and reduction of RT volumes is becoming the standard of care. Arguments in favour of this policy are the late morbidity of long-term paediatric survivors and the high rate of responses to CT before starting RT. However, these alternative approaches should aim at preserving the high cure rates achieved by RT alone.

Nevertheless, large RT volumes as in craniospinal irradiation (CSI) with a boost to the tumour bed are still valid in patients with disseminated germinomas [23, 26]; and for nongerminomatous cases as well [23]. In particular, patients from an adult series with long follow-up have shown that they are able to work and maintain normal social activities after high dose whole brain irradiation (WBI) [29]. An MD Anderson report [16] found that the 10-year local control rate in the brain for patients who received only focal RT was 59% compared with 100% for patients treated with CSI (non significant trend, $p=.08$). However, the rate of distant control in the spine at 5 years was statistically significant (62% for patients who received focal RT and 100% for patients who received CSI).

On the other hand, small RT volumes (partial RT, only in tumoral bed) or whole ventricular radiotherapy (WVRT) seem to be indicated in mature teratoma cases [23] and some even advocate that they can also be safely managed with surgery alone. According to several series [13, 18, 26], CSI was no better for overall survival (OS) compared to partial volume RT for localised germinomas. In the particular case of the Haas-Kogan et al report [13], they recommended WVRT (32.4 Gy) followed by primary tumour boost to a total dose of 45-50 Gy. In fact, one of three patients failed with as low a dose as 11.6 Gy to the tumour bed but was rescued by surgery, chemotherapy (CT) and new focal RT. Stereotactic RT is becoming an alternative for final boost to the tumour bed [10].

Low dose RT is defined as

1. WBI using a dose of 25.5 Gy or less,
2. Less than 50 Gy (or only 24 Gy after CT) to the primary site,
3. Less than 22 Gy to the spine [12, 22, 24].

Final RT doses for germinomas should also be determined by responses to neoadjuvant CT [7, 8, 22]. Series with higher RT dose (tumour bed 48-57.6 Gy, WBI 36-45 Gy, CSI 24-36 Gy) have been published with good results in terms of OS [23, 29]. CSI was considered in a combined CT-RT schedule only for highly malignant tumours. The other cases were treated by using involved-field RT alone [3]. Again, the lack of randomized trials means that no large body of evidence is available on which to base decisions concerning RT, but orientational guidelines can be suggested (Table 3).

Table 3 – Orientate guidelines of radiotherapy delivering according histological subtypes of germ cell tumours of the central nervous system (CNS)

Radiotherapy	Type of Germ Cell Tumour of CNS
Involved field, high dose, without CT	Focal germinoma, mature teratoma, mixed (G-MT)
IF+ ventricular RT (low/high dose) with CT	Focal germinoma, mixed Germinoma-mature teratoma, immature teratoma (high RT dose)
Low/high dose, large volume CSI without CT	Disseminated germinoma, immature teratoma
IF+ low dose CSI with CT	Disseminated germinoma
High dose and large volume with CT	Mixed tumours with malignant components Yolk sac Embryonal carcinoma Choriocarcinoma

Abbreviations: RT: radiotherapy; CT: chemotherapy; G: germinoma; MT: mature teratomas; IF: involved field; CSI: craniospinal irradiation

Chemotherapy

Many drugs have been explored in the treatment of GCT-CNS, mainly in children. Classical cisplatin-based schedules have become the most common type of neoadjuvant approach prior to starting RT and have formed the basis of several phase II trials. Eleven germinoma patients were entered in a New York series [2] using carboplatin alone in the neoadjuvant setting prior to RT. Carboplatin was administered 150 mg/m^2 weekly for 4 consecutive weeks with a 2-week break. Complete remission (CR) was achieved in 7 patients. These results have led to a decrease in RT dose of CSI and of involved field (tumour bed) irradiation. Other series [4] recruited more cases (71 patients), 45 patients with germinomas. CT was used alone (carboplatin 500mg/m^2/d days 1 and 2, etoposide 150 mg/m^2/d days 1 and 2, and bleomycin 15 mg/m^2) without RT. Of these patients, 84% had CR but more than 50% (20 patients) relapsed and were rescued using chemo-radiation or RT alone (3 patients died of disease). Eighteen non-germinomatous tumours were explored in a different setting [20]. After intent of radical surgery, a "sandwich" scheme was proposed (CT-RT-CT). Neoadjuvant CT consisted of 3-4 cycles of cisplatin (100mg/m^2/cycle) and etoposide (500 mg/m^2/cycle). Nine of 12 evaluable patients achieved response (5 CR and 4 PR). An adjuvant CT approach was based on 4 cycles with vinblastine (6.5 mg/m^2/cycle), bleomycin (15 mg/m^2/cycle), etoposide (300 mg/m^2/cycle) and carboplatin (450 mg/m^2/cycle). Four patients died (3 of progressive disease and 1 of metabolic failure). Sawamura *et al.* [22] included 22 patients with both histologies (16 patients with germinoma and 6 with nongerminomatous tumours). Cisplatin and etoposide with or without ifosfamide were administered as a neoadjuvant scheme. Low dose RT after CT (only 24 Gy to the tumoral bed) was delivered. A phase II schedule from Mayo clinic [7] was delivered in 17 patients (9 germinomas and 8 nongerminomatous). A conventional neoadjuvant dose of etoposide (100 mg/m^2/day) and CDDP (20 mg/m^2/day) daily for 5 days/3 weeks for 4 cycles were administered. It should be noted that two different doses of dextrose and manitol were taken into account for both children and adults. Fourteen out of the 17 patients received more than 90% of CT for 4 cycles. Alternative CT schedules were explored by the French group [5]: carboplatin and etoposide in alternative combination with ifosfamide and etoposide for 4 courses (carboplatin 600 mg/m^2 on day 1; etoposide 150 mg/m^2/day, ifosfamide 1.8 g/m^2). Aoyama and colleagues [3] changed the CT schedule according histological variants. For pure germinoma, they administered etoposide and cisplatin, and for nongerminomatous cases they added ifosfamide.

An interesting non-randomized study by Haas-Kogan *et al.* [13] analyzed 93 patients receiving RT (germinoma, nongerminomatous, and non-biopsied lesions). Twenty-four of them received CT as part of the initial treatment in the neoadjuvant setting. The addition of CT did not influence either progression free survival or overall survival.

As has been said previously, reports of specific adult series with CNS-GTC are very scarce in the literature. Calugaru and colleagues [8] published very recently a retrospective report of 10 patients with pure germinoma using neoadjuvant CT (cisplatin 100 mg/m^2/day 1 and etoposide 100 mg/m^2/days 1-3) (1 case with bleomycin) for 3-4 cycles following high dose of RT (CSI 30-36 Gy and tumour bed 50-54 Gy) in patients at risk of dissemination. This RT dose was decreased for patients with CR after CT. A further series with patients with median age of 20 years comes from England [14]. They used a “central nervous system-friendly” chemo-radiotherapy regimen in 8 mainly non-germinomatous patients, using drugs such as vincristine 2mg, carboplatin 200-300 mg/m^2/day for 3 days and etoposide 100 mg/m^2/daily for 3 days by 1-2 cycles. The RT dose was conventional (CSI 30 Gy, tumour bed 50 Gy). Another series of exclusively adults patients was published recently by Silvani *et al.* [26] administering the PVB scheme (cisplatin 20 mg/m^2 for 5 days, vinblastine 4 mg/m^2 days 1 and 8 and bleomycin 10 mg/m^2 on days 1,8 and 15) every 3 weeks for 3 courses.

Treatment side effects

It is not easy to ascribe side effects to any single factor in these patients. Improvement of surgical techniques is the reason for reduced post-surgery morbidity and mortality over the last two decades. A Japanese series [22] included patients over a long period (1970-1995) and showed operative mortality of 3.6% and post-surgical morbidity of 19%. Toxicities such as palsy of the cranial nerves have been observed [29].

It is important to note that many deficits, damage and symptoms are present at diagnosis. In the Boston series [12], 22/40 patients studied had evidence of at least one endocrine abnormality. No new abnormalities at follow-up were seen but an increase in hormonal deficits was observed. Fourteen patients at presentation showed growth retardation but were not observed at follow-up, a fact also seen in other series [7, 13, 18]. However, there was a greater than 50% chance of additional endocrine abnormalities developing in the previously affected patients over time. On the other hand, Haas-Kogan *et al.* [13] found that 48 patients out of 93 did not need any hormone replacement. Also memory deficit prior to RT was seen in 8 patients. At the follow-up only one patient showed increased memory problems following treatment, and in 5 patients it improved. Tumour location (tumour not involving neurohypophyseal region *vs* involved- 92% *vs* 71%) influenced attending school or ability to work at the follow-up. In summary, the treatment toxicity faced by CNS germinoma patients appears to be less than anticipated.

In spite of these considerations, RT itself can cause different late effects.

Several series have described endocrinopathies after high dose RT [13, 22, 29]. Hormone replacement was needed in over 65% of patients having received more than a dose of 35 Gy [22]. Auditory and visual dysfunctions, without the presence of disease, are also noted but not very well analyzed [22]. Memory loss and mental retardation could be important late effects [29]. These effects are influenced again by volume and total dose of RT. In the Sawamura *et al.* series [22], 7 out of 19 patients studied showed varying degrees of neurocognitive damage. Vascular deficits have also been emphasised in the literature with significant deterioration of quality of life [13, 22]. The estimated incidence of occlusive vasculopathy was 11.7% in one series [22]. Radiation necrosis has been seen in patients mainly treated before the new RT techniques were available [22].

Regarding second cancers, several series found some cases of gliomas and meningiomas after more than 6 years post RT [12, 13, 22]. The analysis of Karnofsky index (KI) in the Japanese series [22] is interesting. With a median follow-up of 99 months in 85 surviving patients, only 11 cases (13%) had KI of 100% but 48 of 85 maintained a KI of 80-90%. Furthermore, tumour location also influences KI in the long term [18].

Combination of CT and RT increased rates of hearing loss [22, 29]. Also, CT can cause progressive multicystic encephalomalacia [22]. In spite of the short median follow-up of phase II trials, two series have shown no more side effects than in the past. Buckner *et al.* [7] did not find significant impairment after psychometric tests in 5 patients followed more than 36 months; nor did the Florida series [24] observe dementia in patients receiving low dose of RT. However, one patient [7] was affected with progressive ataxia, dysartria and tremors. Another patient suffered ischemic attacks (considered to be radiation vasculopathy). One second cancer (AML), related probably to CT, was seen in the Florida series [24].

Chemotherapy per se causes damage. Cisplatin is considered to be an indispensable drug but it may cause renal damage, ototoxicity, peripheral neuropathy, and sterility, while etoposide is associated with an excess frequency of secondary neoplasms [6, 18]). In the international phase II trial without RT [4], 10% of patients died of CT-related toxic effects. Grade III-IV myelosupression is frequent [7, 26]. In adult patients included in CT-RT regimens, less relevant adverse effects of radiation would be expected in comparison with those observed in younger patients after the same treatment. In fact, patients in the Italian trial had no change in their professional activities [26].

In summary, the potential benefit of prophylactic spinal irradiation must be carefully balanced against the potential toxicity in patients requiring platinum-based chemotherapy [23].

Outcome and survival

Median follow-up of the main series ranged from 36 to 122 months [18, 23]. The main areas of tumour spread after treatment are in the local tumour bed or in CSF. Other failures are from abdominal contamination via ventriculo-peritoneal spread or haematogenous dissemination (bone and lung) [21, 23]. These relapses lead to increased distant metastases and are correlated with histological subtypes [22, 23].

Neoadjuvant CT achieved complete remissions in a significant group of patients (18/24 in two series) [7, 8]. Patients without CR after CT achieved that after completing RT [8].

For germinoma cases, progression free survival (PFS) and overall survival (OS) are significantly better than for nongerminomatous cases. PFS in patients with germinoma ranged from 80% to 100% at 5 years, and reach 80% at 10 years [12, 14, 22, 23]. In a series with low dose RT (21 Gy) [24] PFS was 94% with a median follow-up of 7 years. OS in patients with germinoma ranged from 79% to 97% at 5 years and reach almost 80% at 10 years [12, 22, 29].

PFS in patients with nongerminomatous histology ranged from 21% to 48% at 5 years and 10 years, but in cases with a highly malignant component, PFS dropped to 13% at 10 years [23]. OS in patients with non-germinomatous tumours depends on tumour histology. In the Japanese series [22], with 111 patients analyzed, OS at 5 years was: 100% for mature teratomas, 67% for immature teratomas, and 69% for immature teratomas mixed with germinoma. Tumours with yolk sac or embryonal components had 38% OS. Schild *et al.* [23] found an OS at 3 years of 86% for mature teratomas, 67% for immature teratomas, 44% for mixed GCT, and 13% for other histological types (statistically significant).

These figures of PFS and OS are very difficult to separate between children and adults, leading us to consider both groups as a whole.

Prognostic factors

Several prognostic factors have been identified. In an old series, neurological performance status at diagnosis was prognostic [9].

Histological subtype, as mentioned before, plays the most important role in terms of outcome [9, 11, 13, 20]. However, specific components of mature teratomas with germinoma did not influence OS [22]. Ogawa *et al.* [17] described a useful prognostic classification according histological subtypes (see Table 1). Five and 10 years OS for all patients were 50% and 34% respectively; while for good prognosis this was 100%, for intermediate 68%, and only 8% for the worst prognostic group.

Surgery has an important role for some authors in non-germinomatous cases [23].

While in some series [22], increased beta-HCG indicates a worse prognosis for progression in germinomas, other authors did not find it significant [18], provided a high dose of RT can be delivered [19].

References

1. **Agranat P, Jedynak P, Epardeau B *et al.* (1995) Cerebral germ cell tumors in adults. A retrospective study of 19 cases. Bull Cancer 82: 650-9**
2. Allen JC, DaRosso RC, Donahue B, Nirenberg A (1994) A phase II trial of pre-irradiation carboplatin in newly diagnosed germinoma of the central nervous system. Cancer 74: 940-4
3. Aoyama H, Shirato H, Ikeda J *et al.* (2002) Induction chemotherapy followed by low-dose involved-field radiotherapy for intracranial germ cell tumors. J Clin Oncol 20: 857-65
4. Balmaceda C, Heller G, Rosenblum M *et al.* (1996) Chemotherapy without irradiation. A novel approach for newly diagnosed CNS germ cell tumors: results of an international cooperative trial. J Clin Oncol 14: 2908-15
5. Bouffet E, Baranzelli MC, Patte C *et al.* (1999) Combined treatment modality of intracranial germinomas: results of a multicentre SFOP experience. Br J Cancer 79:1199-204

6. Brandes AA, Pasetto LM, Monfardini S (2000) The treatment of cranial germ cell tumours. Cancer Treat Rev 26: 233-42
7. **Buckner JC, Peethambaram PP, Smithson WA *et al.* (1999) Phase II trial of primary chemotherapy followed by reduced-dose radiation for CNS germ cell tumors. J Clin Oncol 17: 933-40**
8. **Calugaru V, Taillibert S, Lang P *et al.* (2007) Chimiothérapie néoadjuvant suivie d'une radiothérapie adaptée à la réponse tumorale dans les tumeurs germinales séminomateuses du système nerveux central: expérience de l'hôpital de la Pitié-Salpêtrière et revue de la littérature. Cancer Radiothérapie 11: 122-8**
9. Dearnaley DP, A'Hern RP, Whittaker S, Bloom HJ (1990) Pineal and CNS germ cell tumors: Royal Marsden Hospital experience 1962-1987. Int J Radiat Oncol Biol Phys 18: 773-81
10. Endo H, Kumabe T, Jokura H, Tominaga T (2005) Stereotactic radiosurgery followed by whole ventricular irradiation for primary intracranial germinoma of the pineal region. Minim Invasive Neurosurg 48: 186-90
11. Fuller BG, Kapp DS, Cox R (1994) Radiation therapy of pineal region tumors: 25 new cases and a review of 208 previously reported cases. Int J radiat Oncol Biol Phys 28: 229-45
12. Hardenbergh PH, Golden J, Billet A *et al.* (1997) Intracranial germinoma: the case for lower dose radiation therapy. Int J Radiat Oncol Biol Phys 39: 419-26
13. Hass-Kogan DA, Misset BT, Wara WM *et al.* (2003) Radiation therapy for intracranial germ cell tumors. Int J Radiat Oncol Biol Phys 56: 511-8
14. **Janmohamed S, Grossman AB, Metcalfe K *et al.* (2002) Suprasellar germ cell tumours: specific problems and the evolution of optimal management with a combined chemoradiotherapy regimen. Clinical Endocrinology 57: 487-500**
15. Kan P, Gottfried ON, Blumenthal DT *et al.* (2006) Primary spinal yolk sac tumor with brain metastasis: case report and review of the literature. J Neurooncol 78: 249-53
16. Nguyen QN, Chang EL, Allen PK *et al.* (2006) Focal and craniospinal irradiation for patients with intracranial germinoma and patterns of failure. Cancer 107: 2228-36
17. Ogawa K, Toita T, Nakamura K *et al.* (2003) Treatment and prognosis of patients with intracranial nongerminomatous malignant germ cell tumors. Cancer 98: 369-76
18. Ogawa K, Shikama N, Toita T *et al.* (2004) Long-term results of radiotherapy for intracranial germinoma: a multi-institutional retrospective review of 126 patients. Int J Radiat Oncol Biol Phys 58: 705-13
19. Ogino H, Shibamoto Y, Takanaka T *et al.* (2005) CNS germinoma with elevated serum human chorionic gonadotropin level: clinical characteristics and treatment outcome. In J Rradiat Oncol Biol Phys 62: 803-8
20. Robertson PL, DaRosso RC, Allen JC (1997) Improved prognosis of intracranial non-germinoma cell tumors with multimodality therapy. J Neurooncol 32: 71-80
21. Roselblum MK, Nakazato Y, Matsutani M. CNS germ cell tumours. In "WHO classification of tumours of the central nervous system". Edited by DN Louis, H Ohgaki, OD Wiestler, and WK Cavenee. International Agency for Research on Cancer. WHO press, Lyon 2007.
22. Sawamura Y, Ikeda J, Shirato H *et al.* (1998) Germ cell tumours of the central nervous system: treatment consideration based on 111 cases and their long-term clinical outcomes. Eur J Cancer 34: 104-10
23. Schild SE, Haddock MG, Scheithauer BW *et al.* (1996) Nongerminomatous germ cell tumors of the brain. Int J Radiat Oncol Biol Phys 36: 557-63
24. Schoenfeld GO, Amdur RJ, Schmalfuss IM *et al.* (2006) Low-dose prophylactic craniospinal radiotherapy for intracranial germinoma. Int J Radiat Oncol Biol Phys 65: 481-5
25. Shirane R, Shamoto H, Umezawa K *et al.* (1999) Surgical treatment of pineal region tumours through the occipital transtentorial approach: evaluation of the effectiveness of intra-operative micro-endoscopy combined with neuronavigation. Acta Neurochir 141: 801-9
26. **Silvani A, Eoli M, Salmaggi A *et al.* (2005) Combined chemotherapy and radiotherapy for intracranial germinomas in adult patients: a single-institution study. J Neuro-Oncol 71: 271-6**

1

27. Surawicz TS, McCarthy BJ, Kupelian V *et al.* (1999) Descriptive epidemiology of primary brain and CNS tumors: results from the Central Brain Tumor registry of the United States, 1990-1994. Neuro-Oncol 1: 14-25
28. Tang J, Ma Z, Luo S *et al.* (2008) The germinomas arising from the basal ganglia and thalamus. Childs Nerv Syst 24: 303-6
29. Villar S, Villà S, Ferrán E *et al.* (1998) Germinal tumours of the pineal region. Radiotherapy and Oncology 48: supp. 1, Abst 615
30. Wellons JC, Reddy AT, Tubbs RS *et al.* (2004) Neuroendoscopic findings in patients with intracranial germinomas correlating with diabetes insipidus. J Neurosurg 100: 430-6

Atypical and malignant meningiomas

D. Pasquier and N. Rezvoy

2

Five Essential Points

1. *The natural history, location and gender ratio differ from those of benign meningiomas.*
2. *Mitotic rate remains an important and reproducible prognostic factor for both anaplastic and malignant meningiomas.*
3. *In future, knowledge of genomic alterations could be useful for evaluating the prognosis and offering more tailored treatments.*
4. *Despite the low level of evidence, adjuvant radiotherapy is generally recommended after excision of an atypical or malignant meningioma – even when this excision is thought to have been complete.*
5. *The value of radiotherapy in general and that of certain techniques in particular (dose escalation in fractionated radiotherapy, fractionated and single-dose stereotactic radiotherapy, proton radiotherapy, etc.) must be evaluated prospectively.*

Introduction

Meningiomas are tumours that arise from the meninges of the brain and the spinal cord. The term meningioma was used for the first time in 1922 by Harvey Cushing. The arachnoidal origin of this type of tumour was also described at that time. By 1938, Cushing and Eisenhardt had already reported unusually aggressive, brain-invading meningiomas and had classified them as malignant [3]. The incidence of meningioma is approximately 6 per 100,000 [16]. These tumours occur primarily in middle-aged or elderly patients but can also occur in younger patients, typically with neurofibromatosis Type 2. Meningiomas constitute approximately 20% of all brain tumours, and at least 90% are histologically benign. A minority of these tumours present with clinical and histological features suggesting aggressive potential (atypical and malignant meningiomas). Atypical (grade II) and malignant (grade III) meningiomas constitute approximately 5-7% and 1-3% of meningiomas, respectively [10,19,38]. A large range of prevalence data for these aggressive forms has been reported, owing to the use of different classification systems in the literature. Benign meningiomas occur most often in women, whereas atypical and malignant forms seem to be more frequent in men and more common in cerebral convexities [10,16,22,33]. Atypical and malignant meningiomas can occur de novo or after reappearance of a previously benign form. Because of the rarity of this disease, optimal management is difficult to establish.

Imaging of atypical and malignant meningiomas

In computed tomography (CT), meningioma typically appears as a homogeneous mass that is spontaneously hyperdense (when compared with brain parenchyma) and presents a meningeal attachment. The mass displaces the adjacent brain parenchyma, rather than invading it. As a result of abundant tumour vascularisation, the meningioma stands out very soon after the injection of contrast agent. Contrast uptake is usually homogeneous and intense. With Magnetic Resonance Imaging (MRI), the tumour is isointense or slightly hypointense on T1-weighted sequences and hyperintense on T2-weighted sequences. It is also characterised by homogeneous, intense contrast uptake that makes the tumour and its dural attachment stand out even more than in CT. The meningeal origin is easier to establish with MRI, by virtue of higher contrast resolution.

Between 10 and 15% of meningiomas have an atypical radiological aspect (heterogeneous aspect, irregular contour, absence of calcification, significant oedema, invasion of the brain parenchyma and/or a poorly visible dural attachment). This radiological feature can orient the physician towards a diagnosis of atypical or malignant meningioma. These atypical radiological forms should also prompt consideration of a differential diagnosis of metastasis or brain glioma. Dufresnes *et al.* [5] studied 76 meningiomas; 51 were benign and 23 were malignant. The authors showed that the presence of necrosis, intratumour cysts, significant oedema, multiple lobes, irregular boundaries and the absence of calcification are more often associated with malignancy. In a series of 230 operated meningiomas, Servo *et al.* [41] also found that multiples lobes, nodular boundaries, cysts and the absence of calcification were more often associated with malignancy. However, neither of the studies found a discriminant criterion for predicting the histological grade with enough sensitivity and specificity. Hence, in anatomical sequences, an atypical radiological presentation is thus just one guiding element for the diagnosis of atypical or malignant meningioma. Progression between two successive examinations is another guiding element.

An increasing number of functional parameters are now accessible, notably thanks to the MR diffusion & perfusion imaging techniques and proton spectroscopy [1]. Diffusion imaging is an MRI technique that makes it possible to study the movements of water molecules in the extracellular space. An increase in cell density induces a decrease in the diffusion of water in the extracellular space and thus in the apparent diffusion coefficient (ADC). Hypercellularity is a characteristic of tumour tissues and this parameter increases with the grade. This is well established for glial tumours: a decrease in the ADC correlates with a high grade [1]. Filippi *et al.* [8] have also reported a significant decrease in ADC for malignant meningiomas, compared with benign meningiomas. However, the latter study dealt with very few cases (17 meningiomas, of which only 4 were malignant). This observation appears to have been confirmed since by other groups [12]. Nagar *et al.* [29] reported the same findings when comparing 25 atypical or malignant meningiomas with 23 benign meningiomas and were even able to determine a normalized ADC threshold for distinguishing atypical or malignant meningiomas from benign meningiomas with 96% sensitivity and 100% specificity.

Magnetic resonance spectroscopy is another functional imaging technique of value. Meningiomas are characterised by low creatine and acetylaspartate levels and by an increase in the choline and alanine peaks. The choline/creatine ratio appears to be higher in atypical meningiomas [4]. In a 37-patient study, Majos *et al.* [23] used spectroscopy to identify 4 out of 5 histologically confirmed atypical meningiomas. All these tumour characterization techniques are promising but must be confirmed in larger, prospective studies.

Pathology

Meningioma grading has long been (and remains) a subject of debate. The first classifications introduced a significant degree of subjectivity, due to the selected criteria. Later, more reproducible factors (such as mitotic rate, macronuclei, prominent nucleoli, sheet-like growth patterns and hypercellularity) were studied. Mitotic rate is a well known prognostic factor in the literature [14,33-35]. Two major retrospective series published by the Mayo Clinic deserve particular attention [34,35]; they aimed at establishing reproducible prognostic factors in large patient cohorts by re-examining histology slides. In the first series [34], 581 consecutive patients were analyzed. Brain invasion, sheeting, absence of nuclear atypia and a maximal mitotic rate greater than 4 per 10 high-power field (HPF) were univariately associated with decreased recurrence-free survival. The investigators recommended that "atypical" meningiomas be defined by the presence of at least three of these features: sheeting, macronuclei, hypercellularity, small-cell formation, or a minimum of 4 mitoses per 10 HPF [34]. In their second study, Perry *et al.* [35] expanded their analysis to 116 patients diagnosed with "malignant" meningioma. On multivariate analysis, histological parameters that remained significant were anaplasia, extent of resection, >20 mitoses per 10 HPF, and nuclear atypia. The median survival for "frankly" anaplastic meningioma was 1.5 years, and the 5-year mortality rate was 68% [35].

The 2000 WHO classification adopted the majority of Perry *et al.*'s results [34-35]. In the 2000 WHO classification [19], a mitotic rate >4 per 10 HPF was considered as the most significant factor for defining atypical meningioma. In patients with a lower mitotic rate, the presence of at least three of the following variables is necessary: increased cellularity, macronuclei, prominent nucleoli, sheet-like growth pattern, and necrosis. Malignant meningioma is defined as the presence of a mitotic rate >20 per 10 HPF or "obvious" malignant cytology, or both. Ho *et al.* [14] found MIB-1 (Ki67) to be a powerful prognostic marker, and a cut-off point of 10% discriminated tumours in patients with different prognoses. In the literature, although a poor prognosis may be associated with a high MIB-1 labelling index, significant overlap exists in the MIB-1 labelling ranges for benign, atypical, and anaplastic meningiomas.

The prognostic role of brain invasion has been widely discussed in the recent literature. Brain invasion used to be a standard criterion for malignancy [2] but pathologists have progressively cast doubt on this idea. In 1993, the WHO classification still considered brain invasion as a malignancy criterion, although the classification's authors already indicated that it could sometimes be displayed by benign-looking meningiomas. Examination of the Mayo Clinic histological series has confirmed this notion [34,35]. The Mayo Clinic group suggested that brain invasion should be a criterion for atypical meningioma. This criterion was not included in the 2000 revision of the WHO classification [19]. However, the classification's authors added that brain invasion should be mentioned in the pathology report as a risk factor for incomplete excision and thus recurrence. Crossing the pia mater thus had to be considered as an element for tumour staging, rather than a histological grade criterion - in line with the adjacent organ invasion criterion found in the TNM classification of many types of neoplasia. In the latest revision of the WHO classification (2007), brain invasion has become a criterion for atypical meningioma [37]. This is the only significant modification for meningioma, compared with the previous edition (Table 1).

Genetic alterations are often present in meningiomas. A mutation of the NF2gene (on the 22q12 chromosome) is found in 60% of sporadic meningiomas, regardless of the grade. Weber *et al.* [43] identified different genomic alterations in benign, atypical, and malignant meningiomas. The 1p, 9q, 10q and 14q deletions are preferentially associated with grades II and III. Murakami *et al.* [28] also suggested that 10q loss may contribute to malignant progression. As in Weber *et al.* [43], 9p deletions were associated with malignant progression and poor prognosis in malignant meningiomas in Perry *et al.* [36]. The genes involved in meningioma carcinogenesis are poorly known. The specific CDKN2A, CDKN2B and ARF genes located on 9p are involved in the G1/S phase cell cycle checkpoint [39]. In the future, genomic alterations could be useful to appraise prognosis and to propose more adapted treatments.

Table 1 – Summary of the 2007 World Health Organization grading scheme for meningiomas [37]. WHO = World Health Organization; HPF= High Power Field.

WHO grade	Histological features	Histological subtype
Benign (grade I)	No criteria for grade II or III	Meningothelial, fibroblastic, transitional, angiomatous, microcystic, secretory, lymphoplasmacytic metaplastic, psammomatous
Atypical (grade II)	4 or more mitoses/10 HPF and/or 3 or more of the following criteria: increased cellularity, small cells, necrosis, prominent nucleoli, sheet-like growth pattern and/or brain invasion in an otherwise Grade I	Chordoid, clear cell
Anaplastic (grade III)	20 or more mitoses/10 HPF and/or obvious malignant cytological characteristics such that tumour cell resembles carcinoma, sarcoma or melanoma	Papillary, rhabdoid

Treatment

As with benign meningiomas, no prospective studies have yet evaluated the results and the respective values of the various modes of therapy for atypical and malignant forms (surgery, conformational and stereotactic radiotherapy, proton radiotherapy and chemotherapy). The therapeutic approaches have thus been established on the basis of retrospective data, with low levels of evidence.

Surgery

As with benign meningiomas, surgery is the benchmark treatment for (operable) lesions. Surgery provides an anatomopathological diagnosis, reduces the effect of the tumour mass and improves the symptoms. The surgical principles are the same as for benign forms and excision should be as complete as possible. The quality of the surgical excision is typically graded according to the system described by Simpson (grades 1 to 5) [42]. Grades 1 and 2 represent complete excision with resection and coagulation of the dural attachment, respectively, and grade 5 corresponds to a simple biopsy.

As in benign forms, completion of resection was associated with outcome in several series. Goyal *et al.* [10] reported that 8 of 22 patients with atypical meningiomas received adjuvant radiotherapy or radiotherapy for relapse. The overall 5- and 10-year survival rates were 91% and 76%, respectively. Patients with gross total resection had 5- and 10-year control rates of 87% and 87%, whereas patients with either subtotal resection or resection of unknown extent had local control rates of 51% and 17%, respectively ($p = 0.02$). In a series reported by Palma *et al.* [32], radical excision was significantly related to prolonged survival on multivariate analysis ($p < 0.0003$). Considering patients with incomplete resection, the survival curve of atypical meningioma was not significantly different from that of malignant meningioma. In a recent series [33] the completion of resection was not a significant prognostic factor, probably because of the difficulty to retrospectively assess the completion of resection. Jääskelainen *et al.* [16] regarded Simpson Grades 1 and 2 as "complete resection" but in a later study Jääskelainen [17] found that simple coagulation of the dura mater (Grade 2) vs. excision (Grade 1) doubled the recurrence rate in that series of benign meningiomas. Clinical prognostic factors (such as age and general patient status) have also been put forward (Tables 2 and 3).

Table 2 – Characteristics and results of the main published series for patients presenting atypical or malignant meningiomas.

Author	N. of patients Atypical/ Malignant	Sex ratio (M/F)	Median age (years)	Surgery (%)	Complete resection (%)	Radio-therapy (%)	Adjuvant radio-therapy (%)	5 years relapse free survival (%)	10 years relapse free survival (%)	5 years overall survival (%)	10 years overall survival (%)
Liu [20]	22 0/22	1.2	52.5	100	100	100	100	27.3	13.6	36.4	22.7
Perry [35]	116 0/116	1.1	60	100	72	31	16			62	47
Milosevic [25]	59		58	93	53	100	41			28	
Goyal [10]	22 22/0	1.75	55,5	100	68	64	36	70	55	91	76
Dziuk [6]	38 0/38	0.6	60	100	58		50	25			
Hug [15]	31 15/16	1.2	49	94	26	100	52	45		70	
Ho [14]	31 31/0			100	100			29	6		
Palma [32]	71 42/29			100	100					95% grade 2 64% grade 3	79% grade 2 35% grade 3
Pasquier [33]	119 82/37	1.3	57.6	100	71	100	79	58	48	65	51

2

Table 3 – Prognostic factors found in the principal published series for patients presenting atypical or malignant meningiomas (multivariate analysis except [10]).

Author	Prognostic factors
Liu [20]	Location; Simpson grade (1 *vs* 2)
Perry [35]	Simpson grade; Anaplasia; Mitotic rate; Nuclear atypia
Milosevic [25]	Age; Radiotherapy after 1975; Radiotherapy dose > 50 Gy
Goyal [10]	Complete resection
Dziuk [6]	Simpson grade; Adjuvant radiotherapy
Hug [15]	RT dose > 60 Gy; Atypical *vs* Malignant
Ho [14]	MIB1; Necrosis; Mitotic rate
Palma [32]	Atypical *vs* Malignant; Simpson grade (1 *vs* 2-3)
Pasquier [33]	Age < 60 years; Karnofsky Performace Status; Mitotic rate

Pre-operative embolization can help reduce tumour volume and blood losses and facilitate the surgical act itself. However, malignant tumours are not necessarily more vascularised than benign forms and the benefit is uncertain. Embolization can also perturb the anatomopathological examination (tumour necrosis).

Radiotherapy

The main indications are (i) adjunct radiotherapy after surgical excision or after relapse and (ii) radiotherapy of non-operable tumours. Adjuvant radiotherapy after incomplete resection (benign or aggressive meningioma) has not been evaluated in a prospective study to date [26]. Some retrospective trials promote adjuvant radiotherapy after incomplete resection in patients with atypical meningioma, and independently of the status of resection in malignant meningioma [6,27]. The role of adjuvant radiotherapy in completely resected (Simpson Grade 1) atypical meningioma is unclear. In our series [33] the outcome was not related to radiotherapy dose, whereas in certain series dose is a prognostic factor [6,25]. In Milosevic *et al.* [25], dose >50 Gy and age <40 years were the two prognostic factors associated with a favourable outcome on multivariate analysis. The use of dose <50 Gy is not optimal in patients with meningioma, as in benign meningioma, in which a dose–response relationship for local control was shown up to 52 Gy in retrospective series but not beyond [9,26]. Despite the fact that no randomized trial has yet specified the value of radiotherapy in the treatment of meningioma, adjuvant radiotherapy is generally recommended after excision of an atypical or malignant meningioma - even when excision is thought to have been complete. The roles of dose escalation (dose >55-60 Gy) and radiosurgery in aggressive meningioma have not been evaluated in a controlled, prospective study. Some retrospective series report benefit in terms of local control after fractionated or single-dose stereotactic radiotherapy or after proton radiotherapy [13,18,31]. It is nevertheless important to prospectively evaluate such techniques in this respect. The recently initiated Phase II 22042 European Organisation for Research and Treatment of Cancer trial is assessing the impact of high-dose radiotherapy on progression-free survival, treatment tolerance and post-treatment global cognitive functioning in patients with resected atypical or malignant meningioma [7].

Chemotherapy and medical treatment

Chemotherapy results have been reported in small series as part of recurrent meningioma or metastatic disease. Extracerebral metastasis can be encountered in patients with atypical or malignant meningiomas. In the Mayo Clinic series [35], 3 out of 27 patients with "frankly" anaplastic meningiomas presented with distant metastases. In the Milosevic *et al.* series [25], 4 of 59 patients with atypical and malignant meningiomas presented pathologically distant bone metastases. In our series 6 patients presented with skin or other distant metastases. Four patients presented skin metastases near the surgical incision. Two patients with Grade 3 meningiomas were found to have histologically proven (biopsy and autopsy) liver metastasis and bone and liver metastases [33].

The results for several compounds have been described retrospectively in the literature. By virtue of the presence of hormone receptors, anti-oestrogen and anti-progesterone treatments such as tamoxifen, megestrone acetate and mifepristone have been used but without success. The negative results of a randomized trial with mifepristone have been reported by Grunberg *et al.* [11]. The results of combination chemotherapy have been described in a small series but hydroxyurea has been more often used in patients presenting a benign or aggressive meningioma, with both favourable [24,40] and unfavourable outcomes [21,30]. Overall, there is no convincing evidence on the efficacy of drug treatments for intracerebral or metastatic recurrence; inclusion in multicentre, prospective trials is desirable. Therapeutics targeting epidermal growth factor (EGF), vascular endothelial growth factor (VEGF) and platelet-derived growth factor (PDGF) are under evaluation.

References

1. Cha S (2006) Update on brain tumor imaging: from imaging to physiology. AJNR Am J of Neuroradiol 27(3): 475-87
2. Commins DL, Atkinson RD, Burnett ME (2007) Review of meningioma histopathology. Neurosurg Focus 23(4): E3
3. Cushing H, Eisenhardt L (1938). Meningiomas: their classification, regional behaviour, life history, and surgical end results. Springfield, IL: Charles C Thomas publishers
4. Demir MK, Iplikcioglu AC, Dincer A *et al.* (2006) Single voxel proton MR spectroscopy findings of typical and atypical intracranial meningiomas. Eur J radiol 60(1): 48-55
5. Dufresne MC, Bedard F (1996) X-ray computed tomographic aspects of malignant meningioma and meningeal hemangiopericytoma. J Can Assoc Radiol 47: 279-87
6. Dziuk TW, Woo S, Butker EB *et al.* (1998) Malignant meningioma: an indication for initial aggressive surgery and adjuvant radiotherapy. J Neurooncol 37(2): 177-88
7. European Organisation for Research and Treatment of Cancer-22042 trial http://www.cancer.gov/clinicaltrials/EORTC-22042
8. Filippi CG, Edgar MA, Ulu AM *et al.* (2001) Appearance of meningiomas on diffusion-weighted images: correlating diffusion constants with histopathologic findings. AJNR Am J of Neuroradiol 22(1): 65-72
9. Goldsmith BJ, Wara WM, Wilson CB *et al.* (1994) Postoperative irradiation for subtotally resected meningiomas. A retrospective analysis of 140 patients treated from 1967 to 1990. J Neurosurg 80: 195-201
10. Goyal L, Suh J, Mohan D *et al.* (2000) Local control and overall survival in atypical meningioma: A retrospective study. Int J Radiat Oncol Biol Phys 46: 57-61
11. Grunberg SM, Rankin C, Townsend J *et al.* (2001) Phase III double-blind randomized placebo controlled study of mifepristone (RU) for the treatment of unresectable meningioma. ASCO Proceedings 20: 56a

2

12. Hakyemez B, Yildirim N, Gokalp G *et al.* (2006) The contribution of diffusion-weighted MR imaging to distinguishing typical from atypical meningiomas. Neuroradiology 48(8): 513-20
13. Harris AE, Lee JYK, Omalu B *et al.* (2003) The effect of radiosurgery during management of aggressive meningiomas. Surg Neurol 60: 298-305
14. Ho D, Hsu C, Ting L *et al.* (2002) Histopathology and MIB-1 labeling index predicted recurrence of meningiomas. A proposal of diagnostic criteria for patients with atypical meningioma. Cancer 94: 1538-47
15. Hug EB, Devries A, Thornton AF *et al.* (2000) Management of atypical and malignant meningiomas: role of high dose, 3D-conformal radiation therapy. J Neurooncol 48(2): 151-60
16. Jääskelainen J, Haltia M, Servo A (1986) Atypical and anaplastic meningiomas: radiology, surgery, radiotherapy and outcome. Surg Neurol 25: 233-42
17. Jääskelainen J. (1986) Seemingly complete removal of histologically benign intracranial meningioma: Late recurrence rate and factors predicting recurrence in 657 patients. A multivariate analysis. Surg Neurol 26: 461-9
18. Kano H, Takahashi JA, Katsuki T *et al.* (2007) Stereotactic radiosurgery for atypical and anaplastic meningiomas. J Neurooncol 84(1): 41-7
19. Kleihues P, Cavenee W (2000) World Health Organization Classification of tumors: Pathology and genetics of tumors of the nervous system. Lyon, France, IARC Press
20. Liu Y, Liu M, Li F *et al.* (2007) Malignant meningiomas: a retrospective study of 22 cases. Bull Cancer 94(10): E27-31
21. Loven D, Hardoff R, Sever ZB *et al.* (2004) Non-resectable slow growing meningiomas treated by hydroxyurea. J Neurooncol 67: 221-6
22. Mahmood A, Caccamo D, Tomecek F *et al.* (1993) Atypical and malignant meningiomas: A clinicopathological review. Neurosurgery 33: 955-63
23. Majos C, Alonso J, Aguilera C *et al.* (2003) Utility of proton MR spectroscopy in the diagnosis of radiologically atypical intracranial meningiomas. Neuroradiology 45(3): 129-36
24. Mason WP, Gentili F, MacDonald DR *et al.* (2002) Stabilization of disease progression by hydroxyurea in patients with recurrent or unresectable meningioma. J Neurosurg 97: 341-6
25. Milosevic MF, Frost PJ, Laperriere NJ *et al.* (1996) Radiotherapy for atypical or malignant intracranial meningioma. Int J Radiat Oncol Biol Phys 34(4): 817-22
26. Mirimanoff RO (2004) New radiotherapy technologies for meningiomas: 3D conformal radiotherapy? Radiosurgery? Stereotactic radiotherapy? Intensity-modulated radiotherapy? Proton beam radiotherapy? Spot scanning proton radiation therapy. Or nothing at all? Radiother Oncol 71: 247-9
27. Modha A, Gutin P (2005) Diagnosis and treatment of atypical and anaplastic meningiomas: A review. Neurosurgery 57: 538-50
28. Murakami M, Hashimoto N, Takahashi Y *et al.* (2003) A consistent region of deletion on 1p36 in meningiomas: Identification and relation to malignant progression. Cancer Genet Cytogenet 140: 99-106
29. Nagar VA, Ye JR, NG WH *et al.* (2008) Diffusion-weighted MR imaging: diagnosing atypical or malignant meningiomas and detecting tumor dedifferentiation. AJNR Am J of Neuroradiol 29(6): 1147-52
30. Newton HB, Slivka MA, Stevens C (2000) Hydroxyurea chemotherapy for unresectable or residual meningioma. J Neurooncol 49: 165-70
31. Noel G, Habrand JL, Mammar H *et al.* (2002) Highly conformal therapy using proton component in the management of meningiomas: Preliminary experience of the Centre de Protontherapie d'Orsay. Strahlenther Onkol 178: 480-5
32. Palma L, Celli P, Franco C *et al.* (1997) Long-term prognosis for atypical and malignant meningiomas: A study of 71 surgical cases. J Neurosurg 86: 793-800
33. **Pasquier D, Bijmolt S, Veninga T *et al.* (2008) Atypical and malignant meningioma: outcome and prognostic factors in 119 irradiated patients. A multicenter, retrospective study of the rare cancer Network. Int J Radiat Oncol Biol Phys 71: 1388-93**
34. Perry A, Stafford SL, Scheithauer BW *et al.* (1997) Meningioma grading: An analysis of histologic parameters. Am J Surg Pathol 21: 1455-65
35. Perry A, Scheithauer BW, Stafford SL *et al.* (1999) "Malignancy" in meningiomas: A clinicopathologic study of 116 patients, with grading implications. Cancer 85: 2046-56

36. Perry A, Banerjee R, Lohse C *et al.* (2002) A role for chromosome 9p21 deletions in the malignant progression of meningiomas and the prognosis of anaplastic meningiomas. Brain Pathol 12: 183-90
37. Perry A (2007) Meningiomas In: Louis D, Ohgaki H, Wiestler OD, Cavenee WK, Burger PC, Jouvet A *et al.* (eds). World Health Organization classification of tumours of the central nervous system, ed 4, Lyon, IARC pp 164-72
38. Pourel N, Auque J, Bracard S *et al.* (2001) Efficacy of external fractionated radiation therapy in the treatment of meningiomas: A 20-year experience. Radiother Oncol 61: 65-70
39. Riemenschneider M, Perry A, Reifenberger G (2006) Histological classification and molecular genetics of meningiomas. Lancet Neurol 5: 1045-54
40. Schrell UMH, Rittig MG, Anders M *et al.* (1997) Hydroxyurea for treatment of unresectable and recurrent meningiomas: II–Decrease in the size of meningiomas in patients treated with hydroxyurea. J Neurosurg 86: 840-4
41. Servo A, Porras M, Jaaskelainen J *et al.* (1990) Computed tomography and angiography do not reliably discriminate malignant meningiomas from beningn ones. Neuroradiology 32(2): 94-7
42. Simpson D (1957) The recurrence of intracranial meningiomas after surgical treatment. J Neurol Neurosurg Psychiatry 20(1): 22-39
43. Weber R, Bostrom J, Wolter M *et al.* (1997) Analysis of genomic alterations in benign, atypical, and anaplastic meningiomas: Toward a genetic model of meningioma progression. Proc Natl Acad Sci USA 94: 14719-24

Primary central nervous system lymphoma

3

Ph. M.P. Poortmans

Five Essential Points

1. *Imaging and histopathology including immunohistochemistry are of utmost importance for confirming the diagnosis of PCNSL.*
2. *High-dose MTX-based chemotherapy, according to a published schedule, followed by consolidating whole-brain radiotherapy is the standard treatment approach for all patients, unless age (>60 years and >65 years if in good condition) or general and neurological condition renders this impossible.*
3. *Participation in clinical trials should be encouraged as much as possible.*
4. *The risk for long term cognitive dysfunction induced by the disease, the chemotherapy and the radiotherapy should be explained to the patients before treatment. Neuropsychological tests should be carried out before and after treatment to monitor this.*
5. *PCNSL is an excellent example of a disease where a broad multidisciplinary approach is of utmost importance.*

Introduction

Primary Central Nervous System Lymphoma (PCNSL) is a relatively rare localisation of non-Hodgkin's lymphoma (NHL) that is confined to the brain, the leptomeninges, the eyes, the cerebrospinal fluid (CSF) or the nerve bundles. PCNSL is, as a primary brain tumour, by definition not diagnosed in the setting of widespread localisations outside the central nervous system (CNS) [37]. Therefore, it should be differentiated from the secondary involvement of the CNS which occurs in 5% to 29% of patients with systemic NHL, usually associated with progressive widespread systemic disease and involving often only the meningeal surface. The prognosis of patients with PCNSL with conventional treatment similar to that for other NHL is very poor, with a 5-year survival rate at usually less than 10%. Some rare but distinctive subtypes of PCNSL should be recognised.

Incidence

PCNSL accounts for about 1 % of all intracranial neoplasms and for about 1 to 2% of all NHL. The highest incidence of non AIDS-related PCNSL is reported in the age group from 45 to 70 with a median age of 60. The incidence is higher in men (male/female ratio 1.7:1). A higher incidence is found in patients with a congenital, acquired or iatrogenic immunodeficiency syndrome, especially in patients with the acquired immunodeficiency syndrome (AIDS). Their risk for developing PCNSL is 2-6%. It increases over time and is found in 12% during post mortem examination, suggesting that the diagnosis is not always suspected. The incidence of AIDS-related PCNSL is decreasing in developed countries after the introduction of highly active antiretroviral therapy (HAART). Over the last decades a marked increase in the incidence of PCNSL was seen, which can however not entirely be explained by the increased incidence of especially AIDS, the use of new diagnostic tools, or better pathological examinations. Notably in the United States, currently up to 5% of all newly diagnosed primary brain tumours are PCNSL [11, 46]. This chapter only deals with PCNSL in immunocompetent patients.

Diagnosis

Clinical signs and symptoms vary considerably and depend on the site of the tumoural involvement. A combination of behavioural changes, focal sensory or muscle function loss, seizures, visual disturbances and signs of elevated intracranial pressure can occur. PCNSL develops preferentially in supratentorial sites, notably the deeper-seated structures including the periventricular white matter, the corpus callosum, the basal ganglia and the thalamus. Typically, up to 50% of the patients present with multifocal cerebral disease. Involvement of the meningeal surface and/or the CSF is reported in at least one-third of the cases [5]. In 7% of the cases, only meningeal involvement without an obvious parenchymal tumour localisation is found [30]. Spinal cord lymphoma is very rare and can occur alone or associated with brain involvement. During careful ophthalmologic examination in about 20% of the patients ocular disease will be found and at follow up of PCNSL patients after treatment, ocular lymphoma will develop in up to one quarter of them.

Optimal imaging of the brain parenchyma requires a gadolinium-enhanced MRI scan (Figure 1). A contrast-enhanced CT scan can be used for patients where MRI is medically contraindicated (e.g. cardiac pacemaker) or unavailable. The appearance on CT and MRI examinations is highly variable, although often rather suggestive for PCNSL. On CT-scanning, isodense or slightly hyperdense lesions typically enhance densely and diffusely after contrast administration. T1-weighted MRI images show

a b

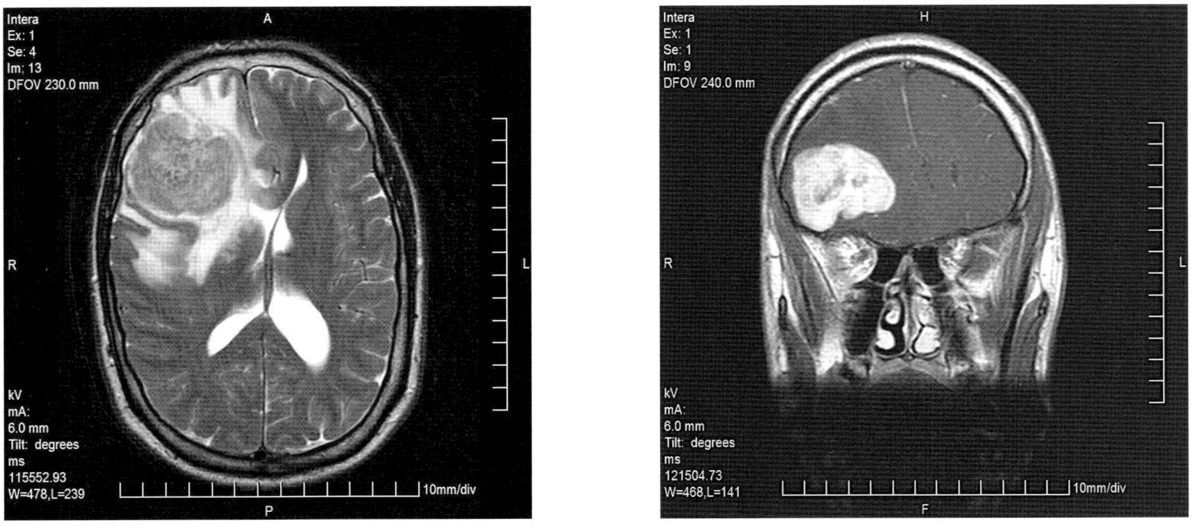

Fig. 1. Pre-treatment MRI images of a male, 25 years old, complaining of headache, nausea and visual disturbances. Treated with combined modality treatment. Disease free after 2.5 years.

most often iso- or hypodense lesions, explicitly enhancing after contrast administration. The appearance on T2-weighted images can be very unspecific and in 5-10% of the cases the lesions do not enhance with contrast at all. A necrotic appearance of the central part of the tumour is often clearly seen in patients with immunodeficiency. The amount of surrounding oedema can be quite variable, further hampering an estimate of the marginal tumour extension which is itself already not well delineated [29, 31]. The radiological differential diagnosis includes other primary CNS tumours, brain metastases, inflammatory and reactive infiltration including toxoplasmosis, histiocytosis, sarcoidosis, multiple sclerosis and leucoencephalopathy [14, 43]. Spontaneous remissions of histology-proven PCNSL are reported in the literature [4].

In the case of suspicion of PCNSL, treatment with corticosteroids should be withheld until the diagnostic biopsy has been performed, unless the patient is in immediate danger due to elevated intracranial pressure. The reason for this is the often rapid response of PCNSL to corticosteroid therapy. Histological or cytological tissue diagnosis is essential to confirm the differential diagnosis with several other intracranial processes, as listed above, which can have a similar appearance and a clear but transient response to corticosteroid treatment. Therefore, the neurosurgeon, neurologist or ophthalmologist should aim at obtaining a representative sample for examination. This can be done by stereotactic biopsy of the radiological demonstrable tumour or by examination of CSF or vitreous material. All patients should undergo a lumbar puncture for CSF cytology unless medically contraindicated. If the CSF contains cytologically abnormal cells or an elevated lymphocyte count, further examination of CSF should consist of immunocytology or flow-cytometry. The presence of cytologically abnormal cells with a B-cell immunophenotype or a monoclonal B-lymphocytosis is highly suggestive for the presence of a PCNSL [50]. Most PCNSL are diffuse large cell B-cell lymphoma.

As occult systemic disease has been reported in up to 8% of patients initially thought to have isolated PCNSL, complete staging is necessary in every patient to rule out the presence of systemic NHL but should never lead to postponement of diagnosis and treatment of confirmed PCNSL. The backbone of this examination is a comprehensive physical and neurological examination with particular attention to the peripheral lymph nodes in all patients and to the testes in men. Baseline laboratory evaluation includes serum LDH and determination of the hepatic and renal function in those who will receive intensive chemotherapy. A creatinine clearance above 50-60 ml/min is necessary to ensure adequate excretion of high-dose methotrexate (HD-MTX). All patients should be tested for human immunodeficiency virus infection given the increased incidence of PCNSL and the possibly different approach in this population. A CT scan of the chest, abdomen and pelvis and a bone marrow biopsy with aspirate are the recommended staging procedures. Based on the signs and symptoms or findings at physical examination, other more specific investigations can be performed. Furthermore, an evaluation of the cognitive function is important at baseline with which to compare the follow up assessments, to gauge the benefit of therapy as well as to monitor treatment-induced neurocognitive decline. Currently, as no accepted standard for neuropsychological testing exists, the Mini Mental State Examination (MMSE) should be scored regularly as a minimum in all patients.

Recently, a consensus paper on standardised guidelines for the baseline evaluation and response assessment of PCNSL was published by an international group of experts (IPCG), aiming at ensuring comparability among clinical trials for newly diagnosed patients. The response guidelines are based on the results of imaging, steroid use, ophthalmologic examination and cerebrospinal fluid cytology. A critical issue that requires further study is the optimal method to assess the neurocognitive impact of therapy and address the quality of life of PCNSL survivors [2].

Prognosis

Median survival with surgery alone is in the range of only 1-5 months, similar to treatment with corticosteroids only. When treated with conventional treatment similar to that for NHL at other disease sites, consisting of radiotherapy alone or of standard chemotherapy with or without radiotherapy, the prognosis of patients with PCNSL is comparable to that of glioblastoma multiforme patients, with a median survival limited to approximately 15 months and a 5-year survival rate rarely exceeding 10%. Potential unfavourable prognostic factors are: age > 60 years; WHO performance status > 2; poor pre-treatment neurologic function; extensive intracerebral tumour spread; no administration of HD-MTX chemotherapy; CSF protein level at diagnosis > 0,6 g/l and steroid-dependence [6, 18]. In a multivariate analysis, only age and performance status (PS) could be identified, enabling the construction of a simple but useful prognostic score with 3 distinct classes: class 1 = age < 50; class 2 = age ≥ 50 and PS 0-1; class 3 = age ≥ 50 and PS > 1 [3].

Treatment

Corticosteroids

The administration of corticosteroids leads to a clinical amelioration for most patients and, in at least 40% of the patients, a significant shrinkage or disappearance of the tumour. Regardless of apparent tumour regression, steroid-induced remission is short lived in the majority of patients, but with isolated reports of patients with a prolonged survival after corticosteroids alone [48]. It is very often used as the initial treatment for patients with distressing tumour-induced symptoms but should be withheld in others to avoid problems in obtaining proper tumour tissue for histological diagnosis.

Surgery

Because of the diffuse nature and the often deeply-seated localisation of PCNSL, aggressive surgical decompression to attempt partial or gross total removal of the tumour is of no benefit to patients and might even induce serious neurological deficits. Therefore, the neurosurgeon should aim at obtaining tumour tissue in a way least likely to cause side effects. Most often, a stereotactic biopsy will be the preferred way [24].

Radiotherapy

Whole brain radiotherapy (WBRT) combined with corticosteroids has been used in many series and for many years as single modality treatment for patients with PCNSL (Figure 2). The initial tumour and subjective response is most often good with a prompt resolution on CT/MRI, but patients almost invariably recur in or nearby the primary site in the brain. An increase of the radiotherapy dose up to 60 Gy or irradiation of the entire craniospinal axis clearly does not clearly improve results [34]. On the other hand, a dose reduction from 45 to 30 Gy after HD-MTX containing chemotherapy led to significantly worse results in 2 successive phase II trials [7].

a b
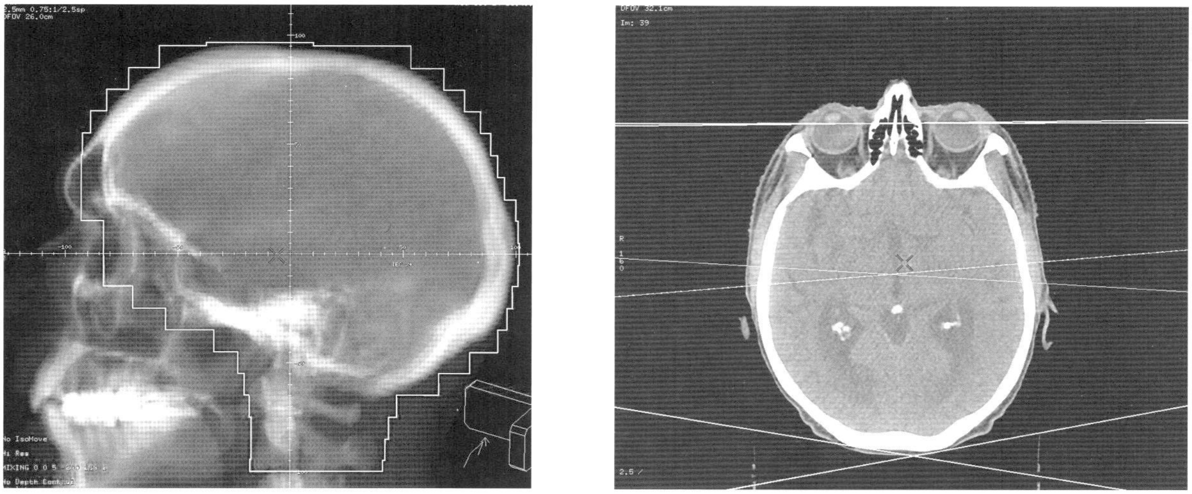

Fig. 2. Typical radiotherapy field including the whole brain, the meningeal surface, the medulla oblongata and the posterior part of the orbital structures.

Standard combined modality treatment

Systemic chemotherapy has been employed in many series [15, 32]. The blood-brain barrier (BBB) prevents hydrophilic compounds, including most chemotherapeutic agents and monoclonal antibodies, from entering the cerebral parenchyma [26]. Standard chemotherapy schedules such as CHOP, even combined with radiotherapy, do not improve the outcome compared to radiotherapy alone.

High dose combined modality treatment

Several attempts have been made to pass or disrupt the BBB. With HD-MTX, followed by leucovorin rescue, therapeutic MTX concentrations are attained in the CSF. Several retrospective and phase II prospective studies showed the efficacy of this approach followed by consolidating WBRT in improving overall median survival to around 3 years [8, 16, 20, 42]. As therapeutic MTX concentrations are attained in the CSF, the use of intrathecal chemotherapy may even been obviated [17]. The role of other chemotherapy compounds including high-dose cytosine arabinoside (HD-AraC), BBB disruption, immunological treatments including rituximab, maintenance chemotherapy and chemotherapy alone remain to be confirmed or have not been proved to be effective [9, 19, 35, 38].

By far the most experience has been obtained with HD-MTX based chemotherapy followed by consolidating radiotherapy for PCNSL. The overall response rate varies between 65 and 95% and the 2-year survival between 22 and 86%. Projections after a longer follow up period are made with an estimated 3-year survival of 45% to 58% and 5-year survival of 30% to 56%. However, we must realise that most series reporting 3- and 5-year survival have a limited number of patients and a rather short follow-up period. Moreover, for a correct interpretation of many of the published results, we have to consider that patients older than 65 and in a poor general or neurological condition were often not eligible for trial participation, thereby excluding the worst patient subset.

Several authors have suggested that adding HD-AraC to HD-MTX might improve outcome. The results of a Dutch trial in which AraC was given before MTX in each cycle were not superior to the results of RT alone [49]. This finding might suggest that if AraC is given in combination with MTX, the latter should be given first. An interesting approach is further intensification of chemotherapy with autologous stem-cell transplantation, with or without consolidating radiotherapy [10, 25].

Treatment for relapse

Prognosis after disease progression or relapse is poor despite high response rates to salvage therapy. In selected patients, high dose salvage chemotherapy with stem cell support leads possibly to an increase in survival. Also radiotherapy, if not given before, can – especially for patients in a good general condition – lead to tumour regression and a limited gain in survival [28, 47].

When cure is not possible

Increasing age is related both to a poor prognosis and to an increased risk of both early and late toxicity induced by aggressive combined modality treatment. An upper age limit of 60 years or possibly 65 years, if the patient is in good general and neurological condition, should be respected for this treatment approach with curative intent. Therefore, most patients above the age of 60 and those that are in such a bad condition, rendering them unsuitable to undergo intensive treatment, can be offered only a palliative approach. Depending on the symptoms, the age and the patient's preference, this could just as well be corticosteroids, WBRT or moderate intensity chemotherapy [41]. Often, corticosteroids can be started, with WBRT or chemotherapy withheld until clinical signs and symptoms of disease recur.

Toxicity

Early toxicity

The acute chemotherapy-induced toxicity is mainly leucocytopenia. Especially for patients already in a suboptimal condition due to the effects of the primary brain tumour, a high rate of severe and even lethal toxicity can be expected. General condition is a well-known important predictive factor for excessive toxicity caused by intensive treatment schedules. Another point of concern is that, due to the limited incidence of PCNSL, hardly any centre can gain significant experience with this disease and its specific treatment. Therefore, hospitalisation and highly specialised care is essential during the administration of chemotherapy due to the need for expert management of grade 3 and 4 toxicity.

Late toxicity

With the improved prognosis after combined HD-MTX and WBRT, long-term treatment-related neurological toxicity has emerged as a potentially serious problem with important implications for cognitive functioning and quality of life (QoL). The most common late neurotoxicity induced by this kind of treatment is leucoencephalopathy, which is initially characterised by neurobehavioral changes (confusion, personality changes, memory loss, apathy), co-ordination problems and gait disturbances and related to white matter abnormalities and cortical atrophy on neuroradiological evaluation (Figure 3). The decline is often but not always progressive and

a
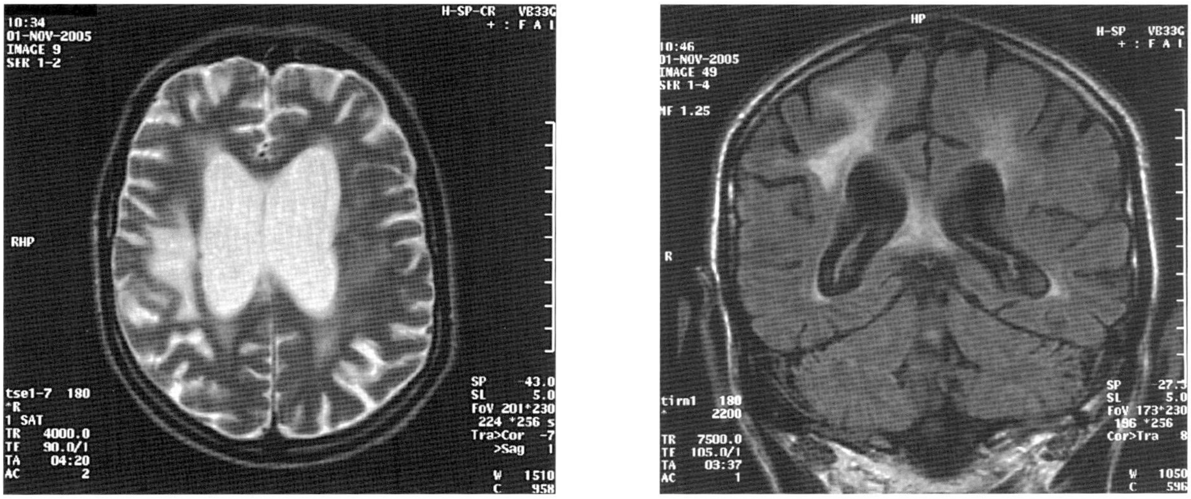

b

Fig. 3. Images of periventricular leucoencephalopathy and cortical atrophy after combined modality treatment for PCNSL in a male, 61 years old at the time of treatment and disease free for 4 years.

can eventually result in dementia, ataxia, paralysis or stupor, even leading to premature death. The impact of treatment-related neurotoxicity on QoL can be very important, as some patients require support in daily life activities, or even institutional care. The reported incidence of late neurotoxicity in PCNSL patients varies, based on the duration of follow-up and the way of measuring this, from 0% to 36%. Risk factors are age > 60, initial poor neurological function, increasing dose of WBRT, HD-MTX given after radiotherapy and prolonged survival after treatment [1,13, 23, 44]. Because the combination of HD-MTX and WBRT increases late neurological toxicity especially when WBRT is given first, combined modality treatment should always start with chemotherapy. Although omitting radiotherapy might decrease the relapse free survival, some authors advocate postponing WBRT until disease recurrence or progression, especially for patients aged > 60.

Careful follow up of neurological function, especially gait and neuroimaging changes, are also important. In the framework of clinical trials, a more thorough evaluation including measures of psychomotor speed, executive, and memory abilities to detect treatment effects in this population should be incorporated [2, 12, 22, 36, 39].

Distinct presentations

Spinal cord PCNSL

Very little is known about this relatively rare presentation of PCNSL. Especially because the risk for late neurotoxicity is low thanks to the location of the disease outside of the intracranial CNS, it seems logical to treat these patients with curative intent with combined modality treatment including HD-MTX containing chemotherapy and consolidating radiotherapy to the involved part of the spinal cord only. This disease presentation should be clearly discriminated from the primary epidural NHL, which should be treated like primary non-CNS extranodal NHL [33].

Ocular PCNSL

In intraocular PCNSL, lymphoma cells can be found in the vitreous cavity and the subretinal epithelial space. In view of the very important therapeutic consequences, the diagnosis should always be confirmed by biopsy. When this is done, the presence of other localisations of PCNSL should always be excluded. When these patients are treated only locally, they will eventually nearly all develop bilateral ocular disease and in up to 80% of the cases intracranial PCNSL, sometimes even after a latency period of many years. Treatment with curative intent should be the same as for other forms of PCNSL but the role of consolidating WBRT can be questioned and may be replaced by ipsilateral ocular irradiation only. Intraocular injections with MTX and rituximab are under investigation [21].

T-cell PCNSL

In the framework of the IPCG, a retrospective study was organised with the aim of describing the demographic and tumour-related characteristics and outcomes for patients with primary T-cell PCNSL [45]. A total of 45 patients with T-PCNSL was collected by twelve cancer centres from seven countries. The male/female ratio was 35/10 and the median age was 60 years (range 3 to 84). Twenty six (58%) had involvement of a cerebral hemisphere and sixteen (36%) had lesions of the deeper structures of the brain. Concerning pathology, the tumour was described as "angiocentric" in 28% of the reviewed cases; the cell size was "small" or "small to medium" in about half of the cases and either "pleomorphic" or "medium to large" cells in the other half. Among these latter, one quarter had features of anaplastic large cell lymphoma and stained positive for CD30 in addition to CD3. The median disease- specific survival (DSS) was 25 months (95% confidence interval [CI] 11-38 months). The two and five-year DSS were 51 % (CI 35-66 %) and 17 % (CI 6-34 %) respectively. In the univariate and multivariate analyses, only performance score and the use of MTX-based chemotherapy were significantly associated with better outcome with hazard ratios (HR) of 0.2 (CI 0.1-0.4) and 0.4 (CI 0.2-0.8) respectively. To conclude, the presentation and outcome of T-PCNSL appears to be similar to that of B-cell PCNS with performance score 0 or 1 and the administration of MTX being associated with a better survival.

Low-grade PCNSL

Also in the framework of the IPCG, a retrospective study was carried out, aimed at the characterisation of a possible distinctive clinical presentation, course and outcome of low-grade PCNSL [27]. Forty patients with a male/female ratio of 18/22 and a median age of 60 years (range 19 to 78), were collected from 18 cancer centres in five countries. Involvement of a cerebral hemisphere or deeper brain structures was seen in 37 patients; only leptomeningeal involvement in two cases, and spinal cord disease in one patient. Concerning pathology, 80% of the patients had a B-cell and 20% a T-cell lymphoma. B-cell histology included lymphoplasmacytic lymphoma (n = 11), follicular grade 1 lymphoma (n = 1), and lymphomas not further classified but described as "small lymphocytic, low-grade", "small lymphocytic", or "poorly differentiated lymphocytic, low-grade" (n = 20). The T-cell cases were described as "angiocentric" (n = 3) and "small lymphocytic, low-grade" (n = 5) and were confirmed by the presence of T-cell and the absence of B-cell markers in immunophenotyping. Combined modality treatment with WBRT was carried out in 15 patients, WBRT alone in 12, chemotherapy alone in 10, and tumour resection alone in two. One patient received no treatment. The median progression-free survival, disease-specific survival and overall survival was 62 (range, 0-204), 130 (range, 1-204), and 79 (range, 1-204) months, respectively. Only age was associated with a worse prognosis in the multivariate analysis, with patients ≥ 60 years performing worse. To conclude, low-grade PCNSL clearly differs from the high-grade subtype in its pathological, clinical and radiological features. It has a better long-term outcome than PCNSL in general with only older age adversely affecting survival.

Discussion

No large-scale prospective randomised trial comparing different treatment approaches in PCNSL patients has been carried out and published. At this time, there is no consensus on a "standard" chemotherapy schedule, although the published results from retrospective studies, phase II trials and small phase III trials strongly support the use of combined modality treatment with an intravenous HD-MTX-based chemotherapy regimen followed by consolidating WBRT.

The general condition at the time of diagnosis is an important predictive factor especially for early toxicity from intensive treatment schedules. However, some investigators state that a selection based on general and neurological function will exclude the last chance for a durable response and prolonged survival for an important subset of the patients who might, be it in a lower percentage, show a good subjective as well as objective reaction to intensive therapy. Alternatively, WBRT alone can be offered to those patients. Even if patients do respond well, chemotherapy should be given with great caution because of the very high risk of neurotoxicity when WBRT is given first. In some cases, a low dose of WBRT, such as 10 Gy in 5 fractions together with corticosteroids, can be given with an evaluation after 1 or 2 weeks, to offer only an intensive combination treatment to patients who respond well.

Neurotoxicity can occur as a result of the original tumour infiltration, high dose chemotherapy, whole brain radiotherapy and especially a combination of these factors. Therefore, some authors advocate postponing WBRT until disease recurrence or progression for patients in whom a complete remission is obtained with chemotherapy alone. However, radiological evaluation of the response of the patients can be difficult. Residual radiological abnormalities may be the result of non-tumour containing residual fibrotic tissue or non-specific tissue reaction, rather than of viable tumour cells. Those radiological abnormalities can disappear slowly over time [31]. This is of importance in view of the strict timetable for combined modality treatment and might also hamper trials evaluating chemotherapy as a single-treatment modality.

Conclusions

PCNSL should be considered as a potentially curable brain tumour. Therefore, an intensive multi-modality treatment should be offered to patients fulfilling the eligibility criteria for this. However, late toxicity, especially neurotoxicity, remains an important point for concern. Remarkably, the important progress in our knowledge and management of PCNSL has not yet translated into the overall patient population [40].

3

As our current therapeutic knowledge of PCNSL is mainly derived from retrospective series and from non-randomised phase II clinical trials, many fundamental issues remain unanswered. These include questions, currently being addressed by the IPCG, regarding the need for consolidating WBRT; the optimal chemotherapy regimen; the causes and prevention of long-term neurotoxicity and the identification of an effective salvage therapy for patients with relapsed or refractory PCNSL.

Acknowledgements

I thank many colleagues from the EORTC Lymphoma Group and from the IPCG for our excellent collaboration in the research in primary central nervous system lymphoma. I want to mention particularly Hanneke C. Kluin-Nelemans, Hanny Haaxma-Reiche, Martin Van den Bent, Gustaaf van Imhoff and Helena Harder for their active contribution.

References

1. Abrey LE, DeAngelis LM, Yahalom J (1998) Long-term survival in primary CNS lymphoma. J Clin Oncol 16:859-63
2. **Abrey LE, Batchelor TT, Ferreri AM *et al.* for the International Primary CNS Lymphoma Collaborative Group (IPCG) (2005) Report of an International Workshop to Standardize Baseline Evaluation and Response Criteria for Primary Central Nervous System Lymphoma. J Clin Oncol 23: 5034-43**
3. **Abrey LE, Ben-Porat L, Panageas KS *et al.* (2006) Primary central nervous system lymphoma: the Memorial Sloan-Kettering Cancer Center prognostic model. J Clin Oncol 24: 5711-5**
4. Al-Yamany M, Lozano A, Nag S *et al.* (1999) Spontaneous remission of primary central nervous system lymphoma: report of 3 cases and discussion of pathophysiology. J Neurooncol 42: 151-9
5. Balmaceda C, Gaynor JJ, Sun M *et al.* (1995) Leptomeningeal tumor in primary central nervous system lymphoma: recognition, significance, and implications. Ann Neurol 38: 202-9
6. Bataille B, Delwail V, Menet E *et al.* (2000) Primary intracerebral malignant lymphoma: report of 248 cases. J Neurosurg 92: 261-6
7. Bessel EM, López-Guillermo A, Villá S *et al.* (2002) Importance of radiotherapy in the outcome of patients with primary CNS lymphoma: an analysis of the CHOD/BVAM regimen followed by two different radiotherapy treatments. J Clin Oncol 20: 231-6
8. Blay J-Y, Bouhour D, Carrie C (1995) The C5R protocol: a regimen of high-dose chemotherapy and radiotherapy in primary cerebral non-Hodgkin's lymphoma with no known cause of immunosuppression. Blood 8: 2922-9
9. Brada M, Dearnaley D, Horwich A *et al.* (1990) Management of primary cerebral lymphoma with initial chemotherapy: preliminary results and comparison with patients treated with radiotherapy alone. Int J Radiat Oncol Biol Phys 18: 787-92
10. Colombat P, Lemevel A, Bertrand P *et al.* (2006) High-dose chemotherapy with autologous stem-cell transplantation as first-line therapy of primary CNS lymphoma in patients younger than 60 years: a multicenter phase II study of the GOELAMS group. Bone Marrow Transplant 38: 417-20
11. Corn BW, Marcus SM, Topham A *et al.* (1997) Will primary central nervous system lymphoma be the most frequent brain tumor diagnosed in the year 2000? Cancer 79: 2409-13
12. **Correa D, Maron L, Harder H *et al.* (2007) Cognitive functions in primary central nervous system lymphoma: literature review and assessment guidelines. Ann Oncol 18: 1145-51**

13. Crossen JR, Garwood D, Glatstein E *et al.* (1994) Neurobehavioral sequelae of cranial irradiation in adults: a review of radiation-induced encephalopathy. J Clin Oncol 12: 627-42
14. DeAngelis LM (1990) Primary central nervous system lymphoma imitates multiple sclerosis. J Neurooncol 7: 177-81
15. DeAngelis L, Seiferheld W, Clifford Schold S *et al.* (2002) Combination chemotherapy and radiotherapy for primary central nervous system lymphoma: Radiation Therapy Oncology Group study 93-10. J Clin Oncol 20: 4643-8
16. Desablens B, Gardembas M, Haie-Meder Ch *et al.* (1999) Primary CNS lymphomas: long term results of the GOELAMS LCP 88 trial with a focus on neurological complications among 152 patients. Ann Oncol 10: 40 (abstract)
17. Ferreri AJM, Reni M, Villa E (2000) Therapeutic management of primary central nervous system lymphoma; lessons from prospective trials. Ann Oncol 11: 927-37
18. Ferreri AJM, Blay J-Y, Reni M *et al.* (2003) Prognostic scoring system for primary CNS lymphomas: the international extranodal lymphoma study group experience. J Clin Oncol 21: 266-72
19. Freilich RJ, Delattre J-Y, Monjour A *et al.* (1996) Chemotherapy without radiation therapy as initial treatment for primary CNS lymphoma in older patients. Neurology 46: 435-9
20. Glass J, Gruber ML, Cher LC *et al.* (1994) Preirradiation methotrexate chemotherapy of primary central nervous system lymphoma: long-term outcome. J Neurosurg 81: 188-95
21. Gündüz K, Pulido JS, McCannel CA, O'Neill BP (2006) Ocular manifestations and treatment of central nervous system lymphomas. Neurosurg Focus 21: E9
22. Harder H, Cornelissen J, Van Gool A *et al.* (2002) Cognitive functioning and quality of life in long-term adult survivors of bone marrow transplantation. Cancer 95: 183-92
23. Harder H, Holtel H, Bromberg JEC *et al.* (2004) Cognitive status and quality of life after treatment for primary CNS lymphoma. Neurology 62: 544-7
24. **Hunt MA, Jahnke K, Murillo TP *et al.* (2006) Distinguishing primary central nervous system lymphoma from other central nervous system diseases: a neurosurgical perspective on diagnostic dilemmas and approaches. Neurosurg Focus 21: E3**
25. Illerhaus G, Marks R, Ihorst G *et al.* (2006) High-dose chemotherapy with autologous stem-cell transplantation and hyperfractionated radiotherapy as first-line treatment of primary CNS lymphoma. J Clin Oncol 24: 3865-70
26. Jahnke K, Doolittle ND, Muldoon LL *et al.* (2006) Implications of the blood-brain barrier in primary central nervouw system lymphoma. Neurosurg Focus 21: E11
27. Jahnke K, Korfel A, O'Neill BP *et al.* (2006) International study on low-grade primary central nervous system lymphoma. Ann Neurol 59: 755-62
28. Jahnke K, Thiel E, Martus P *et al.* (2006) Relapse of primary central nervous system lymphoma: clinical features, outcome and prognostic factors. J Neurooncol 80: 159-65
29. Johnson BA, Fram EK, Johnson PC *et al.* (1997) The variable MR appearance of primary lymphoma of the central nervous system: comparison with histopathologic features. Am J Neuroradiol 18: 563-72
30. Lachance DH, O'Neill BP, Macdonald DR *et al.* (1991) Primary leptomeningeal lymphoma. Report of 9 cases, diagnosis with imunocytochemical analysis, and review of the literature. Neurology 41: 95-100
31. Lanfermann H, Heindel W, Schaper J *et al.* (1997) CT and MR imaging in primary cerebral non-Hodgkin's lymphoma. Acta Radiol 38: 259-67
32. Mead GM, Bleehen NM, Gregor A *et al.* (2000) A Medical Research Council randomized trial in patients with primary cerebral non-Hodgkin lymphoma: cerebral radiotherapy with and without cyclophosphamide, doxorubicin, vincristine and prednisone chemotherapy. Cancer 89: 1359-70
33. Monnard V, Sun A, Epelbaum R *et al.* (2006) Primary spinal epidural lymphoma: patients' profile, outcome, and prognostic factors: a multicenter Rare Cancer Network study. Int J Radiat Oncol Biol Phys 65: 817-23
34. Nelson DF, Martz KL, Bonner H *et al.* (1992) Non-Hodgkin's lymphoma of the brain: can high-dose, large volume radiation therapy improve survival? Report on a prospective trial by the Radiation Therapy Oncology Group (RTOG): RTOG 8315. Int J Radiat Oncol Biol Phys 23: 9-17

35. Neuwelt EA, Goldman DL, Dahlborg SA *et al.* (1991) Primary CNS lymphoma treated with osmotic blood-brain barrier disruption: Prolonged survival and preservation of cognitive function. J Clin Oncol 9: 1580-90
36. Neuwelt EA, Guastadisegni PE, Várallyay P *et al.* (2005) Imaging changes and cognitive outcome in primary CNS lymphoma after enhanced chemotherapy delivery. Am J Neuroradiol 26: 258-65
37. O'Neill BPO, Dinapoli RP, Kurtin PJ *et al.* (1995) Occult systemic Non-Hodgkin's lymphoma in patients initially diagnosed as primary central nervous system lymphoma: how much staging is enough? J Neurooncol 25: 67-71
38. O'Neill BP, Wang CH, O'Fallon JR (2001) Primary central nervous system non-hodgkin's lymphoma (PCNSL): survival advantages with combined initial therapy? A final report of the north central cancer treatment group. Int J Radiation Oncology Biol Phys 43: 559-63
39. Osoba D, Aaronson N, Muller M *et al.* (1997) Effect of neurological dysfunction on health-related quality of life in patients with high-grade glioma. J Neurooncol 34: 263-78
40. Panageas KS, Elkin EB, DeAngelis LM *et al.* (2005) Trends in survival from primary central nervous system lymphoma, 1975-1999: a population-based analysis. Cancer 104: 2466-72
41. Panageas KS, Elkin EB, Ben-Porat L *et al.* (2007) Patterns of treatment in older adults with primary central nervous system lymphoma. Cancer 110: 1338-44
42. **Poortmans PMP, Kluin-Nelemans HC, Haaxma-Reiche H *et al.* (2003) High-dose methotrexate-based chemotherapy followed by consolidating radiotherapy in non–AIDS–related primary central nervous system lymphoma: EORTC Lymphoma Group phase II trial 20962. J Clin Oncol 21: 4483-8**
43. Postler E, Bornemann A, Skalej M *et al.* (1999) Intracranial inflammatory tumors: a survey of their various etiologies by presentation of 5 cases. J Neurooncol 43: 209-17
44. Relling MV, Fairclough D, Ayers D *et al.* (1994) Patient characteristics associated with high-risk Methotrexate concentrations and toxicity. J Clin Oncol 12: 1667-72
45. Shenkier TN, Blay JY, O'Neill BP *et al.* (2005) Primary CNS lymphoma of T-cell origin: a descriptive analysis from the international primary CNS lymphoma collaborative group. J Clin Oncol 23: 2233-9
46. Schabet M (1999) Epidemiology of primary CNS lymphoma. J. Neurooncol 43: 199-201
47. Soussain C, Suzan F, Hoang-Xuan K *et al.* (2001) Results of intensive chemotherapy followed by hematopoietic stem-cell rescue in 22 patients with refractory or recurrent primary CNS lymphoma or intraocular lymphoma. J Clin Oncol 19: 742-9
48. Van den Bent M, Vanneste JAL and Ansink BJJ (1992) Prolonged remission of primary central nervous system lympoma after discontinuation of steroid therapy. J Neurooncol 13: 257-9
49. van Imhoff GW, Haaxma-Reiche H *et al.* for the Dutch Neuro-Oncology Group (1996) High-dose ARA-C and MTX before radiotherapy in primary central nervous system lymphoma (PCNSL). Eur J Cancer 7: 452 (abstract)
50. Wildemann B, Jansen O, Haas J *et al.* (2001) Rapid distinction of acute demyelinating disorders and central nervous system lymphoma by molecular analysis of cerebrospinal fluid cells. J Neurol 248: 127-30

Treatment of medulloblastoma in adults

4

N. Penel, C. Ferte, É. Le Rhun and Y. Belkacémi

Five Essential Points

1. *In adults with medulloblastoma, prognostic factors are not clearly established.*
2. *Surgery is the cornerstone of curative intent treatment. Post-surgical residue leads to poor outcome.*
3. *Whole cranio-spinal irradiation therapy is the second component of curative intent treatment.*
4. *New radiation therapy techniques need to be better evaluated.*
5. *The role of chemotherapy is debated.*

Introduction

Medulloblastoma (M) is an aggressive posterior fossa tumour that probably originates from germinative neuroepithelial cells in the fourth ventricle (however, histogenesis is very controversial). Medulloblastoma accounts for 1% of all adult brain tumours and 25% of brain tumours in children. It is exceptional in patients aged over 16 years, while the median age of adult medulloblastoma is about 28 [1]. The most common revealing symptoms are: intra-cranial hypertension, cerebellar disorders and palsy of cranial nerves. In adults, the MRI findings show an homogeneous tumour predominantly located in the cerebellar hemisphere, poorly defined with weak contrast enhancement, with hypersignal flair and hypo-signal T1. Laterally located tumours are most common in adults compared to children (30% *versus* 7%). The WHO histological classification distinguishes 4 classical subtypes (classic M, extensive nodulary M, desmoplastic M and large cell M) and 2 rare subtypes (melanocytic M and medullomyoblastoma). The desmoplastic subtype is more frequent in adults than in children (40% *versus* 15%). Metastasis is more common in adults than in children: initial spinal or cerebral metastasis in about 30% of cases, cerebrospinal fluid involvement in about 30% of cases and metastasis outside the CNS (bone) in 5% of cases [1,3,7]. A specific TNM classification has been described by [3].

Prognosis

The prognostic factors are clearly defined in children with two main prognostic groups:

- average risk group: complete resection, age $\leq$ 4 years without distant metastases;
- high-risk group: post-surgical residue, age < 4 or distant metastases [2].

4

Conversely, the prognostic factors in adults are not clearly established. In a large retrospective study, Padovani and colleagues have identified 3 prognostic factors:

- brainstem involvement;
- VIth ventricular floor involvement;
- Radiation therapy dose delivered to the posterior fossa, less than 50 Gy [7].

Surgery

Surgery is the cornerstone of medulloblastoma treatment. Post-surgical residue had a very poor prognostic value. Surgery should be as radical as possible and is complete is about 2/3 of cases, while extensive surgery may induce severe neurological sequellae. Resection of CNS metastases should be discussed [1,2,7]. The presence of a macroscopic residue is a major unfavourable prognostic factor in children [2]. Within the 72 hours following resection, a new cranio-spinal MRI is recommended to detect residue and discuss the possibility of a new surgical procedure. Moreover, surgery plays a major role in symptomatic treatment – a ventriculo-peritoneal shunt can reduce the symptoms of intra-cranial hypertension.

A complete work-up must be realised 2 weeks after surgery including cranio-spinal MRI, CSF fluid examination and bone scan in symptomatic patients.

Cranio-spinal radiotherapy

Efficacy

This is the second step in the treatment with curative intent, including:

- Whole cranio-spinal axis irradiation delivering 36 Gy using a standard fractionation of 1.8 to 2 Gy per fraction.
- Boost to the posterior fossa delivering a dose of 20 Gy in 10 fractions.

Radiation technique generally consists of:

1. posterior field (patient on supine position) for the vertex;
2. lateral-opposed fields for the cranial area and the two first cervical vertebrae.

The treatment is performed using photons and electrons (with an adapted energy) for cranial and spinal volumes, respectively.

The radiotherapy effectiveness in adults is dependent on at least three parameters:

- the total dose of radiation therapy delivered to the posterior fossa;
- the time interval between surgery and radiotherapy;
- the total duration of treatment.

Padovani and colleagues found that a dose inferior to 50 Gy delivered to the posterior fossa is associated with poor outcome (5-year overall survival: 76 *versus* 32%, $p<0.0001$) in multivariate analysis [7]. Brandes and colleagues reported total dose as the major prognostic factor. The 10-year disease free survival was 71% for patients who received more than 55 Gy *versus* 34% if the total dose was < 52 Gy [2].

Abacioglu and colleagues found that 5-year overall survival depends on the interval between surgery and radiotherapy, with 85%, 75% and 0% for < 3 weeks, 3-6 weeks and more than 6 weeks respectively [1].

Paulino and colleagues found that duration of radiotherapy influences the outcome. The 5-year disease control rate is 81% with radiotherapy administered in less than 48 days and 49% if the radiotherapy is administered in more than 48 days [9].

New techniques

In terms of RT technique, the use of protons is under investigation. Because of improved physical dose distribution, proton radiotherapy allows dose escalation to improve local tumour control in anatomic sites and histologies where local control is suboptimal with photons. The improved dose localization also reduces normal tissue doses with an anticipated reduction in acute and late toxicity. Clinical treatment protocols, developed to exploit the dosimetric advantages of protons over photons, have been grouped into two broad categories. In the first, dose is escalated for anatomic sites where local control with conventional radiation doses has been suboptimal. In the second, normal tissue sparing with protons is designed to minimize acute and late toxicity. Treatment of patients in clinical research protocols has been encouraged. According to the Boston experience, the results to date indicate that proton radiation therapy offers several potential treatment advantages to patients that can be studied in the clinical trial setting [4]. For normal tissue sparing, intensity-modulated radiotherapy (IMRT) has been also considered as a valid treatment option for spinal axis irradiation. Parker and colleagues showed recently that IMRT results in sparing of organs at risk without a significant increase in integral dose [8].

Adjuvant chemotherapy

The benefit of adjuvant chemotherapy has been clearly established in children with high-risk medulloblastoma. In adults, although there is no clear evidence, most experts currently feel that adjuvant chemotherapy in adults is beneficial, at least in patients considered at high-risk (given that prognostic factors are not clearly established).

Moreover, the issue of adjuvant chemotherapy is debatable regarding its timing and the best regimen.

Most published data favours post-irradiation adjuvant chemotherapy rather than pre-irradiation chemotherapy [5,6]. Pre-irradiation adjuvant chemotherapy delays radiotherapy and is associated with more local relapse [5,6]. However, no agreed protocol exists. Given its rarity, no randomised studies have been performed in adults with medulloblastoma. A randomised clinical trial in children has clearly shown the superiority of the association vincristine-lomustine-prednisone compared with the protocol "eight drugs in one day" (5-year progression free survival 63% *versus* 45%) [10].

Outcome

The largest retrospective study estimates 5- and 10-year overall survival at 72% and 55% respectively [7]. In adults, late relapses (> 2 years) appear more frequently, occurring in the posterior fossa in most cases, while the median overall survival after recurrence is 6 months.

Moreover, in cured children, late neurological, psychological and neuroendocrine sequellae remain a serious problem, which alters durably the quality of life [2]. There is no clear policy concerning follow-up.

Conclusions

Role and conditions of surgery and cranio-spinal irradiation are well-established in the treatment of adult medulloblastoma. Prognostic factors, modality and role of adjuvant chemotherapy need further evaluation.

References

1. **Abacioglu U, Uzel O, Sengoz M *et al.* (2002) Medulloblastoma in adults: treatment results and prognostic factors. Int J Radiation Oncol Biol Phys 54: 855-60**
2. **Brandes AA, Paris MK (2004) Review of the prognostic factors in medulloblastoma of children and adults. Crit Rev Onco Hematol 50: 121-8**
3. Chang CH, Horton J, Schoenfeld D *et al.* (1983) Comparison of postoperative radiotherapy and combined postoperative radiotherapy and chemotherapy in the multidisciplinary management of malignant gliomas. A joint Radiation Therapy Oncology Group and Eastern Cooperative Oncology Group Study. Cancer 52: 997-1007
4. Delaney TF (2007) Clinical proton radiation therapy research at the Francis H Burr Proton Therapy Center. Technol Cancer Res Treat 6: 61-6
5. Hartsell WF, Guijar A, Heidemann RL *et al.* (1997) Patterns of failure in children with medulloblastoma: effects of preradiation chemotherapy. Int J Radiat Oncol Biol Phys 39: 15-24
6. Kortmann RD, Kuhl J, Timmerman B *et al.* (2000) Postoperative chemotherapy before radiotherapy as compared to immediate radiotherapy followed by maintenance chemotherapy in the treatment of medulloblastoma in childhood: results of the German prospective randomised trial HIT '91. Int J Radiat Oncol Biol Phys 46: 269-79
7. **Padovani L, Sunyach MP, Perol D *et al.* (2007) Common strategy for adult and pediatric medulloblastoma: a multicenter series of 253 adults. Int J Radiat Oncol Biol Phys 68: 433-40**
8. **Parker W, Filion E, Roberge D *et al.* (2007) Intensity-modulated radiotherapy for craniospinal irradiation: target volume considerations, dose constraints, and competing risks. Int J Radiat Oncol Biol Phys 69: 251-7**
9. Paulino AC, Wen BC, Mayr NA *et al.* (2003) Protracted radiotherapy treatment duration in medulloblastoma. Am J Clin Oncol 26: 55-9
10. **Zeltzer PM, Boyett JM, Finlay JL *et al.* (1999) Metastasis stage, adjuvant treatment, and residual tumor are prognostic factors for medulloblastoma in children: conclusions from the Children's Cancer Group 921 randomized phase III study. J Clin Oncol 17: 832-45**

Cerebellar glioblastoma multiforme

D.C. Weber

5

Five Essential Points

1. *Patients with cerebellar GBM typically present with manifestation of obstruction of the fourth ventricular outlet and raised intra-cerebral pressure.*
2. *Cerebellar GBM should be treated identically as their cerebral counterpart, namely with optimal surgery and postoperative chemo-radiation therapy, followed by adjuvant chemotherapy using temozolomide.*
3. *Conformal radiotherapy should be administered, with no whole brain or cranio-spinal irradiation.*
4. *The outcome of these tumours is similar to cerebral GBM.*
5. *The pattern of failure is local in all cases.*

Introduction

In 1928, the English physician Edward Carmichael provided the first documented account of cerebellar glioblastoma (GBM) [1]. This tumour localization is uncommon and all but one series [33] have included small numbers (≤ 8 cases; Table 1). No prospective data are available for this tumour localization and cerebellar GBM patients are not eligible in GBM prospective cooperative trials. As such, the radiotherapy techniques for this tumour are ill defined and the outcome of these exceptional patients is somewhat unclear.

Incidence

The incidence of GBM in the general population varies between 2 and 3 per 100,000 people in European and American countries. Supratentorial GBM is the most frequent malignant brain tumour and accounts for 10-15% of all intracranial neoplasms and 50-60% of all astrocytic tumours in adults. They generally occur in the fifth and sixth decade. GBM are infiltrating tumours located in the deep white or grey matter, mainly in the cerebral hemispheres. Infrequently, these tumours can be located in the cerebellum or brainstem, the former localization accounting for less than 0.5-1% of all intracranial GBMs [23]. The majority of these tumours occurs in adults, although they have occasionally been reported in children [7, 13, 29]. In a retrospective analysis of 488 children with a central nervous system neoplasm, 43 (8.8%) presented GBM, 2 (0.4%) of which were located in the cerebellum [6].

5

Table 1 – Overview of the literature reporting cerebellar glioblastoma.

Study, First author [ref]	Patients included	Age (years)	Type of treatment
Weber *et al.* [33]	45*	21 - 82	Best supportive care/surgery, radiotherapy/chemotherapy/ chemo-radiation therapy
Mattos *et al.* [15, 25]	1	46	Surgery and RT[a]
Nishioka *et al.* [19]	1	26	Surgery and chemo-RT[a]
Demir *et al.* [5]	2	17 and 28	Surgery and chemo-RT[a]/ Surgery and RT[a]
Levine *et al.* [14]	1	80	NS[b]
Pato-Pato *et al.* [23]	1	55	Surgery and chemo-RT[a]
Gupta *et al.* [8]	3	[b]NS	[b]NS
Yang *et al.* [34]	1*	15	Surgery
Tamaki *et al.* [32]	1	74	Surgery and chemo-RT[a]
Kopelson *et al.* [11] [10]	8	10 - 67	Surgery/Surgery and RT[a]
Chamberlain *et al.* [2]	5	4 - 46	Surgery/Surgery and RT[a]
Katz *et al.* [9]	1	4.5	Surgery
Kulkarni *et al.* [13]	4	0.9 - 15	Surgery/chemotherapy only/ Surgery and chemo-RT[a]/ Surgery and RT[a]

[a] RT, Radiotherapy. [b]NS, Not specified. * Includes radiation-induced cerebellar glioblastoma.

Pathology

Identical to their cerebral counterpart, the majority of these tumours are primary GBM, but some secondary GBM has been reported in younger patients [33]. Radiation-induced cerebellar GBM (Table 1) has been reported occasionally [33, 34]. In the 2000 WHO classification, two GBM variants have been described. Giant cell glioblastoma (ICD-O 9441/3) and gliosarcoma (ICD-O 9442/3) are grade IV tumours presenting with multinucleated giant cells and mesenchymal differentiation, respectively. However, these tumours are infrequent, with cases being reported only occasionally and accounting for approximately < 5% of all supratentorial GBMs [17, 21]. Likewise, these histological variants have been rarely reported for cerebellar GBM; both Queiroz *et al.* [25] and Demir *et al.* [5] reported on one patient with a giant cell GBM. In a large multicentric retrospective study of the Rare Cancer Network, Weber *et al.* reported on the outcome of 45 adults with cerebellar GBM [33]. In this cohort, only one (2%) patient with a giant cell-variant was included in the analysis. No gliosarcoma variant has been reported in a cerebellar localization.

The histopathological criteria defining GBM, namely astrocytic cells with marked nuclear atypia, high mitotic index, glomeruloid capillary endothelial proliferation and necrosis with pseudopalisading apply indiscriminately to supra- and infratentorial tumours alike. The immunochemistry for cerebellar GBM has been reported by a Canadian group in children [13]. A strong immunostaining positivity of tumour cells to glial fibrillary acidic protein was observed in all cases, associated with a weaker vimentin staining. Nuclear immunopositivity quantitative MIB-1 analysis ranged from 32 to 73% in this series. These characteristics are identical to those found in their supratentorial counterpart. Non-GFAP or non-vimentin reactivity, such as EGFR, MDM2 and PDGF-receptor α, and molecular biology or cytogenetics has not been reported for cerebellar GBM.

Clinical presentation

Patients with cerebellar GBM typically present with headache, vomiting and ataxic gait [5, 32]. These symptoms are manifestation of obstruction of the forth ventricular outlet. Papilledema can be observed in a substantial number of patients [13]. As such, a majority of these patients (>70%) receive steroids [33]. In the Rare Cancer Network study, all but 1 patient presented with ataxia [33]. Headache and nausea was observed in approximately 60% and 25% of cases, respectively [33]. In this study, physical examination revealed nystagmus in roughly one half of the patients. As nystagmus occurs with brainstem or cerebellar lesion alike, this symptom was observed in patients with (80%) or without (36%) brainstem invasion. Some authors have also reported neck pain or disturbance of consciousness as presenting symptoms [13, 19]. Progressive awkwardness and clumsiness, with difficulty standing or walking alone, has been reported in children [9]. Cranial nerve dysfunction has not been reported in a large retrospective series [33], but it has been reported in some patients in case report forms [9, 23].

Radiological evaluation

The MRI radiological features are non-specific to the cerebellar location, not limited to but including isointense to grey matter on long repetition time (TR) and long echo time (TE) sequences, with Gadolinium inhomogeneous enhancement on the periphery of the lesion on T1-weighted sequences. Due to the peri-lesional edema, compression of the fourth ventricle can be frequently observed [9], although not infrequently the associated edema can be moderate or absent [13]. It should be noted that the tumour can be multi-focal in a substantial number of cases. Mutifocality was observed in one third of the patients in the Rare Cancer Network cohort [33]. This rate of mutlifocality is much higher than usually reported for supratentorial GBMs, with < 5% of patients presenting with multi-focal supratentorial GBM in the University of California-San Francisco series [22]. Likewise, brainstem invasion can also be commonly observed [33]. T1-weighted hyperintensity within a hypointense tumour may be observed, suggesting the possibility of intra-tumoral hemorrhage [13, 19]. The location of the GBM has been reported to be mainly hemispheric [5]. Only 27% of cerebellar GBMs were of vermian localization in the Rare Cancer Network series [33], while others have observed an equal number of cases with midline and hemispheric lesions [13]. In the cerebellar localization, the GBM volume may be smaller when compared to the cerebral location. Maximum tumour diameter, as determined by MRI, was between 5-10 cm for 361/645 (56%) patients with cerebral GBM [30], whereas this size range was observed in only 9 and 25% of patients with cerebellar GBM in two retrospective studies [13, 33]. In the Rare Cancer Network series, the mean tumour volume was 14.1 ml (range 2.4 to 82.1) [33].

Treatment

Neurosurgical management is the cornerstone of the initial management of this tumour. The surgical intervention has at least three goals: (a) to establish a definite diagnosis for this uncommon localization, (b) to reduce the mass effect and consequential neurological symptoms and (c) to reduce the tumour bulk. However, optimal cytoreduction cannot be achieved in a majority of cases. Only a minority of cases (20-25%) had a complete resection in the two largest retrospective series [11, 33], due to the diffuse infiltrating nature of malignant glioma and the direct vicinity of critical structures. This rate of gross total resection is identical to the one achieved in cerebral GBM. Simpson *et al.* reported on 645 patients treated on three consecutive phase III Radiation Therapy Oncology Group trials comparing radiotherapy alone *vs* radio-chemotherapy [30]. Nineteen percent of patients in this retrospective analysis underwent gross total resection.

Radiation therapy (RT) has been shown to be the single most effective therapy in the treatment of GBM in prospective randomized trials. As such, postoperative RT should be administered in all cases with appropriate performance status, age and cognitive function. With regard to this treatment modality, some authors have recommended whole brain [26] or cranio-spinal irradiation [27]. However, this concept has to be questioned, as no patients presented non-posterior fossa recurrences only in the two largest published series [11, 33]. In the Rare Cancer Network cohort, approximately one patient out of four presented an extra-cerebellar component with, however, always a concomitant local recurrence [33]. As such, the irradiation volume should encompass partially the posterior fossa, with a planning target volume defined as the gross tumour volume/resection cavity plus a margin of 2-3 cm [3].

The role of chemo-radiation therapy has been clearly established for cerebral GBM [31]. Temozolomide, an oral alkylating agent, has demonstrated antitumour activity as a single agent in the treatment of malignant glioma [18, 24]. Both in primate models and in melanoma–glioma patients, the concentration of this agent measured in CSF is approximately 20% to 40% of that measured in plasma [20, 35]. Moreover, this drug may preferentially concentrate in both microscopic and macroscopic disease, when compared with levels achieved in the normal brain [16]. Given the identical histology and possibly also the outcome, this chemotherapy agent should also be implemented for cerebellar tumours. A strong caution should however be emphasized with chemotherapy delivered before radiation therapy. Weber *et al.* reported on two patients treated with chemotherapy alone [33]. Both patients progressed, one locally and the other one locally with an extra-cerebellar component during non-temozolomide chemotherapy (carmustine only and procarbazine, lomustine and vincristine chemotherapy treatment respectively). Only one of these patients could be efficiently salvaged. As a result, concomitant chemo-(temozolomide) radiation therapy with adjuvant chemotherapy should be administered to these patients.

Outcome

The results of the Rare Cancer Network study suggest that the outcome of cerebellar GBM appears to be identical to that of supratentorial tumours [33]. In this series, the 1- and 2-year overall survival was 38% and 14%, respectively. The observed 10 months median survival compares to the survivorship reported with cerebral GBM patients treated with radiotherapy [4]. Some authors have reported an increase survival of patients with cerebellar tumour, when compared with brainstem or spinal cord GBM. Kopelson *et al.* reported on 8, 5 and 2 patients with cerebellar, intramedullary and brainstem GBM [11]. In this series, GBM was however defined as grade III and IV glioma. This incremental survivorship for cerebellar tumours resulted from one long term anaplastic astrocytoma survivor (> 8 years) with an infratentorial tumour. Most case reports have reported patient survival between 3 and 15 months (Table 1) [5, 14, 19, 25].

Major prognostic factors are age, neurological function, performance and mental status. The small sample size of 45 patients limited the statistical power to detect associations between these prognosticators and outcome in the largest retrospective study [33]. In this series, brainstem invasion was a major independent prognostic factor for survival. The 2-year overall survival was 0% and 19% for patients, with and without brainstem invasion ($p = 0.02$). Less than half of the patients presenting with brainstem invasion could be treated, as a result of tumour progression, postoperative complications or sudden death, resulting in a dismal survivorship. Likewise, the extent of surgery was significant for the 2-year overall survival in both the univariate ($p < 0.02$) and multivariate ($p = 0.03$) analyses. The prognostic impact of maximum tumour resection is much debated for cerebral GBM, with some studies showing an improved outcome [30], with other series showing no benefit [12, 28] after gross total resection. This factor will be assessed prospectively in future phase III trials for cerebral GBM.

References

1. Carmichael E (1928) Cerebral gliomata. J Path Bact 31:493-510
2. Chamberlain MC, Silver P, Levin VA (1990) Poorly differentiated gliomas of the cerebellum. A study of 18 patients. Cancer 65: 337-40
3. **Chang EL, Akyurek S, Avalos T *et al.* (2007) Evaluation of peritumoral edema in the delineation of radiotherapy clinical target volumes for glioblastoma. Int J Radiat Oncol Biol Phys. 68: 144-50**
4. **DeAngelis LM (2001) Brain tumors. N Engl J Med 344: 114-23**
5. Demir MK, Hakan T, Akinci O *et al.* (2005) Primary cerebellar glioblastoma multiforme. Diagn Interv Radiol. 11: 83-86
6. Dohrmann GJ, Farwell JR, Flannery JT (1976) Glioblastoma multiforme in children. J Neurosurg 44: 442-8
7. Fresh CB, Takei Y, O'Brien MS (1976) Cerebellar glioblastoma in childhood. Case report. J Neurosurg. 45: 705-8
8. Gupta V, Goyal A, Sinha S *et al.* (2003) Glioblastoma of the cerebellum. A report of 3 cases. J Neurosurg Sci. 47: 157-164; discussion 164-155
9. Katz DS, Poe LB, Winfield JA *et al.* (1995) A rare case of cerebellar glioblastoma multiforme in childhood: MR imaging. Clin Imaging 19:162-4
10. Kopelson G (1982) Cerebellar glioblastoma. Cancer 50: 308-11
11. Kopelson G, Linggood R (1982) Infratentorial glioblastoma: the role of neuraxis irradiation. Int J Radiat Oncol Biol Phys 8: 999-1003
12. Kowalczuk A, Macdonald RL, Amidei C *et al.* (1997) Quantitative imaging study of extent of surgical resection and prognosis of malignant astrocytomas. Neurosurgery. 41: 1028-1036; discussion 1036-1028
13. Kulkarni AV, Becker LE, Jay V *et al.* (1999) Primary cerebellar glioblastomas multiforme in children. Report of four cases. J Neurosurg 90: 546-50
14. Levine S, McKeever P, Greenberg H (1987) Primary cerebellar glioblastoma multiforme. J Neurooncol 5: 231-6
15. Mattos JP, Marenco HA, Campos JM *et al.* (2006) Cerebellar glioblastoma multiforme in an adult. Arq Neuropsiquiatr 64: 132-5

5

16. Meikle SR, Matthews JC, Brock CS *et al.* (1998) Pharmacokinetic assessment of novel anti-cancer drugs using spectral analysis and positron emission tomography: a feasibility study. Cancer Chemother Pharmacol 42: 183-93
17. Meis JM, Martz KL, Nelson JS (1991) Mixed glioblastoma multiforme and sarcoma. A clinicopathologic study of 26 radiation therapy oncology group cases. Cancer 67: 2342-9
18. Newlands ES, O'Reilly SM, Glaser MG *et al.* (1996) The Charing Cross Hospital experience with temozolomide in patients with gliomas. Eur J Cancer 32A: 2236-41
19. Nishioka H, Saito F, Haraoka J *et al.* (1991) [Glioblastoma of the cerebellum: report of an autopsy case associated with intratumoral hemorrhage and CSF seedings]. No Shinkei Geka 19: 547-52
20. Ostermann S, Csajka C, Buclin T *et al.* (2004) Plasma and cerebrospinal fluid population pharmacokinetics of temozolomide in malignant glioma patients. Clin Cancer Res 10: 3728-36
21. Palma L, Celli P, Maleci A *et al.* (1989) Malignant monstrocellular brain tumours. A study of 42 surgically treated cases. Acta Neurochir (Wien) 97: 17-25
22. Parsa AT, Wachhorst S, Lamborn KR *et al.* (2005) Prognostic significance of intracranial dissemination of glioblastoma multiforme in adults. J Neurosurg. 102: 622-8
23. Pato-Pato A, Cimas-Hernando I, Lorenzo-Gonzalez JR *et al.* (2004) [Cerebellar glioblastoma multiforme: a case report]. Rev Neurol 38: 839-42
24. Plowman J, Waud WR, Koutsoukos AD *et al.* (1994) Preclinical antitumor activity of temozolomide in mice: efficacy against human brain tumor xenografts and synergism with 1,3-bis(2-chloroethyl)-1-nitrosourea. Cancer Res 54: 3793-9
25. Queiroz LS, Faria AV, Zanardi VA *et al.* (2005) Lipidized giant-cell glioblastoma of cerebellum. Clin Neuropathol 24: 262-6
26. Salazar OM, Rubin P (1976) The spread of glioblastoma multiforme as a determining factor in the radiation treated volume. Int J Radiat Oncol Biol Phys 1: 627-37
27. Salazar OM, Rubin P, McDonald JV *et al.* (1976) Patterns of failure in intracranial astrocytomas after irradiation: analysis of dose and field factors. AJR Am J Roentgenol 126: 279-92
28. Sandberg-Wollheim M, Malmstrom P, Stromblad LG *et al.* (1991) A randomized study of chemotherapy with procarbazine, vincristine, and lomustine with and without radiation therapy for astrocytoma grades 3 and/or 4. Cancer 68: 22-9
29. Sgouros S, Fineron PW, Hockley AD (1995) Cerebellar astrocytoma of childhood: long-term follow-up. Childs Nerv Syst 11: 89-96
30. **Simpson JR, Horton J, Scott C *et al.* (1993) Influence of location and extent of surgical resection on survival of patients with glioblastoma multiforme: results of three consecutive Radiation Therapy Oncology Group (RTOG) clinical trials. Int J Radiat Oncol Biol Phys 26: 239-44**
31. **Stupp R, Mason WP, van den Bent MJ *et al.* (2005) Radiotherapy plus concomitant and adjuvant temozolomide for glioblastoma. N Engl J Med 352: 987-96**
32. Tamaki T, Eguchi T, Sakamoto M *et al.* (2004) Glioblastoma multiforme of the cerebellum in an elderly man. J Chin Med Assoc 67: 301-4
33. Weber DC, Miller RC, Villa S *et al.* (2006) Outcome and prognostic factors in cerebellar glioblastoma multiforme in adults: a retrospective study from the Rare Cancer Network. Int J Radiat Oncol Biol Phys 66: 179-86
34. Yang S, Wang K, Cho B *et al.* (2005) Radiation-induced cerebellar glioblastoma at the site of a treated medulloblastoma: case report. J Neurosurg 102: 417-22
35. Yung WK, Prados MD, Yaya-Tur R *et al.* (1999) Multicenter phase II trial of temozolomide in patients with anaplastic astrocytoma or anaplastic oligoastrocytoma at first relapse. Temodal Brain Tumor Group. J Clin Oncol 17: 2762-71

Chordoma and chondrosarcoma of the skull base

6

A. Pica and R.-O. Mirimanoff

Five Essential Points

1. *Chordoma and chondrosarcoma are very rare tumours of the base of skull with an incidence of less than 0.1 per 100.000 per year.*
2. *Although relatively similar in their presentation, chordoma and chondrosarcoma present important histological and immuno-histochemical differences.*
3. *Prognosis is significantly better for chondrosarcoma compared to chordoma. Women with chordoma have the worst prognosis.*
4. *Surgery is the mainstay of treatment and should be as extensive as reasonably possible.*
5. *Postoperative RT is indicated in most situations. High-dose and high-precision techniques (proton, FSRT) are required and offer a good local control.*

Chordoma: general features

Chordomas are very rare, slowly growing tumours of the bone with an incidence rate of <0.1 per 100,000 per year. They represent about 1% to 4% of all primary malignant bone tumours [17]. The median age at presentation is around 60 years; however, presentation with skull base tumours may occur at a younger age and has been reported in children and adolescents [21]. Chordomas arise from embryonic remains of notochord and show a dual epithelial-mesenchymal differentiation. Its epithelial phenotype is manifested through expression of positive markers for cytokeratin (CK) and epithelial membrane antigen (EMA). They also are positive for S-100 and vimentin. After obliteration of the notochord and its displacement from the central to the cranial and caudal positions, microscopic foci may persist in the vertebral bodies at the cranial and caudal ends of the embryo. The sacrococcygeal bones (50%) and clivus (in 25% to 36% of cases) are the preferential sites for chordomas. Malignant transformation typically occurs between the third and fourth decade for spheno-occipital lesions and between the fifth and sixth decade for the sacrococcygeal type [14,23]. Chordomas are lobular grey, semitranslucent tumours of varying size. They are usually soft and gelatinous, sometimes with foci of calcification. They may invade the dura to stretch cranial or spinal nerves, or displace blood vessels and the brain stem. In typical chordoma, the cells tend to be arranged in cords set in a pale matrix of mucopolysaccharide with a characteristic physaliphourous appearance (Fig. 1) [20]. Mitoses are infrequent, even in specimens from recurrent or metastasized chordomas. In chondroid chordomas, the stroma resembles hyaline cartilage with neoplastic cells in lacunae. The chondroid histology, commonly seen in the skull base, exhibits low-grade behaviour and

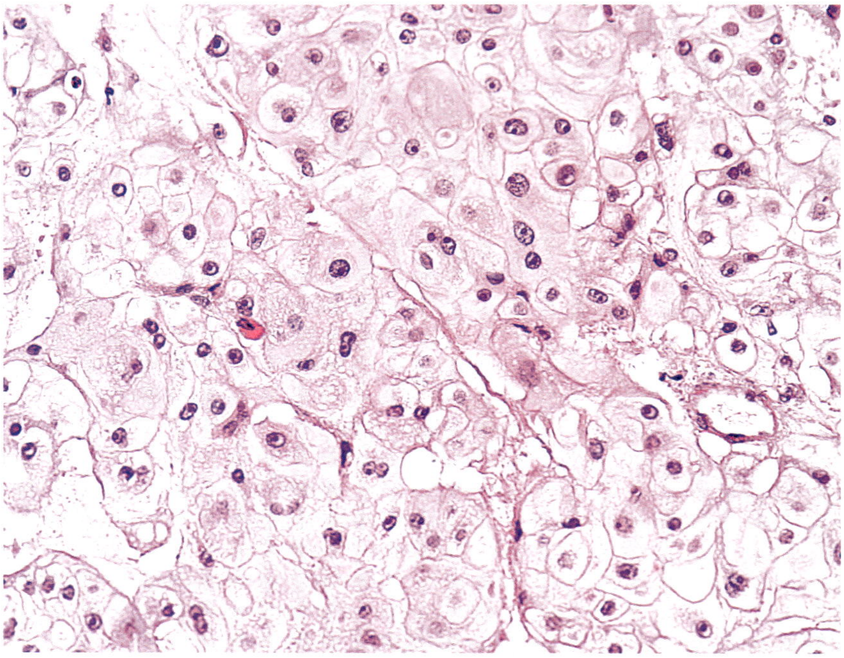

Fig. 1. Histopathological aspect of a typical chordoma: cells are arranged in chords set in a matrix of mucopolysaccharide.

favourable long-term outcome. Conversely, dedifferentiated chordoma is observed in < 5% of cases, has features of high grade spindle cell sarcoma and demonstrates an aggressive clinical course [3]. Clinical presentation depends on the specific sites of their extension. Pain is the main symptom followed by visual disturbances and lower cranial nerve palsies, based on the location of the lesion. Intracranial chordoma typically arises from the clivus and can invade the dura, extend in any direction, for example towards the foramen magnum, compress the brainstem or infiltrate anteriorly the cavernous sinus [16]. Among cranial nerves, the abducens nerve is the most commonly affected. Headache is usually reported in an occipital or retro-orbital location.

Chondrosarcomas: general features

Chondrosarcomas are generally slow growing, malignant tumours of bone that are characterized by the formation of cartilaginous neoplastic tissue. They account for only 0.16% of all intracranial tumours and the majority of these occurs at the base of the skull. Chondrosarcomas are believed to arise from primitive mesenchymal cells or from embryonic remains of the cartilaginous matrix in the cranium. They are sometimes mistakenly diagnosed as chordoma, but it is important to distinguish them from the latter since they have a better prognosis [13,24]. More than 90% are designated as conventional chondrosarcomas. Classic chondrosarcoma, the most common type, is a low grade to intermediate-grade tumour (grade 1 or 2), which has an indolent clinical behaviour and low metastatic potential [7]. Mesenchymal chondrosarcomas are composed of areas of undifferentiated mesenchymal cells and areas of cartilage. Histologically, they are similar to Ewing's sarcoma with foci of cartilaginous differentiation. Dedifferentiated chondrosarcoma is a tumour in which a low grade chondrosarcoma transforms into a high grade sarcoma, most frequently exhibiting features of osteosarcoma, fibrosarcoma, or malignant fibrous histiocytoma. Compared with chordomas, chondrosarcomas lack cytokeratin and EMA expression and they are positive for S-100 and vimentin. Like chordoma, chondrosarcoma tends to invade local structures. Metastatic sites (lungs, bone and liver) usually occur late in the course of the disease. Local disease is the main problem, with local recurrences frequent in a follow up of more than 15 years.

Imaging characteristics

Chordoma and chondrosarcoma have a similar radiological appearance. Both CT and MR imaging are usually required for pretreatment evaluation. At high-resolution CT, chordoma appears as a centrally-located, well-circumscribed, expansive soft-tissue mass that arises from the clivus with associated extensive lytic bone destruction and intratumoral calcifications. There is moderate to marked enhancement following administration of iodinated contrast material. The typical appearance of chondrosarcoma on CT scan is a destructive lesion with scalloped erosive borders. Calcification within the tumour matrix is occasionally present. The chordoma and the chondrosarcoma exhibit similar MRI features. MR imaging is actually the best modality for radiological evaluation of intracranial chordomas [15]. On conventional spin-echo T1-weighted MR images, intracranial chordoma has intermediate to low signal intensity and is easily recognized within a high signal intensity of the fat of the clivus. Classical intracranial chordoma has high signal intensity on T2-weighted images. This reflects the high fluid content of the vacuolated cellular components. Also, T2-weighted imaging is excellent for differentiating tumour from adjacent neural structures [25]. The majority of intracranial chordomas demonstrate moderate to marked enhancement following contrast material injection. Despite the finding that chondrosarcomas have a similar appearance on MRI, they can occasionally be distinguished from chordomas due to their more lateral location along the petroclival fissure [8]. Chondrosarcomas start laterally and grow towards the midline, whereas chordomas are tumours that originate from the midline and grow laterally.

Prognostic factors

Heffelfinger *et al.* found that the variant chondroid of the chordoma have a more benign issue [12]. However, Colli *et al.* did not find significant difference between survival and recurrence-free survival (RFS) for patients with typical chordomas and chondroid chordomas [4]. The age of the patient has been suggested as having an important role in the prognosis of skull base chordomas. Forsyth *et al.* have reported that the 5- and 10-year survival rates for the younger population were 75% and 63% respectively, compared with 30% and 11% for the older population [10].

Female sex has been shown to have a negative prognostic impact, especially in chordoma: in the Massachusetts General Hospital series, the 10-year local control rate was 65% for males *versus* 42% only for females [22].

Standard treatment of chordoma and chondrosarcoma

Surgery

Although chordoma and chondrosarcoma of the skull base present with important differences in histopathology, biological behaviour and outcome, they have a good number of features in common and their overall management is relatively similar. Surgical resection is a very effective treatment for chordomas and chondrosarcomas. Longer survival rates have been associated with more extensive tumour removal [1]. However, a complete resection in the skull base region is rarely possible because of the anatomical location of the tumour at the base of the skull and the close proximity of critical anatomical structures. Total or near-total tumour resection of craniocervical chordomas and chondrosarcomas ranges from 62 to 78.5% [11,19]. However, the recurrence rate, even after radical resection, remains high for chordomas [18]. If maximal surgical cytoreduction is performed either for chordoma or chondrosarcoma, then survival can be improved; with extensive surgery, Crockard *et al.* have reported 5-year survival rates of 77% and 93% respectively, for chordoma and chondrosarcoma [5]. However, in most current situations, even in chondrosarcoma, surgery alone is insufficient. At the present time, most patients still present with gross residual disease after surgical resection, as evidenced by postoperative imaging.

Radiotherapy

For many decades, chondrosarcoma and chordoma were considered to have a low radiosensitivity, although a favourable and even prolonged effect could be demonstrated [2]. In fact, these tumours can be controlled, provided a sufficiently high dose (more than 70 Gy) can be administered. With conventional techniques, this can be rarely achieved because of the proximity of sensitive structures such as the brainstem, optic pathways, the temporal lobes, etc. Particle therapy (proton, helium) is particularly suited because of its extreme precision and a fairly high total dose (70-80 Gy) can be delivered safely in many cases. The experience at the Massachusetts General Hospital, the University of Loma Linda, the Centre d'Orsay and the Paul Scherer Institute has demonstrated that doses of 67-74 CGE (cobalt-Gray equivalent) can be given in these tumours [9,13,22,24,26,27].

With postoperative proton-beam radiotherapy, a 3- to 5-year local control rate of between 50 and 80% for chordoma and between 70 and 100% for chondrosarcoma was achieved with an acceptable level of complications [9,13,22,24,26,27]. At this moment, proton-beam radiotherapy is considered by many specialists to be the standard treatment for chordoma and chondrosarcoma. However, radiosurgery and fractionated stereotactic radiotherapy (FSRT) are reasonable alternatives to particle therapy (Fig. 2). In a German series, FSRT delivered 65-67 Gy to 45 patients with a 4-year local control rate of 50% for chordoma and 100% for chondrosarcoma [6].

Conclusion

Chordoma and chondrosarcoma are very rare tumours of the base of skull, with similarities in their location, behaviour and treatment. However, there are also substantial differences in the pathology, in the recurrence rate and overall prognosis, with a more favourable outcome for chondrosarcoma. High-precision therapy with protons or possibly with FSRT yield good overall local control rates.

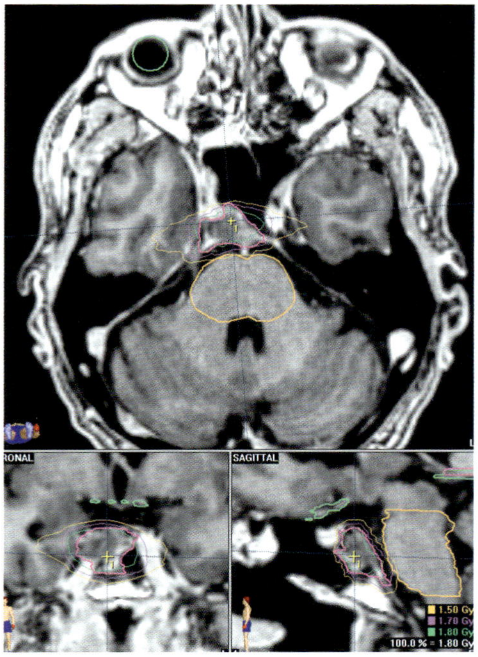

Fig. 2. Fractionated stereotactic radiotherapy: dose distribution for a patient with a chordoma of the clivus.

References

1. Al-Mefty O, Borba LA (1997) Skull base chordomas: a management challenge. J Neurosurg 86: 182-9
2. Catton C, O'Sullivan B, Bell R *et al.* (1996) Chordoma: long-term follow-up after radical photon irradiation. Radiother Oncol 41: 67-72
3. Chugh R, Tawbi H, Lucas DR *et al.* (2007) Chordoma: the nonsarcoma primary bone tumor. The Oncologist 12: 1344-50
4. Colli BO, Al-Mefty O (2001) Chordomas of the skull base: follow-up review and prognostic factors. Neurosurg Focus 10 (3): 1-11
5. **Crockard HA, Steel T, Plowman N *et al.* (2001) A multidisciplinary team approach to skull base chondrosarcomas. J Neurosurg 95: 175-83**
6. **Debus J, Schultz-Erntner D, Schad L *et al.* (2000) Stereotactic fractionated radiotherapy for chordoma and chondrosarcoma of the skull base. Int J Radiat Oncol Biol Phys 47: 591-6**
7. Dorfman HD, Czerniak B (1998) Bone tumors. Mosby Inc., St Louis, MO, USA: 353-440
8. Erdem E, Angtuaco EC, Van Hemert R *et al.* (2003) Comprehensive review of intracranial chordoma. Radiographics 23: 995-1009
9. **Fagundes MA, Hug EB, Liebsch NJ *et al.* (1998) Radiation therapy for chordomas of the base of skull and cervical spine: patterns of failure and outcome after relapse. Int J Radiat Oncol Biol Phys 15: 579-84**
10. Forsyth PA, Cascino TL, Shaw EG *et al.* (1993) Intracranial chordoma: a clinicopathological and prognostic study of 51 cases. J Neurosurg 78: 741-7
11. Gay E, Sekhar LN, Rubinsten E, *et al.* (1995) Chordomas and chondrosarcomas of the cranial base: results and follow-up of 60 patients. Neurosurgery 36: 887-97
12. Heffelfinger MJ, Dahlin DC, MacCarty CS *et al.* (1973) Chordomas and cartilaginous tumors at the skull base. Cancer 32: 410-20
13. **Hug EB, Slater JB (2000) Proton radiation therapy for chordomas and chondrosarcoma of the skull base. Neurosurg Clin N Am 11: 627-38**

14. Korten AGC, Ter Berg HJ, Spincemaille GH *et al.* (1998) Intracranial chondrosarcoma: review of the literature and report of 15 cases. J Neurol Neurosurg Psychiatry 65: 88-92
15. Larson TC, Houser W, Laws ER (1987) Imaging of cranial chordomas. Mayo Clin Proc 62: 886-93
16. Maire JP, Liguoro D, San Gelli F (2001) Volume tumoral macroscopique (GTV) et volume-cible anatomoclinique (CTV) dans la radiothérapie des tumeurs bénignes de la base du crane. Cancer Radiother 5: 581-96
17. McMaster ML, Goldstein AM, Bromles CM *et al.* (2001) Chordoma: incidence and survival pattern in the United States, 1973-1995. Cancer Causes Control 12: 1-11
18. Menezes AH, Traynelis VC. Tumors of the craniocervical junction. In: Youmans JR (ed) (1996) Neurological Surgery, Edn 4. WB Saunders, Philadelphia, USA, Vol IV, pp 3041-72
19. Menezes AH, Gantz BJ, Traynelis VC *et al.* (1997) Cranial base chordoma. Clin Neurosurg 44: 491-509
20. Mindell ER (1981) Chordoma. J Bone Joint Surg Am 63: 501-5
21. Mirra J (2002) Pathology and genetics of tumours of soft tissue and bone. Lyon, France: IARC press; pp 316-7
22. Munzenrider JE, Liebsch NH (1999) Proton therapy for tumors of the skull base. Strahlenther Onkol 175(S2): 57-63
23. Neff B, Sataloff RT, Storey L *et al.* (2002) Chondrosarcoma of the skull base. Laryngoscope 112: 131-5
24. **Noel G, Habrand JL, Mammar H *et al.* (2001) Combination of photon and proton radiation therapy for chordoma and chondrosarcoma of the skull base: the Centre de Protonthérapie d'Orsay experience. Int J Radiat Oncol Biol Phys 51: 392-8**
25. Oot RF, Melville GE, New PJ *et al.* (1998) MR and CT in evaluating clival chordomas and chondrosarcomas. AJR Am J Roentgenol 151: 567-75
26. Rutz HP, Weber DC, Goitein G *et al.* (2008) Post-operative spot-scanning proton radiation therapy for chordoma and chondrosarcoma in children and adolescents: initial experience at the Paul Scherrer Institute. Int J Radiat Oncol Biol Phys 71: 220-5
27. Weber DC, Rutz HP, Pedroni ES *et al.* (2005) Results of spot-scanning proton radiation therapy for chordoma and chondrosarcoma of the skull base: the Paul Scherrer Institute experience. Int J Radiat Oncol Biol Phys 63: 401-9

Primary spinal epidural lymphoma

7

V. Monnard and R.-O. Mirimanoff

Five Essential Points

1. *Primary spinal epidural lymphoma (PSEL) is a rare and distinct form of NHL and one of the many causes of spinal cord compression.*
2. *Diagnosis is established in the majority of cases during an emergency laminectomy and surgery should be limited to surgical decompression.*
3. *Radiation therapy (RT) (35-40 Gy) plays a central role and is followed by an excellent local control.*
4. *Chemotherapy should be associated to RT in intermediate and high-grade PSEL.*
5. *Overall prognosis after combined modality is relatively good, especially in younger patients.*

Introduction

Lymphomas primarily occurring in the epidural space in the absence of other previously detected lymphomatous foci, represent a very rare entity in non-Hodgkin's lymphoma (NHL). Nodal localization of NHL is by far the most frequent one and is encountered in about 60% of all cases. NHL can present as an isolated lesion in about 35% of cases or accompanied by other localizations in about 30% of cases. The most frequent extra-nodal localisations, either purely extra-nodal or concomitant with a nodal involvement, are the bone marrow, the head and neck region, the intestinal tract and the skin.

Incidence

Epidural localization is a rare presenting site both in Hodgkin's disease and in NHL, accounting for 10% of spinal epidural tumours [1] and for 0,1 to 3,3% of all lymphomas [12,19]. Median age at diagnosis is in the sixties with a range from 21 to 96 years [15]. There is a sex prevalence for men (male-to-female ratio of 2 : 1) [15].

Anatomy and Pathology

The adult spinal cord can be between 42 and 45 cm in length. It extends from the foramen magnum in the occipital bone to the level of the second lumbar vertebra. In the vertebral canal, it is embedded in the spinal meninges (dura mater, arachnoid mater and pia mater). The virtual cavity between the bony and ligamentous walls of the vertebral canal and the dura mater (the outermost covering membrane of the spinal cord) is called the epidural space. Usually, the thoracic region of the epidural space is the most commonly affected site probably because it corresponds also to the longest part of the spine. The origin of primary spinal epidural lymphoma (PSEL) remains unknown. Rubinstein states that it stems from the lymphatic tissue present in the epidural space and proposes a theory of antigenic stimulation with a transformation cascade, which under appropriate conditions can produce primary spinal lymphoma from mesodermal cells lining the epidural space [18]. Other authors support the hypothesis that primary spinal epidural lymphoma originates from the paravertebral lymph nodes or from the vertebral body, which later extends onto the epidural space [9,13]. Recent immunochemical and electron microscopic studies have identified that the PSEL most frequently originates from B lymphocytes [3,10]. The most widely used histologic classification for NHL in Europe is the Kiel classification system [11]. However the Working Formulation is often used because it is thought to be the most reproducible classification [20] whereas in the United States, the World Health Organisation (WHO) classification system is the one most often used.

Table 1 – Ann-Arbor classification for lymphoma [2].

	Clinical stage (CS)
Stage I	Involvement of a single lymph node region (I), or localized involvement of a single extralymphatic organ or site (Ie)
Stage II	Involvement of two or more lymph node regions on the same side of the diaphragm (II), or localized involvement of a single extralymphatic organ or site an its regional lymph node(s) with or without involvement of other lymph node regions on the same side of the diaphragm (IIe) *Note: the number of lymph node regions involved may be indicated by a subscript (ex : II2)*
Stage III	Involvement of lymph node regions on both side of the diaphragm(III), which may also be accompanied by localized involvement of an associated extralymphatic organ or site (IIIe), or by involvement of the spleen (IIIs), or both (IIIes)
Stage IV	Disseminated (multifocal) involvement of one or more extralymphatic organs, with or without associated lymph node involvement; or isolated extralymphatic organ involvement with distant (non regional) nodal involvement.

Table 2 – Kiel Classification of Non-Hodgkin's lymphoma [11].

Low grade malignant lymphomas	B-cell chronic lymphocytic leukemia T-cell chronic lymphocytic leukemia Prolymphocytic leukemia Hairy cell leukemia Mycosis fungoides/Sezary's syndrome T-zone lymphoma Lymphoplasmacytic/cytoid immunocytoma Plasmocytic (plasmacytoma) Centrocytic lymphoma Centroblastic/centrocytic lymphoma
High grade malignant lymphomas	Centroblastic lymphoma Lymphoblastic lymphoma Burkitt type (B) Convoluted-cell type (T) Unclassified Immunoblastic lymphom

Table 3 – The Working Formulation [20].

Low grade	Small lymphocytic lymphoma	4% of all lymphoma, does not have a follicular architecture
	Follicular small cleaved cell lymphoma	Together with follicular mixed lymphoma constitute 40% of adult NHL
	Follicular mixed (small cleaved and large cell)	
Intermediate grade	Follicular, predominantly large cell	15% of all follicular lymphoma
	Diffuse, small cleaved cell	5-10%
	Diffuse mixed small and large cell	
	Diffuse large cell	Large cell immunoblastic, diffuse large cell and diffuse mixed lymphomas represent together 40-50% of all lymphoma
High grade	Large cell immunoblastic lymphoma	
	Lymphoblastic lymphoma	Constitutes less than 5% of all NHL
	Small noncleaved lymphoma (Burkitt)	Constitute less than 1% of all NHL

Clinical presentation

The symptoms depend mainly on the localization along the spinal canal, knowing that the thoracic region is the most affected diseased site (65% of patients). In the Rare Cancer Network (RCN) experience, the most common symptoms are varying degrees of lower limb weakness (88%), back pain (79%), sensory deficit (71%), bladder dysfunction (23%), sphincter dysfunction (19%), bowel dysfunction (17%), neck pains (11%) and upper limb weakness (9%) [15]. The occurrence of "B symptoms", namely weight loss, night sweats and fever is rare, as those symptoms are usually associated with extensive NHL disease. In our series for example, only two patients out of 52 patients had unexplained weight loss and one presented with night sweats [15].

Staging procedure

In the vast majority of cases (92%), the diagnosis of this lymphoma is established during an emergency decompressive laminectomy [15]. Work up should include, in the acute phase, an MRI (or CT scan if the former is not available or contra-indicated). Sagittal and axial T1 and T2-weighted images with and without gadolinium should be obtained. MRI enables the study of the spinal cord in 3D, the study of the adjacent structures, and allows determination of the topography of the lesion with precision (i.e. skeletal, epidural, intradural - either extra-medullar or intramedullar). It allows the rapid study of the whole vertebral column and the estimation of the degree of medullary suffering and to pinpoint the aetiology of the lesion. Tissue sampling for a definite pathologic diagnosis should be obtained in most situations. Elective work up should consist of a complete medical history and physical examination, full blood counts, blood chemistry including serum electrophoresis, cerebrospinal fluid examination, whole-body CT scan or MRI, bone marrow aspiration and/or biopsy and, when available, a positron emission tomography. Currently in most situations, MRI has replaced myelography and computed tomography in the examination of epidural neoplasms. Da-Chung *et al.* have determined the MRI characteristics of these lesions [3]. An epidural infiltration of spinal lymphoma is relatively homogeneous on MRI. Most lymphomas show a lower signal intensity than that of fat and a slightly higher signal intensity than that of muscle on T1W1; they are isointense or have a lower signal intensity than that of fat and higher signal intensity than that of muscle on T2W1. A homogeneous enhancement is found following the administration of gadolinium on the infiltration, which extends along the epidural space. These observations suggest that lymphomas have a characteristic appearance on MRI, and therefore can be differentiated from other epidural tumours [3].

Treatment

Surgery

Epidural spinal cord compression is an emergency condition that requires prompt and adequate diagnosis and treatment. In malignancies compressing the spinal cord, the first therapeutic approach is generally surgery, which should consist of decompressive laminectomy with or without partial removal of the tumour mass, which immediately alleviates the spinal cord compression and enables the clinician to establish the correct histological diagnosis. However, because lymphomas are very chemo- and radiosensitive tumours, surgery should ideally be limited to decompressive laminectomy or biopsy only, leaving the major role to radiotherapy (RT) and chemotherapy [6,8,15]. So after surgery, and as soon as the correct diagnosis is established, further treatment with radiation and chemotherapy should be administered to ensure both a high probability of local control and to prevent further dissemination.

Radiation therapy

RT plays a central role in the treatment of localised lymphomas. In PSEL, our data support the treatment of a relatively large volume, encompassing the epidural mass with two to three vertebral bodies both above and below the lesion [15]. However, it may be that with the advent of new imaging modalities, such as PET-CT, the volume could be reduced and limited only to the identifiable residual lesion. Another argument in favour of a limited irradiation volume is that more and more, chemotherapy is also administered and may efficiently treat subclinical extent of PSEL. The radiation doses employed by various authors vary widely, with ranges between 20 and 60 Gy [8,21]. Generally, doses of at least 25 Gy are recommended [14]. It appears though from the RCN experience that a dose of at least 36 Gy at 2 Gy per fraction, or its equivalent, should be considered. RT should be given with at least 3D conformal techniques and if possible IMRT.

Chemotherapy

Although Oviatt *et al.* reported on two patients with epidural compression secondary to NHL, who were successfully treated by chemotherapy alone [16], most authors have opted for a treatment based on surgery followed by RT [5,6,12,17]. Chemotherapy is now generally added to radiation therapy using four to six cycles of cyclophosphamide, doxorubicin, vincristine and prednisone (CHOP) or CHOP-like regimes, especially in young patients and in patients who have an intermediate or a high grade lymphoma [15].

Combined modality treatment and treatment results

There are relatively few large series on PSEL, therefore outcome is not so easy to assess. However combined modality treatment including RT and chemotherapy seems to be the most efficient treatment for primary spinal epidural lymphoma. In the RCN series, the local control was 88% and the 5-year overall survival 69% [15]. Di Marco *et al.* treated 9 patients with PSEL, and reported a long-term survival only in two patients who received a complete chemotherapeutic course after RT [4]. Epelbaum *et al.* with intensive combined therapy, using RT and chemotherapy, achieved an actuarial 5-year survival rate of 66% [6]. Rathmell *et al.* in their series of 22 patients reported a significant difference between patients treated with RT alone and those treated with a combination of RT and chemotherapy with an overall actuarial survival of 33% and 86% respectively [17]. In our series, on multivariate analysis, combined modality treatment was superior to RT alone (p = 0.01), since among the 20 patients who received RT alone, 11 suffered a systemic relapse, from which 7 died, 2 survived with disease, respectively 4 and 9 years after treatment and 2 are alive without disease, 4 and 15 years after treatment [15]. In addition, of those patients treated with RT alone, one patient had a local relapse and died 8 months after the end of the treatment. Among the 32 patients who received a combined modality treatment, 19 (59%) are still alive without disease 2 to 13 years after treatment, 8 had a systemic relapse and 5 a local relapse. The outcome depends on the neurological status after treatment. In our series, a complete neurological response was observed in 25% of patients who presented initially with motor weakness. Even if it takes several months to achieve a complete recovery, complete neurological response was the most significant favourable prognostic factor in the multivariate analysis with regard to overall survival (p = 0.001). Other series also found that the outcome depends on the neurological status after treatment [5,17]. In the RCN series, with regard to the outcome, the overall prognosis for patients with PSEL was relatively good as amongst the 52 patients, 25 are alive without disease 2-17 years after treatment, 3 are alive with disease after 4-9 years, 6 died without disease 10-89 months after treatment and 18 died with disease 6-121 months after treatment [15].

Similar findings have also been made by others [6,8]. Rathmell *et al.* found an excellent local control of 88% at 10 years, with only 2 patients failing to achieve a permanent local control [17]. In our series, 42% of patients suffered from a systemic relapse, mainly in the lymph nodes. Among the 10 patients of Epelbaum *et al.* with spinal cord presentation of NHL, 70% achieved a complete remission after initial treatment. Four who were treated by combined modality treatment relapsed after a median time of 15 months with relapse in bone, bone marrow, CNS and mediastinum. Three remained free of disease and three progressed while on initial treatment [6].

Prognostic factors

In our study, we determined that sex and tumour grade did not influence the prognosis. However, age did have an impact on univariate analysis with a significant survival and DFS advantage for patients aged less than 63 years (p = 0.001 and 0.006 respectively) [15]. However it should be noted that younger patients tended to be treated more aggressively than older ones, both with radiation therapy and chemotherapy. We also found that the volume of the radiotherapy (more than focal), the total dose given (>36 Gy) and combined modality treatment (radiotherapy and chemotherapy) influenced the overall survival (p = 0.001, 0.01 and 0.005, respectively), by multivariate analysis [15].

Conclusion

Spinal epidural lymphoma is obviously a very rare entity and for this reason, we should be very cautious in drawing too firm conclusions, especially with regard to therapy. However, regarding diagnosis and work-up, it is safe to say that one should include in the acute phase an MRI (or if not available, a CT scan) of the entire spine and tissue sampling during the emergency surgery, for a definitive pathological diagnosis. Elective workup should consist of a complete medical history and physical examination, full blood counts, blood chemistry including serum electrophoresis, CSF examination, whole-body CT scan or MRI and bone marrow aspiration or biopsy. Positron emission tomography or positron emission tomography-CT scan should also be part of the work-up if available.

Treatment will almost always include in the acute phase some form of emergency decompressive surgery, with or without resection, followed by RT and chemotherapy. RT plays a central role and should be given to a volume encompassing the epidural mass, with margins that will depend on the type of available imaging, at a dose of at least 36 Gy at 2 Gy per fraction or its equivalent. Chemotherapy should almost always be added to RT in high- or intermediate-grade PSEL, using four to six cycles of cyclophosphamide, doxorubicin, vincristine and prednisone or cyclophosphamide, doxorubicin, vincristine and prednisone-like regimes.

References

1. Boukobza M, Mazel C, Touboul E (1996) Primary vertebral and spinal epidural non- Hodgkin's lymphoma with spinal cord compression. Neuroradiology 38: 333-7
2. Carbone PP, Kaplan HS, Mushoff K *et al.* (1971) Report of the committee on Hodgkin's disease staging classification. Cancer Res 31: 1860-1
3. Da-Chung L, Jung-Mao C (2007) MRI of primary spinal epidural lymphoma: case report. Chin J Radiol 32: 147-51
4. Di Marco A, Campostrini F, Garusi GF (1989) Non-Hodgkin's lymphoma presenting with spinal epidural involvement. Acta Oncol 28: 485-8
5. **Eeles RA, O'Brien P, Horwich A *et al.* (1991) Non-Hodgkin's lymphoma presenting with extradural spinal cord compression: Functional outcome and survival. Br J Cancer 63: 126-9**
6. **Epelbaum R, Haim N, Ben-Shahar M *et al.* (1986) Non-Hodgkin's lymphoma presenting with spinal epidural involvement. Cancer 58: 2120-4**
7. Grant JW, Kaech D, Jones DB (1986) Spinal cord compression at first presentation of lymphoma-A review of 15 cases. Histopathology 10: 1191-202
8. Haddad P, Thaell JF, Kiely JM *et al.* (1976) Lymphoma of the spinal extradural space. Cancer 38: 1862-6
9. Iwanow G, Remodanowsky K (1972) Primary extradural non-Hodgkin's lymphoma and cord compression. Exp Med: 56-9
10. **Kapoor R, Kumar V, Sharma SC (2006) Primary extradural Non-Hodgkin's lymphoma. JK Science 1: 45-8**
11. Lennert K, Feller AC (1990) Histopathology of non-Hodgkin's lymphoma (based on the updated Kiel classification). Berlin. Heidelberg. New York. Springer
12. Lim CCT, Chong BK (1996) Spinal epidural non-Hodgkin's lymphoma: Case reports of three patients presenting with epidural cord compression. Singapore Med J 37: 497-500

13. Liznka H, Nakamun T (1989) Malignant lymphoma of the epidural space. Report of three cases. Neurol Med Chair (Tokyo) 29: 307-11
14. Lyons MK, O'Neill BP, Marsh WR *et al.* (1992) Primary spinal epidural lymphoma: Report of 8 patients and review of the literature. Neurosurgery 30: 675-9
15. Monnard V, Sun A, Epelbaum E *et al.* (2006) Primary spinal epidural lymphoma: patients'profile, outcome and prognostic factors: a multicentre rare cancer network study. Int J Radiat Oncol Biol Phys 65(3): 817-23
16. Oviatt DL, Kirshner HS, Stein RS (1982) Successful chemotherapeutic treatment of epidural compression in non-Hodgkin's lymphoma. Cancer 49: 2446-8
17. Rathmell AJ, Gospodarowicz MK, Sutcliffe SB *et al.* (1992) Localized extradural lymphoma: Survival, relapse pattern and functional outcome. Radiother Oncol 24: 14-20
18. Rubinstein LJ (1972) Pathology of Tumors of the Nervous System. Arch. of tumour pathology. Facide 6. Tumour of the lymphorect. System. AFIP 66: 13
19. Salvati M, Cervoni L, Artico M *et al.* (1996) Primary spinal epidural non-Hodgkin's lymphomas: a clinical study. Surg Neurol 46: 339-44
20. The non-Hodgkin's lymphoma pathologic classification project (1982) National Cancer Institute sponsored study of classifications of non-Hodgkin's lymphomas. Summary and description of Working Formulation for clinical usage. Cancer 49: 2112-35
21. Vasudev Rao T, Narayanaywamy KS, Shankar SK *et al.* (1982) Primary spinal epidural lymphomas: A clinico-pathological study. Acta neurochir 62: 307-17

Section 2
Head and neck tumours

Esthesioneuroblastoma

1

O. Matzinger

Five Essential Points

1. *Esthesioneuroblastoma (ENB), or olfactory neuroblastoma, is a rare malignancy thought to arise from the olfactory epithelium.*
2. *Because of the uncommon nature of the disease, its clinical characteristics and it's the best treatment regimen remain difficult to study.*
3. *Standard treatment modalities include radiotherapy (RT) alone, combined RT and craniofacial resection (CFR), and CFR alone.*
4. *Experience at several institutions using various chemotherapeutic regimens has suggested that this tumour is sensitive to chemotherapy. Cisplatin-based combination regimens (particularly cisplatin and etoposide) have often been chosen.*
5. *The most important factor influencing outcome in patients with ENB is the extent of disease at diagnosis.*

Introduction

Esthesioneuroblastoma (ENB), or olfactory neuroblastoma, first described in 1924 by Berger *et al.* is a rare malignancy thought to arise from the olfactory epithelium. It accounts for approximately 6% of nasal cavity/paranasal sinus cancers [39]. Because of the uncommon nature of the disease, its clinical characteristics and its impact on survival remain difficult to study. A review of the world literature up to 1997 found only 945 described cases[4].

Clinical presentation

ENB has a bi-modal age distribution: between the age of 10 and 20 years and later between the age of 50 and 60 years [4]. There appears to be no sex predilection for the disease [37]. No etiological agent or exposure has been documented in human beings [40].

This tumour typically presents with advanced stage at the time of diagnosis, which is attributed to the nonspecific symptoms associated with the disease [28]. It can extend locally to involve the surrounding paranasal sinuses, cribriform plate, and orbits [10]. The course of development is highly variable and not necessarily predictable. The tumour can show varied biological activity that ranges from indolent growth, with patients surviving with known tumour for more than 20 years, to a highly aggressive course [34]. The most common site of metastasis are the cervical lymph nodes (10%-33% of patients), while sites of distant metastasis, including the lungs, brain, and bone, are less common [15,4,13].

The most common symptoms at presentation include (unilateral) nasal obstruction, epistaxis, anosmia, and headache [7]. Because of these nonspecific symptoms, ENB is often initially mistaken for benign disease of the nasal cavity. Further rare symptoms include frontal headache and diplopia. These symptoms are related both to the site and local extent of the tumour: anosmia is caused by involvement of the cribriform plate, while epistaxis reflects the marked vascularity of the tumour. Pain, proptosis, and excessive lacrimation are secondary to orbital extension. Ear pain and otitis media result from obstruction of the eustachian tube. Frontal headache suggests involvement of the frontal sinus [4,34].

Physical examination usually reveals a polypoid mass located high in the nasal cavity [7].

Imaging

Advances in pre-therapeutic imaging have significantly contributed to the management of sino-nasal tumours. CT and MR imaging play complementary roles in the assessment and staging of these malignancies by determining the presence or absence of extension of disease into the skull base and the orbit [23]. CT provides the best information about local invasion into surrounding bony structures and allows detailed assessment of bony erosion or destruction, particularly of the cribriform plate [24]. MRI is more accurate for defining the margins of intracranial tumour extension into adjacent soft tissue areas, such as the anterior cranial fossa and the retromaxillary space [6,36].

However, CT and MRI alone are insufficient to make a definite diagnosis which requires pathological examination and confirmation with immunohistochemistry [3].

Staging

There is no uniformly accepted staging for ENB. Kadish *et al.* developed the first and most commonly referenced staging system from Stage A to C (see Table 1) [18].

Table 1 – Staging system of ENB by Kadish [18].

Stage A	Limited to the nasal cavity
Stage B	Involve the nasal cavity and one or more paranasal sinuses
Stage C	Extends beyond the nasal cavity and paranasal sinuses

Morita *et al.* have added a group D for tumours with regional (cervical lymph node) or distant metastases [31].

Other staging systems have also been used, but no single staging classification has been universally adopted for this tumour to date, as the prognostic utility of each system has not been validated [9,12,17,30].

Pathology

On gross examination, the tumour is polypoid, soft, and hemorrhagic. Microscopically, it is composed of small round cells slightly larger than lymphocytes with hyperchromatic nuclei, small or indistinct nucleoli, and uniform chromatin distribution. The stroma is typically pink, neurofibrillary or edematous, and well-vascularized. Mitoses are rare. Flexner type rosettes (composed of tumour cells surrounding a central lumen) are rare and Homer-Wright pseudorosettes (composed of tumour cells surrounding a central pink fibrillar material) are noted in approximately 50% of cases. Necrosis, dystrophic calcification, and vascular or lymphatic invasion are not uncommon [2,26].

Hyams developed a pathological grading system classifying ENB into four grades based on histological features such as mitotic activity and necrosis. This grading scheme reportedly provides prognostic information, with grade I patients having a uniformly good outcome and grade IV patients all dying of disease [16] (see Table 2).

Table 2 – Grading system of ENB by Hyams [16].

Grade I	Tumours are characterized by a prominent fibrillary matrix, tumour cells with uniform nuclei and absence of nuclear pleomorphism, mitotic activity, or necrosis
Grade II	Tumours have some fibrillary matrix and exhibit moderate nuclear polymorphism with some mitotic activity. There is no necrosis
Grade III	Tumours have minimal fibrillary matrix and Flexner type rosettes are present. There is prominent mitotic activity and nuclear polymorphism and some necrosis may be seen
Grade IV	Tumours have no fibrillary matrix or rosettes and show marked nuclear pleomorphism and increased mitotic activity with frequent necrosis

Most studies report a good correlation of Hyams grade with prognosis [30].

A variety of other small cell tumours can present in the sinonasal region (eg, sinonasal undifferentiated carcinoma, neuroendocrine carcinoma, melanoma, lymphoma, plasmacytoma, embryonal rhabdomyosarcoma, Ewing sarcoma, peripheral primitive neuroectodermal tumours, and vascular tumours) [3,30].

There is general agreement that a diagnosis of ENB by light microscopy is not difficult when the tumour is well differentiated and consists of homogenous small cells with uniform round to oval nuclei, with rosette or pseudorosette formation, and eosinophilic fibrillary intercellular background material. However when the tumour is undifferentiated with anaplastic hyperchromatic small cells that show many mitotic figures and scant cytoplasm, differentiation from other small-cell nasal neoplasms by light microscopy becomes difficult and the diagnosis can be based only on the results of antigen expression using a panel of antibodies by immunohistochemistry [2] and, if necessary, confirmed by electron microscopy.

Treatment

The assessment of therapeutic efficacy of treatment of ENB is complicated by several factors: the rarity of the tumour, the lack of a universally accepted staging system, and a lack of consistency of treatment as a result of significant advances in this field over time. Management has evolved but, as in most rare tumours, there are no randomized trials to guide treatment decisions. As a result, there is no consensus as to the optimal treatment either for localized or advanced disease.

Standard treatment modalities include radiotherapy (RT) alone, combined RT and craniofacial resection (CFR), and CFR alone [28,37,41]. Despite the lack of support for the use of single-modality treatment regimens, a substantial number of patients are still treated by surgery or radiotherapy alone [11]. As the location of the primary tumour makes it difficult to obtain negative margins, postoperative radiation has been advocated to decrease the risk of local recurrence [1,5,8]. Some recent studies have suggested a potential benefit of adding chemotherapy to the combined approach of surgery and postoperative radiotherapy [21,22,35].

Surgery plus radiotherapy

Most institutions favour surgery as the first treatment modality, followed by radiotherapy [10, 25,32]. The theoretical advantage that preoperative radiotherapy could reduce an unresectable tumour to a resectable size has never been clearly demonstrated [1]. Newer radiotherapy techniques, such as proton beam therapy [33] and intensity modulated radiation therapy (IMRT) [8] are more effective at sparing normal structures. Endoscopic resection followed by radiotherapy, appears promising in patients with localized ENB[5,38]. The usual recommended dose ranges from 55 to 65 Gy – actually in most cases above 60 Gy [5,10,18, 25,28,32,38].

Chemotherapy

Despite definitive local treatment, local recurrence and distant metastases are often reported [9,17]. Chemotherapy is therefore often also implemented in patients with advanced ENB. Experience at several institutions using various chemotherapeutic regimens has suggested that this tumour is chemo-sensitive [19,21,25,28,29].

Cisplatin-based combination regimens (particularly cisplatin and etoposide) [21,35] have often been chosen, predominantly because this combination has proven its efficacity for the treatment of small cell lung carcinoma (SCLC), the most common malignancy derived from neuroendocrine cells (ENB has many similar histologic characteristics of neuroendocrine tumours) and because of their success in the treatment of head and neck squamous cell cancer. Non-platinum combinations, such as irinotecan plus docetaxel may, however, also be active [22].

Neoadjuvant chemotherapy has been reported to reduce tumour burden in order to achieve better surgical resection to increase progression free survival in advanced stage patients [10,14,19,25]. Some retrospective analysis have also found efficacy of chemotherapy for high grade tumours in the adjuvant setting [27,35].

It can be concluded that high grade ENB is sensitive to platinum-based chemotherapy and that associated to surgery and/or radiotherapy it is probably effective in prolonging time to tumour relapse. However, the optimal chemotherapy regimen for ENB is still difficult to ascertain due to the fact that the disease incidence is low, that there is no universal staging system, that no treatment approach has been consistently used between studies, and that institutional reports frequently include other sinonasal neoplasms.

Prognosis

A meta analysis by Dulguerov [11] found a 5-year survival of 45%. The most frequent recurrence was local, with rates around 30%. Craniofacial resection followed by radiotherapy seemed to result in fewer recurrences – around 10%. Salvage after local recurrence was possible in 33–50% of cases. Regional recurrence, when the primary site was controlled, occurred in 15-20% of cases and was salvageable by further treatment in a third of the cases. Distant metastases with locoregional control were not very common (8%) and carried a very poor prognosis. Other authors [17,20] have confirmed those results.

The most important factor influencing outcome in patients with ENB is the extent of disease at diagnosis. Improved disease-specific survival at ten years correlated with limited disease according to the modified Kadish staging system (83%, 49%, 39%, and 13% for stages A, B, C, and D, respectively).

References

1. Bachar G, Goldstein DP, Shah M *et al.* (2008) Esthesioneuroblastoma: The Princess Margaret Hospital experience. Head Neck 30:1607-1614.
2. Bellizzi AM, Bourne TD, Mills SE, Stelow EB (2008) The cytologic features of sinonasal undifferentiated carcinoma and olfactory neuroblastoma. Am J Clin Pathol 129: 367-76
3. Bradley PJ, Jones NS, Robertson I (2003) Diagnosis and management of esthesioneuroblastoma. Curr Opin Otolaryngol Head Neck Surg 11: 112-8
4. Broich G, Pagliari A, Ottaviani F (1997) Esthesioneuroblastoma: a general review of the cases published since the discovery of the tumour in 1924. Anticancer Res 17: 2683-706
5. Castelnuovo P, Bignami M, Delù G *et al.* (2007) Endonasal endoscopic resection and radiotherapy in olfactory neuroblastoma: our experience. Head Neck 29: 845-50
6. Chirico G, Pergolizzi S, Mazziotti S *et al.* (2003) Primary sphenoid esthesioneuroblastoma studied with MR. Clin Imaging 27: 38-40
7. Constantinidis J, Steinhart H, Koch M *et al.* (2004) Olfactory neuroblastoma: the University of Erlangen-Nuremberg experience 1975-2000. Otolaryngol Head Neck Surg 130: 567-74
8. Daly ME, Chen AM, Bucci MK *et al.* (2007) Intensity-modulated radiation therapy for malignancies of the nasal cavity and paranasal sinuses. Int J Radiat Oncol Biol Phys 67: 151-7
9. Dias FL, Sa GM, Lima RA *et al.* (2003) Patterns of failure and outcome in esthesioneuroblastoma. Arch Otolaryngol Head Neck Surg 129: 1186-92
10. Diaz EM, Johnigan RH, Pero C *et al.* (2005) Olfactory neuroblastoma: the 22-year experience at one comprehensive cancer center. Head Neck 27: 138-49
11. **Dulguerov P, Allal AS, Calcaterra TC (2001) Esthesioneuroblastoma: a meta-analysis and review. Lancet Oncol 2: 683-90**
12. Dulguerov P, Calcaterra T (1992) Esthesioneuroblastoma: the UCLA experience 1970-1990. Laryngoscope 102: 843-9
13. Elkon D, Hightower SI, Lim ML *et al.* (1979) Esthesioneuroblastoma. Cancer 44: 1087-94
14. Fitzek MM, Thornton AF, Varvares M *et al.* (2002) Neuroendocrine tumors of the sinonasal tract. Results of a prospective study incorporating chemotherapy, surgery, and combined proton-photon radiotherapy. Cancer 94: 2623-34
15. Ghaffar S, Salahuddin I (2005) Olfactory neuroblastoma: a case report and review of the literature. Ear Nose Throat J 84: 150-2
16. **Hyams VJ, Batsakis JG, Michaels L (US) AFIOP. Tumors of the upper respiratory tract and ear. Armed Forces Institute of Pathology; 1988**

1

17. Jethanamest D, Morris LG, Sikora AG, Kutler DI (2007) Esthesioneuroblastoma: a population-based analysis of survival and prognostic factors. Arch Otolaryngol Head Neck Surg 133: 276-80
18. Kadish S, Goodman M, Wang CC (1976) Olfactory neuroblastoma. A clinical analysis of 17 cases. Cancer 37: 1571-6
19. Kim DW, Jo YH, Kim JH *et al.* (2004) Neoadjuvant etoposide, ifosfamide, and cisplatin for the treatment of olfactory neuroblastoma. Cancer 101: 2257-60
20. Kim HJ, Cho HJ, Kim KS *et al.* (2008) Results of salvage therapy after failure of initial treatment for advanced olfactory neuroblastoma. J Craniomaxillofac Surg. 36: 47-52
21. Kim HJ, Kim CH, Lee BJ *et al.* (2007) Surgical treatment versus concurrent chemoradiotherapy as an initial treatment modality in advanced olfactory neuroblastoma. Auris Nasus Larynx 34: 493-8
22. Kiyota N, Tahara M, Fujii S *et al.* (2008) Nonplatinum-based chemotherapy with irinotecan plus docetaxel for advanced or metastatic olfactory neuroblastoma: a retrospective analysis of 12 cases. Cancer 112: 885-91
23. Lloyd G, Lund VJ, Howard D, Savy L (2000) Optimum imaging for sinonasal malignancy. J Laryngol Otol 114: 557-62
24. Loevner LA, Sonners AI (2002) Imaging of neoplasms of the paranasal sinuses. Magn Reson Imaging Clin N Am 10: 467-93
25. Loy AH, Reibel JF, Read PW *et al.* (2006) Esthesioneuroblastoma: continued follow-up of a single institution's experience. Arch Otolaryngol Head Neck Surg 132: 134-8
26. Mahooti S, Wakely PE (2006) Cytopathologic features of olfactory neuroblastoma. Cancer 108: 86-92
27. McElroy EA, Buckner JC, Lewis JE (1998) Chemotherapy for advanced esthesioneuroblastoma: the Mayo Clinic experience. Neurosurgery 42: 1023-7; discussion 1027-8.
28. McLean JN, Nunley SR, Klass C *et al.* (2007) Combined modality therapy of esthesioneuroblastoma. Otolaryngol Head Neck Surg 136: 998-1002
29. Mishima Y, Nagasaki E, Terui Y *et al.* (2004) Combination chemotherapy (cyclophosphamide, doxorubicin, and vincristine with continuous-infusion cisplatin and etoposide) and radiotherapy with stem cell support can be beneficial for adolescents and adults with estheisoneuroblastoma. Cancer 101:1437-44
30. Miyamoto RC, Gleich LL, Biddinger PW, Gluckman JL (2000) Esthesioneuroblastoma and sinonasal undifferentiated carcinoma: impact of histological grading and clinical staging on survival and prognosis. Laryngoscope 110: 1262-5
31. Morita A, Ebersold MJ, Olsen KD *et al.* (1993) Esthesioneuroblastoma: prognosis and management. Neurosurgery 32: 706-14; discussion 714-5
32. Nakao K, Watanabe K, Fujishiro Y *et al.* (2007) Olfactory neuroblastoma: long-term clinical outcome at a single institute between 1979 and 2003. Acta Otolaryngol Suppl 113-7
33. Nishimura H, Ogino T, Kawashima M *et al.* (2007) Proton-beam therapy for olfactory neuroblastoma. Int J Radiat Oncol Biol Phys 68: 758-62
34. Olsen KD, DeSanto LW (1983) Olfactory neuroblastoma. Biologic and clinical behavior. Arch Otolaryngol 109: 797-802
35. Porter AB, Bernold DM, Giannini C *et al.* (2008) Retrospective review of adjuvant chemotherapy for esthesioneuroblastoma. J Neurooncol 90: 201-4
36. Raghavan P, Phillips CD (2007) Magnetic resonance imaging of sinonasal malignancies. Top Magn Reson Imaging 18: 259-67
37. Simon JH, Zhen W, McCulloch TM *et al.* (2001) Esthesioneuroblastoma: the University of Iowa experience 1978-1998. Laryngoscope 111: 488-93
38. Suriano M, De Vincentiis M, Colli A *et al.* (2007) Endoscopic treatment of esthesioneuroblastoma: a minimally invasive approach combined with radiation therapy. Otolaryngol Head Neck Surg 136: 104-7
39. Svane-Knudsen V, Jørgensen KE, Hansen O *et al.* (1998) Cancer of the nasal cavity and paranasal sinuses: a series of 115 patients. Rhinology 36: 12-4
40. Wang SL, Li SH, Chen WT, Chai CY (2007) Absence of Epstein-Barr virus in olfactory neuroblastoma. Pathology 39: 565-6
41. Zafereo ME, Fakhri S, Prayson R *et al.* (2008) Esthesioneuroblastoma: 25-year experience at a single institution. Otolaryngol Head Neck Surg 138: 452-8

Extranodal NK/T-cell lymphoma, nasal-type

2

Y.X. Li

Five Essential Points

1. *Extranodal nasal-type NK/TCL is highly radiosensitive, with complete response rate of more than 80%. The 5-year overall survival with primary radiotherapy range from 40% to 86%.*
2. *Nasal NK/TCL is resistant or refractory to conventional chemotherapy, with complete response rate of 5-50% and stable/progressive disease rate of 40-50%. The 5-year overall survival with primary chemotherapy range from 0% to 50%.*
3. *Primary or up-front radiotherapy results in superior outcomes compared to chemotherapy alone or primary chemotherapy. The addition of chemotherapy to radiotherapy does not provide further benefit in overall survival.*
4. *Patients with limited stage I nasal NK/TCL should receive radiotherapy alone with curative intent, and patients with extended stage I or II disease should be treated with radiotherapy followed by consolidation chemotherapy.*
5. *Extended field and a radical radiation dose of 50 Gy is recommended. Prophylactic neck irradiation is not necessary for patients with stage I nasal NK/TCL.*

Introduction

Extranodal natural killer (NK)/T-cell lymphoma, nasal-type, is a distinct clinicopathologic entity according to the Revised European American Lymphoma (REAL)/World Health Organization (WHO) classification of lymphoid tissue [5, 9]. Clinically, this entity is characterized by a predominance in males, young age of onset, a large proportion of early stage diseases, frequent systemic symptoms, good performance, low-risk international prognostic index (IPI), and a propensity for extranodal spread [7, 30, 31, 50]. Extranodal nasal-type NK/T-cell lymphoma (NK/TCL) is highly sensitive to radiotherapy but refractory to doxorubicin-based chemotherapy.

The management of extranodal nasal-type NK/TCL has been based largely on extrapolation from the experience with aggressive non-Hodgkin's lymphoma (NHL) or diffuse large B-cell lymphoma. The prognosis and optimal therapy of this particular disease have been largely undetermined, due to the small series, heterogeneous treatments, and variable diagnostic criteria. Reported overall survival displays wide variations between the series [2, 4, 6, 7, 10-12, 15-21, 30-31, 38, 50]. The aim of this chapter is to review the clinical features and advances in treatment for this relatively uncommon disease.

Incidence

Extranodal NK/TCL, nasal-type, shows variations in incidence in different populations and geographic locations. It is a rare disease in the United States and Europe [4, 37], but it is relatively common in Asian and Latin American countries such as China, Korea and Mexico [2, 23-27, 29-32]. Extranodal nasal-type NK/TCL accounts for 2-10% of all NHL cases in China [6, 10, 27-32, 38].

Pathology

Extranodal nasal-type NK/TCL represents a heterogeneous group of lymphomas based on the major site of involvement, of which the nasal cavity is the most common site [20, 24-26, 30]. The term "nasal NK/T-cell lymphoma" is used only for those cases presenting in the nasal cavity with or without involvement of adjacent organs or tissues. The histological features of extranodal nasal-type NK/TCL are similar irrespective of the anatomical sites involved [22]. Tumours with an identical morphology and phenotype occur in the extra-nasal sites, mostly in the Waldeyer ring, skin, gastrointestinal tract and soft tissue, are referred to as nasal-type NK/T-cell lymphoma. Extranodal nasal-type NK/TCL was formerly called angiocentric T-cell lymphoma in the REAL classification in 1994, and many other terms including lethal midline granuloma, malignant granuloma, midline malignant reticulosis, and angiocentric immunoproliferative lesion have been clinically used before 1994 [5, 9].

The morphology of this disease shows several typical features including angiocentricity, angioinvasion, zone-necrosis, and polymorphism of individual cells. It is characterized by a broad cytologic spectrum with small or medium size of tumour cells and polymorphous inflammatory infiltrate. Repeated biopsy is usually required for pathologic diagnosis, due to extensive necrosis and the small size of specimens.

The typical phenotype is CD2+, surface CD3-, cytoplasmic CD3+, CD56+, CD20-/CD79a-, cytotoxic molecules (T-cell Intracellular Antigen-1 [TIA-1], Granzyme B, Perforin)+ and Epstein-Barr virus (EBV) +. CD43, CD45RO, Fas (CD95) and Fas ligand are commonly expressed [5, 9]. Other NK-cell and T-cell markers are usually negative: CD4, CD8, CD16, CD57, and T-cell receptor (TCR). The criteria of immunopathological diagnosis include CD2+CD56+, surface CD3- and cytoplasmic CD3+ (NK-cell origin). Additionally, many studies include cytotoxic T-cell lymphomas expressing CD3ε+, CD56-, cytotoxic molecule (TIA, Gram B, Perforin)+ and EBV+. However, nasal or other extranodal lymphomas that are CDε+CD56-, but negative for cytotoxic molecules and EBV should be diagnosed as peripheral T-cell lymphoma. Extranodal nasal-type NK/TCL is postulated to originate from immature (activated) NK-cells or rarely, from a subset of cytotoxic T-cell lymphocytes. There is no difference in survival or clinicopathologic features between the true NK-cell lymphomas and their T-cell counterparts.

TCR and immunoglobulin gene rearrangements are usually absent. EBV genomes are usually present and are detectable in the majority of patients by in-situ hybridization for EBER-1. EBV infection is observed in more than 90% of nasal NK/T-cell lymphoma cases [12, 22]. In contract, EBV expression is relatively low (40-76%) for patients with extranasal NK/TCL [8, 22]. Loss of heterozygosity within chromosome 6q, overexpression of matrix metalloproteinase 9, and interleukin-9 have been observed in this disease [4, 35, 43]. The inactivation or mutation of p53 is a common occurrence in NK/TCL [39].

Clinical presentation

Extranodal nasal-type NK/TCL, has variable presentations depending on the major site of involvement. It consists of three distinct subgroups: nasal NK/TCL, Waldeyer ring NK/TCL and NK/TCL of the extra-upper aerodigestive tract, with important differences in clinical features, prognosis and treatment strategy [3, 24, 29-31, 33]. The main clinical characteristics and treatment of three subgroups are summarized in Table 1.

Table 1 – Variable clinical presentations of extranodal nasal-type NK/T-cell lymphoma.

	Nasal NK/T-cell lymphoma	**Waldeyer ring NK/T-cell lymphoma**	**NK/T-cell lymphoma of the extra-upper aerodigestive tract**
Primary site	Nasal cavity, often direct extension to the ethmoid sinus, maxillary sinus and nasopharynx	Waldeyer ring, often involving adjacent multiple sites, mainly involving upper aerodigestive tract sites. Nasopharynx and tonsil are the most common sites of primary involvement	Extra-upper aerodigestive tract, often involving skin, soft tissue and gastro-intestinal tract
Age	Usually adults, median age of 40-50 years old	Usually adults, median age of 38-50 years old	Usually adult, median age of 50 years old
Sex	Male predominance, M:F=2-4:1	Male predominance, M:F=2.6:1	Male predominance, M:F=1.5-2.3:1
Stage	Usually presenting with stage I (60-80%); uncommon with stage III and IV	Usually involving lymph nodes and extranodal sites Stage I: 18% Stage II-IV: >80%	Usually presenting with disseminated lesions and advanced stage disease Stage III-IV: 50%
Performance	Good performance, ECOG 0-1: >80%	Good performance, ECOG 0-1: 95%	Usually poor performance, ECOG ≥ 2
Elevated LDH	High frequency: 30-50%	Low frequency: 19%	High frequency: 50-70%
Common sites of nodal involvement	Submandibular and cervical lymph nodes	Cervical lymph node	Regional lymph nodes
IPI	Usually low risk, IPI 0-1: >90%	Usually low risk, IPI 0-1: ≥80%	Usually high risk, IPI 0-1: 25-58%
Patterns of failure	Major failures are extra-nodal organs. The most common site of systemic involvement is skin	Major failures are both systemic lymph nodes and extranodal organs, usually involving skin	Extranodal organs
Initial response for chemo-therapy or radiotherapy	Chemoresistance. Usually CR<40%, SD/PD 46%; Highly sensitive to radiotherapy, CR≥80%	Intermediate chemosensitivity. CR 34%, PR 55%, SD/PD 11%; Highly sensitive to radiotherapy, CR≥76%	Chemoresistance. Usually CR <25%; Sensitive to radiotherapy
Clinical behaviour	Aggressive	Aggressive	Highly aggressive
Prognosis	Favourable in stage I patients with appropriate radiotherapy; poor for stage II-IV patients	Relatively favourable compared to nasal and extra-upper aerodiges tive tract variant	Extremely poor; median survival of 3.5-19 months
Treatment suggestion	Primary radiotherapy for stage I and II; more effective systemic therapy for advanced disease.	Combined radiotherapy and chemotherapy for stage I and II; chemotherapy with consolidation radiotherapy for advanced disease	Recommend innovative systemic therapy; radiotherapy for localized disease

Abbreviations: LDH, lactate dehydrogenase; ECOG, Eastern Cooperative Oncology Group; IPI, International Prognostic Index; CR, complete response; PR, partial response; SD, stable disease; PD, progression disease.

The most frequent presenting symptom of nasal NK/TCL is nasal obstruction. Locally advanced disease is more likely to be associated with aggressive signs and symptoms including facial swelling, epistaxis, proptosis, hard palate perforation and cranial nerve palsy [29]. Nasal NK/TCL more commonly affects men and the median age is 40-50 years old. The male to female ratio is 2-4:1. This disease is characterized by good performance status, high frequency of B symptoms, elevated lactate dehydrogenase (LDH) and low-risk IPI [20, 30]. The majority (67-98%) of patients present with stage I disease whereas involvement of regional lymph nodes or distant extranodal organs is uncommon at presentation. However, these early stage tumours often present with a bulky primary tumour and directly extend into the neighbouring organs or tissues. Approximately 42-60% of patients have an involvement of multiple organs or tissues within the vicinity of the primary tumour. The most frequently involved sites are the maxillary and ethmoid sinuses, followed by the nasopharynx. The major pathway of lymph node spread for nasal NK/TCL is to the submandibular and cervical lymph nodes. Distant extranodal dissemination is the primary pattern of failure and the most involved extranodal sites are the skin, lung and liver. The propensity for disease spread to the extranodal organs, especially the skin at presentation or during progression and recurrence is related to the homing capacity of NK/T-cell lymphocytes.

Nasal-type NK/TCL occurring outside the nasal cavity has different clinical features and prognosis [3, 20, 25, 31]. The most frequent presenting symptoms for patients with Waldeyer ring disease are odynophagia, dysphagia and cervical lymphadenopathy [31]. B symptoms are observed in one-third of the patients. The pattern of regional nodal spread appears to be consistent with the primary drainage of Waldeyer ring as a lymphoid tissue, i.e. the cervical lymph nodes rather than submandibular nodes. Patients are more likely to present with a good performance status, regional nodal involvement, more advanced stages, low elevated LDH, intermediate chemosensitivity and have a relatively favourable prognosis [31]. However, patients with nasal-type NK/TCL of the extra-upper aerodigestive tract such as skin, soft tissue, gastrointestinal tract and other sites usually present with a poor performance status, high frequency of elevated LDH, disseminated and advanced stage disease and extremely poor prognosis [3, 20, 25, 33].

Staging procedure

Initial Evaluation

Clinical evaluations include a complete history and physical examination. All patients should be examined with special attention to the upper aerodigestive tract including the nasal cavity, nasopharynx, oropharynx, tonsil, hard palate, oral cavity, base of the tongue, hypopharynx and larynx for determination of disease extent. A careful and systemic examination of the skin is warranted, as this disease shows a propensity for skin involvement both at presentation and recurrence. Initial blood tests should include a complete blood count, biochemistry, liver and renal function tests and LDH. EBV serology and bone marrow biopsy are useful for predicting the prognosis for patients with EBV+ nasal NK/TCL [8].

MRI and CT scan of the head and neck area are recommended in all cases, as a soft tissue mass in the nasal cavity with bone erosion or destruction, extension of adjacent organs, or involvement of multiple organs can be detected. However, the findings on MRI and/or CT scan are usually non-specific [36]. CT scans of the chest, abdomen and pelvis are recommended for possible systemic disease.

The value of PET or PET/CT for local and distant disease has been studied in several studies. 18F-FDG-PET identified all involved sites (100%) in two small studies [14, 46]. Moreover, a high tumour 18F-FDG uptake was associated with poor prognosis in a study of 21 patients with extranodal NK/TCL of the head and neck [44].

Stage

The Ann Arbor staging system is not easily applied to extranodal lymphomas, especially for extranodal nasal-type NK/TCL, as the extent of primary tumour is an important prognostic factor for extranodal NHL. Therefore, a modified Ann Arbor staging system is suggested for patients with nasal NK/TCL at the Cancer Hospital of Chinese Academy of Medical Sciences (CAMS) and Peking Union Medical College (PUMC), Beijing, China. Ann Arbor stage IE is subclassified into Limited Stage IE and Extensive Stage IE [29, 30]. Limited Stage IE tumours are confined to the nasal cavity, whereas Extensive Stage IE tumours extend beyond the nasal cavity and into the neighbouring structures, without any sign of nodal or distant dissemination.

Treatment

Stage I and II

Radiotherapy is the primary treatment for early stage nasal NK/TCL. For patients with limited stage IE or stage IE disease without any adverse factors, radiotherapy alone should be considered for curative-intent treatment. Radiotherapy followed by consolidation chemotherapy should be considered for patients with extensive stage I and stage II disease. Chemotherapy is not recommended for primary treatment in early stage nasal NK/TCL due to its chemoresistance and poor prognosis.

Recently, six large retrospective studies have demonstrated that the outcome with primary or up-front radiotherapy is superior to chemotherapy alone or initial chemotherapy [7, 10, 11, 27, 38, 50]. On the other hand, another five studies have confirmed that the addition of chemotherapy with doxorubicin-based regimens to radiotherapy does not provide additional survival benefit for patients with stage I and II nasal disease [6, 16, 17, 30, 32] (Table 2).

Radiotherapy

A definite advantage of primary radiotherapy has been confirmed in recent years. In a large series of 105 patients with stage I and II nasal disease receiving primary radiotherapy, the 5-year overall survival (OS) and progression-free survival (PFS) were 71% and 59% for stage I and II disease altogether. OS and PFS were 78% and 63% for stage I disease, and 46% and 40% for stage II disease, respectively [30]. In the study from Mexico with 108 patients with early stage and treated with radiotherapy followed by 4 cycles of CHOP-bleo, the 8-year OS was 86% [2]. Additionally, six studies have reported that primary radiotherapy resulted in superior initial response and survivals compared with chemotherapy alone or primary chemotherapy [7, 10, 11, 27, 38, 50] (Table 2). Chim *et al.* reported a series of

Table 2 – Comparison of initial response and survivals of nasal and nasal-type NK/T-cell lymphoma treated with primary radiotherapy or primary chemotherapy in large series of publications.

Authors	Time	No	Primary sites in nasal cavity No (%)	Stage	Treatment	*CR after initial therapy (%)	5-year OS (%)	P
Primary RT versus initial CT±RT								
Chim *et al.* [7]	2004	67	67 (100)	I-IV	RT: 7 cases	100	83.3 (10-year)	
					CT+ RT: 59 cases	59 (CT+RT)	32	0.03
You *et al.* [50]	2004	46	46 (100)	I-II	RT: 6 cases	-	83.3	
					CT ± RT: 40 cases	-	28.5	0.027
Li CC *et al.* [27]	2004	56	43/77 (56)	I-II	RT: 11 cases	55	50	
					RT + CT: 27 cases	74	59	
					CT: 18 cases	50	15	0.01
Pan ZH *et al.* [38]	2005	93	NA	I-IV	CT: 34 cases	41	About 0	
					CT + RT: 54 cases	83 (CT+RT)	About 30	<0.05
Huang *et al.* [11]	2008	82	66 (80)	I-II	RT ± CT: 74 cases	88-100	62.1 (3-year)	0.000
					CT: 8 cases	25	12.5 (3-year)	
He YF *et al.* [10]	2006	108	108 (100)	I-II	CT + RT: 81 cases		60	
					CHOP: 27 cases	29.6	20	<0.001
RT versus RT plus CT								
Cheung *et al.* [6]	2002	79	79 (100)	I-II	RT ± CT: 18 cases	78	29.8	
					CT ± RT: 61 cases	49 (CR+PR)	40.3	0.693
Kim GE *et al.* [16]	2001	143[B]	74 (52)	I-II	RT: 104 cases	69	35	
					CT + RT: 39 cases	8	38	0.93
Kim K *et al.* [17]	2005	53	29 (55)	I-II	RT: 33 cases	52	76	
					CT + RT: 20 cases	38	59	0.27
Li YX *et al.* [30]	2006	105	105 (100)	I-II	RT: 31 cases	97	66	
					RT + CT: 34 cases	71	77	
					CT + RT ± CT: 37 cases	19	74	0.518
Ma FF *et al.* [32]	2008	71	71 (100)	I/II: 64	RT + CT: 41 cases (Stage I-II)		61.5	0.469
				III/IV: 7	RT: 23 cases (Stage I-II)		57.9	
Others								
Aviles *et al.* [2]	2000	108	108 (100)	I-II	RT + CHOP-Bleo: 108 cases	92	86 (8-year)	
Kim BS *et al.* [15]	2003	59	45 (76)	I-IV	CT ± RT: 59 cases	35.6	44 (2-year)	
Kim *et al.* [19]	2006	43	29 (67)	I-II	CHOP-Bleo±RT: 43 cases	44.2		
Bossard *et al.* [4]	2007	48	48 (100)	I-IV	CT (4 with RT): 48 cases	50	49	

*defined as CR rate after radiotherapy or chemotherapy without any combination of radiotherapy and chemotherapy; NA, not available. Abbreviations: CHOP, cyclophosphamide, doxorubicin, vincristine, and prednisone; RT, Radiotherapy; CT, Chemotherapy; OS, overall survival; CR, complete response; PR, partial response.

67 patients, 7 of whom were treated with radiotherapy alone, and 59 with chemotherapy followed by radiotherapy. The 10-year OS and DFS for all patients was 42.5% and 52% [7]. All (100%) seven patients treated with radiotherapy achieved a complete response, whereas only 35 of 59 (59.3%) patients with initial chemotherapy achieved a complete response (p=0.04). The 10-year OS is 83.3% with radiotherapy and 32% with chemotherapy and salvage radiotherapy, respectively (p=0.03). You *et al.* reported that in 46 patients with stage I and II, 6 patients were treated with radiotherapy alone, 22 with chemotherapy alone and 18 patients were salvaged with radiotherapy after chemotherapy. The 5-year OS was 83.3% for primary radiotherapy and 28.5% for primary chemotherapy (P=0.0269) [50]. Li *et al.* reported that of 56 patients with stage I-II nasal and nasal-type NK/T-cell lymphoma, 11 patients received radiotherapy alone, 27 radiotherapy followed by chemotherapy, and 18 chemotherapy alone. Radiotherapy with or without chemotherapy resulted in significantly better survival than chemotherapy alone,

with a 5-year OS of 50% for radiotherapy alone, 59% for radiotherapy plus chemotherapy, and 15% for chemotherapy alone, respectively (P=0.01) [27]. In a recent study of 82 patients with stage I disease, the 18 patients receiving up-front radiotherapy (radiotherapy alone or radiotherapy followed by chemotherapy) had a significantly better OS and DFS than the 28 patients receiving initial chemotherapy (5-year OS 90% *versus* 48.9%, p=0.012; 5-year DFS 78.7% *versus* 39.9%, p=0.021) [11]. He *et al.* reported that in 108 patients, 81 patients received a combination of radiotherapy and chemotherapy, and 27 patients received chemotherapy alone. The 5-year OS was 60% and 20%, respectively (p<0.001) [10].

Patients with Waldeyer ring NK/TCL also had a better complete response to radiotherapy than to chemotherapy [31]. However, only 8% of patients had stable or progressive disease after initial chemotherapy. This phenomenon may reflect an intermediate sensitivity to conventional chemotherapy. Compared to radiotherapy alone, combined modality therapy tended to improve survival for stages I and II disease. Moreover, patients who received radiotherapy had a low rate of locoregional failure compared with those who received chemotherapy alone. Additionally, patients who received chemotherapy had a low rate of systemic failure compared with those receiving radiotherapy alone [31]. Therefore, patients with Waldeyer ring disease may benefit from a combination of chemotherapy and radiotherapy.

Chemotherapy

As discussed above, conventional combination chemotherapy (CHOP or CHOP like-based regimens) plays a limited role in the definitive treatment of nasal NK/TCL. The reported complete response rate ranged from 5% to 50% after chemotherapy, most of which being lower than 40% [4, 6, 11, 12, 16-19, 27, 30, 31, 38, 49]. The low response rate and poor prognosis after chemotherapy alone reflect the resistance to conventional chemotherapy, which may be associated with p53 mutation and expression of P-glycoprotein [39, 45, 47].

Several recent large series have reported no convincing clinical benefit by adding conventional chemotherapy to radiotherapy in early stage disease [6, 16, 17, 30, 32] (Table 2). Radiotherapy and chemotherapy resulted in the similar outcome compared to radiotherapy alone. Li *et al.* reported that in 105 patients with stage I and II nasal NK/T-cell lymphoma, 31 patients were treated with radiotherapy alone, 34 with radiotherapy followed by chemotherapy, 37 patients with short course of chemotherapy followed by radiotherapy and only 3 patients with chemotherapy alone. There was no statistically significant difference in survivals between radiotherapy alone and radiotherapy plus chemotherapy. The 5-year overall survival and progression-free survival were 76% and 61% for combined modality therapy compared with 66% and 61% for radiotherapy alone (p=0.643 for OS, p=0.839 for PFS) [30]. Cheung *et al.* also reported that in the 79 patients with stage I and II nasal disease, the 5-year OS and DFS rates were 40.3% and 35.8% for combined modality therapy compared with 29.8% and 30.5% for radiotherapy (p=0.693 for OS, p=0.795 for DFS) [6]. Kim *et al.* also reported that, in a series of 143 patients with stage I and II angiocentric lymphoma of the head and neck area, no statistically significant difference in 5-year OS was observed between radiotherapy alone and the combined modality therapy (35% *versus* 38%) [16]. In another study from Korea with 53 patients with stage I and II, the 5-year OS was 76% for radiotherapy alone and 59% for the combined modality therapy, respectively (P=0.27) [17]. Ma *et al.* reported that in a total of 71 patients, 64 with stage I and II disease received radiotherapy plus chemotherapy (n=41) or radiotherapy alone (n=23) and the

5-year OS was 61.5% for the combined modality therapy and 57.9% for radiotherapy alone, respectively (p=0.469) [32].

Thus a high local progression or relapse after chemotherapy alone or initial chemotherapy was observed in several of these studies [6, 19]. Some patients with locoregional failure after initial chemotherapy can be successfully salvaged with radiotherapy. Cheung *et al.* reported that, of 61 patients receiving initial chemotherapy, 31 (51%) had disease progression and 14 of them progressed in distant extranodal organs. Nine of the remaining 17 patients with locoregional failure were successfully salvaged with radiotherapy. In contrast, of 18 patients receiving radiotherapy, 14 patients (78%) achieved a complete response whereas none of the remaining 4 patients, who had disease progression, were salvaged with chemotherapy [6].

Stage III and IV

CHOP or CHOP-like based chemotherapy is considered to be the primary treatment for patients with advanced stage extranodal nasal-type disease; however patients with advanced stage nasal disease or disease of the extra-upper aerodigestive tract carry an extremely poor prognosis and survival for more than 5 years is rare [4, 7, 38].

New chemotherapeutic regimens such as IMEP (ifosfamide, methotrexate, etoposide and prednisolone) or SMILE (dexamethasone, methotrexate, ifosfamide, L-asparaginase, and etoposide) have been evaluated recently. In a phase I study of chemotherapy with SMILE for advanced-stage, refractory or relapsed extranodal NK/TCL and leukemia, the complete response rate was 50% [48]. CHOP-based chemotherapy combined with L-asparaginase or oral nitrosourea was evaluated in a few studies. Its value was not confirmed as these patients received salvage radiotherapy following initial chemotherapy [49].

Successful treatment with autologous stem cell transplantation has been reported in several small studies [1, 40]. However, the data is limited and further investigation is needed.

Radiation Technique

Clinical Target Volume

Extended fields are recommended for irradiation of early stage disease. In general, CTV includes all gross tumour (or GTV) and adjacent organs and structures. For patients with limited stage I nasal disease, CTV encompasses the bilateral nasal cavity, hard plate, ipsilateral or bilateral maxillary sinus, bilateral anterior ethmoid sinuses. It also includes the nasopharynx when the primary tumour is close to the posterior nasal aperture, or extends into the nasopharynx. For patients with extensive stage I and stage II disease, CTV is extended to the involved paranasal organs/tissues or cervical lymph nodes.

Several techniques can be successfully used, however three-dimensional conformal radiotherapy (3D-CRT) or intensity modulated radiotherapy (IMRT) definitely offer a much better dose distribution (Fig. 1).

The clinical target and radiation fields have been investigated previously [13, 16, 23, 30]. A higher local failure with small CTV was observed in several retrospective studies. In a study of 35 patients with stage I and II nasal and nasal-type disease who were treated with radiotherapy, 27 patients were treated with a generous CTV (as described above) while the remaining 8 patients received a smaller volume treatment: the 5-year local control probability was 71.9% *versus* 41.7%

A

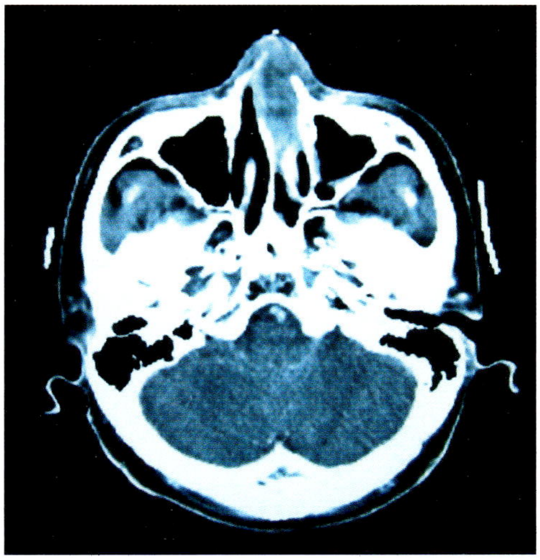

B

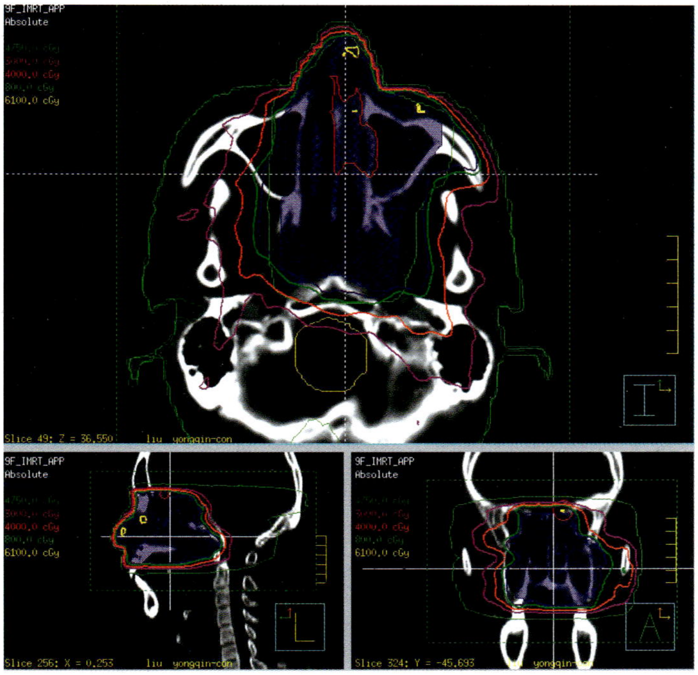

Fig 1. A. Computed tomogram from a patient with nasal NK/T-cell lymphoma shows a mass in the left nasal cavity; B. Clinical target volume (CTV) includes the nasal cavity, left maxillary sinus, bilateral anterior ethmoid sinuses, and nasopharynx (blue area).

respectively (p=0.007) [13]. Similarly, Li *et al.* reported that in 56 patients with stage I and II, the radiation fields included the involved primary with small margins: 24 (43%) of these patients later developed local failure [27].

Prophylactic neck radiation

Cervical lymph node should not be irradiated electively for patients with stage I nasal NK/T-cell lymphoma, due to its rare involvement [23, 29, 30]. In a study of 133 patients with stage I nasal lymphoma (majority of them are NK/T-cell type), prophylactic neck irradiation was not used in 106 and only 2 of them (2%) developed a progression or a relapse in the cervical lymph nodes [29]. In another study, only 1 of 46 (2%) stage IE patients with nasal and nasal-type disease who did not receive elective neck radiotherapy developed regional lymph node recurrence [23]. Shikama *et al.* reported that in 37 patients with stage I nasal lymphoma who did not receive prophylactic neck radiotherapy, only 1 patient developed relapse in the cervical lymph node [41].

For patients with Waldeyer ring disease, a large radiation field is used to cover the clinical target volume including Waldeyer ring, neighbouring organs or structures, and cervical lymph nodes [31].

Radiation Dose

A total dose of 50 Gy to the primary tumour is considered as a radical irradiation dose for nasal and nasal-type disease. An additional 5-10 Gy is to be administered as a boost to the residual disease. Total doses of irradiation lower than 50 Gy have resulted in higher local failure rates in several studies [6, 11, 13].

With high doses (median dose of 50 Gy) to the nasal cavity and neighbouring organs or structures, a local failure of only 7.8% was observed in 102 patients with nasal disease receiving radiotherapy [30]. Similarly, Li *et al.* have also observed a very low local (6.5%) and low locoregional failure rates (7.8%) in 77 patients with Waldeyer ring disease receiving radiotherapy [31]. You *et al.* have administered higher radiotherapy doses of 54-60 Gy and achieved a 5-year failure-free survival rate of 83.3% [50]. Several studies have observed a dose-response relationship for local control. Among 102 patients with stage I-II nasal and nasal-type disease of the head and neck areas, a median dose of 45 Gy was given. The complete response rate was 72%, however the ultimate local failure was as high as 47%. Local failure was 64% for doses less than 45 Gy compared with 38% for doses of 45 Gy or above (p=0.02) [23]. This study has demonstrated in particular a dose-response relationship within the range of 20-54 Gy, with a plateau at doses in excess of approximately 54 Gy. The vast majority of the patients (90%) had a local failure within the radiation field or at the margins. Furthermore, Huang *et al.* reported that in 74 patients with stage I and II, the 5-year OS and DFS were 75.5% and 46.1% with a dose of more than 54 Gy, as compared to 60.3% and 33.4% if less than 54 Gy was applied ($p<0.05$) [11]. Consistently, Isobe *et al.* reported a local failure of 67% with less than 50 Gy and 27% with more than 50 Gy in 35 patients with nasal and nasal-type disease (p=0.038) [13].

Prognosis

Prognosis of early stage extranodal nasal-type NK/TCL varies from series to series, with 5-year overall survival ranging from 20% to 86%. As discussed before, this discrepancy of outcome could be due to the fact that chemotherapy was given as initial therapy in some series, but also to the high proportion of advanced stage and high local failure after low radiation dose and small field. The 5-year overall survival of stage I and II nasal disease treated with primary radiotherapy were in the range of 40-86%, whereas those treated with chemotherapy as primary treatment were less than 50% [2, 4, 7, 15, 30, 50].

Ann Arbor Stage and its modification is one of the most important prognostic factors for nasal disease. Patients with stage I disease had much better prognosis compared with those with stage II disease. The 5-year overall survival is about 70% for stage I and less than 50% for stage II, respectively [2, 6, 7, 11, 16, 22, 23, 30, 50]. Paranasal extension, B symptoms, performance status, elevated LDH and IPI are independent prognostic factors. The prognostic value of the international prognostic index (IPI) or modified IPI (stage II as adverse factor) was confirmed in many recent studies [7, 15, 21, 27, 34, 30, 37], but not in other studies [2, 6, 18]. Recently, Lee *et al.* analyzed 262 patients with extranodal nasal-type disease and proposed a prognostic model based on B symptoms, advanced stage, elevated LDH and regional lymph nodes as adverse prognostic factors for survival [26].

Patients with nasal and Waldeyer ring NK/TCL showed a plateau in their survival curves after treatment. Conversely, survival of patients with disease of the extra-upper aerodigestive tract continued to decline, this particular disease of the extra-upper aerodigestive tract being associated with a highly aggressive clinical behaviour, with a median survival time of only 3.5-19 months [20, 26, 33]. This extremely poor prognosis is also validated by other studies in patients with cutaneous disease [3, 33].

The expression of EBV, Ki-67 and COX-2 and p53 mutation were associated with poor outcome [8, 22, 18, 42].

References

1. Au WY, Lie AKW, Liang R *et al.* (2003) Autologous stem cell transplantation for nasal NK/T-cell lymphoma: a progress report on its value. Ann Oncol 14: 1673-6
2. Aviles A, Diaz NR, Neri N *et al.* (2000) Angiocentric nasal T/natural killer cell lymphoma: a single center study of prognostic factors in 108 patients. Clin Lab Haematol 22: 215-20
3. Bekkenk MW, Jansen PM, Meijer CJLM *et al.* (2004) CD56+ hematological neoplasms presenting in the skin: a retrospective analysis of 23 new cases and 130 cases from the literature. Ann Oncol 15: 1097-108
4. Bossard C, Belhadj K, Reyes F *et al.* (2007) Expression of the granzyme B inhibitor PI9 predicts outcome in nasal NK/T-cell lymphoma: results of a Western series of 48 patients treated with first-line polychemotherapy within the Groupe d'Etude des Lymphomes de l'Adulte (GELA) trials. Blood 109: 2183-9
5. Chan JKC, Quintanilla-Martinez L, Ferry JA, Peh SC (2008) Extranodal NK/T-cell lymphoma, nasal type. In Jaffe ES, Harris NL, Stein H, Vardiman JW, eds. World Health Organization Classification of Tumours: Pathology and Genetics of Tumours of Haematopoietic and Lymphoid Tissues. Lyon, France: IARC Press 285-8
6. Cheung MMC, Chan JK, Lau WH *et al.* (2002) Early stage nasal T/NK-cell lymphoma: clinical outcome, prognostic factors, and the effect of treatment modality. Int J Radiat Oncol Biol Phys 54: 182-90
7. Chim CS, Ma SY, Au WY *et al.* (2004) Primary nasal natural killer cell lymphoma: long-term treatment outcome and relationship with the international prognostic index. Blood 103: 216-21
8. Hahn JS, Lee ST, Min YH *et al.* (2002) Therapeutic outcome of Epstein-Barr virus positive T/NK cell lymphoma in the upper aerodigestive tract. Yonsei Med J 43: 175-82
9. Harris NL, Jaffe ES, Stein H *et al.* (1994) A revised European-American classification of lymphoid neoplasms: a proposal from the International Lymphoma Study Group. Blood 84: 1361-92
10. He YF, Zhang YJ, Li YH *et al.* (2006) Primary non-Hodgkin's lymphoma of the nasal cavity at early stage: Long-term treatment outcomes and prognostic analyses of 108 cases. Chin J Cancer 25: 1538-42
11. Huang MJ, Jiang Y, Liu WP *et al.* (2008) Early or up-front radiotherapy improved survival of localized extranodal NK/T-cell lymphoma, nasal-type in the upper aerodigestive tract. Int J Radiat Oncol Biol Phys 70: 166-74
12. **International T-Cell Lymphoma Project (2008) International peripheral T-Cell and natural killer/T-cell lymphoma study: Pathology findings and clinical outcomes. J Clin Oncol 26: 4124-30**
13. Isobe K, Uno T, Tamaru JI *et al.* (2006) Extranodal natural killer/T-cell lymphoma, nasal type. Cancer 106: 609-15
14. Kako S, Izutsu K, Ota Y *et al.* (2007) FDG-PET in T-cell and NK-cell neoplasms. Ann Oncol 18: 1685-90
15. Kim BS, Kim TY, Kim CW *et al.* (2003) Therapeutic outcome of extranodal T/NK-cell lymphoma initially treated with chemotherapy. Result of chemotherapy in T/NK-cell lymphoma. Acta Oncol 42: 779-83
16. Kim GE, Lee SW, Chang SK *et al.* (2001) Combined chemotherapy and radiation versus radiation alone in the management of localized angiocentric lymphoma of the head and neck. Radiother Oncol 61: 261-9
17. Kim K, Chie EK, Kim CW *et al.* (2005) Treatment outcome of angiocentric T-cell and NK/T-cell lymphoma, nasal type: radiotherapy versus chemoradiotherapy. Jpn J Clin Oncol 35: 1-5
18. Kim SJ, Kim BS, Choi CW *et al.* (2007) Ki-67 expression is predictive of prognosis in patients with stage I/II extranodal NK/T-cell lymphoma, nasal type. Ann Oncol 18: 1382-7
19. Kim SJ, Kim BS, Choi CW *et al.* (2006) Treatment outcome of front-line systemic chemotherapy for localized extranodal NK/T cell lymphoma in nasal and upper aerodigestive tract. Leuk Lymph 47: 1265-73
20. **Kim TM, Lee SY, Jeon YK *et al.* (2008) Clinical heterogeneity of extranodal NK/T cell lymphoma, nasal type: a national survey of the Korea Cancer Study Group. Ann Oncol 19: 1477-84**

2

21. Kim TM, Park YH, Lee SY *et al.* (2005) Local tumor invasiveness is more predictive of survival than International Prognostic Index in stage IE/IIE extranodal NK/T cell lymphoma, nasal type. Blood 106: 3785-90
22. Ko YH, Cho EY, Kim JE *et al.* (2004) NK and NK-like T-cell lymphoma in extranasal sites: a comparative clinicopathological study according to site and EBV status. Histopathology 44: 480-9
23. Koom WS, Chung EJ, Yang WI *et al.* (2004) Angiocentric T-cell and NK/T-cell lymphomas: radiotherapeutic viewpoints. Int J Radiat Oncol Biol Phys, 59: 1127-37
24. Lee J, Kim WS, Park YH *et al.* (2005) Nasal-type NK/T cell lymphoma: clinical features and treatment outcome. Brit J Caner 92: 1226-30
25. Lee J, Park YH, Kim WS *et al.* (2005) Extranodal nasal type NK/T-cell Lymphoma: Elucidating clinical prognostic factors for risk-based stratification of therapy. Eur J Cancer 41: 1402-8
26. **Lee J, Suh C, Park YH *et al.* (2006) Extranodal natural killer/T-cell lymphoma, nasal-type: a prognostic model from a retrospective multicenter study. J Clin Oncol 24: 612-8**
27. Li CC, Tien HF, Tang JL *et al.* (2004) Treatment outcome and pattern of failure in 77 patients with sinonasal natural killer/T-cell or T-cell lymphoma. Cancer 100: 366-75
28. Li T, Hongyo T, Syaifudin M *et al.* (2000) Mutations of the p53 gene in nasal T/NK-cell lymphoma. Lab Invest 80: 493-9
29. Li YX, Coucke PA, Li JY *et al.* (1998) Primary non-Hodgkin's lymphoma of the nasal cavity: Prognostic significance of paranasal extension and the role of radiotherapy and chemotherapy. Cancer 83: 449-56
30. **Li YX, Yao B, Jin J *et al.* (2006) Radiotherapy as primary treatment for stage IE and IIE nasal natural killer/T-cell lymphoma. J Clin Oncol 24:181-189.**
31. **Li YX, Fang H, Liu QF *et al.* (2008) Clinical features and treatment outcome of nasal-type NK/T cell lymphoma of Waldeyer ring. Blood 112: 3057-64**
32. Ma HH, Zhang HY, Qian LT *et al.* (2008) Prognostic factors and long term treatment outcome of 71 cases of nasal NK/T cell lymphoma. Chin J Radiat Oncol 17: 7-10
33. Mraz-Gernhard S, Natkunam Y, Hoppe RT *et al.* (2001) Natural killer/natural killer-like T-cell lymphoma, CD56+, presenting in the skin: an increasingly recognized entity with an aggressive course. J Clin Oncol 19: 2179-88
34. Na II, Kang HJ, Park YH *et al.* (2007) Prognostic factors for classifying extranodal NK/T cell lymphoma, nasal type, as lymphoid neoplasia. Eur J Haematol 79: 1-7
35. Nagato T, Kobayashi H, Kishibe K *et al.* (2005) Expression of interleukin-9 in nasal natural killer/T-cell lymphoma cell lines and patients. Clin Cancer Res, 11: 8250-7
36. Ooi GC, Chim CS, Liang R *et al.* (2000) Nasal T-cell/natural killer cell lymphoma: CT and MR imaging features of a new clinicopathologic entity. Am J Roentgenol 174: 1141-5
37. Pagano L, Gallamini A, Trape G *et al.* (2006) NK/T-cell lymphomas 'nasal type': an Italian multicentric retrospective survey. Ann Oncol 17: 794-800
38. Pan ZH, Huang HQ, Lin XB *et al.* (2005) Prognostic analysis of patients with nasal-type NK/T-cell non-Hodgkin's lymphoma: a report of 93 cases. Chin J Cancer 24: 1493-7
39. Quintanilla-Martinez L, Kremer M, Keller G *et al.* (2001) p53 mutations in nasal natural killer/T-cell lymphoma from Mexico: Association with large cell morphology and advanced disease. Am J Pathol 159: 2095-105
40. Sasaki M, Matsue K, Takeuchi M *et al.* (2000) Successful treatment of disseminated nasal NK/T cell lymphoma using double autologous peripheral blood stem cell transplantation. Int J Hematol 71: 75-8
41. Shikama N, Ikeda H, Nakamura S *et al.* (2001) Localized aggressive non-Hodgkin's lymphoma of the nasal cavity: a survey by the Japan Lymphoma Radiation Therapy Group. Int J Radiat Oncol Biol Phys 51: 1228-33
42. Shim SJ, Yang WI, Shin E *et al.* (2007) Clinical significance of cyclooxygenase-2 expression in extranodal natural killer (NK)/T-cell lymphoma, nasal type. Int J Radiat Oncol Biol Phys 67: 31-8
43. Siu LL, Wong KF, Chan JK, Kwong YL (1999) Comparative genomic hybridization analysis of natural killer cell lymphoma/leukaemia. Recognition of consistent patterns of genetic alterations. Am J Pathol 155: 1419-25
44. Suh C, Kang YK, Roh JL *et al.* (2008) Prognostic Value of Tumor 18F-FDG Uptake in Patients with Untreated Extranodal Natural Killer/T-Cell Lymphomas of the Head and Neck. J Nucl Med, 49: 1783-9

45. Takahara M, Kishibe K, Bandoh N *et al.* (2004) P53, N- and K-Ras, and -Catenin gene mutations and prognostic factors in nasal NK/T-cell lymphoma from Hokkaido, Japan Hum Pathol 35: 86-95.
46. Tsukamoto N, Kojima M, Hasegawa M *et al.* (2007) The usefulness of ^{18}F-fluorodeoxyglucose positron emission tomography (^{18}F-FDG-PET) and a comparison of ^{18}F-FDG-pet with ^{67}gallium scintigraphy in the evaluation of lymphoma. Cancer 110: 652-9
47. Yamaguchi M, Kita K, Miwa H *et al.* (1995) Frequent expression of P-glycoprotein/MDR1 by nasal T-cell lymphoma cells. Cancer 76: 2351-6
48. Yamaguchi M, Suzuki R, Kwong YL *et al.* (2008) Phase I study of dexamethasone, methotrexate, ifosfamide, L-asparaginase, and etoposide (SMILE) chemotherapy for advanced-stage, relapsed or refractory extranodal natural killer (NK)/T-cell lymphoma and leukemia. Cancer Sci
49. Yong W, Zheng W, Zhu J *et al.* (2006) Midline NK/T-cell lymphoma nasal-type: treatment outcome, the effect of L-asparaginase based regimen, and prognostic factors. Hematol Oncol 24: 28-32
50. You JY, Chi KH, Yang MH *et al.* (2004) Radiation therapy versus chemotherapy as initial treatment for localized nasal natural killer (NK)/T-cell lymphoma: a single institute survey in Taiwan. Ann Oncol 15: 618-25

Uncommon tumours of the nasopharynx

3

E. Özyar and M. Gültekin

Four Essential Points

1. *Concurrent chemoradiotherapy is the standard treatment for locoregionally advanced nasopharyngeal cancer.*
2. *Radiotherapy alone is accepted as standard for solitary plasmacytoma with a dose threshold greater than 40 Gy.*
3. *Nasopharyngeal angiofibroma presents in young men and treatment options are surgery, radiation therapy or a combination of both, depending on stage.*
4. *Surgery with acceptable morbidity and postoperative radiotherapy is accepted as the mainstay of treatment for nasopharyngeal salivary gland carcinoma.*

Introduction

The main purpose of this chapter is to summarize the current treatment options in patients with uncommon nasopharyngeal tumours where surgical intervention is difficult because of the anatomic localisation. For these cases, radiotherapy is preferred as a treatment option due to surgical difficulty. With that scope, treatment options of nasopharyngeal carcinomas, plasmacytomas, angiofibromas, and minor salivary gland tumours will be discussed.

Nasopharyngeal Carcinoma

Epidemiology

Being different from other head and neck tumours by its particular histology, its geographic distribution and its close relationship to the Epstein-Barr virus (EBV), nasopharyngeal carcinoma (NPC) is accepted as a major tumour of the nasopharyngeal epithelium. While NPC is an endemic malignancy in south-eastern Asia, it is rarely seen in the United States or Western Europe [60]. Even though the undifferentiated carcinoma (WHO type 2 and 3) is the most frequent subtype in endemic areas, squamous cell carcinoma (WHO type 1) is more common in North America and Europe and has a worse prognosis. The histological subtype may be accepted as a prognostic factor with undifferentiated carcinoma having a higher local control rate after treatment with radiotherapy (RT) with a higher propensity for development of distant metastases [51]. Although NPC is present, mostly in the fourth to fifth decade, the classic age incidence graph is bimodal, with an initial peak in the second decade [46]. Recently, tumour volume, pre-treatment serum lactate dehydrogenase level and plasma EBV DNA levels have been acknowledged as the important prognostic factors which may have an effect on the staging system in the future [9, 34, 56].

Combined treatment

Compared with other head and neck cancers, endemic NPC is the one most responsive to chemotherapy and RT [61]. Due to the anatomical location of the primary tumour, external beam RT is standard treatment for patients with non-metastatic NPC. The standard treatment of stage I disease is RT resulting in a 10-year survival rate of 98% [11]. However, RT alone fails with unsatisfactory survival rates in >60% of loco-regionally advanced NPC patients [22]. In patients with locally advanced disease, RT alone provides an overall survival rate of 32% to 52% in 5 years [1]. Since the disease is highly chemo-sensitive, several studies have been performed to combine chemotherapy with RT for better results [7, 26]. Even the real benefit is still not clear. Six randomized trials and two meta-analyses have shown that concomitant chemotherapy and RT are more effective than RT alone, in terms of relapse-free and overall survival [27]. The RTOG trial has shown an overall survival increase from 54% to 78% by the combination of RT and 3-weekly concurrent platinum and with 3 cycles of adjuvant platinum-5FU combination [2]. According to the result of the recent meta-analysis of MAC-NPC collaborative group, additional chemotherapy allows a small but significant benefit on overall survival (6% in 5 years) and event-free survival (10% in 5 years) [4]. It is confirmed with this meta-analysis that concurrent chemo-RT can be applied as standard treatment for locoregionally advanced (≥ T2b and/or N+ patients) NPC.

Neoadjuvant and adjuvant chemotherapy

The integration of neoadjuvant [37] or adjuvant chemotherapy [10] beside RT showed no improvement in overall survival. Four phase III trials and a recent meta-analysis have shown adding induction chemotherapy to RT failed to show an improvement in overall survival even though a significant reduction was observed in local and distant failures in the neoadjuvant chemotherapy arm [37]. Neoadjuvant chemotherapy, so far, is the only recommended treatment for patients with bulky intracranial tumours close to the optic nerves, chiasm or brainstem. Neoadjuvant chemotherapy followed by concurrent chemo-RT studies are ongoing [8]. Among these three approaches (neoadjuvant, concurrent, and adjuvant chemotherapy), it is concluded by several studies that concurrent chemoradiotherapy is the most effective treatment [61].

Radiotherapy techniques

Significant limitations of 2D planning have led many authors to study the effect of high-precision radiotherapy in NPC. Studies have shown that there is a correlation between tumour control for NPC and higher doses of radiation delivered to the tumour. In order to increase local control rates in NPC, several types of strategies such as chemotherapy, stereotactic RT, posterior parapharyngeal boost, three-dimensional (3D) conformal RT, altered fractionation, brachytherapy (BRT) and intensity-modulated RT (IMRT) have been incorporated by several groups [29]. However, hyperfractionated RT for nasopharyngeal carcinoma must be carefully applied. An increase in radiation damage to the CNS with no improvement in tumour control has been reported from a study of accelerated hyperfractionation with two-dimensional RT planning [59].

BRT can be applied in the treatment of local recurrence of primary NPC, local persistence (residual tumour after external beam RT [EBRT]) and as an adjuvant after EBRT [58]. It has been reported that adjuvant BRT after EBRT improved local control rates in early T-stage NPC patients [58]. The role of adjuvant BRT after RT has not yet been evaluated due to lack of prospective randomized trials. A boost dose by use of intracavitary BRT for T1 and T2 tumours provides 16% improvement in tumour control in one study [33]. Dose gradient of BRT cannot be effective in advanced T disease [47].

To improve the dose differential between the tumour and the dose-limiting organs, IMRT is definitely preferable to 3D conformal planning and gives a higher rate of local control and decrease in salivary gland toxicity [65]. Allowing treatment of the primary tumour and the upper neck nodes in one volume throughout and providing excellent locoregional control of NPC, IMRT also renders possible the delivery of treatment with a secure dose and target volume at the junction between the primary tumour and the lymphatics of the neck [24] (Fig. 1). Both cone-down field treatment [66] and BRT [31] give good results for residual tumours of the nasopharynx. The dose should not exceed the initial radiation dose [57]. For patients with small localized tumours of the nasopharynx, stereotactic RT, BRT and surgical resection can be applied. Use of stereotactic RT resulted in a 2-year local tumour control rate of 72% in patients with residual and recurrent tumour [12]. A second course of external RT is required for more advanced and infiltrative tumours [32].

Despite significant risk of major late toxicities, a 5-year actuarial overall survival rate of 26% was obtained [48].

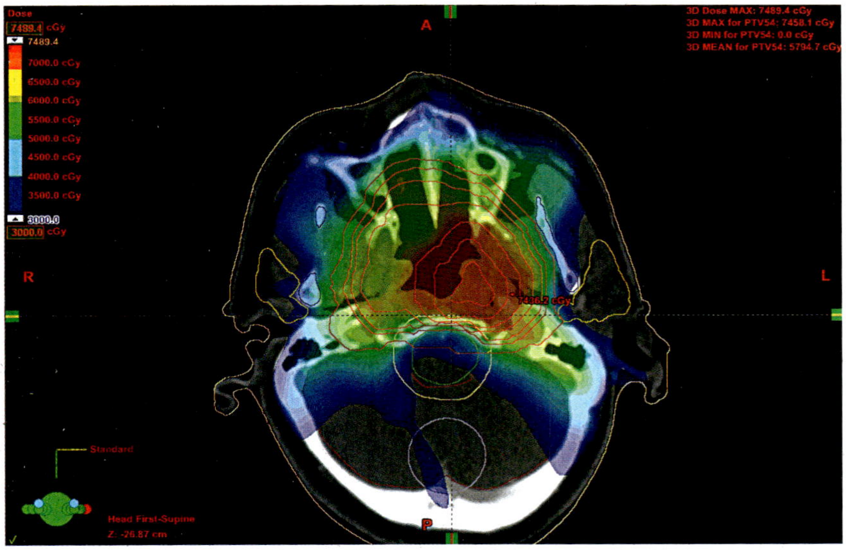

Fig. 1. An example of high precision radiotherapy (IMRT – Intensity Modulated Radiotherapy) for an early stage NPC patient. Sparing of salivary glands is clearly seen (salivary glands received less than 3,000 cGy) while a high dose was applied with simultaneous integrated boost IMRT technique (dose painting).

Being too extensive for BRT or extending into the paranasopharyngeal space, residual or recurrent tumour in the nasopharynx can be treated by nasopharyngectomy for patients with localized disease [57]. It is also reported that the 5-year actuarial control of tumours in the nasopharynx is about 65% and the 5-year disease-free survival rate is around 54% in selected patients [19].

Role of surgery

There is no role for planned neck dissection in NPC. Three months after completion of therapy if the neck nodes do not regress entirely, there is probable residual disease in these lymph nodes. When the neck nodes are the only site with disease, further salvage treatment should be instituted to eradicate the malignancy. Having 66% of 5-year tumour control rate in the neck and 38% of 5-year actuarial survival, radical neck dissection is the frequently performed surgical salvage procedure for persistent or recurrent neck disease. Interstitial BRT can additionally be applied for patients with close resection margins after radical neck dissection [62].

Management of M1 disease

In case of distant metastases, platinum-based regimens are accepted as standard chemotherapy and the combination of cisplatin and 5-fluorouracil remains as the most used in first-line chemotherapy [36]. It is also reported that newer agents including taxanes and gemcitabine have showed high response rates and a favourable toxicity profile when combined with cisplatin or carboplatin. Evaluation of the role of targeted therapies such as cetuximab is still continuing [6]. Gene therapy and immune therapy are included in strategies targeted at EBV, and the proof-of-principle studies have been performed in laboratories accordingly.

Nasopharyngeal Plasmacytomas

Nasopharyngeal extramedullary plasmacytomas (EMP) have positive prognosis with several treatment options. EMP represents about 3% of all plasma cell neoplasms and is associated with a long survival [15]. Constituting 0.5% of all the upper respiratory tract malignancies, 80% of EMP occurs in the head-and-neck region [43]. Presenting as a vascular, soft tissue mass, these tumours usually involve the submucosal lymphoid tissue of the paranasal sinuses, nasal cavities, nasopharynx and pharyngeal areas. Approximately 50% of EMP occurs as a solitary mass but 20% may present in multiple areas [64]. Mostly detected at ages between 50 and 60, EMPs are more common in males [64].

Pathologically confirmed tissue samples and demonstration of monoclonal plasma cell infiltration, with no indication of systemic myeloma, are needed to diagnose EMP [42, 43]. RT is accepted as standard treatment for solitary plasmacytoma since EMP is highly radiosensitive. With a dose threshold greater than 40 Gy, a total dose of 35 to 60 Gy is recommended [40].

Five-year myeloma-free survival rates range between 60% and 70% and local control rates range between 80% and 95% [35]. At diagnosis, cervical-node invasion rates vary from 7% to 30% for EMP. However, no general guideline exists for elective neck irradiation [35, 54]. Some authors support a similar policy of nodal irradiation applied for squamous cell carcinomas in the same site [35]. Use of elective neck irradiation has been advised in bulky tumours [59] or tumours with a high risk of cervical-node metastasis (oral cavity, oropharynx, or nasopharynx) [55, 59]. The recommended dose should be ≥ 36 Gy for elective neck irradiation. According to a national guideline, the optimal current evidence-based recommendations seems to be a RT dose of 40 Gy in 20 fractions for tumours < 5 cm and up to 50 Gy in 25 fractions for tumours ≥ 5 cm with a minimal 2 cm margin encompassing the primary tumour and cervical nodes [21]. Surgical salvage is left as an option for patients with recurrent or persistent tumour despite primary chemotherapy or radiation.

To obtain complete resection of nasopharyngeal EMPs either as a primary therapeutic or salvage modality, various well-described anterior skull base approaches may be considered [63]. Adjuvant chemotherapy has not been reported as reducing relapse or improving survival rates in the primary management of EMP [43]. Due to the lack of published data regarding the use of adjuvant chemotherapy, the use of adjuvant chemotherapy and/or novel therapeutic agents has not been verified outside a clinical trial. In recurrence or dissemination of disease, adjuvant chemotherapy can be used.

Nasopharyngeal Angiofibromas

Nasopharyngeal angiofibroma (NA) is a rare highly vascular tumour of the nasopharynx and is found in young men – these being most likely androgen dependent – explaining its almost exclusive presentation in males [52]. Treatment options are surgery, RT or a combination of both depending on stage. Combined therapy is frequently needed for intermediate and advanced stages. Surgical excision alone is the treatment of choice for early tumours. The most frequently used surgical procedures are transpalatal and medial maxillectomy. Providing a good alternative to wide and open surgical approaches, transnasal endoscopy has lately emerged as a new modality [44, 49]. Because of its reduced mutilation, fewer postoperative complications and shorter hospitalization period, the endoscopic approach has become preferable [18, 23]. Preoperative arterial embolization is accepted as part of the standard management. However, its role to decrease operative blood loss is still controversial.

Unlike RT-treated patients, patients who had surgery alone have a high recurrence rate [5]. The effectiveness of RT is confirmed by other studies when used as primary treatment in advanced stages, as well as in persistent and recurrent cases [30, 39, 50]. For residual disease, routine RT is also supported by some reports [14]. On the other hand, many others observe the disease radiologically for several years, until tumour progression [45].

In cases with invasion into cavernous sinuses, orbit and multiple recurrences or persistence with intracranial extension, IMRT and stereotactic RT should be considered [14]. For patients with extensive disease involving the cavernous sinus and skull base, IMRT can be applied with doses of 34-45 Gy [25]. This can result in a reduction in tumour size in follow-up imaging. For decades, RT has been a primary modality in the management of unresectable tumours.

Long-term local control of 80% using 30 to 35 Gy was described for a series of 55 patients and salvage using surgery or a second course of RT eventually controlled all patients [13].

It was reported that visible abnormalities vanished in 50% of irradiated patients at 12 months and in 90% at 36 months. Adjuvant RT was required for patients with incomplete resection, inoperable tumours and tumours with intracranial extension.

The use of RT has also been suggested as a primary treatment method [38]. Two recent large series using conventional RT reported local tumour control rates of more than 85% [30, 50]. The patient and the family must be notified before treatment as long-term complications including growth impairment, endocrine hypofunction and secondary malignant neoplasms may occur even though RT provides good control rates.

On condition that angiofibroma is detected by CT and/or MRI scans, angiography together with embolisation should be performed and the least invasive surgical procedure should be applied to remove tumour. Intermediate dose RT should be applied as treatment for patients with progressive disease while advanced disease is not suitable for surgery. Because of controversial effects on response rates, hormonal therapy and chemotherapy are not suggested as treatment options [52]. An alternative approach in unresectable tumours is the 'wait and scan policy' where spontaneous regression may be observed [16].

Nasopharyngeal Minor Salivary Gland Tumours

Approximately 2% of the all head and neck minor salivary gland tumours occurs in the nasopharynx and the most common histological subtype is adenoid cystic carcinoma (ACC), accounting for 65% of the total [20]. It has a tendency to invade and spread along nerves and metastasize at a distance [3]. Early recurrences regularly occur at the base of skull and along cranial nerves. Mucoepidermoid carcinoma, adenocarcinoma and acinic cell carcinoma are other common variants. Because of the well-defined difficulties in accessing the nasopharynx surgically and the high degree of morbidity with these procedures, radiation therapy is accepted as the mainstay of treatment for nasopharyngeal salivary gland carcinoma. Locoregional control with photon-based RT (x-rays, gamma rays) or neutron beam RT is reported to be 56% and 57% at 5 years, respectively [41, 17]. Some other studies still support the use of primary surgical management with postoperative radiation therapy for nasopharyngeal salivary gland carcinoma [53].

Covering the nerve pathways up to and including base of skull, surgical resection followed by RT is another treatment option. By using neutron RT instead of conventional radiation, a randomized trial has shown better results in ACC. However, neutron therapy is not available at this time [28]. Chemotherapy, on the other hand, is comparatively ineffective in ACC. Not explored as primary therapy, chemo-RT can be used as a treatment option to improve on radiation therapy for patients with nasopharyngeal ACC.

References

1. Ali H, Al-Sarraf M (2000) Chemotherapy in advanced nasopharyngeal cancer. Oncology (Huntingt) 14: 1223-30
2. Al-Sarraf M, LeBlanc M, Giri PG *et al.* (1998) Chemoradiotherapy versus radiotherapy in patients with advanced nasopharyngeal cancer: phase III randomized Intergroup study 0099. J Clin Oncol 16: 1310-7
3. Anderson J, Beenken S, Crowe R *et al.* (1995) Prognostic factors in salivary gland cancer. Head Neck 17: 480-6
4. Baujat B, Audry H, Jean Bourhis J *et al.* (2006) Chemotherapy in locally advanced nasopharyngeal carcinoma: an individual patient data meta-analysis of eight randomized trials and 1753 patients. Int J Radiat Oncol Biol Phys 64: 47-56

5. Carrillo JF, Albores O, Ramirez-Ortega MC *et al.* (2007) An audit of nasopharyngeal fibromas. Eur J Surg Oncol 33: 655-61
6. Chan AT, Hsu MM, Goh BC *et al.* (2005) Multicenter, phase II study of cetuximab in combination with carboplatin in patients with recurrent or metastatic nasopharyngeal carcinoma. J Clin Oncol 23: 3568-76
7. Chan AT, Leung SF, Ngan RK *et al.* (2005) Overall survival after concurrent cisplatin-radiotherapy compared with radiotherapy alone in loco-regionally advanced nasopharyngeal carcinoma. J Natl Cancer Inst 97: 536-9
8. Chan AT, Ma BB, Lo YM *et al.* (2004) Phase II study of neoadjuvant carboplatin and paclitaxel followed by radiotherapy and concurrent cisplatin in patients with locoregionally advanced nasopharyngeal carcinoma: Therapeutic monitoring with plasma Epstein-Barr virus DNA. J Clin Oncol 22: 3053-60
9. Cheng SH, Yen KL, Jian JJ *et al.* (2001) Examining prognostic factors and patterns of failure in nasopharyngeal carcinoma following concomitant radiotherapy and chemotherapy: impact on future clinical trials. Int J Radiat Oncol Biol Phys 50: 717-26
10. Chi KH, Chang YC, Guo WY (2002) A phase III study of adjuvant chemotherapy in advanced nasopharyngeal carcinoma patients. Int J Radiat Oncol Biol Phys 52: 1238-44
11. Chua DT, Sham JS, Kwong DL *et al.* (2003) Treatment outcome alter radiotherapy alone for patients with stage I-II nasopharyngeal carcinoma. Cancer 98: 74-80
12. Chua DT, Sham JS, Kwong PW *et al.* (2003) Linear accelerator-based stereotactic radiosurgery for limited, locally persistent, and recurrent nasopharyngeal carcinoma: efficacy and complications. Int J Radiat Oncol Biol Phys 56: 177-83
13. Cummings BJ, Blend R, Keane T *et al.* (1984) Primary radiation therapy for juvenile nasopharyngeal angiofibroma. Laryngoscope 94: 1599-605
14. Dare AO, Gibbons KJ, Proulx GM *et al.* (2003) Resection followed by radiosurgery for advanced juvenile nasopharyngeal angiofibroma: report of two cases. Neurosurg 52: 1207-11
15. Dimopoulos MA, Kiamouris C, Moulopoulos LA (1999) Solitary plasmacytomas of bone and extramedullary plasmacytoma. Hematol Oncol Clin N Am 13: 1249-57
16. Dohar JE, Duvall AJ III (1992) Spontaneous regression of juvenile nasopharyngeal angiofibroma. Ann Otol Rhinol Laryngol 101: 469-71
17. Douglas JG, Laramore GE, Austin-Seymour M *et al.* (2000) Treatment of locally advanced adenoid cystic carcinoma of the head and neck with neutron radiotherapy. Int J Radiat Oncol Biol Physics 46: 551-7
18. El-Banhawy OA, El-Dien AE, Amer T (2004) Endoscopic-assisted midfacial degloving approach for type III juvenile angiofibroma. Int J Pediatr Otolaryngol 68: 21-8
19. Fee Jr WE, Moir MS, Choi EC *et al.* (2002) Nasopharyngectomy for recurrent nasopharyngeal cancer: a 2- to 17-year follow-up. Arch Otolaryngol Head Neck Surg 128: 280-4
20. Garden AS, Weber RS, Ang KK *et al.* (1994) Postoperative radiation therapy for malignant tumors of minor salivary glands. Cancer 73: 2563-9
21. **Guidelines Working Group of the UK Myeloma Forum (UKMF) (2004) Guidelines on the diagnosis and management of solitary plasmacytoma of bone and solitary extramedullary plasmacytoma. Br J Haemato 124: 717-26**
22. Heng DM, Wee J, Fong K *et al.* (1999) Prognostic factors in 677 patients in Singapore with nondisseminated nasopharyngeal carcinoma. Cancer 86: 1912-20
23. Herman P, Lot G, Chapot R *et al.* (1999) Long-term follow-up of juvenile nasopharyngeal angiofibromas: analysis of recurrences. Laryngoscope 109: 140-7
24. Kam MK, Chau RM, Suen J *et al.* (2003) Intensity-modulated radiotherapy in nasopharyngeal carcinoma: dosimetric advantage over conventional plans and feasibility of dose escalation. Int J Radiat Oncol Biol Phys 56: 145-57
25. Kuppersmith RB, Theo BS, Donavan DT *et al.* (2000) The use of intensity modulated radiotherapy for the treatment of extensive and recurrent juvenile angiofibroma. Int J Pediatr Otolaryngol 52: 261-8
26. Kwong DL, Sham JS, Au GK *et al.* (2004) Concurrent and adjuvant chemotherapy for nasopharyngeal carcinoma: a factorial study. Clin Oncol 22: 2643-53
27. **Langendijk JA, Leemans R, Buter J *et al.* (2004) The additional value of chemotherapy to radiotherapy in locally advanced nasopharyngeal carcinoma: a meta-analysis of the published literature. J Clin Oncol 22: 4604-12**

3

28. Laramore GE, Krall JM, Griffin TW *et al.* (1993) Neutron versus photon irradiation for unresectable salivary gland tumors: final report of an RTOG-MRC randomized clinical trial. Int J Radiat Oncol Biol Phys 27: 235-40
29. Le QT, Tate D, Koong A *et al.* (2003) Improved local control with stereotactic radiosurgical boost in patients with nasopharyngeal carcinoma. Int J Radiat Oncol Biol Phys 56: 1046-54
30. Lee JT, Chen P, Safa A *et al.* (2002) The role of radiation in the treatment of advanced juvenile angiofibroma. Laryngoscope 112: 1213-20
31. Leung TW, Tung SY, Sze WK *et al.* (2000) Salvage brachytherapy for patients with locally persistent nasopharyngeal carcinoma. Int J Radiat Oncol Biol Phys 47: 405-12
32. Leung TW, Tung SY, Sze WK *et al.* (2000) Salvage radiation therapy for locally recurrent nasopharyngeal carcinoma. Int J Radiat Oncol Biol Phys 48: 1331-8
33. Levendag PC, Lagerwaard FJ, Pan C *et al.* (2002) High-dose, high-precision treatment options for boosting cancer of the nasopharynx. Radiother Oncol 63: 67-74
34. Liaw CC, Wang CH, Huang JS *et al.* (1997) Serum lactate dehydrogenase level in nasopharyngeal carcinoma. Acta Oncol 36: 159-64
35. Liebross RH, Ha CS, Cox JD *et al.* (1999) Clinical course of solitary extramedullary plasmacytoma. Radiother Oncol 52: 245-49
36. Ma BB, Chan AT (2005) Recent perspectives in the role of chemotherapy in the management of advanced nasopharyngeal carcinoma. Cancer 103: 22-31
37. Ma J, Mai HQ, Hong MH (2001) Results of a prospective randomized trial comparing chemotherapy plus radiotherapy with radiotherapy alone in patients with locoregionally advanced nasopharyngeal carcinoma. J Clin Oncol 19: 1350-7
38. Marshall AH, Bradley PJ (2006) Management dilemmas in the treatment and follow-up of advanced juvenile nasopharyngeal angiofibroma. ORL J Otorhinolaryngol Relat Spec 68: 273-8
39. McAfee WJ, Morris CG, Amdur RJ *et al.* (2006) Definitive radiotherapy for juvenile nasopharyngeal angiofibroma. Am J Clin Oncol 29: 168-70
40. Mendenhall WM, Mendenhall CM, Mendehall NP (2003) Solitary plasmacytoma of bone and soft tissues. Am J Otolaryngol 24: 395-9
41. Mendenhall WM, Morris CG, Amdur RJ *et al.* (2004) Radiotherapy alone or combined with surgery for adenoid cystic carcinoma of the head and neck. Head Neck 26: 154-62
42. Michalaki VJ, Hall J, Henk JM *et al.* (2003) Definitive radiotherapy for extramedullary plasmacytomas of the head and neck. Br J Radiol 76: 738-41
43. Miller FR, Lavertu P, Wanamaker JR, *et al.* (1998) Plasmacytomas of the head and neck. Otolaryngo Head Neck Surg 119: 614-8
44. Nicolai P, Berlucchi M, Tomenzoli D *et al.* (2003) Endoscopic surgery for juvenile angiofibroma: when and how. Laryngoscope 113: 775-82
45. Onerci TM, Yucel OT, Ogretmenoglu O (2003) Endoscopic survey in treatment of juvenile nasopharyngeal angiofibroma. Int J Pediatr Otolaryngol 67: 1219-25
46. Ozyar E, Selek U, Laskar S *et al.* (2006) Treatment results of 165 pediatric patients with non-metastatic nasopharyngeal carcinoma: A Rare Cancer Network study. Radiother Oncol 81: 39-46
47. Ozyar E, Yıldız F, Akyol F *et al.* (2002) Adjuvant high-dose-rate brachytherapy after external beam radiotherapy in nasopharyngeal carcinoma. Int J. Radiat Oncol Biol Phy 52: 101-8
48. Poon D, Yap SP, Wong ZW *et al.* (2004) Concurrent chemoradiotherapy in locoregionally recurrent nasopharyngeal carcinoma. Int J Radiat Oncol Biol Phys 59: 1312-8
49. Pryor SG, Moore EJ, Kasperbauer JL (2005) Endoscopic versus traditional approaches for excision of juvenile nasopharyngeal angiofibroma. Laryngoscope 115: 1201-7
50. Reddy KA, Mendenhall WM, Amdur RJ *et al.* (2001) Long-term results of radiation therapy for juvenile nasopharyngeal angiofibroma. Am J Otolaryngol 22: 172-5
51. Reddy SP, Raslan WF, Gooneratne S *et al.* (1995) Prognostic significance of keratinization in nasopharyngeal carcinoma. Am J Otolaryngol 16: 1038
52. Schick B, Urbschat S (2004) New aspects of pathogenesis of juvenile angiofibroma. Hosp Med 65: 269-73
53. Schramm VL, Imola MJ *et al.* (2001) Management of Nasopharyngeal Salivary Gland Malignancy. Laryngoscope 111(9): 1533-44

54. Soutar R, Lucraft H, Jackson G *et al.* (2004) Guidelines on the diagnosis and management of solitary plasmacytoma of bone and solitary extramedullary plasmacytoma. Clin Oncol (R Coll Radiol) 16: 405-13
55. Strojan P, Soba E, Lamovec J, *et al.* (2002) Extramedullary plasmacytoma: Clinical and histopathologic study. Int J Radiat Onco Biol Phys 53: 692-701
56. Sze WM, Lee AW, Yau TK *et al.* (2004) Primary tumor volume of nasopharyngeal carcinoma: prognostic significance for local control. Int J Radiat Oncol Biol Phys 59: 21-7
57. Teo PM, Leung SF, Chan AT *et al.* (2000) Final report of a randomized trial on altered-fractionated radiotherapy in nasopharyngeal carcinoma prematurely terminated by significant increase in neurologic complications. Int J Radiat Oncol Biol Phys 48: 1311-22
58. Teo PM, Leung SF, Lee WY *et al.* (2000) Intracavitary brachytherapy significantly enhances local control of early T-stage nasopharyngeal carcinoma: The existence of a dose-tumour-control relationship above conventional tumoricidal dose. Int J Radiat Oncol Biol Phys 46: 445-58
59. Tournier-Rangeard L, Lapeyre M, Graff-Caillaud P *et al.* (2006) Radiotherapy for solitary extramedullary plasmacytoma in the head-and-neck region: A dose greater than 45 Gy to the target volume improves the local control. Int J Radiat Oncol Biol Phys 64: 1013-7
60. Turen S, Ozyar E, Altundag K *et al.* (2007) Serum Lactate Dehydrogenase Level is a Prognostic Factor in Patients with Locoregionally Advanced Nasopharyngeal Carcinoma Treated with Chemoradiotherapy. Cancer Invest 25: 315-21
61. Wei WI, Sham JS (2005) Nasopharyngeal carcinoma. Lancet 365: 2041-54
62. Wei WI, Mok VW (2007) The management of neck metastases in nasopharyngeal cancer. Curr Opin Otolaryngol Head Neck Surg 15: 99-102
63. Wein OR, Popat SR *et al.* (2002) Plasma cell tumors of the skull base: Four case reports and literature review. Skull Base: An Interdisciplinary Approach 12: 77-86
64. Windfyhn J, Ott G (2002) Extramedullary plasmacytoma manifesting a palpable mass in the nasal cavity. Ear Nose Throat J 81(2): 110-14
65. Wu WW, Kwong DL, Sham JS (2004) Target dose conformity in 3 dimensional conformal radiotherapy and intensity modulated radiotherapy. Radiother Oncol 71: 201-6
66. Yan JH, Xu GZ, Hu YH *et al.* (1990) Management of local residual primary lesion of nasopharyngeal carcinoma: II. Results of prospective randomized trial on booster dose. Int J Radiat Oncol Biol Phys 18: 295-8

Uncommon tumours of the oral cavity and oropharynx

4

A. Şefik Hoşal

Five Essential Points

1. *Treatment of unusual oral tumours presents a unique challenge because of the low incidence and lack of a staging system.*
2. *The majority of the rare neoplasms consists of mucosal malignant melanoma, minor salivary gland tumours, sarcomas, lymphomas and metastatic cancers.*
3. *Unlike squamous cell carcinoma, cervical lymph node metastases is not a characteristic feature of these tumours.*
4. *Surgery is the main treatment modality in most tumours, except for lymphomas and oral metastases.*
5. *Treatment of most sarcomas consists of wide surgical excision combined with chemotherapy. Postoperative radiation therapy is given to increase local control.*

Introduction

The rare non-squamous tumours of the oral cavity and oropharynx consist of a different variety of malignancies which are no less significant than squamous cell carcinoma. They pose a challenging problem in differential diagnosis and appropriate treatment. Clinicians should be aware of these unusual neoplasms. This article is an overview of different histologic types along with their clinical presentations, findings, and treatment modalities.

Squamous cell carcinoma represents 90% of all malignant lesions in the oral cavity and oropharynx. Non-squamous cell tumours, however, are relatively rare and encompass a wide variety of neoplasms, including malignant melanoma, minor salivary gland neoplasms, soft tissue sarcomas, lymphomas, and metastatic cancers.

The diagnosis of these rare tumours often presents a dilemma due to similar presentations and non-diagnostic radiologic features. Management is dictated by histological examination and extent or stage of the disease. The treatment of some neoplasms, however, presents a unique challenge because of the low incidence and lack of a staging system. In most tumours, surgery is the main treatment modality, except for lymphomas and oral metastases.

Mucosal Malignant Melanoma

Oral malignant melanoma (MM) is a rare clinical condition and accounts for 0.5% of all oral malignancies, representing 0.2-8% of all melanomas [19]. The palate is the most common location for oral MM, and the maxillary gingiva is the second most frequently encountered site [17]. Oral MM is very uncommon under the age of 20. Overall, middle-aged and older patients are more often affected with a slight male preponderance [16]. The clinical presentation of a MM is usually pigmented swelling with our without ulceration. Pigmentation has a wide range of coloration from black, brown, purple even to reddish. Rarely, some tumours are amelanotic. Amelanotic MMs have no pigmentation, making diagnosis difficult [15]. The tumour surface may be smooth with an intact mucosa, or may be ulcerated, or nodular [12]. Bone invasion is characteristic of aggressive cancer, and in 78% cases, there is an extensive destruction of underlying bone [15]. The majority of patients present with disease confined to the primary site, 10 to 30% have clinically positive cervical lymph nodes [13].

Most MMs arise *de novo* in the normal mucosa. However, pre-existing oral pigmentations occur in about 30% cases [12,16]. If a pigmented lesion is detected in the oral cavity or in the oropharynx, a biopsy or a prophylactic excision is recommended, because of uncertain behavior. If the pathology confirms benign melanosis, the lesion should be watched periodically. Any change in size or increase in pigmentation, or particularly any ulceration, indicates the need for complete excision [18]. On the other hand, excisional biopsy with adequate margins may not be feasible in the oral cavity, particularly near the teeth. Therefore, incisional biopsy is usually preferred. Since small biopsies cannot provide a precise diagnosis, an incisional biopsy should be performed through the most suspicious, thickest and ulcerated part of the lesion. Clark's classification applied for cutaneous melanoma cannot be used in mucosal melanomas because of the lack histologic dermal landmarks.

The main treatment modality of oral MM is surgery. Surgery consists of wide radical excision of the mucosa. As most lesions arise in the palate and maxillary gingiva, partial or total resection of the palate and the alveolar bone is required in patients when the underlying bone is involved. However, true radical surgery is sometimes impracticable because of anatomic considerations. Radical or modified radical neck dissection is indicated in positive cervical lymph nodes, but the role of elective neck dissection in clinically N_0 neck is still controversial.

The use of primary radiation therapy as a therapeutic approach is uncertain, since MM is classically thought not to be very radiosensitive. However, favourable response can be obtained in some selected patients, particularly in early lesions. Unresectable, locally advanced disease may also be treated with definitive radiotherapy for palliation. Otherwise, postoperative irradiation is recommended in order to diminish local recurrence. Although postoperative radiotherapy does not seem to increase survival, it is associated with improved local control [12]. Another irradiation modality is brachytherapy. The author's group has been using intra-oral mould brachytherapy at the Hacettepe University, as the treatment of choice in palate and gingival melanomas.

Chemotherapy has been used in metastatic melanoma for palliation, but does not influence survival [12]. Other therapies, such as interferon and vaccine therapy have been suggested in cutaneous melanomas but are still investigational. Approximately 10% survival advantage with interferon has been reported in cutaneous MM. According to these findings, the author's group recommends using interferon in mucosal melanomas with an adjuvant regime. Prognosis is poor in mucosal melanomas. The local control rates range between 40 to 60% at 5-years [13]. Clinical stage, tumour thickness, nodal metastases, ulceration and anatomic sites have been reported as independent risk factors. The overall 5-year survival rate of oral malignant melanoma is 15%, with a median of 25 months. Gingival location has a better survival than palate: 46 months *versus* 22 months, respectively [12]. Most of the patients die of distant metastases. Average rate of distant metastases varies from 8 to 10% at presentation, and 51 to 60% after treatment. Almost half of distant metastases occurs in patients without any local and regional recurrences [19].

Minor Salivary Gland Tumours

Neoplasms of minor salivary glands are rare, and represent 0.3-1.5% of all oral pathologies [14]. The incidence of malignancy in these tumours varies from 37-45%. The palate is the most common site, followed by the lips and cheek. They occur mostly between the fifth and seventh decade of life and are more common in females [2]. The majority of malignant tumours are mucoepidermoid carcinoma (MEC), adenoid cystic carcinoma (ACC), and polymorphous low-grade adenocarcinoma. The tumours present as painless submucosal enlarging masses. Ulceration may occur, and suggest malignancy. If there is ulceration, incisional biopsy is used for diagnosis. In patients without ulceration, the method of biopsy is controversial. Fine needle aspiration cytology may help distinguish benign from malignant tumours. However, clinical behaviour depends on grade and histologic type of each tumour. Histological grading is a crucially important prognostic parameter in treatment planning particularly in MECs. Therefore, incisional biopsy is preferred in the diagnosis. Alternatively, excisional biopsy can be done in small, circumscribed lesions which seem to be benign or in low-grade tumours.

Mucoepidermoid carcinoma

Mucoepidermoid carcinoma represents the most common malignant tumour in minor salivary glands. However, some studies from various countries around the world have revealed that ACC is the predominant tumour [2]. In MEC, clinical behaviour and prognosis are closely related to histological grade, though grading is subjective. Low-grade tumours have an excellent 5-year survival of 90-100%. Conversely, intermediate and high-grade mucoepidermoid carcinomas tend to be aggressive and have a propensity for recurrence with a 5-year cure rate of about 50% [20].

Adenoid cystic carcinoma

Adenoid cystic carcinoma is characterized by infiltration, perineural invasion, local recurrences and late distant metastases. Palatal location has more favourable outcome when compared with other minor salivary gland sites. Again, histologic pattern is closely related to prognosis. High-grade ACCs have a tendency to recur locally and to develop metastases. On the other hand, low-grade tumours are slow growing with infrequent distant metastases [6]. The 5-year survival rate is approximately 70%, but the 20-year survival varies from 20 to 30% [4].

Polymorphous low-grade adenocarcinoma

Polymorphous low-grade adenocarcinoma is the third most common malignant salivary gland tumour. In some series, it is the second most common. Before its first description in 1983, this histologic entity was been categorized under adenocarcinoma, or adenoid cystic carcinoma. This tumour mostly occurs in minor salivary glands and at the junction between the hard and soft palate. It is a low-grade malignancy with uncommon metastases and has a local recurrence rate of up to 17% [4].

The other malignant tumours of minor salivary glands are acinic cell carcinoma, malignant mixed tumour, adenocarcinoma, epithelial myoepithelial carcinoma and clear cell carcinoma. These tumours are extremely rare in the oral cavity and the oropharynx.

Surgery is the treatment of choice in the malignant tumours of minor salivary glands. Low-grade carcinomas should be treated with wide local excision with a surrounding normal tissue. Enucleation and preservation the overlying mucosa should not be done because of the risk of recurrence. The frozen section of surgical margins is not reliable. When the tumour is large and involves the bone, the bone should be also removed. Adequate resection is crucial as high recurrence rates have been reported in the presence of positive surgical margins [1,6]. High-grade tumours require wide radical resection. Partial maxillectomy and marginal or segmental mandibulectomy are indicated in case of bony invasion. In tumours that have a tendency to spread via the neural spaces, such as ACCs, wider resection and frozen section of nerves should be performed in order to obtain clear margins. However, radical excision is sometimes impossible due to adjacent vital structures. There is no indication for elective neck dissection in the N_0 neck. Neck dissection should be reserved for clinically positive cervical lymph node metastases. Adjuvant radiation therapy is indicated in patients with positive or close surgical margins (<3mm), in high-grade carcinomas, recurrent tumours, advanced stage, perineural invasion and neck node metastases [10].

Oral Sarcomas

Oral sarcomas are quite rare, with an estimated annual incidence of about one per million. These account for less than 1% of all oral malignancies [21]. There are different types of sarcomas, all rarely encountered in the oral cavity or oropharynx, including fibrosarcoma, liposarcoma, rhabdomyosarcoma, leiomyosarcoma, angiosarcoma and neurosarcoma. Besides these soft tissue sarcomas, osteosarcoma, Kaposi's sarcoma, and malignant fibrous histiocytoma may occur in the oral cavity and oropharynx. Clinical findings are not specific and even histologic diagnosis can sometimes be difficult. Immunhistochemical studies are usually needed for further differentiation of mesenchymal origin. Treatment consists of wide surgical excision combined with either neoadjuvant or adjuvant chemotherapy. Radical resection with a cuff of normal tissue around the tumour is the preferred therapy. Tumour recurrence is common if complete resection has not been achieved. Postoperative radiation therapy is given to increase local control. However, the efficacy of radiation has yet to be defined.

Fibrosarcoma

Fibrosarcoma represents 2% of malignant mesenchymal tumours in the oral cavity. It usually affects patients around their fifth decade and the cheek, body of the mandible and the maxilla are the most common sites. Although the degree of differentiation is important in the outcome, the prognosis is better than other sarcomas. It seems to be radioresistant, and surgery is the preferred treatment modality [3].

Angiosarcoma

Angiosarcoma is very rare, and mostly seen in the palate of patients during the middle decades. Only 4-5% of head and neck angiosarcomas develop in the oral cavity and pharynx. It is characterized by aggressive, rapid growth, with regional and distant metastases. Treatment is combined therapy, including surgery, radiotherapy and chemotherapy, but prognosis is very poor. Radiation followed by radical surgery has been suggested as the most effective modality, however, 5-year survival is approximately 12% [5].

Leiomyosarcoma

Leiomyosarcoma is extremely uncommon, because of the lack of smooth muscle tissue in the oral and oropharyngeal area. It is mostly encountered in the fifth and sixth decades of life. The maxilla and the mandible are the most commonly involved sites. Leiomyosarcomas rarely occur in the pharynx. However, many tumours originating in the oral cavity extend into the pharynx. Prognosis is poor with more than half of the reported cases in the literature resulting in death [22].

Rhabdomyosarcoma

Rhabdomyosarcoma is more common than smooth muscle sarcoma. It is most frequent in children, and the palate and the cheek are major locations. Primary treatment is surgery followed by chemotherapy and radiation [3].

Liposarcoma

Liposarcoma is also rare; the patients are usually above the age of 40. The cheek and the floor of the mouth are the sites of preference. The lesions are most often slow growing.

Neurogenic sarcoma

Neurogenic sarcoma is derived from Schwann cells, either occurring as primary neurogenic malignant tumour or resulting from malignant degeneration of neurofibroma. It is characterized by neural invasion, which is a poor prognostic indicator. Treatment is wide surgical excision with a 50% cure rate.

Osteosarcoma

Osteosarcoma of the jaw is an aggressive malignant tumour that constitutes approximately 5% of skeletal osteosarcomas. The main clinical presentation is bony hard swelling either painless or painful. Most tumours are high grade, but distant metastases occur in about approximately 20% of patient. Distant metastases are usually located in the lungs, in other bones and in the liver. Radical excision is the main treatment modality. If surgically clear margins are obtained, the outcome is favorable. Segmental mandibulectomy is more often required, since osteosarcoma has a tendency for bone marrow infiltration. Otherwise, uncontrolled local disease is a major cause of death. Local recurrence may occur in up to 70% the tumours. Postoperative radiation has been shown to be ineffective and does not improve outcome in patients with positive margins. However, adjuvant chemotherapy is thought to be better in controlling local disease, although it does not improve prognosis. Chemotherapy can be given on a neo-adjuvant basis. Since cervical metastases are uncommon, elective neck dissection is not required. However, in the presence of lymph node metastases, modified radical neck dissection should be performed [11].

Malignant fibrous histiocytoma

Malignant fibrous histiocytoma is another rare lesion of the oral cavity. It is frequently seen in middle age or older, mainly in the mandible and cheek. Clinical presentation is usually firm swelling mass, which is not characteristic. Treatment is radical resection. Radiation and chemotherapy do not seem to be effective. Metastases are common through lymphatic or hematogenous dissemination. Recurrence and metastases occur in approximately 40% of patients [3,4].

Kaposi's sarcoma

Kaposi's sarcoma is a malignant tumour of endothelial cells. It is a variant of angiosarcoma, which is less malignant. Clinical presentation is that of purplish lesions on the oral mucous membranes. Radiation therapy is to be considered because of its radiosensitivity. There is another type of Kaposi'sarcoma that presents in HIV+ patients. Multifocal red nodules are the main presenting symptoms. The palate and the gingiva are the most common sites, and bony invasion may occur. Lymph node involvement and distant metastases are frequent. Treatment consists of radiation and chemotherapy, but the prognosis is poor due to dissemination of disease [3,4].

Oral Lymphoma

Lymphoma is the most common non-epithelial malignant tumour of the oral cavity, the third most frequent malignancy, after squamous cell carcinoma and minor salivary gland tumours [9].

Non-Hodgkin's lymphoma

Oral lymphoma is often associated with disseminated disease, but it may arise in oral mucosa as primary extranodal lesions. Two to three percent of extranodal non-Hodgkin's lymphomas occur in the oral cavity and jaws [8]. In the oropharynx, the tonsil is the most common site while in the oral cavity, the most frequent location is the palatal mucosa. The majority of oral lymphomas are of the B-cell type, with a predominance of the diffuse large B cell lymphoma. Fever and weight loss are uncommon. Most lesions are high-grade or intermediate, and they are considered to have an aggressive clinical course [4,8,9]. The treatment consists of a combination of radiation and chemotherapy. Age of above 60 years, advanced stage, extranodal involvement in more than one site, performance status, increased levels of serum lactate dehydrogenase, and the type of lymphoma are poor prognostic indicators. Low-grade tumours have a favourable outcome, with median survival of 8 to 10 years. In contrast, 5-year survival is about 40% in high-grade lesions [4,21].

Oral Hodgkin's lymphoma

Hodgkin's lymphoma of the oral cavity is extremely rare. There are only eight reports in the international literature on Hodgkin's lymphoma arising primarily in the oral mucosa in the absence of disseminated disease. There is no site of predilection in the oral cavity. Extranodal oral Hodgkin's lymphoma seems to have a good prognosis with radiotherapy or a combination of radiation with chemotherapy [23].

Oral Metastatic Tumours

Metastases to the oral cavity are uncommon. They occur either in the bone or in the soft tissues. In the jawbones, the posterior part of the mandible is the most frequent site. Among oral soft tissues, the gingiva is mostly the involved location followed by the tongue. In men, the lung, kidney, liver, and prostate are the most common primary organs. In women, breast, genital organs, kidney, and colon are major locations that have a propensy to develop metastases in the oral region. Oral metastases are characterized by rapid growth, pain and numbness. The majority of bone metastases are osteolytic. The initial clinical presentation of the gingival involvement may not differ from inflammatory lesions, such as pyogenic granuloma. In this regard, it should be noted that approximately 25% of oral metastases is the first finding of metastatic spread. The treatment of oral metastases is generally palliative radiation and chemotherapy. Prognosis is particularly poor with expected survival of less than one year [7].

References

1. Brandwein, MS, Ivanov K, Wallace DI *et al.* (2001) Mucoepidermoid carcinoma – A clinicopathologic study of 80 patients with special reference to histological grading. Am J Surg Pathol 25(7): 835-45
2. Buchner A, Merrell PW, Carpenter WM (2007) Relative frequency of intra-oral minor salivary gland tumors: a study of 380 cases from northern California and comparison to reports from other parts of the world. J Oral Pathol Med 36: 207-14
3. **Chow JM, Skolnik EM (1986) Nonsquamous tumors of the oral cavity. Otolaryngologic Clin N Am 19(3): 573-607**
4. **Daley T, Darling M (2003) Nonsquamous cell malignant tumours of the oral cavity: An overview. J Can dent Assoc 69(9): 577-82**
5. Favia G, Muzio LL, Serpicio R, Maiorano E (2002) Angiosarcoma of the head and neck with intra-oral presentation. A clinico-pathological study of four cases. Oral Oncology 38: 757-62
6. Gluckman JL, Barrord J, Snow GB, Van der Waal I (1986) Non-squamous cell tumors of the minor salivary glands. Otolaryngologic Clin N Am 19(3): 497-505
7. Hirshberg A, Shapiro AS, Kaplan I, Berger R (2008) Metastatic tumours to the oral cavity-Pathogenesis and analysis of 673 cases. Oral Oncology 44: 743-52
8. Kemp S, Gallagher G, Kabani S, Noonan V, O'Hara C (2008) Oral non-Hodgkin's lymphoma: review of the literature and World Health Organization classification with reference to 40 cases. Oral Pathol Oral Radiol Endod 105: 194-201
9. Kolokotronis A, Konstantinou N, Christakis I *et al.* (2005) Loçalized B-cell non-Hodgkin's lymphoma of oral cavity and maxillofacial region: A clinical study. Oral Surg Oral Med Oral Pathol Oral Radiol Endod 99: 303-10
10. Le QT, Birdwell S, Terris DJ *et al.* (1999) Postoperative irradiation of minor salivary gland malignancies of the head and neck. Radiotherapy Oncology 52: 165-71

11. Mardinger O, Givol N, Talmi YP, Taicher S (2001) Osteosarcome of the jaw. The Chaim Sheba medical center experience. Oral Surg Oral Med Oral Pathol Oral Radiol Endod 91: 445-51
12. **Meleti MM, Leemans CR, Mooi WJ *et al.* (2007) Oral malignant melanoma: A review of the literature. Oral Oncology 43: 116-21**
13. Mendenhall WM, Amdur RJ, Hinerman RW *et al.* (2005) Head and neck mucosal melanomas. Am J Clin Oncol 28(6): 626-30
14. **Pires FR, Pringle GA, Almeida OP, Chen SY (2007) Intra-oral minor salivary gland tumors: A clinicopathological study of 546 cases. Oral Oncology 43: 463-70**
15. Pour H (2008) Malignant melanoma of the oral cavity: A review of literature. Indian J Dent Res 19(1): 47-51
16. Rapini RP, Golitz LE, Greer RO *et al.* (1985) Primary malignant melanoma of the oral cavity. Cancer 55(7): 1543-51
17. Snow GB, Van der Waal I (1986) Mucosal melanomas of the head and neck. Otolaryngologic Clin N Am 19(3): 537-47
18. Stal S, Loeb T, Spira M (1986) Melanoma of the head and neck. Otolaryngologic Clin N Am 19(3): 549-64
19. Tanaka N, Mimura M, Ogi K, Amagasa T (2004) Primary malignant melanoma of the oral cavity: assessment of outcome from the clinical records of 35 patients. Int J Oral Maxillofac Surg 33: 761-5
20. Triantafillidou K, Dimitrakopoulos J, Iordanidis F, Koufofgiannis D (2006) Muco-epidermoid carcinoma of minor salivary glands: a clinical study of 16 cases and review of the literature. Oral Diseases 12: 364-70
21. **Van der Waal R, Van der Waal I (2007) Oral non-squamous malignant tumors; diagnosis and treatment. Med Oral Patol Oral Cir Bucal 12(7): 486-91**
22. Wertheimer-Hatch L, Hatch III GF, Hatch KF *et al.* (2000) Tumors of the oral cavity and pharynx. World J Surg 24: 395-400
23. Whitt JC, Dunlap CL, Martin KF (2007) Oral Hodgkin lymphoma: a wolf in wolf's clothing. Oral Pathol Oral Radiol Endod 104: e45-e51

Rare malignant tumours of the larynx and hypopharynx

5

C. Ikonomidis and L. Bron

Five Essential Points

1. *Non-epithelial pharyngo-laryngeal malignant tumours are rare. They represent about 5% of all laryngeal malignant tumours. The histology is highly variable and remains the principal guide to treatment options and prognosis. The clinical behaviour of these tumours is not always similar to the other body locations of the same histologic type.*
2. *The specific anatomopathological diagnosis and the correct classification require a systematic open biopsy which is an essential point for treatment planning. Therefore, tumour and nodal stage influence survival rates more than histology alone.*
3. *Appropriate treatment should be based on well-documented similar cases, when a sufficient experience is provided by the medical literature.*
4. *Surgery remains the initial treatment of choice for the majority of these cases and can preserve the organ function in most type of tumours, depending on the extension and aggressiveness of the primary.*
5. *To gain more experience on these rare tumours, well-conducted multicentric studies appear to be the only solution.*

Introduction

Squamous cell carcinomas (SCC) represent about 95% of all laryngeal-hypopharyngeal malignant tumours [4,5,7,10,15,22]. This chapter focuses on the classification, the clinical specification and the various treatment options of the remaining 5% which are considered as rare laryngeal and hypopharyngeal malignant tumours.

These tumours mainly originate from sub-mucosal tissues, presenting as a submucosal mass, thus the diagnosis is often difficult and disease at an advanced stage. Prior irradiation has been clearly implicated in the pathogenesis of some tumour types, such as soft tissue malignant tumours. Professional exposure to toxic substances such as asbestos is also mentioned as a risk factor. Some tumour types remain of unknown pathogenesis [4,10,13,26,45].

Tumours are mainly located in the glottic and supraglottic region. Some subglottic location mainly for adenoid cystic carcinoma has been described. Patients usually present with hoarseness or swallowing difficulties. Similarly to SCC, they present a higher male prevalence and they mainly occur in the 5th to 7th decade [4,5,10,14,19,22,26,27,29,31,45].

Due to very small series, both the clinical and the pathological classification of many of these tumours have been modified over time following research and new observation. Therefore some degree of confusion regarding the different anatomopathologic classifications has been noticed in the medical literature, mainly in the past. Some published old cases have been re-evaluated by pathologists and the final diagnosis was changed according to recent criteria and up-to-date classifications,

5

thus modifying the initial impression of the behaviour and incidence of some tumours [4,10,18,26,45]. The limited number of non-squamous cell malignancies published, added to the variability of their behaviour depending on the primary site, sometimes results in controversial therapies [29,31]. Chondrosarcomas are an example. These tumours are very aggressive when located in the extremities and skeleton. Conversely, they are slow growing and have a good prognosis when localised in the larynx [24,36,43]. Surgical treatment should therefore aim at preservation of function and does not need to be as radical and mutilating as for other sites of the same primary tumour [4,10,18,24,26,36,45].

The anatomo-pathological classification of this chapter is based on the 2005 World Health Organisation (WHO) Classification of Tumours as published by the International Academy of Pathology (IAP) (Table 1) [4]. The following text focuses on malignant tumours only, excluding the precursor forms of carcinoma as well as the benign tumours. Incidence and other epidemiological parameters are given when the number of published cases is considered sufficient.

The purpose of this chapter is to underline the pathologic characteristics and the clinical behaviour of these rare malignant tumours along with the main lines of treatment, according to the recent knowledge published in the international literature.

Table 1 – 2005 WHO Classification modified for *malignant* laryngeal and hypopharyngeal tumours.

Epithelial tumours *Squamous cell carcinoma (SCC)* Variants: - Verrucous carcinoma - Basaloid SCC - Papillary SCC - Spindle cell Carcinoma - Acantolytic SCC - Adenosquamous Carcinoma Lymphoepithelial Carcinoma Giant cell Carcinoma	***Soft tissue tumours*** - Fibrosarcoma - Malignant fibrous histiocytoma - Liposarcoma - Leiomyosarcoma - Rhabdomyosarcoma - Angiosarcoma - Kaposi sarcoma - Malignant peripheral nerve sheath tumour - Synovial sarcoma
Salivary Gland Type Tumours - Muco-epidermoid carcinoma - Adenoid cystic carcinoma - Acinic cell carcinoma - Myoepithelial carcinoma - Salivary duct carcinoma - Papillary adenocarcinoma - Mucinous adenocarcinoma - Clear Cell carcinoma	***Tumours of bone and cartilage*** - Chondrosarcoma - Osteosarcoma
Neuroendocrine tumours - Typical carcinoid - Atypical carcinoid - Small cell carcinoma neuroendocrine type - Combined small cell carcinoma neuroendocrine type	***Hematolymphoid tumours*** - *Non Hodgkin Lymphoma*
Mucosal malignant melanoma	***Secondary tumours (metastases)***

Squamous cell carcinoma variants

These tumours are composed of squamous cells and an additional cellular component. Even though some types of these tumours are considered rare, the pathogenesis, location and treatment options are generally similar to SCC of the same extent, thus they are not presented in this chapter [4,10,26,44,45].

Lymphoepithelial carcinoma

Definition, characteristics

Undifferentiated carcinoma with major reactive, lymphoplastic infiltrate along with the identification in some cases of a squamous cell component. Its morphological aspect is generally identical to nasopharyngeal carcinoma with EBV aetiology rarely demonstrated. Regional lymph node metastases are generally present and distant metastases exist in around 30% of cases [30].

Synonyms

Lymphoepithelioma, nasopharyngeal type undifferentiated carcinoma, undifferentiated carcinoma with lymphoid stroma.

Incidence

Extremely rare, these tumours account for less than 0, 5% of all laryngeal cancers [4,30].

Treatment

Conservative with combined radio-chemotherapy.

Prognosis

Aggressive tumours with high metastatic potential. Mortality rate is around 30% in a reported 21 months follow–up series [4,30,45].

Giant cell carcinoma

Definition, characteristics

Mostly poorly differentiated carcinoma composed of irregular, multinucleated giant cells, these tumours show similarities to giant cell carcinoma of the lung. They can exist in pure or mixed form along with SCC, adenocarcinoma or spindle cell components.

Synonyms

Large cell carcinoma, pleomorphic carcinoma, anaplastic carcinoma.

5

Incidence

Less than 10 cases reported [23].

Treatment

Surgical excision with adjuvant radiotherapy in cases of local infiltration.

Prognosis

It is highly dependent on the differentiation stage and is mostly favourable for well differentiated types [4,26,45].

Malignant minor salivary gland-type tumours

Less than 1% of tumours of the pharyngo-larynx arise from accessory salivary gland tissue, scattered on the surface or the sub-mucosa [1,4,19].

In the majority of the cases, tumours are adenoid cystic or mucoepidermoid carcinomas. Their anatomopathological characteristics and clinical behaviour are similar to the lesions arising in major salivary glands [1,4,19].

Adenoid Cystic Carcinoma

Approximately 150 cases of adenoid cystic carcinoma of the larynx are reported in the literature. This represents 0,1-0,25% of all laryngeal carcinomas [4,19,32]. Contrary to tumours found in major salivary gland, the incidence of regional nodal metastases is high (50%) [4,19].

Incidence

About 40% of malignant salivary gland tumours of the larynx [4,19].

Treatment

Surgical excision with neck dissection if clinically positive lymph nodes are present. Radiotherapy is the main line of adjuvant treatment and has a proved beneficial for microscopic disease clearance [19,32].

Prognosis

Good, with up to 75% 5-years survival rate reported [19,32].

Mucoepidermoid Carcinoma

It accounts for almost the second half of tumours of salivary tissue origin in the hypopharynx and larynx. Approximately 100 cases are reported in the literature. The incidence of regional lymph node metastases is fairly high with up to 50 % of regional node involvement [9,10,19,20].

Incidence

About 33% of malignant salivary gland tumours of the larynx [4,9,26]

Treatment

Surgical excision is dependant on the tumour grade and can remain conservative. High grade tumours require more radical surgery along with a neck dissection when clinical positive neck nodes are present. Based on histopathological final diagnosis, adjuvant treatment is advisable [4,19,26].

Prognosis

The prognosis is mostly dependant on the initial grade of the tumour and the extent of resection but it sometimes seems unpredictable [4,7,9,10,19,26,45].

The incidence of all the other histological types of malignant salivary gland-type tumours in the pharyngo-laryngeal area as mentioned in Table 1, remains extremely low with mainly isolated case reports found in the literature. In all cases surgical treatment appeared to be the best solution [4,7,8,9,10,18,26,45].

Neuroendocrine tumours

Neuroendocrine tumours are a heterogeneous group of cancers that vary from benign to highly malignant. They form the largest group of non-squamous cell tumours of the larynx. About 500 cases have been reported in the literature among which, atypical carcinoid appears to be the most frequent histological type described [4,17,37]. They are characterized by the presence of cells which are similar to Kultchitsky cells found in the bronchi, or the endobronchial stem cells. The common histopathological picture shows the presence of both epithelial and neuroendocrine cells. The potential of distant metastases rises with the grade of malignancy and is often accompanied by a clinical carcinoid syndrome [4,17,45]. The classification, clinical behaviour and prognosis of these tumours are summarized in Table 2. Some mixed forms of SCC along with a squamous or adenocarcinomatous component are mentioned in the literature as "Combined Small Cell Carcinomas, Neuroendocrine type". They are very rare with around 14 cases reported [4].

Table 2 – Neuroendocrine tumours.

Classification:	**Typical carcinoid**	**Atypical carcinoid**	**Small cell carcinoma neuroendocrine type**
Synonyms:	Well differentiated (grade I) neuroendocrine Carcinoma	Malignant carcinoid, moderately differentiated (Grade II) neuroendocrine carcinoma, large cell carcinoma, pleomorphic or anaplastic	Small cell (or oat cell) neuroendocrine carcinoma, poorly differentiated (grade III) neuroendocrine carcinoma
Incidence:	3%	54%	34%
Aggressiveness:	Low	High	Very high, metastatic in early stages
Treatment:	Conservative surgery	Radical surgery, neck dissection	Radical surgery if still possible. Otherwise alternative radiochemotherapy protocols
Prognosis:	Generally favourable	5 year survival rate: 48% 10 year rate: 30%	Poor. 5 year rate: 16%.

Treatment

Radio-chemotherapy is generally considered of limited benefit and surgery is therefore the treatment of choice. It should be conservative when possible; radical if the tumour shows an aggressive behaviour. A neck dissection is not mandatory and is usually indicated according to the degree of malignancy of the primary tumour and the presence of regional lymph node metastases. It is always indicated for aggressive tumours such as atypical and small cell carcinomas [4,17,37,39,45].

Small cell carcinomas are usually highly metastatic in early stages and therefore surgical treatment is rarely indicated and should be replaced by conservative treatment. The protocol for chemotherapy and radiotherapy is often based on the experience in treatment of the pulmonary location of the same tumour [4,17,37,39,45].

Malignant soft tissue tumours

These tumours are of mesenchymatous origin and totally represent less than 1% of all laryngeal malignant tumours. They are often considered to be radiation-induced. Due to a high rate of local recurrence and a very unpredictable behaviour, malignant fibrous histiocytoma, angiosarcoma and all types of radiation-induced sarcoma are considered the most aggressive and their prognosis remains poor. The treatment of choice always includes complete surgical excision with large margins, when possible. Adjuvant radio-chemotherapy has proven to be beneficial for non radiation-induced tumours [4,7,12,13,25,38,45].

Fibrosarcoma

Many soft tissue tumours have been classified as fibrosarcomas in the past. According to recent pathologic criteria, this tumour's pure form is very rare [4,34].

Malignant fibrous histiocytoma

With less than 50 cases reported in the literature, the experience is low but the overall prognosis is generally considered poor [4,35,38].

Liposarcoma

Presenting usually as a low-grade tumour. Its prognosis is globally favourable provided adequate surgical removal [3,4,47].

Leiomyosarcoma

This tumour arises from the smooth muscle of blood vessels or from the undifferentiated mesenchymal tissue. Its prognosis depends on the initial stage of the tumour. Elective neck dissection is not routinely recommended for low grade tumours [41,42].

Rhabdomyosarcoma

Mostly found in the paediatric population, the tumour is clearly less aggressive when found in the pharyngo-larynx, compared to other locations [4,13,40].

Angiosarcoma

With less than 40 cases reported in the current literature, it is considered very aggressive locally, notably when radiation-induced [4,25,28].

Kaposi sarcoma

The laryngeal occurrence of this tumour is documented mostly on immunocompromised patients with advanced HIV disease. It is very rare and the treatment of choice seems to be non-surgical. The response rate to radio-chemotherapy is satisfactory [4].

Malignant peripheral nerve sheath tumours

Of very rare occurrence, these cancers must be distinguished from Schwannoma and Neurofibroma, their benign counterparts [4].

Synovial sarcoma

Primary Synovial Sarcoma of the laryngo-hypopharynx is extremely rare. Secondary extension from the prevertebral connective tissue space or other neck locations is more common [4].

Malignant tumours of bone and cartilage

Chondrosarcoma

Definition, characteristics

Chondrosarcomas originate from the neoplastic transformation of hyaline cartilage. The primary predilection sites are the posterolateral parts of the cricoid cartilage. The thyroid cartilage is the second predilection site. Some other very rare locations such as the epiglottis or the arytenoids have also been described. They present as submucosal masses without breech of the overlying mucosa (Fig. 1) and are characterized by a low growth rate without metastatic potential. Nevertheless, undifferentiated tumours of high histological grade will eventually metastasize [24,36,43].

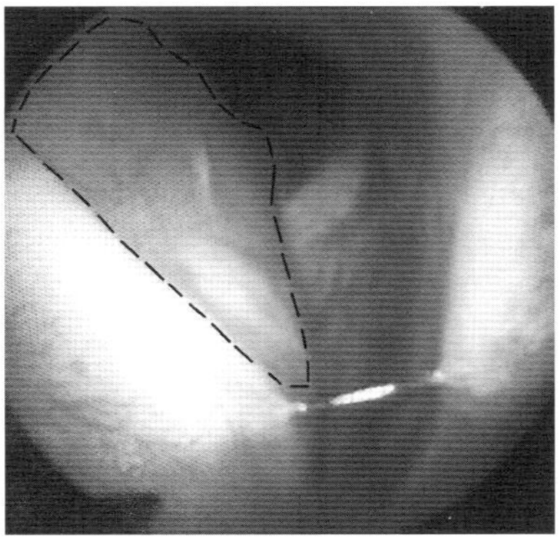

Fig. 1. Sub-mucosal mass aspect of a cricoid cartilage chondrosarcoma.

Incidence

Chondrosarcomas are the most common non-epithelial malignancy of the larynx. About 300 cases have been reported in the medical literature. They represent about 1% of all cartilaginous tumours of the body, 0, 5% of all laryngeal malignant tumours and 75% of all laryngeal sarcomas [4,24,36,43]. These tumours are often reported by multiple individual case reports which give the impression that the real tumour incidence is underestimated.

Histologic types

Chondrosarcomas are classified in grades I, II, III and undifferentiated, but low grade chondrosarcomas are by far the most common and represent 95% of all described cases [24,36,43,45].

Treatment

Due to this large preponderance of low grade tumour as well as to its general non-aggressive behaviour, function-preserving surgery is indicated [24,36,43,45]. Radio-chemotherapy is generally ineffective but has been tried in some inoperable patients with favourable effects[11,21].

Prognosis

Provided excision is complete, chondrosarcomas have an excellent prognosis with a very low mortality [4,24,36,43,45].

Osteosarcoma

Definition, characteristics

These highly malignant tumours are characterized by the direct formation of osteoid by neoplastic cells. They usually arise from the endolaryngeal soft tissue rather than from the laryngeal framework [4,33].

Incidence

It is a rare tumour with around 20 cases reported in the literature [4,33].

Treatment

Excision is the only therapeutic option with usually very poor response to non-surgical treatment [4,33].

Prognosis

These aggressive tumours recur locally and generally tend to present with distant metastases. According to the small number of reported cases, the prognosis is very poor with a mortality rate of around 50% within the first year of diagnosis [4,33].

Mucosal malignant melanoma

Definition, characteristics

Primary laryngeal melanoma has been described. It originates from melanocytes scattered in the upper aerodigestive tract mucosa. As for other locations, it is an aggressive cancer with a high potential for regional and distant metastases with its own biological behaviour completely different from skin melanoma [4,46].

Incidence

About 60 cases are reported, but it represents only a very small portion of melanomas in all sites (<1%) [4,46].

Treatment

Radical surgery is the only therapeutic option as primary or adjuvant radiochemotherapy has shown some disappointing results.

Prognosis

As for other mucosal melanoma, 5-years survival rate [4,46].

Lymphomas

Non-Hodgkin Lymphoma (NHL)

Primary laryngeal-hypopharyngeal NHL have been described but this very rare location is more commonly secondary. Primary NHL of the larynx accounts for 1% of all extranodal disease, B-cell type being the commonest.

Treatment

The treatment is non surgical with a very good response to radio-chemotherapy [2,4].

Secondary tumours

Metastases to the larynx are uncommon and generally associated with terminal, widespread disease. Less than 150 cases reported in the literature [4,6,16].

Some of the commonest reported laryngeal metastases concern primary tumours of skin and melanoma. Less common primary tumours metastasizing to the larynx include kidney, breast, lung, prostate and colon [4, 6,16].

Prognosis

Not surprisingly, prognosis is quite poor in this setting. Palliative therapies with radiation or chemotherapy can be applied in isolated and well localised metastases [6,16].

References

1. Alavi S, Namazie A, Calcaterra TC, Blackwell KE (1998) Glandular carcinoma of the larynx: the UCLA experience. Ann Otol Rhinol Laryngol 108: 485-9
2. Ansell SM, Habermann TM, Hoyer JD *et al.* (1997) Primary laryngeal lymphoma. Laryngoscope 107: 1502-6
3. Archaki A, Sahraoui S, Benider A *et al.* (1999) Liposarcome du larynx. Revue de la littérature à propos d'un cas. Cancer/Radiother 3: 245-8
4. **Barnes L *et al.* (2005) The WHO and TNM Classification of head and neck tumors. International Academy of Pathology. IARC Press 108-62**
5. Batsakis J, Luna MA, El-Naggar AK (1992) Nonsquamous Carcinomas of the Larynx. Ann Otol Rhinol Laryngol 101: 1024-6
6. Batsakis JG, Luna MA, Bryers RM (1985) Metastases to the larynx. Head Neck Surg 7: 458-60
7. Becker M *et al.* (1998) Non-squamous Cell Neoplasms of the Larynx: Radiologic-Pathologic Correlation. Radiographics 18: 1189-209
8. Boscolo-Rizzo P, Da Mosto MC, Marchiori C, Boccato P (2004) Transglottic Acinic Cell Carcinoma. ORL 66: 286-9
9. Calis AB, Coskun BU, Seven H *et al.* (2006) Laryngeal mucoepidermoid carcinoma: Report of two cases. Auris Nasus Larynx 211-4
10. Crotty KA, Grassi TD, Grygiel J (1999) Rare tumors of the larynx. Textbook of uncommon Cancer, 2nd edition, pp 131-143
11. Dailiana T *et al.* (2002) Chondrosarcoma of the larynx: Treatment with Radiotherapy. Skeletal Radiol 31: 547-9
12. Davis RK, Waner M (1988) Soft Tissue Sarcomas of the Head and Neck. Textbook of uncommon cancer, pp 1007-1017
13. De Bree R *et al.* (2006) Prognostic factors in adult soft tissue sarcomas of the head and neck: A single center experience. Oral Oncology 42: 703-9
14. Ferlito A, Rinaldo A, Marioni G (1999) Laryngeal malignant neoplasms in children and adolescents. Intern J Ped Otorhinol 49: 1-14
15. Ferlito A (1993) The WHO revised classification of tumours of the larynx, hypopharynx and trachea. Ann Otol Rhinol Laryngol 102: 666-9
16. Ferlito A, Caruso G, Recher G (1998) Secondary laryngeal tumours. Report of seven cases with review of the literature. Arch Otolaryngol Head Neck Surg 114: 635-9
17. Ferlito A, Shaha AR, Rinaldo A (2002) Neuroendocrine neoplasms of the larynx: diagnosis, treatment and prognosis. ORL J Otorhinolaryngol Relat 64: 108-13
18. Fernandez-Acenero MJ, Larach F, Ortega-Fernandez C (2008) Non-epithelial lesions of the larynx: review of the 10-year experience in a tertiary Spanish hospital. Acta Oto-Laryngologica 1-5
19. Ganly I, Patel SG, Coleman M *et al.* (2006) Malignant Minor Salivary Gland Tumours of the larynx. Arch Otolaryngol Head Neck Surg 132: 767-70
20. Gomes V, Costarelli L, Cimino G *et al.* (1990) Mucoepidermoid carcinoma of the larynx. Eur Arch Otorhinolaryngol 248: 31-4
21. Gripp S, Pape H, Schmitt G (1998) Chondrosarcoma of the larynx. The role of radiotherapy revisited. A case report and review of the literature. Cancer 82: 108-15
22. **Harrison WL, Bhattacharyya N (2008) Staging and Survival Analysis for Nonsquamous Cell Carcinomas of the Larynx. Laryngoscope 118: 1003-13**
23. Gurbuz Y, Kose N, Aydin O, Ozturk M (2007) An immunohistochemical profile of giant cell carcinoma of the larynx. Auris Nasus Larynx 34: 413-6
24. Ikonomidis C, Konu P, Meier D (2008) Chondrosarcome de bas degré du cartilage cricoïde. Présentation d'un cas. Revue de la littérature. Orl aktuell 31, sup. no 40 Forum Médical Suisse: 68-70

25. Katsutoshi M, Yoonseup K, Han G, Tsutsui Y (2003) Radiation- induced laryngel angiosarcoma after cervical tuberculosis and squamous cell carcinoma: Case report and review of the literature. Pathology International 53: 710-5
26. Khariwala S, Strome M (2006) Rare tumours of the larynx. Textbook of Uncommon Cancer, 3rd edition. Wiley, pp 102-112
27. Lin HW, Bhattacharyya N (2008) Staging and Survival Analysis for Non-squamous Cell Carcinomas of the Larynx. Laryngoscope 118: 1003-13
28. Loos BM, Wieneke JA, Thompson LD (2001) Laryngeal angiosarcoma: a clinico-pathologic study of five cases with a review of the literature. Laryngoscope 111: 1197-202
29. Lucioni M, Marioni G, Della Libera D *et al.* (2008) Treatment of unusual or rare laryngeal nonsquamous primary malignancies: radical (total/extended total laryngectomy) or conservative surgery? Am J Otolaryngol 29: 106-12
30. MacMillian C, Kapadia SB, Finkelstein SD *et al.* (1996) Lymphoepithelial carcinoma of the larynx and hypopharynx: study of eight cases with relationship to Epstein-Barr virus and p53 gene alterations, and review of the literature. Hum Pathol 27: 1172-9
31. Marioni G, Marchese-Ragona R, Cartei G *et al.* (2006) Current opinion in diagnosis and treatment of laryngeal carcinoma. Cancer treatment reviews 32: 504-15
32. Moukarbel R *et al.* (2008) Adenoid cystic carcinoma of the larynx: a 40- years experience. Head and neck – DOI 10.1002/hed: 919-24
33. Mysiiorek D, Patel M, Wasserman P, Rofeim O (1998) Osteosarcoma of the larynx. Ann Otol Rhinol Laryngol 107: 70-4
34. Nishimura G *et al.* (2006) Myxofibrosarcoma of the hypopharynx. Auris Nasus Larynx 33: 93-6
35. Nakazimo M, Yokoshima K, Sugisaki Y (2004) Malignant Fibrous Histiocytoma of the Hypopharynx: A Case Report in a Young Adult. J Nippon Med Sch 71(4): 301-4
36. Olsen KD, Lewis JE, Inwards CY (1997) Cartilaginous tumors of the Larynx: Clinicopathologic review of 47 cases. Ann Otol Rhinol Laryngol 106: 94-100
37. Procopio G *et al.* (2006) Neuroendocrine tumors of the larynx: A clinical report and literature review. Tumori 92: 72-5
38. Resta L, Pennella A, Fiore MG, Botticella MA (2000) Malignant fibrous histiocytoma of the larynx after radiotherapy for squamous cell carcinoma. Eur Arch Otorhinolaryngol 257: 260-2
39. Sano M, Kitahara N, Toma M (2005) Hypopharyngeal small cell carcinoma: A case report. Auris Nasus Larynx 32: 319-22
40. Schrock A, Jacob M, Zhou H, Bootz F (2007) Laryngeal pleomorphic rhabdomyosarcoma. Auris Nasus Larynx 34: 553-6
41. Skoulakis CE, Stavroulaki P, Moschotzopoulos P *et al.* (2006) Laryngeal leiomyosarcoma: a case report and review of the literature. Eur Arch Otorhinolaryngol 263: 929-34
42. Takahashi T, Higo R, Nakata H, Sugasawa M (2008) Leiomyosarcoma of the hypopharynx: A case report. Auris Nasus Larynx 35: 304-7
43. Thompson LD, Gannon FH (2002) Chondrosarcoma of the larynx: a clinicopathologic study of 111 cases with a review of the literature. Am J Surg Pathol 26: 836-51
44. Thompson LD, Wieneke J, Miettinen M, Heffner D (2002) Spindle Cell (Sarcomatoid) Carcinomas of the Larynx. Am. J Surg Pathol 26(2): 153-70
45. Wenig BM (2007) Atlas of Head and Neck Pathology. 2nd edition. Saunders, pp 207-68
46. Wenig BM (1995) Laryngeal mucosal malignant melanoma. A clinicopathologic, immunohistochemical and ultrastructural study of 4 patients and a review of the literature. Cancer 75: 1568-77
47. Wenig BM Heffner DK (1995) Liposarcomas of the larynx and hypopharynx: a clinicopathologic study of eight new cases and review of the literature. Laryngoscope 105: 747-56

Primary Orbital Lymphoma

G. Ugurluer, A. Zouhair and M. Ozsahin

6

Five Essential Points

1. *Primary orbital non-Hodgkin's lymphoma (NHL) is a rare presentation of extranodal NHL, accounting for less than 1% of cases.*
2. *The extranodal marginal zone lymphoma, mucosa associated lymphoid tissue (MALT) type is the most common subtype.*
3. *Primary orbital lymphomas are thought to be isolated to the orbit so by definition they are stage IE, but a complete staging workup is essential.*
4. *Radiotherapy is the most effective treatment for local disease either as the sole treatment for low grade lymphoma or in combination with chemotherapy for intermediate and high grade lymphoma.*
5. *A multicenter prospective study may bring further clarification to this rare type of tumour.*

Introduction

Primary orbital non-Hodgkin's lymphoma (NHL) is a rare presentation of extranodal NHL accounting for less than 1% of cases [13]. A marked increase in the incidence has been observed over the last decade [35]. However, with a few exceptions, almost all reported studies have included a relatively small number of patients from one institution; therefore, a reasonably meaningful estimate of pretherapeutic or therapeutic prognostic factors has been difficult to establish [33]. Various subsites within the orbit may be involved, including the conjunctiva, lacrimal apparatus, eyelids and musculature. Although many histologic subtypes of NHL may be encountered, the extranodal marginal zone lymphoma, mucosa associated lymphoid tissue (MALT) type is the most common subtype [21]. Several prognostic factors such as age, anatomical location of tumour, stage, histological subtype, grade, lactate dehydrogenase level, complete response to treatment, have been identified that could be used when considering the overall management of this uncommon site of primary lymphoma [11, 33]. Radiotherapy (RT) is the most effective treatment for local disease either as the sole treatment for low grade lymphoma or in combination with chemotherapy for intermediate and high grade lymphoma [15]. In the recent years, targeted therapy has become an important additional treatment modality for NHL and rituximab is the most commonly used [17].

Clinical characteristics

The presenting symptoms of primary orbital lymphoma (POL) vary according to the site of involvement. Common symptoms are diplopia, ptosis, pain, changes in visual acuity, or restriction of eye movement; signs may include soft tissue swelling arising from the conjunctiva, eyelids or lacrimal gland or proptosis due to the orbital tumour [37]. With the exception of pain with associated bone erosion on radiological examination (most often observed in so-called high-grade lymphomas), there are few symptoms or signs that aid the clinical distinction between reactive lymphoid hyperplasia and malignant lymphoma [11]. Very few studies have systemically assessed the implications of these symptoms on outcome [6]. POL can be seen at all ages, but it is most commonly diagnosed in patients in the fifth to seventh decades of life [16]. POL tends to affect women more often than men, and occurs most frequently in the orbit and the conjunctiva [19]. Approximately 10–17% of cases demonstrate bilateral involvement, with the bilaterality occurring either simultaneously or subsequently [11]. The non-ophthalmic findings discovered on physical examination depend on the presence or absence of systemic malignant lymphoma.

Diagnosis, histopathological classification and staging

A detailed investigation as in other lymphoma sites is necessary, and the diagnosis of POL requires appropriate imaging studies. The CT scans and magnetic resonance imaging (MRI) are usually the primary diagnostic tools in the evaluation and both are of use to determine the size, the number and the degree of infiltration of these lesions. However, neither CT scans nor MRI can reliably differentiate lymphoid hyperplasia from malignant lymphoma [20, 40]. The final diagnosis is usually established through histopathological examination, which also helps with the histological classification of lymphoma. A thorough staging workup is necessary to identify those patients who may have additional foci of lymphoma. The staging of the disease includes complete blood count, bone-marrow biopsy, immunophenotyping, CT scans of the neck, chest, abdomen and pelvis and should now include positron emission tomography (PET) [5]. The role of PET was shown in detecting systemic disease compared to traditional total body scans [46]. A limitation of PET however is the low sensitivity in detecting orbital lesion, markedly lower than with traditional imaging, but this could be overcome by the advent of PET/CT, which combines the advantages of both techniques [41]. The majority of orbital lymphomas are B-cell NHL, which are predominantly extranodal marginal zone B-cell lymphomas [11], according to the Revised European American Lymphoma (REAL) classification [24] but they can also include diffuse large cell B-cell lymphomas and follicular lymphomas as well as less common B-cell lymphoma subtypes. Orbital lymphomas of non-B-cell type are rare in these sites [26]. Hodgkin's disease of the ocular adnexa is exceptionally rare, with only a few cases being reported in the literature [27]. POL is thought to be isolated to the orbit as the only extranodal site of involvement, thus by definition POL is stage I. Approximately 60–80% of POL are limited in their extension at the time of diagnosis and represent stage IE disease [2, 12, 42]. Bilateral involvement without systemic lymphoma is reported in about 10-17% of the cases but no consensus has been reached with regard to the classification of bilateral disease and depending on the author, it can be referred to as Stage I, II, IE, IEE or IIEE [33].

Prognosis

Various prognostic factors have been described as having an influence on the clinical course of the patients with orbital lymphoma. Major documented prognostic factors for POL include anatomic location of the tumour (the best prognosis is associated with conjunctiva); stage of disease at first presentation; lymphoma subtype (extranodal marginal zone B-cell lymphoma shows a better prognosis), immunohistochemical markers determining factors such as tumour growth rate; and the serum lactate dehydrogenase level (LDH) [11, 23, 28, 29]. In a Rare Cancer Network study of 90 patients, the statistically significant factors on univariate analyses were younger age, low grade, normal erythrocyte sedimentation rate, absence of muscular infiltration, complete response to treatment, conjunctival localization, and normal LDH for overall survival, disease-free survival and freedom from treatment failure [33]. In multivariate analyses, the favorable factors were younger age and low grade for overall survival and disease-free survival; a favorable response, conjunctival localization and complete staging were highly significant for disease-free survival and freedom from treatment failure. The International Prognostic Index (IPI) was documented as a prognostic factor by Sjo, which includes the age (<60 or >60), performance status, Ann-Arbor stage (I-II *vs.* II-IV), extra-nodal sites (<1 *vs.* >1) and LDH level (normal or above normal) [43].

Treatment

The initial step in the treatment of a patient with a diagnosis of POL is to determine the extent of disease at the time of presentation or diagnosis. Several criteria must be considered in the initial assessment of the disease to clearly define optimal treatment, they are: (i) the histopathologic subtype of lymphoma, (ii) extension of the disease (in the ocular region and systemically), (iii) prognostic factors related to the patient and to the disease and (iv) the impact of the lymphoma on the eye(s) and visual function. Thus, treatment decision may vary from patient to patient, and uniform guidelines for treatment of orbital lymphoma do not exist [43]. The extension of disease is given in terms of a clinical stage usually according to the Ann-Arbor Classification [10]. Most POLs are limited in their extension at the time of diagnosis and represent stage IE. Various treatment modalities have been used for POL, including external beam radiotherapy, which is viewed as the gold standard for primary stage IE extranodal lymphoma of the orbit [7, 9, 33], single-agent or combination systemic chemotherapy regimens [4, 44], and combinations of radiotherapy and systemic chemotherapy, whereas bacteria eradicating antibiotic therapy, anti-CD20 therapy and intralesional interferon represent experimental strategies. Pure surgical therapy is not usually recommended in stage IE ocular adnexal lymphoma, as tumour microinfiltration into surrounding tissue is usually present [3]. During the last 10 years, targeted monoclonal antibody (mAb) therapy has become an important additional treatment modality for NHL. Highly specific monoclonal antibodies, such as rituximab and alemtuzumab, directed at lymphoma cells are used for initial treatment and recurrence of some types of non-Hodgkin lymphoma, as are antibodies linked to a radioactive atom, such as ibritumomab tiuxetan and iodine I 131 tositumomab [1]. Esmaeli et al. has reported the use of mAbs for the treatment of orbital lymphoma in four patients in 2002 [18]. They, also, prospectively evaluated systemic targeted radioimmunotherapy, and reported that this latter is an effective and safe front-line treatment for early-stage extranodal indolent B-cell lymphoma of the ocular adnexa [17]. A wait-and-see policy for stage IE extranodal marginal zone lymphoma following excisional biopsy has also been adopted but such a policy is, however, to be discouraged due to the risk of developing either local recurrence or systemic disease [36]. Finally, systemic corticosteroids, which may produce an initial decrease in tumour size, have been proven to be ineffective for long-term control of POL [11].

The dose of localized radiotherapy for primary orbital lymphomas remains controversial given the rarity of condition and varies between a total dose from 28-36 Gy for low-grade lymphomas and 30-40 Gy for intermediate to high-grade lymphomas [3]. A total dose of less than 28 Gy has been reported to result in an increase in tumour recurrence rates [34], whereas those greater than 36 Gy result only in an increase in side effects which include xerophthalmia, corneal ulceration, cataract formation, and vasculopathy of the retina and the optic nerve [15, 25, 30]. At the recommended dose of 30 Gy most patients achieve complete tumour control, and the 5-year survival approaches 90–100%, with minimal local side effects [14, 33, 45]. In the Rare Cancer Network multicenter study, in which 90 patients were analysed, the local control was achieved in 97% of patients and the 5-year disease-free survival, overall survival and cause-specific survival rate was 65%, 78%, and 87%, respectively [33]. Some investigators have recommended doses from 36-40 Gy for intermediate- and high-grade lesions [9, 15]. Regarding the adequate radiotherapy dose to be given in high-grade NHL, because almost all of these are currently also treated with chemotherapy, a total dose of 30 Gy should be sufficient after a complete response to CHOP or CHOP-like chemotherapy. However, a dose of 40 Gy should be considered after partial remission [9]. In additional to local disease control, treatment of orbital lymphoma should aim at the functional preservation of the eye [8]. The delivery of radiotherapy to the orbit is technically challenging given the critical structures within the treatment field such as lens, lacrimal gland, retina and their relatively low tolerance levels. Intensity modulated radiotherapy is an option when treating orbital lymphoma, and can reduce the dose to critical structures while providing excellent dose coverage of the target volumes [22]. It has also been shown that patients with orbital lymphoma should be treated on the entire orbit not the partial orbit [39].

Should disseminated disease be demonstrated in POL, systemic chemotherapy is required. However, the role of chemotherapy in the treatment of indolent stage IE orbital lymphoma is limited [15, 32, 38]. On the one hand, systemic therapy alone is not sufficient for local control, whereas on the other hand, long-term survival is not influenced by adjuvant chemotherapy directly after radiation treatment [15]. Recently, the worse outcome of patients with high grade histology has led to the more frequent use of neoadjuvant chemotherapy prior to radiotherapy [37]. Most regimens are based on the CHOP scheme, although COMP was additionally administered and combined radiotherapy and chemotherapy can be used in rare cases in which the tumours are bulky or vision-threatening [11].

Previous studies suggest that the development of systemic disease occurs usually within the first 6 months after presentation [11]. However it may occur many years after primary treatment and it is, therefore, recommended that systemic evaluation be repeated every 6 months at least for the first 5 years [29, 31].

Conclusions

Primary orbital lymphoma is a rare presentation of NHL. Recent advances in knowledge of the clinical and pathological features of POL have provided a number of new prognostic factors that could be used when considering the overall management of this uncommon site of primary lymphoma. For POL limited to the adnexa on systemic workup and staging, 30 Gy of radiotherapy in standard fractions has shown efficacy in eradicating the lesions without recurrence. A full staging workup is warranted in these patients. A multicenter prospective study should bring further clarification to this rare type of tumour.

References

1. American Cancer Society: Cancer Facts and Figures 2008. Atlanta, Ga: American Cancer Society, page 15, 2008, available online
2. Auw-Haedrich C, Coupland SE, Kapp A *et al.* (2001) Long term outcome of ocular adnexal lymphoma subtyped according to the REAL classification. Revised European and American Lymphoma. Br J Ophthalmol 85(1): 63-9
3. Baldini L, Blini M, Guffanti A *et al.* (1998) Treatment and prognosis in a series of primary extranodal lymphomas of the ocular adnexa. Ann Oncol 9(7): 779-81
4. Ben Simon GJ, Cheung N, McKelvie P *et al.* (2006) Oral chlorambucil for extranodal, marginal zone, B-cell lymphoma of mucosa-associated lymphoid tissue of the orbit. Ophthalmology 113(7): 1209-13
5. **Bernardini FP, Bazzan M (2007) Lymphoproliferative disease of the orbit. Curr Opin Ophthalmol 18(5): 398-401**
6. Bessell EM, Henk JM, Wright JE, Whitelocke RA (1988) Orbital and conjunctival lymphoma; treatment and prognosis. Radiother Oncol 13(4): 237-44
7. Bhatia S, Paulino AC, Buatti JM *et al.* (2002) Curative radiotherapy for primary orbital lymphoma. Int J Radiat Oncol Biol Phys 54(3): 818-23
8. Bischof M, Karagiozidis M, Krempien R *et al.* (2007) Radiotherapy for orbital lymphoma. Strahlenther Onkol 183(1): 17-22
9. Bolek TW, Moyses HM, Marcus RB Jr *et al.* (1999) Radiotherapy in the management of orbital lymphoma. Int J Radiat Oncol Biol Phys 44(1): 31-6
10. Carbone PP, Kaplan HS, Musshoff K *et al.* (1971) Report of the Committee on Hodgkin's Disease Staging Classification. Cancer Res 31(11): 1860-1
11. **Coupland SE, Hummel M, Stein H (2002) Ocular adnexal lymphomas: Five case presentations and a review of the literature. Surv Ophthalmol 47(5): 470-90**
12. Coupland SE, Krause L, Delecluse HJ *et al.* (1998) Lymphoproliferative lesions of the ocular adnexa. Analysis of 112 cases. Ophthalmology 105(8): 1430-41
13. Coupland SE (2004) Lymphoproliferative lesions of the ocular adnexa. Differential diagnostic guidelines. Ophtalmologe 101(2): 197-215
14. Ejima Y, Sasaki R, Okamoto Y (2006) Ocular adnexal mucosa-associated lymphoid tissue lymphoma treated with radiotherapy. Radiother Oncol: 78(1): 6-9
15. Esik O, Ikeda H, Mukai K, Kaneko A (1996) A retrospective analysis of different modalities for treatment of primary orbital non-Hodgkin's lymphoma. Radiother Oncol 38(1): 13-8
16. Esmaeli B, Faustina M (2005) Orbital Lymphoma In: editor Karcioaeglu ZA. Orbital Tumours: Diagnosis and Treatment. New York: Springer
17. Esmaeli B, McLaughlin P, Pro B *et al.* (2009) Prospective trial of targeted radioimmunotherapy with Y-90 ibritumomab tiuxetan (Zevalin) for front-line treatment of early stage extranodular adnexal lymphoma. Ann Oncol Jan 15. [Epub ahead of print]
18. Esmaeli B, Murray JL, Ahmadi MA *et al.* (2002) Immunotherapy for low-grade non-Hodgkin secondary lymphoma of the orbit. Arch Ophthalmol 120(9): 1225-7
19. **Ferry JA, Fung CY, Zukerberg L *et al.* (2007) Lymphoma of the ocular adnexa: A study of 353 cases. Am J Surg Pathol 31(2): 170-84**
20. Flanders AE, Espinosa GA, Markiewicz DA, Howell DD (1987) Orbital lymphoma. Role of CT and MRI. Radiol Clin North Am 25(3): 601-13
21. Fung CY, Tarbell NJ, Lucarelli MJ *et al.* (2003) Ocular adnexal lymphoma: Clinical behavior of distinct World Health Organisation classification subtypes. Int J Radiat Oncol Biol Phys 57(5): 1382-91
22. Goyal S, Cohler A, Camporeale J *et al.* (2008) Intensity modulated radiotherapy for orbital lymphoma. Radiat Med 26(10): 573-81
23. Gverovic-Antunica A, Markovic I, Bohac M *et al.* (2007) Primary orbital non-Hodgkin's lymphoma: case report. Acta Clin Croatica 46(1): 113-6
24. Harris NL, Jaffe ES, Stein H *et al.* (1994) A revised European-American classification of lymphoid neoplasms: a proposal from the International Lymphoma Study Group. Blood 84(5): 1361-92
25. Hempel M, Hinkelbein W (1993) Eye sequelae following external irradiation. Recent Results Cancer Res 130: 231-6

26. Jaffe ES, Harris NL, Stein H *et al.* (2001) World Health Organization Classification of Tumours. Tumours of Haematopoietic and Lymphoid Tissues. Pathology and Genetics. Lyon: IARC Press

27. Jakobiec FA (1989) Orbital Hodgkin's disease: clinicopathologic conference. N Eng J Med 320: 447-57

28. Jakobiec FA (2008) Ocular adnexal lymphoid tumours: Progress in need of clarification. Am J Ophthalmol 145(6): 941-50

29. Jenkins C, Rose GE, Bunce C *et al.* (2000) Histological features of ocular adnexal lymphoma (REAL classification) and their association with patient morbidity and survival. Br J Ophthalmol 84(8): 907-13

30. Jereb B, Lee H, Jakobiec FA, Kutcher J (1984) Radiation therapy of conjunctival and orbital lymphoid tumours. Int J Radiat Oncol Biol Phys 10(7): 1013-9

31. Knowles DM, Jakobiec FA, McNally L, Burke JS (1990) Lymphoid hyperplasia and malignant lymphoma occurring in the ocular adnexa (orbit, conjunctiva, and eyelids): a prospective multiparametric analysis of 108 cases during 1977 to 1987. Hum Pathol 21(9): 959-73

32. Lee JL, Kim MK, Lee KH *et al.* (2005) Extranodal marginal zone B-cell lymphoma of mucosa-associated lymphoid tissue-type of orbit and ocular adnexa. Ann Hematol 84(1): 13-8

33. Martinet S, Ozsahin M, Belkacémi Y *et al.* (2003) Outcome and prognostic factors in orbital lymphoma: A rare cancer network study on 90 consecutive patients treated with radiotherapy. Int J Radiat Oncol Biol Phys 55(4): 892-8

34. Minehan KJ, Martenson JA Jr, Garrity JA *et al.* (1991) Local control and complications after radiation therapy for primary orbital lymphoma: a case for low-dose treatment. Int J Radiat Oncol Biol Phys 20(5): 791-6

35. Moslehi R, Devesa SS, Schairer C, Fraumeni JF Jr (2006) Rapidly increasing incidence of ocular non-Hodgkin lymphoma. J Natl Cancer Inst 98(13): 936-9

36. Nakata M, Matsuno Y, Katsumata N *et al.* (1999) Histology according to the Revised European-American Lymphoma Classification significantly predicts the prognosis of ocular adnexal lymphoma. Leuk Lymphoma 32(5-6): 533-43

37. Nutting CM, Jenkins CD, Norton AJ *et al.* (2002) Primary orbital lymphoma. Hematol J 3(1): 14-6

38. Ott OJ, Roedel C, Gramatzki M *et al.* (2003) Radiotherapy for stage I-II low-grade non-Hodgkin's lymphoma. Strahlenther Onkol 179(10): 694-701

39. Pfeffer MR, Rabin T, Tsvang L *et al.* (2004) Orbital lymphoma: is it necessary to treat the entire orbit? Int J Radiat Oncol Biol Phys 60(2): 527-30

40. Polito E, Leccisotti A, Galieni P (1996) Clinical and radiological presentation of 95 lymphoid tumours. Graefe Arch Clin Exp Ophtalmol 234(8): 504-9

41. Roe RH, Finger PT, Kurli M *et al.* (2006) Whole-body positron emission tomography/computed tomography imaging and staging of orbital lymphoma. Ophthalmology 113(10): 1854-58

42. Shields CL, Shields JA, Carvalho C *et al.* (2001) Conjunctival lymphoid tumours: clinical analysis of 117 cases and relationship to systemic lymphoma. Ophthalmology 108(5): 979-84

43. Sjo LD (2009) Ophthalmic lymphoma: Epidemiology and pathogenesis. Acta Ophthalmol thesis1: 1-20

44. Song EK, Kim SY, Kim TM *et al.* (2008) Efficacy of chemotherapy as a first-line treatment in ocular adnexal extranodal marginal zone B-cell lymphoma. Ann Oncol 19(2): 242-6

45. Suh CO, Shim SJ, Lee SW *et al.* (2006) Orbital marginal zone B-cell lymphoma of MALT: radiotherapy results and clinical behavior. Int J Radiat Oncol Biol Phys 65(1): 228-33

46. Valenzuela AA, Allen C, Grimes D *et al.* (2006) Positron emission tomography in the detection and staging of ocular adnexal lymphoproliferative disease. Ophthalmology 113(12): 2331-7

Primary MALT lymphoma of the salivary glands

7

Y. Anacak and S. Kamer

Five Essential Points

1. *MALT lymphoma of the salivary glands may develop after Sjögren's syndrome.*
2. *Multiple salivary glands are often involved either at the time of diagnosis or through the course of the disease.*
3. *Staging poses a problem in case of multi-gland involvement.*
4. *Surgery resulting in organ loss should be avoided. Moderate dose (25-30 Gy) radiotherapy is very effective in controlling local disease. Chemotherapy is the treatment of choice in disseminated disease.*
5. *Survival is quite good (>90% at 5 years) despite rather frequent relapses and dissemination.*

Introduction

Mucosa-associated lymphoid tissue (MALT) lymphoma is a distinct entity with specific clinical and pathologic features. The most common site of MALT-lymphoma is the stomach, but it may arise in other organs, the salivary glands being amongst them. Gastric MALT lymphoma tends to remain localized for a long period of time. However MALT lymphoma of the salivary glands usually involves all salivary glands, and has a relatively high rate of multiorgan involvement. There seems to be a strong connection with autoimmune Sjögren's disease as well. In this chapter we summarize clinical features and treatment options for this unique disease with reference to recent literature.

MALT lymphoma is defined as non-encapsulated clusters of lymphocytes. It is typically found throughout the mucosal tissues of the aerodigestive tract and plays an important role in the immune system of the body. Lymphoma arising from MALT was first described by Isaacson and Wright in 1983 [5]. This tumour is a low grade B-cell lymphoma that may involve a variety of extranodal sites, where the most common is stomach, followed by other gastrointestinal organs, respiratory tract and skin. Salivary glands do not contain MALT, but may acquire it as a result of chronic inflammation associated with autoimmune disorders [3, 13]. This involvement is rare and available data is scarce and confined to small series and isolated case reports, thus characteristics of this unique presentation are largely unknown.

MALT lymphoma occurs at a frequency of about 1.5 cases per 100,000 people per year and accounts for about 10% of all non-Hodgkin's lymphomas. It may develop during the course of an autoimmune disease or after a local inflammatory process; gastric MALT lymphoma associated with *Helicobacter pylori* infection is the best example. Theoretically, a malignant clone appears during a prolonged lymphoid proliferation, and is followed by a lymphoma. Autoimmune diseases such as Hashimoto's Thyroiditis and Sjögren's Syndrome are other examples linked with development of MALT lymphoma in the thyroid and salivary glands [9,17,20].

Unlike other tumours, MALT lymphoma may regress following the eradication of the primary cause. The initial therapy against gastric MALT lymphoma is usually directed against Helicobacter pylori using antibiotics, those with persistent tumours being treated with anti-cancer therapies. However there is no similar approach reported for the treatment of MALT lymphoma of other organs.

MALT lymphoma of salivary glands: a unique disease

Malignant lymphoma may occur in the salivary glands as a primary tumour or a metastasis from disseminated disease [2,16]. About 5-10% of NHLs are found in the salivary glands, most frequently in the parotid gland, followed by the submandibular gland, minor salivary glands and sublingual glands; NHLs represent only 1.7% of salivary gland malignancies [12].

The most common subtype is a low-grade B-cell lymphoma categorized in the REAL classification as marginal-zone B-cell lymphoma, extranodal, MALT-type [4]. MALT lymphoma of the salivary glands is predominantly a tumour of adults older than 50 years with a marked female predominance – F/M ratio is around 3/1. The reason for female predominance has not yet been analyzed. However regarding the high rate of Sjögren's syndrome among women (9 out of 10 patients with Sjögren's syndrome are women) and the association of this syndrome with MALT lymphoma, female predominance is not surprising.

As noted above, many patients have a history of Sjögren's syndrome – a chronic autoimmune disorder characterized by lymphocyte-mediated destruction of exocrine glands producing the classical symptoms of dry eyes and dry mouth. Patients with Sjögren's syndrome show a 4.3% prevalence of non-Hodgkin lymphoma (NHL) with a median age at lymphoma diagnosis of 58 years and a median time from Sjögren's syndrome diagnosis to lymphoma diagnosis of 7.5 years [19]. MALT lymphoma constitutes the majority of these lymphomas. The risk of developing a NHL is 44 times and of developing a MALT lymphoma is 28 times higher than in the general population among the patients with Sjögren's syndrome [8, 14].

Frequently both parotids and submandibular glands, even minor salivary glands are affected through the course of the disease, confirming the relation with autoimmune disease [9]. A similar finding is reported for orbital MALT lymphomas, where both eyes are frequently involved. Therefore it should be kept in mind that all salivary glands are at risk, and should be checked for tumour involvement at the time of diagnosis and thereafter. As for all lymphomas, the Ann Arbor system is used, and further management is based on this system. However, it seems inappropriate to classify disease confined to paired organs such as salivary glands and orbits, which could potentially be cured with a local therapy even in advanced disease. MALT lymphoma confined to paired organs has been suggested to be considered a special case of stage II disease [10].

The tendency for multi-gland involvement diminishes the role of surgery for this tumour. Surgery usually results in the loss of a parotid gland unnecessarily, where still tumour deposits are present at the contralateral parotid and other glands. Thus, we recommend avoiding parotidectomy in the management of MALT lymphoma.

Although gastric MALT lymphoma is well known to be an indolent neoplasm without any regional or distant spread for a prolonged period of time, extragastric presentations are rather aggressive. Raderer *et al.* analyzed relapse patterns of MALT lymphomas, where 8 of 36 patients with gastric lymphoma *versus* 24 of 50 nongastric MALT lymphomas (P = 0.02) relapsed, suggesting a higher risk of relapse for extragastric MALT lymphoma [11]. The involvement of regional lymph nodes is quite frequent and distant spread is not unusual. A recent study analyzed 44 new cases of MALT lymphoma of the head and neck region; 23 patients had disseminated disease at the multiple sites and/or lymph node involvement [15].

Management

Until recently, surgery was the standard treatment of MALT lymphomas providing a local control rate of 90%. However the price was the loss of an organ – total gastrectomy, parotidectomy, thyroidectomy etc. For salivary glands in addition to functional loss, tendency to multi-gland involvement means that the tumour may relapse in the other glands despite unilateral parotidectomy, thus surgery should not be the first line treatment. Recently, radiotherapy replaced surgery in the treatment of almost all sites of MALT lymphomas. In a study of 80 patients with MALT lymphoma of various sites, moderate-dose radiotherapy (25-30 Gy) has been shown to be a safe and effective method for early stage (I-II) MALT lymphomas, providing a control rate of 97% [18]. A multicentric phase-II study of the Japan Radiation Oncology Group evaluated the role of radiotherapy in extragastric MALT lymphomas [6]. Complete remission (CR) or CR/unconfirmed was achieved in 34 patients (92%). The 3-year overall survival, progression-free survival, and local control probability were 100%, 91.9%, and 97.3%, respectively. Kalpadakis *et al.* reported 76 patients with extragastric MALT lymphomas, where the tumour was in the salivary glands in 20. Lymph node and bone marrow involvement were noticed in 5/20 and 3/20 patients, respectively. Five patients had an involvement of multiple MALT sites. Half of the patients had a preceding history of Sjögren's syndrome. Cause-specific survival at 5 years was 94% in the whole group despite a 5-year progression-free survival rate of 56% [7].

In a multi-institutional Rare Cancer Network (RCN) study, 62 cases of salivary gland MALT lymphomas from 12 centres were analyzed retrospectively; 21 patients were treated with a single modality and 40 patients were treated with combined modalities where surgery was performed in 45 patients, radiotherapy was given to 41, and chemotherapy to 21 patients. The use of radiotherapy was associated with longer disease-free survival in this study [1]

Chemotherapy has also become another therapeutic option for MALT lymphoma. CHOP-like chemotherapy regimens and the addition of anti-CD20 rituximab is frequently used either alone or in combination with surgery and/or radiotherapy.

MALT lymphoma involving salivary glands may disseminate during its course. In the above mentioned RCN study 37% of the tumours relapsed (22 out of 59). Relapses were local in 4 patients, regional in 8, and distant in 10; tumour spread to other salivary glands occurred in 9 patients (41% of all relapses). Although disease-free survival at 5 years was 53%, disease-specific survival was 92.4% thanks to the indolent nature of this tumour [1]. It is clear that relapses may be late and lifelong observation is required. Transformation to a more aggressive lymphoma occurs rarely, warranting a more aggressive treatment.

7

References

1. **Anacak Y, Miller R, Constantinou N *et al.* (2006) MALT Lymphoma of the Salivary Glands: A Multicenter Rare Cancer Network Study of 59 Patients. Int J Radiat Oncol 66: Suppl-1: S500**
2. Colby TV, Dorfman RF (1979) Malignant lymphomas involving the salivary glands. Pathol Annu 2: 307-24
3. **Harris NL (1999) Lymphoid proliferations of the salivary glands. Am J Clin Pathol 111: S94-S103**
4. Harris NL, Jaffe ES, Stein H *et al.* (1994) A revised European-American classification of lymphoid neoplasms: A proposal from the International Lymphoma Study Group. Blood 84: 1361-92
5. Isaacson PG, Wright DH (1983) Malignant lymphoma of mucosa associated lymphoid tissue. A distinctive of B-cell lymphoma. Cancer 52: 1410-6
6. Isobe K, Kagami Y, Higuchi K *et al.* (2007) A multicenter phase II study of local radiation therapy for stage IEA mucosa-associated lymphoid tissue lymphomas: a preliminary report from the Japan Radiation Oncology Group (JAROG). Int J Radiat Oncol Biol Phys 69: 1181-6
7. Kalpadakis C, Pangalis GA, Vassilakopoulos TP *et al.* (2008) Non-gastric extranodal marginal zone lymphomas – a single centre experience on 76 patients. Leuk Lymphoma 49: 2308-15
8. Kassan SS, Thomas TL, Moutspoulos HM *et al.* (1978) Increased risk of lymphoma in sicca syndrome. Ann Intern Med 89: 888-92
9. **Kojima M, Shimizu K, Nishikawa M *et al.* (2007) Primary salivary gland lymphoma among Japanese: A clinicopathological study of 30 cases. Leuk Lymphoma 48: 1793-8**
10. Mac Manus MP, Ryan G, Lau E *et al.* (2007) Positron emission tomography of stage IV mucosa-associated lymphoid tissue lymphoma confined to the four major salivary glands. Australas Radiol 51: 68-70
11. Raderer M, Streubel B, Woehrer S *et al.* (2005) High relapse rate in patients with MALT lymphoma warrants lifelong follow-up. Clin Cancer Res 11: 3349-52
12. **Roh JL, Huh J, Suh C (2008) Primary non-Hodgkin's lymphomas of the major salivary glands. J Surg Oncol 97: 35-9**
13. Schmid U, Helbron D, Lennert K (1982) Development of malignant lymphoma in myoepithelial sialadenitis (Sjogren's syndrome). Virchows Arch Pathol Anat 395: 11-43
14. Smedby KE, Hjalgrim H, Askling J *et al.* (2006) Autoimmune and chronic inflammatory disorders and risk of non-Hodgkin lymphoma by subtype. J Natl Cancer Inst 98: 51-60
15. Suh C, Huh J, Roh JL (2008) Extranodal marginal zone B-cell lymphoma of mucosa-associated lymphoid tissue arising in the extracranial head and neck region: A high rate of dissemination and disease recurrence. Oral oncology 44: 949-55
16. Tagnon BB, Theate I, Weynand B *et al.* (2002) Long-standing mucosa-associated lymphoid tissue lymphoma of the parotid gland: CT and MR imaging findings. Am J Roentgenol 178: 1563-5
17. Troch M, Woehrer S, Streubel B *et al.* (2008) Chronic autoimmune thyroiditis (Hashimoto's thyroiditis) in patients with MALT lymphoma. Ann Oncol 19: 1336-9
18. Tsang RW, Gospodarowicz MK, Pintilie M *et al.* (2001) Stage I and II MALT lymphoma: results of treatment with radiotherapy. Int J Radiat Oncol Biol Phys 50: 1258-64
19. Voulgarelis M, Dafni UG, Isenberg DA *et al.* (1999) Malignant lymphoma in primary Sjogren's syndrome: a multicenter, retrospective, clinical study by the European Concerted Action on Sjogren's Syndrome. Arthritis Rheum 42: 1765-72
20. **Voulgarelis M, Moutsopoulos H (2008) Mucosa-Associated Lymphoid Tissue Lymphoma in Sjögren's Syndrome: Risks, Management, and Prognosis. Rheum Dis Clin North Am 34: 921-33**

Section 3
Gastro-intestinal tumours

Mucosal melanoma of the upper aero-digestive tract

1

M. Krengli, L. Masini and F. Pia

Five Essential Points

1. *Surgery represents the standard treatment of mucosal melanoma of the upper aero-digestive tract.*
2. *Neck lymph node dissection should be performed in case of oral or pharyngeal location.*
3. *Radiotherapy is recommended as postoperative treatment for macroscopic or microscopic residual disease and when surgery is not feasible.*
4. *Hypofractionation should be considered especially in case of radiotherapy for macroscopic disease to overcome the radioresistance of melanoma cells. In case of 4 Gy/fraction the estimated total dose could be around 50 Gy.*
5. *Systemic therapy (chemotherapy, immunotherapy and targeted therapy) can be useful as palliative treatments in case of advanced unresectable or recurrent disease.*

Introduction

Mucosal melanoma of the upper aero-digestive tract is a rare tumour representing less than 2% of all melanoma cases and 0.4%-10% of head and neck melanomas. The incidence is higher in the population older than 50 years with a slight predominance for male gender. The most common anatomic sites of the upper respiratory tract are the nasal septum, turbinates, lateral wall of the nasal fossae and maxillary and ethmoid sinuses while hard palate and alveolus are the most frequent locations in the oral cavity. Very rare mucosal melanomas are those of the pharynx, larynx and oesophagus [16, 28]. Sinonasal melanoma seems to have better prognosis than oral and pharyngeal melanoma [23, 32]. The general prognosis is related to the risk of both local recurrence and distant metastases that occur approximately in 20%-55% [10, 15, 20-22, 31, 32, 35] 20%-55% and [7, 10, 15, 21, 22, 31, 32] 25%-65% of cases respectively. This chapter is devoted to a description of the clinical and diagnostic aspects and the treatment strategy for the management of mucosal melanoma of the upper aero-digestive tract.

Diagnosis

Biopsy is necessary for diagnosis and possibly for the assessment of thickness and penetration of the primary lesion. The diagnosis of mucosal melanoma is generally based on identification of intracellular melanin detectable in 50%-70% of biopsy and surgical specimens [15]. Recently, immunochemistry has greatly improved the accuracy of diagnosis thanks to the use of S-100, NKI/C-3, HBM-45, and vimentin (Fig. 1). Three types of mucosal melanoma can be distinguished based on cell features: spindle cell, polygonal cell, and mixed cell. Advanced disease stage, tumour invasion deeper than 5-7 mm, and multicentricity are associated with a worse prognosis. A variant of melanoma called desmoplastic melanoma was described and found, although less frequently than in the skin, also in the mucosae, with higher potential of local recurrence and lower frequency of distant metastases [25].

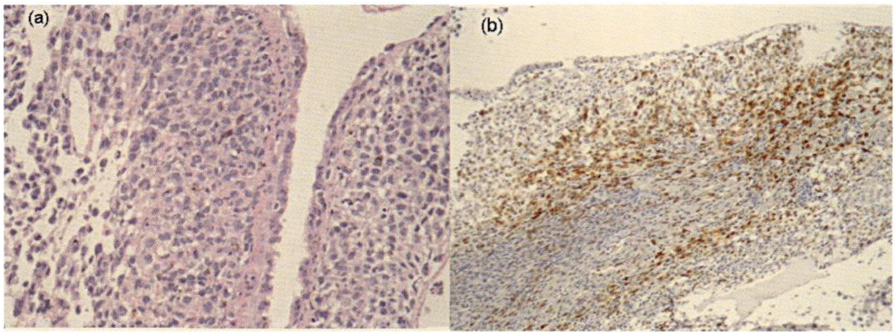

Fig. 1. Mucosal melanoma cells invading the mucosa of the respiratory tract; H&E, o.m. 20x (a). Atypical cells at the basal layer of the squamous epithelium positive for S100 protein at immunochemistry; H&E, o.m. 10x (b).

The staging procedure should include accurate physical examination and fiberoptic endoscopy (Fig. 2) to assess extent of local and regional disease. CT and/or MR are recommended to better define the involvement of bone and soft tissues in depth (Fig. 3). Metastastic workup should be completed with chest x-rays, liver US, and bone-scan. CT-scan of chest and brain are optional and necessary in case of doubt at chest x-rays or presence of symptoms. PET has recently gained interest in the staging as well as for cutaneous melanoma. Several staging criteria have been used with the Ballantyne's system being the most commonly applied (stage I, primary localized lesion; stage II, cervical lymph node metastasis; stage III, distant metastasis) [1, 15, 22, 35].

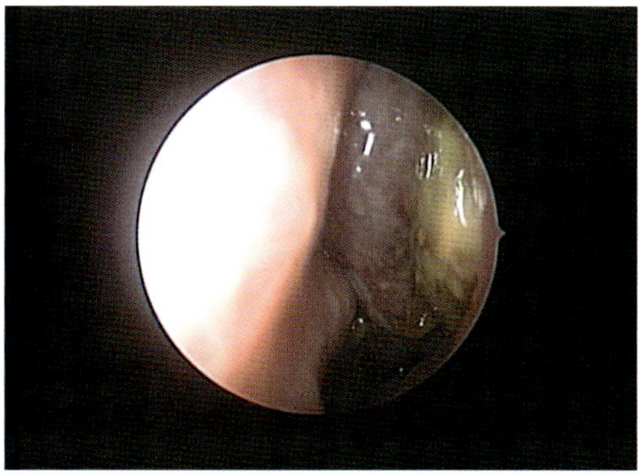

Fig. 2. Fibre endoscopy showing an irregular area of dark pigmented mucosa between nasal septum (left) and turbinate (right) corresponding to the ethmoid region.

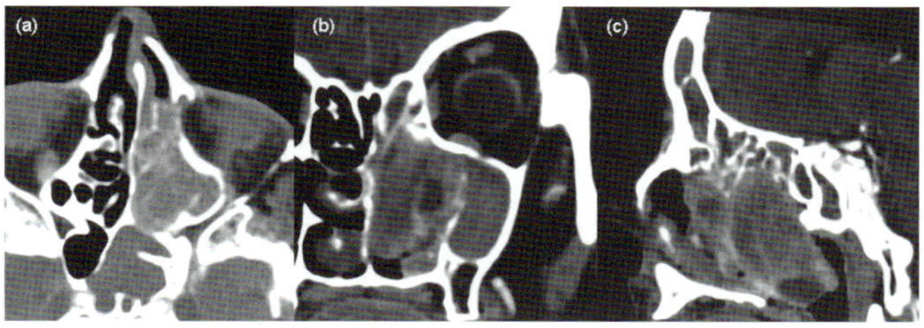

Fig. 3. Axial (a), coronal (b) and sagittal (c) post-contrast computer tomography images showing a mass arising from the nasal cavity with compression of turbinates and invasion of the ethmoid cells. The lateral wall of the maxillary sinus is deformed and partially invaded.

Treatment modality

Traditionally, surgery represents the fundamental treatment modality of mucosal melanoma of the upper aero-digestive tract. Radiotherapy can be used in combination with surgery or as sole treatment modality in case of inoperable disease. Systemic treatment using chemotherapy and immunotherapy has mainly a palliative role in case of advanced, unresectable and metastatic disease.

Surgery

Current knowledge about the results of treatment for mucosal melanoma of the upper aero-digestive tract comes from retrospective studies based on a limited number of cases.

Most authors agree on the primary role of surgery in local control of the disease [3, 4, 14, 15, 17, 22, 23]. The type of surgical approach has not been well defined and remains strictly correlated to the involved sub-site and the size and stage of the tumour. However, there is a general consensus that surgery should achieve a wide resection with possibly wide negative margins.

Nasal cavity and paranasal sinuses

Alongside traditional "open" surgery, recent surgical methods have included endoscopic sinus surgery, typically used in the early tumour stages. This type of surgery is based on the use of rigid endoscopes with optics set at varying angles, giving different views, associated with the use of diode laser equipment which allows surgeons to carry out subpericondral and subperiostium dissections thus minimising local bleeding. Such endoscopic methods can be used with success on early-stage lesions located in the nasal septum, on the lower and middle turbinates and on small peduncolated melanomas on the lateral nasal walls and in the nasopharynx: in case of peduncolated lesions, a dissection with wide macroscopic margins of healthy tissue must be carried out. In case of local recurrence, a radical resection using open techniques should be performed. Endoscopic treatment should not be used when melanomas have infiltrated into the deeper tissues. Therefore, when melanoma is deeply rooted, wide and/or multi-centric, surgery should be more extensive by using degloving resection or lateral rhinotomy [19].

Oral cavity

The most frequently affected sub-sites are the hard palate, the maxillary alveolus and the lip whereas occurrence in the tongue and the floor of the mouth are rarer. Patel *et al.* [22] underline that in oral locations there is greater incidence of multifocality (22%) and regional nodal involvement at diagnosis (25%). Currently, surgery with clear margins offers the best probability for cure and local control [15, 23].

Surgery should obtain wide and deep free margins and therefore a resection of the hard palate with reconstruction using endo-prosthesis should be performed in case of hard palate lesions and partial resection of the upper maxillary bone should be planned for gum melanomas. In other sites, on-demand surgery should be carried out and the use of diode laser equipment should be preferred whenever possible.

Neck lymph nodes

There is no general consensus on prophylactic treatment of clinically negative lymph nodes in mucosal melanoma of the oral cavity. However, considering that

1

local failures are reported as high as 51% and nodal failure as 42% for lesions originating from the oral cavity, it seems appropriate in such cases to carry out a wide tumour resection associated with selective neck dissection for levels I-II-III in deeply rooted or widely extended cases or in case of stage II disease [22].

Recent studies addressed the issue of sentinel node biopsy in the management of head and neck melanoma arising from both skin and mucosae. In some series, the sentinel node status was correlated to thicker and ulcerated tumours and was seen as predictor of disease-free survival [13] whereas in others was associated with an early haematogenous dissemination [30]. Therefore the sentinel lymph node status might be useful in the treatment decision, although further studies are warranted to confirm its role.

Radiotherapy combined with surgery

For several years, melanoma has been considered a typical radio-resistant tumour and very few literature studies using radiotherapy can be found. More recent radiobiological data, shows that melanoma cells have a large range of radiosensitivity suggesting that radiation may have a more relevant role in the treatment of this disease possibly using high dose per fraction [34].

The high rate of loco-regional recurrence of mucosal melanoma after surgical resection varying in most series from 40% to 55% [9, 10, 15, 20-22] justifies the use of radiotherapy in the postoperative setting. Analyzing the published studies, most authors recommend the use of radiotherapy in case of high risk of tumour remnants such as for deep tumour infiltration, close or positive margins and/or anatomic sites requiring difficult and elaborate surgical approaches such as for sinonasal tumour location.

Over the last 20 years, only few retrospective series can be found with a relevant number of cases treated by postoperative radiotherapy (Table 1). These series report on both sinonasal and oral tumour locations treated with doses ranging from 14 to

Table 1 – Retrospective studies over the last 20 years with at least 15 cases in which patients were treated with postoperative radiotherapy.

Author	N° of patients treated with postoperative RT/total	Total RT dose	Outcome
Nandapalan *et al.* 1998[20]	23/259	NA	5-yr DFS = 45% 10-yr DFS = 28% LR = 52%
Patel *et al.* 2002[22]	18/59	NA	5-yr OS = 35% 5-yr DSS = 44% LR = 51%
Owens *et al.* 2003[21]	24/48	30 - 60 Gy	5-yr OS = 26% LR = 17%
Temam *et al.* 2003[32]	39/69	50 - 70 Gy	5-yr OS = 20% LR = 54%
Krengli *et al.* 2006[10]	42/74	14 - 70 Gy	5-yr OS = 28% 5-yr DSS = 47% 5-yr DFS = 28% LR = 31%

Abbreviations: NA not available; OS overall survival; DSS disease specific survival; DFS disease free survival; LR local recurrence; RT radiotherapy.

70 Gy, depending on the fractionation scheme to a quite inhomogeneous target volume mainly limited to the primary tumour site and extended to the lymph node regions in a few cases of oral location. The overall and disease-free survival rates at 5 years range from 20% to 35% and from 28% to 45%, while the local relapse rate was 17% to 54% respectively.

Radiotherapy is currently recommended in case of positive or close excision margins for invasive melanoma which are considered unfavourable prognostic factors in most recent literature series [17, 23]. In some reports, postoperative irradiation is more often used in the sinonasal than oral tumour localizations because of the inherent difficulty in obtaining satisfactory surgical clearance in sinonasal tumours [4].

Radiotherapy alone

In case of unresectable disease, radiotherapy represents the most effective treatment modality. Very different radiotherapy approaches have been used for the treatment of macroscopic disease including external photon radiotherapy, brachytherapy and also neutron and ion therapy. The most relevant retrospective literature studies are reported in Table 2. Overall survival rates at 5 years range from 15% to 28% with local control of 61%-85%. External beam radiotherapy seems to be more efficacious by using a dose per fraction of ≥ 4 Gy giving a local control rate of up to 86% [8]. Shibuya *et al.* report on the use of brachytherapy and electron beam radiotherapy by intra-oral cone with a local control rate of 75% and 5-year overall survival of 25% [29].

In order to overcome the alleged radioresistance, alternative treatments with high linear energy transfer (LET) radiation such as neutrons and light ions were tested. The first experience with neutron radiotherapy in the treatment of melanoma was performed at the Hammersmith Hospital, UK. In a series of 48 melanomas, 4 of them arising from the mucosa, local control was obtained in 71% of cases, with only 9% local recurrence rate after initial complete regression [2]. A subsequent study of Tsunemoto *et al.* [33] is reported in table 2.

Carbon ion radiotherapy was used at the National Institute for Radiological Sciences in Chiba, Japan, to treat 72 patients mainly with mucosal melanoma from sinonasal origin to a total dose of 52.8-64.0 GyE with fractions of 3.6-4.0 Gy. The results were very encouraging with a 5-year local control and overall survival rates of 84.1% and 27.0% respectively [36].

Table 2 – Retrospective studies in which patients were treated with radiotherapy alone.

Author	N° of patients treated with RT alone/total	Type of radiation	Total RT dose	Outcome
Tsunemoto *et al.* 1989[33]	20/20	neutrons	16.2 Gy	5-yr OS = 15% 10-yr OS = 8%
Gilligan *et al.* 1991[6]	28/28	photons	50 - 55 Gy	LC = 61% 5-yr OS = 18%
Shibuya *et al.* 1992[29]	28/28	photons	50 - 76 Gy (EBRT) 50 - 120 Gy (BRT)	LC = 75% 5-yr OS = 25%
Wada *et al.* 2004[35]	21/66	photons	32 - 64 Gy	3-yr DSS = 33%
Yanagi *et al.* 2005[36]	76/76	carbon ions	57.6 - 64.0 Gy	5-yr LC = 84% 5-yr OS = 27%

Legend: OS: overall survival; LC: local control; RT: radiotherapy; EBRT: external beam radiotherapy; BRT: brachytherapy.

It can be concluded from these studies that high local tumour control rates can be achieved with radiotherapy alone and there are some preliminary indications that the results could be improved by using high-LET radiation.

Systemic treatment

Currently, no standard systemic therapeutic regimen exists for metastatic mucosal melanoma and the rarity of the disease makes it difficult to assess the clinical efficacy of systemic therapy. Chemotherapy and immunotherapy have been quite frequently used in a non-controlled fashion mainly with palliative and in some cases with adjuvant intent. Many agents have been investigated for antitumour activity in melanoma, but few showed promising response rates. The most frequently used chemotherapy agents are dacarbazine, carmustine, epidoxorubicin, cisplatin, vinblastine and vindesine. Dacarbazine is the most widely used chemotherapy drug for the treatment of metastatic melanoma, although the response rate is only 14% to 20%, the median response duration is 4 to 6 months and less than 2% of patients survives at least 6 years. [12, 18]. More recently, temozolomide has demonstrated efficacy equal to that of dacarbazine in a randomized phase III trial with the additional benefit of being a convenient oral treatment that penetrates the blood-brain barrier [26, 27]. High dose IL-2 showed response rates similar to those observed with standard chemotherapy. However, unlike chemotherapy, IL-2 achieved low but durable complete response rates that may lead to years of benefit for patients with metastatic melanoma. Data from the randomized trials demonstrated that single-agent IL-2, when given in high dose, can elicit an objective response rate of 5%-27%, with a complete response in 0%-4% of patients and a long-term response rates ranging from 6 to 66 months [5, 24]. Another possible approach deserving further investigation may be represented by the combination of systemic drugs and radiation. The recent progresses in targeted therapy showing its positive interaction with radiation for squamous cell head and neck carcinoma may open interesting perspectives for other tumour types such as melanoma [11].

References

1. Ballantyne AJ (1970) Malignant melanoma of the skin and the head and neck. Am J Surg 4: 425-31.
2. Blake PR, Catteral M, Errington RD (1985) Treatment of malignant melanoma by fast neutrons. Br J Surg 72: 517-9
3. Bradley PJ (2006) Primary malignant mucosal melanoma of the head and neck. Curr Opin Otolaryngol Head Neck Surg 14: 100-4
4. Bridger AG, Smee D, Baldwin MA *et al.* (2005) Experience with mucosal melanoma of the nose and paranasal sinuses. ANZ J Surg 75: 192-7
5. Eton O, Legha SS, Bedikian AY *et al.* (2002) Sequential biochemotherapy versus chemotherapy for metastatic melanoma: results from a Phase III randomized trial. J Clin Oncol 20: 2045-52
6. Gilligan D, Slevin NJ (1991) Radical radiotherapy for 28 cases of mucosal melanoma in the nasal cavity and sinuses. Brit J Radiol 64: 1147-50
7. Guzzo M, Grandi C, Licitra L *et al.* (1993) Mucosal malignant melanoma of head and neck: forty-eight cases treated at Istituto Nazionale Tumori of Milan. Eur J Surg Oncol 19: 316-9
8. Harwood AR, Cummings BJ (1982) Radiotherapy for mucosal melanoma. Int J Radiat Oncol Biol Phys 8: 1121-1126
9. Kingdom TT, Kaplan MJ (1995) Mucosal melanoma of the nasal cavity and paranasal sinuses. Head Neck 17: 184-9
10. Krengli M, Masini L, Kaanders JHAM *et al.* (2006) Radiotherapy in the treatment of mucosal melanoma of the upper aero-digestive tract. A rare cancer network study. Int J Radiat Oncol Biol Phys 65: 751-9

11. Krengli M, Jereczek-Fossa BA, Kaanders JHAM *et al.* (2008) What is the role of radiotherapy in the treatment of mucosal melanoma of the head and neck? Crit Rev Oncol Hematol 65(2): 121-8

12. Lengyel E, Gilde K, Remanar E, Esik O (2003) Malignant Mucosal Melanoma of the Head and Neck – a Review. Pathology Oncology Research 9: 7-12
13. Leong SP, Accortt NA, Essner R *et al.* (2006) Impact of sentinel node status and other risk factors on the clinical outcome of head and neck melanoma patients. Arch Otolaryngol Head Neck Surg 132: 370-3
14. Lund VJ, Howard DJ, Harding L, Wei WI (1999) Management options and survival in malignant melanoma of the sinonasal mucosa. Laryngoscope 109: 208-11

15. Manolidis S, Donald PJ (1997) Malignant mucosal melanoma of the head and neck. Review of the literature and report of 14 patients. Cancer 80: 1373-86

16. McLaughlin CC, Wu XC, Jemal A *et al.* (2005) Incidence of noncutaneous melanomas in the U.S. Cancer 103: 1000-7

17. Mendenhall WM, Amdur RJ, Hinerman RW *et al.* (2005) Head and neck mucosal melanoma. Am J Clin Oncol 28: 626-30

18. Middleton MR, Grob JJ, Aaronson N *et al.* (2000) Randomized phase III study of Temozolamide versus Dacarbazine in treatment of patients with advanced metastatic malignant melanoma. J Clin Oncol 18: 158-66
19. Nakaya M, Mochiki M, Takeuchi S *et al.* (2004) Malignant melanoma of nasal cavity: report of 16 Japanese patients. Auris Nasus Larynx 31: 233-7
20. Nandapalan V, Roland NJ, Helliwell TR *et al.* (1998) Mucosal melanoma of the head and neck. Clin Otolaryngol 23: 107-16
21. Owens JM, Roberts DB, Myers JN (2003) The role of postoperative adjuvant radiation therapy in the treatment of mucosal melanomas of the head and neck region. Arch Otolaryngol Head Neck Surg129: 864-8

22. Patel SG, Prasad ML, Escrig M *et al.* (2002) Primary mucosal malignant melanoma of the head and neck. Head Neck 24: 247-57

23. Penel N, Mallet Y, Mirabel X *et al.* (2006) Primary mucosal melanoma of head and neck: prognostic value of clear margins. Laryngoscope 116: 993-5
24. Petrella T, Quirt I, Verna S and the members of the Melanoma Disease Site Group of Cancer Care Ontario' Program in Evidence-Based Care (2007) Single-agent interleukin 2 in the treatment of metastatic melanoma. Curr Oncol 14: 21-6
25. Prasad ML, Patel SG, Busam KJ (2004) Primary mucosal desmoplastic melanoma of the head and neck. Head Neck 26: 373-7
26. Quirt I, Verma S, Petrella T *et al.* (2007) Temozolamide for the treatment of metastatic melanoma: a systematic review. Oncologist 12: 1114-23
27. Quirt I, Verna S, Petrella T, Bak K, Charette M and the members of the Melanoma Disease Site Group of Cancer Care Ontario' Program in Evidence-Based Care (2007) Temozolamide for the treatment of metastatic melanoma. Curr Oncol 14: 27-33
28. Rapini RP, Golitz LE, Greer RO *et al.* (1985) Primary malignant melanoma of the oral cavity. A review of 177 cases. Cancer 55: 1543-51
29. Shibuya H, Takeda M, Matsumoto S *et al.* (1992) The efficacy of radiation therapy for a malignant melanoma in the mucosa of the upper jaw: an analytic study. Int J Radiat Oncol Biol Phys 25: 35-9
30. Starek I, Koranda P, Benea P (2006) Sentinel lymph node biopsy: a new perspective in head and neck mucosal melanoma? Melanoma Res 16: 423-7
31. Stern SJ, Guillamondegui OM (1991) Mucosal melanoma of the head and neck. Head Neck 27: 13-22
32. Temam S, Mamelle G, Marandas P *et al.* (2005) Postoperative radiotherapy for primary mucosal melanoma of the head and neck. Cancer 103: 313-9
33. Tsunemoto H, Morita S, Moris (1989) Characteristics of malignant melanoma cells in the treatment with fast neutrons. Pigment Cell Res 2: 372-8
34. Van den Aardweg GJMJ, Naus NC, Verhoeven ACA *et al.* (2003) Cellular radiosensitivity of primary and metastatic human uveal melanoma cell lines. Invest Ophthalmol Vis Sci 44: 4660-4
35. Wada H, Nemoto K, Ogawa Y *et al.* (2004) A multi-institutional retrospective analysis of external radiotherapy for mucosal melanoma of the head and neck in northern Japan. Int J Radiat Oncol Biol Phys 59: 495-500
36. Yanagi T, Mizoe J, Hasegawa A *et al.* (2009) Mucosal melanoma of the head and neck treated by carbon ion radiotherapy. Int J Radiat Oncol Biol Phys 74: 15-20

Gastrointestinal stromal tumours[1]

2

M. Montemurro, J.-Y. Blay and S. Leyvraz

Five Essential Points

1. *GIST are malignant mesenchymal tumours caused by a pathogenetic mutation in the KIT or* PDGFRA *gene which is probably the initial oncogenic molecular event.*
2. *Localized GIST can be cured by surgery only, with tumour-free resection margins being of utmost importance. Adjuvant treatment with imatinib reduces the risk of recurrence. Advanced GIST should be treated with TKIs until progression or intolerance. First-line treatment is imatinib 400 mg/d, with the exception of GIST with* KIT *Exon 9 mutation where 800 mg/d is the suggested starting dose.*
3. *Upon progression, imatinib dose should be increased to 800 mg/d where applicable, then treatment switched to sunitinib, sequentially followed by nilotinib. Sorafenib and trial drugs are additional options.*
4. *TKI treatment in metastatic patients should never be stopped for reasons other than progression, intolerance or patient refusal.*
5. *Staging and follow-up of GIST can be cumbersome, and CT should be liberally supplemented by MRI and PET if necessary. Choi-criteria should be used instead of RECIST for TKI response monitoring.*

Introduction

Gastrointestinal stromal tumours (GIST) are rare mesenchymal tumours derived from the interstitial cells of Cajal. Mutations in the *KIT* gene leading to a constitutively activated KIT receptor protein are the most frequent pathogenetic aberration causing clinical GIST. Diagnosis is based on a typical histomorphological appearance and the immunohistochemical detection of the KIT receptor protein (synonym CD117).

Size of tumour, mitotic count, anatomic tumour location and underlying mutation determine the prognosis.

Tyrosine kinase inhibitors (TKI), e.g. imatinib, sunitinib and nilotinib, inhibit the activity of this receptor (or this family of receptors) by blocking the tyrosine kinase domain which phosphorylates downstream signalling molecules.

The selection of treatment depends on extent of disease: surgery is the curative treatment of choice for localised GIST. The role of adjuvant treatment with TKIs is currently being investigated, with 3 ongoing randomized trials and the ACOSOG Z9001 trial that showed a significant increase of recurrence-free survival with adjuvant treatment.

---

1. Many thanks to Annick van den Abbeele for critical comments. We gratefully acknowledge kind provision of figures by Annick van den Abbeele and Gerhard Goerres.

For advanced or metastatic GIST, TKIs are the treatment of choice, considerably extending overall survival to 4.5 years in all studies with sufficient follow-up. Imatinib is used in first-line, sunitinib in 2nd-line and nilotinib is currently investigated in 3rd-line treatment of GIST. Median progression-free survival is 18-24 months in first-line imatinib treatment and 24 weeks for second-line sunitinib. Progression occurs due to secondary mutations, selection of resistant clones or activation of alternative signal transduction pathways, therefore research aims at increasing tyrosine kinase inhibition or blockade of alternate signal transduction pathways and targets.

Selected patients with advanced or metastatic GIST might benefit from preoperative ("neoadjuvant") treatment with TKIs followed by surgery, in particular those in whom complete resection is uncertain or in whom mutilating surgery is foreseen.

Size-based response assessments (RECIST) have their flaws and should be used together with density measurements (Choi criteria). Positron emission tomography might add useful information and should be considered for selected patients. Regular, risk adapted follow-up is recommended.

This chapter will provide insight into the epidemiology, pathogenesis, diagnosis and treatment of the disease and give some advice on follow-up for sporadic GIST in adult patients.

A long history of tyrosine kinase inhibitor development

Several findings were critical for the establishment of current standards for diagnosis and treatment of GIST today. Chromosomal alterations became a recognized feature of malignant disease when Nowell and Hungerford [43] discovered in 1960 the later-termed Philadelphia Chromosome. Only in 1990 was its potent tyrosine kinase function [35] identified and some years later its successful *in vitro* inhibition shown [22]. Druker *et al.* [23] then reported the clinical efficacy of imatinib as therapy for chronic myelogenous leukemias. In 1998 Hirota *et al.* [30] described a pathogenetic gain-of-function KIT mutation in GIST. This together with data of successful *in vitro* KIT inhibition [28] led to the first imatinib treatment of a patient with GIST by Joensuu *et al.* [31] in 2001 being the starting point of targeted therapies in GIST.

Epidemiology

Unknown first then underestimated in the past, a recent population-based study determined the incidence of gastrointestinal stromal tumours (GIST) as 15 per million [42]. Small asymptomatic GISTs, a few millimeters in size, seem to be extremely frequent, identified in approximately 30% of cases in recent pathology series [12]. These GIST carry the same histological and molecular characteristics as the symptomatic larger GIST [12], suggesting that additional molecular events are critical to the development of full GIST [14]. Occurrence of GIST is usually sporadic, and only rarely familial, paediatric, related to neurofibromatosis type I or associated to disease syndromes [14, 38]. Sporadic GISTs are diagnosed at a median age of 59-63 years, ranging from neonates to the oldest, with no gender predominance [19].

Clinical presentation and clinical diagnosis

Two thirds of patients with GISTs present with symptoms such as gastrointestinal bleeding, intra-abdominal haemorrhage, dysphagia or abdominal pain, rarely obstruction, while 20% of GISTs are incidentally found at endoscopy, radiological imaging or surgery for other reasons. Most GISTs arise from the stomach (50-60%), small bowel (25%) or colon/rectum (10%). Half of all patients are affected with metastatic disease at presentation. Liver metastases and/or dissemination inside the abdominal cavity are frequent, while lymph node metastases are extremely rare [19].

Current guidelines [10, 19] propose contrast-enhanced triphasic CT-scan as the imaging modality of choice for both staging and surgical planning of patients with GIST. Magnetic resonance imaging (MRI) might be especially useful for pelvic disease or if radiation exposure is of concern. 18-Fluorodeoxyglucose-positron emission tomography (FDG-PET) combined with CT is more sensitive than CT alone in the detection of GIST.

A sufficient amount of tissue is needed to histologically confirm GIST. Small tumours suspicious of GIST should therefore be resected without biopsy. The use of preoperative biopsies is controversial: generally considered as standard in sarcoma, some experts advocate their avoidance as GISTs are vascularized, fragile tumours and the risk of haemorrhage and tumour dissemination needs to be considered. No consensus on this point is provided by the 2008 guidelines [10]. Biopsy should be performed if the diagnosis is uncertain or before preoperative treatment with TKIs. Endoscopic biopsy is preferred to percutaneous biopsy, where applicable [10, 19].

Histology

GISTs are thought to emerge from the interstitial cells of Cajal or its precursors [24]. Histologically, spindle cell morphology is most frequent; much less common are GISTs with epitheloid or mixed spindle-epitheloid cell morphology [38]. The diagnosis is confirmed upon immunohistochemical detection of the receptor protein KIT, which remains the single most specific marker, positive in 95% of cases [24, 38]. If staining is negative for KIT, diagnosis can be confirmed by mutational analysis: half of these tumours carry oncogenic *KIT* and a third *PDGFRA (platelet-derived growth-factor alpha)* gene mutations [14]. In tumours negative for both KIT and mutational analysis, diagnosis is based on exclusion, e.g. leiomyosarcoma and leiomyoma stain positive for desmin and negative for KIT [38].

The terms c-kit, CD117, kit, CD117-antigen, SCFR, KIT-antigen are often used synonymously in different typing for both receptor and corresponding gene. The official nomenclature is "KIT" for the receptor protein and *"KIT"* in italics for the corresponding gene.

Pathogenesis

Oncogenic mutations in the *KIT* or (*PDGFRA*) gene are probably an initial or very early molecular event for the development of GIST. Close homologues, KIT and PDGFRA receptors belong to the family of receptor tyrosine kinases (RTK). Physiologically, extracellular ligand binding leads to phosphorylation of tyrosine residues in the cytoplasmatic domain of RTKs activating in turn multiple downstream signalling pathways [32]. But, in GIST these receptors are constitutively activated as a consequence of underlying gain-of-function mutations. Two-thirds of GIST harbour mutations in *KIT* exon 11, 10% in *KIT* exon 9 and 5% in *PDGRFA* exon 18, with *KIT* and *PDGFRA* mutations being mutually exclusive. Wild-type GISTs (10%) show no detectable mutation [14]. Deletions or deletion-insertions, missense (point) mutations and (tandem) duplications have been determined by DNA sequencing as being most frequent [33], mapped and correlations of distinct mutations to histology, location of primary tumour and prognosis established [2, 36]. Mutant *KIT* receptors are stabilized by heat shock protein 90 (HSP) increasing their half-life [5]. Oncogenic pathways involved in GIST signalling and cytogenetic profiles differ between different mutations and additional chromosomal alterations occur in GIST progression [14].

TKI, such as imatinib, sunitinib or nilotinib, impair the phosphorylation of the tyrosine kinase domain interrupting the oncogenic signalling [32].

Localised disease - surgery, prognosis and adjuvant therapy

Surgery

Localized GISTs should be resected with negative microscopic margins, strictly avoiding tumour rupture [10, 19]. Resections of choice are wedge for gastric, segmental for intestinal and preferably wide resections for esophageal, duodenal and rectal GIST. Lymph node dissection is usually not warranted as hematologic hepatic spread is the main route of dissemination. Laparoscopic surgery can be considered for small to intermediate tumours if principles of oncologic surgery are met [10, 19].

Prognosis

After complete resection of localized primary GIST median overall survival (OS) is 66 months *vs*. 22 months if incompletely resected (R2) [15]. While survival of low-risk patients equals that of the normal population [42], unfortunately 40% of all [15] and the majority of high-risk patients [37] will relapse. Relapse risk depends on tumour size, mitotic index [24] (so called Fletcher, consensus or NIH criteria; Table 1) and tumour location [37] (Miettinen-classification; Table 2). High-risk GISTs are either gastric GIST with > 5 cm size **plus** a mitotic index > 5 ("double 5") or non-gastric GIST with > 5 mitotic index **or** >10 cm of size ("5 or 10").

Table 1 – Prognosis of GIST (pre-imatinib era) by tumour size and mitotic activity [24].

Risk	Tumour size [cm]	Mitotic count/50 HPF
Very low	> 2	< 5
Low	2-5	< 5
Intermediate	< 5 5-10	6-10 < 5
High	> 5 > 10 Any	> 5 Any > 10
	Resected metastases at diagnosis	

Table 2 – Prognosis of GIST by mitotic rate, tumour size and anatomic tumour localization (pre-imatinib era) – risk of progressive disease and death [37].

Mitotic count per 50 HPFs	Tumour size [cm]	Gastric	Small intestine: Duodenum	Small intestine: Jejunum or ileum	Rectum
≤ 5	≤ 2	None	None	None	None
	2-5	Very Low (2%)	Low (4%)	Low (8%)	Low (8%)
	5-10	Low (4%)	Intermediate (24%)	NA	NA
	> 10	Intermediate (10%)	High (52%)	High (34%)	High (57%)
> 5	≤ 2	None†	High†	NA	High (54%)
	2-5	Intermediate (16%)	High (73%)	High (50%)	High (52%)
	5-10	High (55%)	High (85%)	NA	NA
	> 10	High (86%)	High (90%)	High (86%)	High (71%)

NA: not available due to insufficient data; † very small case number.
(Table modified from Miettinen *et al.*[37]).

Mutational status did not retain a prognostic value on multivariate analysis, but correlations of outcome, primary tumour site and subtypes of mutations (e.g. within exon 11 *KIT* mutations) may still need to be further explored [17].

Adjuvant treatment

Adjuvant treatment with imatinib is currently being investigated in 3 randomized trials, the intergroup EORTC 62024 (400 mg/d imatinib for 2 years *vs.* no treatment), the SSG/AIO trial for high-risk GIST (400 mg/d imatinib 1 year *vs.* 3 years duration of treatment), and a Japanese sarcoma group trial (randomizing imatinib 400 mg/d 1 year *vs.* 6 months).

Today's information on adjuvant treatment stems mostly from the terminated ACOSOG Z9001 trial [16], which randomized patients with primary, KIT expressing GIST of at least 3 cm size to adjuvant imatinib of 1 year duration *vs.* placebo. Planned interim analysis had shown a significant improvement of recurrence-free survival for imatinib patients which has led to an early trial stop after 644 of 708 patients randomized. One year RFS was 98% *vs.* 83% for all patients, the benefit increasing with risk. As cross-over was allowed no differences in OS were seen. Adjuvant imatinib is now recommended and registered in many countries for patients at risk of relapse. It should be given for at least one year and prolongation should be re-evaluated upon release of new data from the EORTC and Scandinavian trials [39].

Advanced disease – tyrosine kinase inhibitors, mutational status and outcome

Definition

Often used synonymously and overlapping, the terms advanced, metastatic or unresectable GIST generally refer to a situation where the tumour has spread beyond the primary tumour site, or where a complete resection (R0) is not achievable at all

2

or only by extensive, mutilating surgery. In this group of patients surgery should be undertaken only after careful consideration or avoided completely. Selected patients might benefit from neoadjuvant TKIs therapy (see below) of 6-12 months duration, ongoing response supposed, which might ultimately allow adequate resection. Neoadjuvant treatment is currently considered investigational but is often used in clinical practice for individual patients to reduce tumour size facilitating future surgery [10, 19, 39].

Prognosis

Median OS for patients with metastatic GIST treated without imatinib was 12 months only according to SEER data [4] and 19 months in a large surgical series [27], with resection status (R0 *vs.* R1/R2 *vs.* no resection) significantly influencing survival.

Tyrosine Kinase Inhibitors

The introduction of the TKI imatinib has considerably improved outcome for these patients. Since then more than 1700 patients have been treated in clinical trials [7, 8, 50] and the efficacy and safety of imatinib clearly demonstrated, with the results being very consistent throughout all studies (Table 3). Assessed with CT, using RECIST, 52-54% of the patients achieved combined complete and partial response (CR, PR) and an additional 28-32% stable disease (SD) [7, 8, 50] to imatinib in first-line metastatic GIST (Table 3). Median time to best response was 107 days [50] and most responses occurred in the first 9 months. Median OS is 51-57 months, while progression-free survival is 18-24 months [7, 8, 50]. Surprisingly, partial response and stable disease resulted in a similar survival benefit.

Response to imatinib depends on the underlying mutation at diagnosis (Table 3).

Table 3 – Overview - Clinical trials in GIST.

	B2222 phase II [7]	**Europe/Austral Asian phase III [49, 50]**	**North American SWOG S0033 [8]**	**Sunitinib phase III [18, 20]**	**Sunitinib treatment trial [41]**
Main design	IM 400 *vs.* 600	IM 400 *vs.* 800, cross over if PD	IM 400 *vs.* 800, cross over if PD	SU 50 *vs.* Placebo	SU 50, open label
N	147	946	746	312	1091
mFU [months]	63	42	54	6	9
mOS [months]	57	49 (all)	55 *vs.* 51 (n.s.)	17	17
mPFS [months]	24 (mTTP)	23	18 *vs.* 20 (n.s.)	6	9
RR (all pts) CR & PR/SD	68%/16%	52%/32%	45%/24%	7%/58%	n.a.
***KIT* Exon 11* CR & PR [44]**	86%	69%	67%	36% (PR/SD) [29]	n.a.
***KIT* Exon 9* CR & PR [44]**	48%	34%	40%	63% (PR/SD) [29]	n.a.

IM = Imatinib; SU = Sunitinib; PD = progressive disease; all doses given were daily doses in mg; SU 50 = 50 mg/d for 4 weeks, 2 weeks off; mFU = median follow-up; mPFS = median progression-free survival; mOS = median overall survival; RR = response rates; n.a. = not available; * = mutational analysis pre-treatment at time of diagnosis.

Negative prognostic factors for both OS and PFS were poor performance status, high neutrophil count, absence of *KIT* exon 11 mutation and male gender, prognostic factors identified for PFS only were small bowel origin and low hemoglobin, and for OS only age, low albumin and large lesion size [49].

Studies EORTC 62005 [50] and S0033 [8] were conceived in parallel to compare different dosages of imatinib (400 mg/d *vs.* 800 mg/d) in the treatment of metastatic GIST. Overall survival was identical for both dosages as cross-over between arms upon progression was allowed. Response rates and PFS did not differ between arms, but toxicity was higher in the 800 mg arm [44]. Dose increase upon cross-over led to a benefit (PR/SD) in one third of patients [44]. A correlation between the most frequently occurring side-effects and some patient characteristics and treatment has been established. Development of anemia was correlated with imatinib dose and baseline haemoglobin level, while occurrence of neutropenia was correlated with baseline neutrophil count and haemoglobin level. The risk of non-haematological toxicities was dose dependent and higher in females (oedema, nausea, and diarrhea), patients of advanced age (oedema, rash, fatigue), poor performance status (fatigue and nausea), prior chemotherapy (fatigue), tumour of gastrointestinal origin (diarrhea) and small lesions (rash) [48].

Subgroup analyses of the combined data of both trials (Meta-GIST) of 772 patients for whom mutational data where available showed that patients with a GIST harbouring a *KIT* exon 9 mutation (n = 92) had a significant PFS benefit from starting with imatinib 800 mg/d as compared to 400 mg/d [49]. Therefore, the recommended starting dose in these patients is 800 mg/d imatinib.

Recently an important correlation between imatinib plasma levels and outcome has been reported [21]. In the 73 patients analysed imatinib trough levels above 1100 ng/ml seemed to confer a significant response and outcome benefit.

Patients with metastatic GIST should never interrupt their treatment, as most patients progress rather rapidly; the BFR14 trial randomized treatment interruption at 1, then 3 years and demonstrated a consistent 6 months median PFS in the group randomized to the STOP arm [1, 9, 45]. Even though there was no difference in overall survival in the 2 arms, it must be noted that this study did not have the statistical power to demonstrate equivalence and therefore a detrimental effect of treatment interruption on overall survival can not be excluded. Therefore, guidelines [39] recommend treatment interruption only for true severe intolerance or patient refusal.

Treatment after progression

In progressing patients – once compliance issues, drug-drug interactions and low imatinib plasma levels [21] have been excluded – imatinib dose-escalation to 800 mg/d [44] should be considered where applicable. This results in a median PFS of 3-4 months and a fifth of these patients still progression free at 1 year in both S0033 and EORTC 62005 trials [44]. Once progression occurs upon imatinib therapy, treatment should be switched to second-line sunitinib. In imatinib-resistant or intolerant patients, sunitinib has led to a response (CR/PR) and SD in 7% and 58% of patients, respectively, achieving 24-35 weeks median PFS [18, 25] and 73-74 weeks median OS [20, 41], results of the phase III trial and data recently reported for 1 091 patients enrolled in a worldwide treatment-use trial. The approved schedule for sunitinib is 50 mg/d for 4 weeks followed by a two-week rest, but continuous administration of 37.5 mg/d may be equally effective (even though no formal randomized comparison has been performed) [25], less toxic and may prevent metabolic tumour rebound in the resting period (Fig. 1). Many experts therefore recommend the continuous regimen [39] or consider it as an option [10].

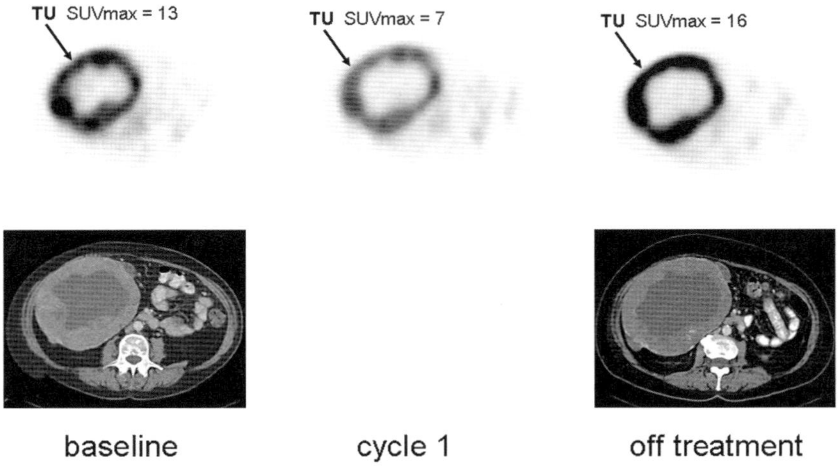

Fig. 1. Axial FDG-PET slices and correlative CT slices in a patient with metastatic GIST prior to sunitinib therapy (left), during cycle 1 (middle), and at the end of the resting period prior to cycle 2 (right) showing a large FDG-avid mass in the right abdomen at baseline prior to sunitinib therapy (straight arrows, TU SUVmax = 13, left) reflecting intense tumour glycolytic activity. The corresponding axial CT slice shows a large abdominal mass with a necrotic center in the right abdomen (lower panel, left). A marked decrease in glycolysis is noted in the tumour mass on FDG-PET as early as 1 week following treatment with sunitinib as reflected by the decrease in FDG uptake and lower SUVmax (TU SUVmax = 7, cycle 1, middle). Note the marked rebound in glycolytic tumour activity at the end of the resting period prior to the next cycle of sunitinib, as reflected by intense FDG uptake and increased SUVmax (TU SUVmax = 16, off treatment, right). Courtesy of Annick D. van den Abbeele, MD and Iryna Rastarhuyeva, MD, Dana-Farber Cancer Institute, Boston, MA [47].

Nilotinib, a second generation TKI, has been investigated in a recently closed worldwide randomized trial in patients progressing on both imatinib and sunitinib. Results of this trial are pending, but recently reported data of a retrospective analysis of 52 patients receiving nilotinib on a compassionate use program show an estimated 34 weeks median OS, with 29% of patients being treated longer than 24 weeks and 12% discontinuing treatment due to toxicity [40].

Patients progressing on imatinib and/or sunitinib treated subsequently with sorafenib, a multitargeted kinase inhibitor, in a phase II trial showed a disease control rate of 78% (PR and SD), 5.7 months median PFS and 8.5 median OS as recently reported [51]. A small retrospective series suggests activity of Sorafenib also in fourth line treatment of GIST [52].

Imaging and follow-up

CT-scans are recommended within 3 months of initiating TKIs therapy, to be repeated at intervals of 3-6 months [19]. Traditional size-based criteria such as RECIST have their limitations in monitoring GISTs treated with TKIs. This is the reason why modified response criteria as proposed by Choi [13] or Antoch [3] that combine tumour density and size measurements should be used instead [6]. Choi-criteria correlate well with PET results. CT combined with ^{18}FDG-PET provides accurate anatomical information and allows for attenuation-correction which reduces statistical noise [46]. Detection of otherwise unknown metastatic sites and response assessment as early as 24 hours after the start of TKIs treatment, with the

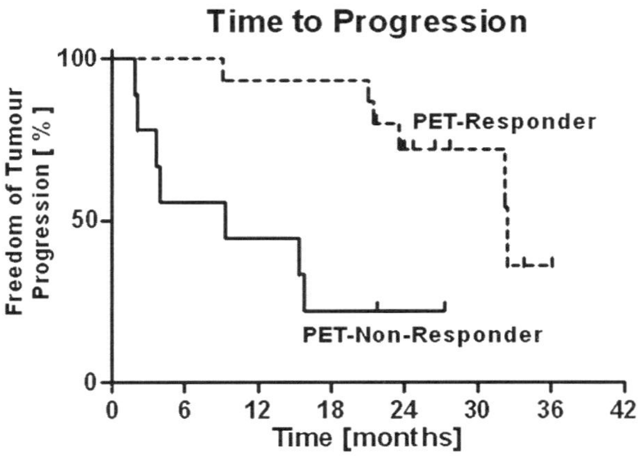

Fig. 2. Time to progression (TTP) according to the result of post-treatment PET or PET/CT scan [26].
Patients with a response on the first post-treatment PET (n = 15) have a median TTP of 32.2 months, while non responding patients (n = 9) have a median TTP of 9.3 months (log-rank test p = 0.002). (Courtesy PD Dr. Gerhard Goerres, Bürgerspital Solothurn, Switzerland).

early PET response being predictive for PFS and OS [26] (Fig. 2), justifies the use of ^{18}FDG-PET, e.g. in a neoadjuvant treatment setting. PET also allows early prediction of response to sunitinib second line treatment [53]. An estimated 10% of patients have PET negative GISTs. Interestingly, contrast-enhanced ultrasound also yields powerful predictive information on response to imatinib, as has been recently reported [11, 34], and is currently being evaluated in a prospective setting.

For follow-up, CT scans should be done every 3-6 months according to individual risk [10, 19]. This proposition is expert opinion only and has not been investigated in a trial. If radiation exposure is an issue MRI might be used instead.

References

1. Adenis A, Cassier PA, Bui BN *et al.* (2008) Does interruption of imatinib (IM) in responding patients after three years of treatment influence outcome of patients with advanced GIST included in the BFR14 trial? ASCO Meeting Abstracts 26(15 suppl): 10522
2. Andersson J, Bumming P, Meis-Kindblom JM *et al.* (2006) Gastrointestinal stromal tumors with KIT exon 11 deletions are associated with poor prognosis. Gastroenterology 130(6): 1573-81
3. Antoch G, Kanja J, Bauer S *et al.* (2004) Comparison of PET, CT, and dual-modality PET/CT imaging for monitoring of imatinib (STI571) therapy in patients with gastrointestinal stromal tumors. J Nucl Med 45(3): 357-65
4. Artinyan A, Kim J, Soriano P, Ellenhorn JD (2008) Survival from metastatic gastrointestinal stromal tumors in the era of imatinib. ASCO Gastrointestinal Cancers Symposium: No 50 (abstract)
5. Bauer S, Yu LK, Demetri GD, Fletcher JA (2006) Heat shock protein 90 inhibition in imatinib-resistant gastrointestinal stromal tumor. Cancer Res 66(18): 9153-61
6. Benjamin RS, Choi H, Macapinlac HA *et al.* (2007) We should desist using RECIST, at least in GIST. J Clin Oncol 25(13): 1760-4
7. Blanke CD, Demetri GD, von Mehren M *et al.* (2008) Long-term results from a randomized phase II trial of standard- versus higher-dose imatinib mesylate for patients with unresectable or metastatic gastrointestinal stromal tumors expressing KIT. J Clin Oncol 26(4): 620-5
8. Blanke CD, Rankin C, Demetri GD *et al.* (2008) Phase III randomized, intergroup trial assessing imatinib mesylate at two dose levels in patients with unresectable or metastatic gastrointestinal stromal tumors expressing the kit receptor tyrosine kinase: S0033. J Clin Oncol 26(4): 626-32
9. Blay JY, Le Cesne A, Ray-Coquard I *et al.* (2007) Prospective multicentric randomized phase III study of imatinib in patients with advanced gastrointestinal stromal

2

tumors comparing interruption versus continuation of treatment beyond 1 year: the French Sarcoma Group. J Clin Oncol 25(9): 1107-13

10. Casali PG, Jost L, Reichardt P *et al.* (2008) Gastrointestinal stromal tumors: ESMO clinical recommendations for diagnosis, treatment and follow-up. Ann Oncol 19(Suppl 2): ii35-8

11. Chami L, Lassau N, Koscielny S *et al.* (2008) Quantitative functional imaging by dynamic contrast enhanced ultrasonography (DCE-US) in patients with GIST treated by thyrosine kinase inhibitor (TKI). ASCO Meeting Abstracts 26(15 suppl): 10552 (abstract)

12. Chetty R (2008) Small and microscopically detected gastrointestinal stromal tumours: an overview. Pathology 40(1): 9-12

13. Choi H, Charnsangavej C, Faria SC *et al.* (2007) Correlation of computed tomography and positron emission tomography in patients with metastatic gastrointestinal stromal tumor treated at a single institution with imatinib mesylate: proposal of new computed tomography response criteria. J Clin Oncol 25(13): 1753-9

14. Corless CL, Heinrich MC (2008) Molecular Pathobiology of Gastrointestinal Stromal Sarcomas. Annu Rev Pathol, Oct 16(epub);3(Feb):557-86

15. Dematteo RP, Lewis JJ, Leung D *et al.* (2000) Two hundred gastrointestinal stromal tumors: recurrence patterns and prognostic factors for survival. Ann Surg 231(1): 51-8

16. DeMatteo RP, Ballman KV, Antonescu CR *et al.* (2009) Adjuvant imatinib mesylate after resection of localised, primary gastrointestinal stromal tumour: a randomised, double-blind, placebo-controlled trial. Lancet 373(9669): 1097-104

17. Dematteo RP, Gold JS, Saran L *et al.* (2008) Tumor mitotic rate, size, and location independently predict recurrence after resection of primary gastrointestinal stromal tumor (GIST). Cancer 112(3): 608-15

18. Demetri GD, van Oosterom AT, Garrett CR *et al.* (2006) Efficacy and safety of sunitinib in patients with advanced gastrointestinal stromal tumour after failure of imatinib: a randomised controlled trial. Lancet 368(9544): 1329-38

19. Demetri GD, Benjamin RS, Blanke CD *et al.* (2009) Imatinib plasma levels are correlated with clinical benefit in patients with unresectable/metastatic gastrointestinal stromal tumours. J Clin Oncol 27(19): 3141-7

20. Demetri GD, Huang X, Garrett CR *et al.* (2008) Novel Statistical Analysis of Long-Term Survival to Account for Crossover in a Phase III Trial of Sunitinib *versus* Placebo in Advanced GIST After Imatinib Failure. J Clin Oncol 26(suppl): 35113 (abstract)

21. Demetri GD, Wang Y, Wehrle E *et al.* (2009) Imatinib plasma levels are correlated with clinical benefit in patients with unresectable/metastatic gastrointestinal stromal tumors. J Clin Oncol 27(19): 3141-7

22. Druker BJ, Tamura S, Buchdunger E *et al.* (1996) Effects of a selective inhibitor of the Abl tyrosine kinase on the growth of Bcr-Abl positive cells. Nat Med 2(5):561-6

23. Druker B, Talpaz M, Resta DJ (1999) Clinical efficacy and safety of an Abl specific tyrosine kinase inhibitor as targeted therapy for chronic myelogenous leukemia. Blood 94: 368a

24. Fletcher CD, Berman JJ, Corless C *et al.* (2002) Diagnosis of gastrointestinal stromal tumors: A consensus approach. Hum Pathol 33(5): 459-65

25. George S, Blay JY, Casali PG *et al.* (2008) Sunitinib (SU) on a continuous daily dosing schedule in pts with advanced GIST. ASCO Gastrointestinal Cancers Symposium: No 39 (abstract)

26. Goerres GW, Stupp R, Barghouth G *et al.* (2005) The value of PET, CT and in-line PET/CT in patients with gastrointestinal stromal tumours: long-term outcome of treatment with imatinib mesylate. Eur J Nucl Med Mol Imaging 32(2): 153-62

27. Gold JS, van der Zwan SM, Gonen M *et al.* (2007) Outcome of metastatic GIST in the era before tyrosine kinase inhibitors. Ann Surg Oncol 14(1): 134-42

28. Heinrich MC, Griffith DJ, Druker BJ *et al.* (2000) Inhibition of c-kit receptor tyrosine kinase activity by STI 571, a selective tyrosine kinase inhibitor. Blood 96(3): 925-32

29. Heinrich MC, Maki RG, Corless CL *et al.* (2006) Sunitinib (SU) response in imatinib-resistant (IM-R) GIST correlates with KIT and PDGFRA mutation status. ASCO Meeting Abstracts 24(18 suppl): 9502 (abstract)

30. Hirota S, Isozaki K, Moriyama Y *et al.* (1998) Gain-of-function mutations of c-kit in human gastrointestinal stromal tumors. Science 279(5350): 577-80

31. **Joensuu H, Roberts PJ, Sarlomo-Rikala M *et al.* (2001) Effect of the tyrosine kinase inhibitor STI571 in a patient with a metastatic gastrointestinal stromal tumor. N Engl J Med 344(14): 1052-6**
32. Krause DS, Van Etten RA (2005) Tyrosine kinases as targets for cancer therapy. N Engl J Med 353(2): 172-87
33. Lasota J, Miettinen M (2006) KIT and PDGFRA mutations in gastrointestinal stromal tumors (GISTs). Semin Diagn Pathol 23(2): 91-102
34. Lassau N, Lamuraglia M, Chami L *et al.* (2006) Gastrointestinal stromal tumors treated with imatinib: monitoring response with contrast-enhanced sonography. Am J Roentgenol 187(5): 1267-73
35. Lugo TG, Pendergast AM, Muller AJ, Witte ON (1990) Tyrosine kinase activity and transformation potency of bcr-abl oncogene products. Science 247(4946): 1079-82
36. Martin J, Poveda A, Llombart-Bosch A *et al.* (2005) Deletions Affecting Codons 557-558 of the c-KIT Gene Indicate a Poor Prognosis in Patients With Completely Resected Gastrointestinal Stromal Tumors: A Study by the Spanish Group for Sarcoma Research (GEIS). Journal of Clinical Oncology 23(25): 6190-8
37. **Miettinen M, Lasota J (2006) Gastrointestinal stromal tumors: pathology and prognosis at different sites. Semin Diagn Pathol 23(2): 70-83**
38. Miettinen M, Lasota J (2006) Gastrointestinal stromal tumors: review on morphology, molecular pathology, prognosis, and differential diagnosis. Arch Pathol Lab Med 130(10): 1466-78
39. Montemurro M, Dirnhofer S, Borner M *et al.* (2008) Diagnose und Behandlung von gastrointestinalen Stromatumoren (GIST) in der Schweiz – Empfehlungen einer multidisziplinären Expertengruppe. Swiss Medical Forum 8(30-31): 544-9
40. Montemurro M, Schöffski P, Reichardt P *et al.* (2009) Nilotinib in the treatment of advanced gastrointestinal stromal tumours resistant to both imatinib and sunitinib. Eur J Cancer (45): 2293-7
41. Morgan JA, Reichardt P, Kang YK *et al.* (2008) Sunitinib (SU) in a worldwide treatment-use trial of patients with GIST: Safety and efficacy. ASCO Gastrointestinal Cancers Symposium: No 31 (abstract)
42. Nilsson B, Bumming P, Meis-Kindblom JM *et al.* (2005) Gastrointestinal stromal tumors: the incidence, prevalence, clinical course, and prognostication in the preimatinib mesylate era – a population-based study in western Sweden. Cancer 103(4): 821-9
43. Nowell PC, Hungerford DA (1960) A minute chromosome in human chronic granulocytic leukemia. Science 132(3438): 1497 (abstract)
44. Patel SR, Zalcberg JR (2008) Optimizing the dose of imatinib for treatment of gastrointestinal stromal tumors: Lessons from the phase 3 trials. Eur J Cancer 44: 501-9
45. Perol D, Domont J, Ray-Coquard IL *et al.* (2008) Does interruption of imatinib (IM) in responding GIST patients after one year of treatment influence the secondary resistance to IM after its reintroduction? Updated results of the prospective French Sarcoma Group randomized phase III trial on long term survival. ASCO Meeting Abstracts 26(15 suppl): 10556
46. Townsend DW (2008) Positron emission tomography/computed tomography. Semin Nucl Med 38(3): 152-66
47. Van den Abbeele A, Melenevsky Y, de Vries D *et al.* (2005) Imaging kinase target inhibition with SU11248 by FDG-PET in patients (pts) with imatinib-resistant gastrointestinal stromal tumors (I-R GIST). Proc Am Soc Clin Oncol: Abstr. 9006
48. Van Glabbeke M, Verweij J, Casali PG *et al.* (2006) Predicting toxicities for patients with advanced gastrointestinal stromal tumours treated with imatinib: A study of the European Organisation for Research and Treatment of Cancer, the Italian Sarcoma Group, and the Australasian Gastro-Intestinal Trials Group (EORTC-ISG-AGITG). EurJ Cancer 42(14): 227-85
49. Van Glabbeke MM, Owzar K, Rankin C *et al.* (2007) Comparison of two doses of imatinib for the treatment of unresectable or metastatic gastrointestinal stromal tumors (GIST): A meta-analysis based on 1,640 patients (pts). J Clin Oncol (Meeting Abstracts) 25(18 suppl): 10004 (abstract)
50. Verweij J, Casali PG, Zalcberg J *et al.* (2004) Progression-free survival in gastrointestinal stromal tumours with high-dose imatinib: randomised trial. Lancet 364(9440): 1127-34
51. Wiebe L, Kasza KE, Maki RG *et al.* (2008) Activity of sorafenib (SOR) in patients (pts) with imatinib (IM) and sunitinib (SU)-resistant (RES) gastrointestinal stromal

tumors (GIST): A phase II trial of the University of Chicago Phase II Consortium. J Clin Oncol (Meeting Abstracts) 26(15 suppl): 10502 (abstract)

52. Montemurro M, Schütte J, Gelderblom H *et al.* (2008) Sorafenib salvage therapy in pretreated metastatic GIST – first experience. Onkologie (Meetings Abstracts) 31(suppl 4): 203
53. Prior J, Montemurro M, Orcurto M *et al.* (2009) Early prediction of response to sunitinib after imatinib failure by 18F-fluorodeoxyglucose positron emission tomography in patients with gastrointestinal stromal tumor. J Clin Oncol 27(3): 439-45

Small cell carcinomas of the gastrointestinal tract

3

M. Shilkrut, A. Peer and A. Kuten

Five Essential Points

1. *SCCGIT is a rare disease, comprising about 1% of all gastrointestinal malignancies. The most frequent site is the esophagus. The major risk factor for development of SCCGIT is a history of smoking.*
2. *Histologicallly, SCCGIT is indistinguishable from SCLC. Similarly, SCCGIT shares common molecular features with SCLC.*
3. *Staging for SCCGIT is based on the VALSG staging system for primary SCC of the lung. Staging is done by chest and abdominopelvic computer tomography, bone scan, brain imaging (for symptomatic patients) and bronchopulmonary lavage to exclude a primary pulmonary origin.*
4. *LS SCCGIT is treated aggressively with a multimodality approach combining local treatment (chemo-radiotherapy or surgery) with chemotherapy. ES SCCGIT is treated palliatively with a combination of platinum-based chemotherapy regimens.*
5. *The role of the PCI is not established in the management of SCCGIT.*

Introduction

Small cell carcinomas of the gastrointestinal tract (SCCGIT) are rare neoplasms with an aggressive course, constituting less than 1% of "conventional" gastrointestinal cancers [3]. While described initially in the esophagus, the most frequent site of SCCGIT, they have been documented in every part of the gastrointestinal system. Histologically they are indistinguishable from pulmonary small cell carcinoma. Similar to small cell lung cancer (SCLC), their clinical course depends heavily on the extension of the disease, and they are characterized by early metastasis and favorable response to chemotherapy and radiotherapy. Unfortunately, because of the rarity of the disease, there are no established treatment guidelines and the current knowledge is based mainly on small series of patients and case reports. The following review attempts to summarize the available clinical and laboratory data on SCCGIT with emphasis on the differences between small cell carcinomas of the different parts of the gastrointestinal tract.

Epidemiology

Since it was first described in 1952, about 700 cases of SCCGIT have been reported in the literature, and several series of site-specific SCCGIT have been published [1,18,23,29]. More than half of these tumours have been described in the esophagus [3]. The incidence rate of SCC of the esophagus ranges from 0.8-2.4% of all esophageal malignancies [29]. The mean age of the patient with SCC of the esophagus is 64 years. Unlike squamous cell carcinoma of the esophagus, there is less male preponderance, with a male-to-female ratio of 1.6:1 [2]. In 48-56% of cases the tumour was located in the lower third of the esophagus, in 40-45.5% in the mid third of the esophagus and in less then 5% in the upper esophagus [29]. Risk factors for the development of SCC of the esophagus are the combination of the risk factors for the development of esophageal squamous and glandular carcinomas. Among the risk factors, heavy smoking was the most consistently reported in the vast majority of patients [1,18,23,29,32]. While the majority of the patients in several series had extensive disease [1,32], other authors have reported limited disease in a vast majority of patients [18,23,29]. This could explain the differences in median survival reported in the published series, from a dismal 7.5 months [32] to 19.8 months in a series where the proportion of patients with limited stage disease was high [23].

Unlike SCC of the esophagus, information on SCC in the remaining areas of the GIT is sparse and is based largely on case reports and small series. Some of the series included patients with other neuroendocrine tumours, complicating any conclusions and generalizations. Most of the 38 cases of SCC of the stomach reported in the literature were diagnosed in Japanese and Chinese patients [27,28,30]. Because of the scarcity of the disease and the fact that information is based on single case-reports rather than on series of patients, no specific risk factors for the disease have been identified.

Fifty three cases of SCC of the gallbladder have been published [13]. SCC of the gallbladder affects the elderly population with a median age of 65 years. More than 70% of patients are female [26]. The majority of cases were diagnosed at late stage. The only risk factor identified for SCC of the gallbladder was cholelithiasis. The median survival for pure SCC of the gallbladder was nine months. Similar to SCC of the stomach, the majority of reports of SCC of the bile ducts were described in Japanese and Korean patients [20,21,24]. No specific risk factors were described.

Fifteen cases of SCC of the ampulla of Vater have been reported [50]. The vast majority of patients were male. In most cases, it was an extremely aggressive disease which was discovered at advanced stage.

SCC of the pancreas is rare and only 12 cases have been documented [35]. This type of carcinoma accounts for about 1% of all pancreatic cancers and is more common in elderly males with a history of smoking. The disease usually progresses rapidly with early metastasis [5].

SCC of the colon and rectum is the second most prevalent SCCGIT [3]. More than 60 cases of the disease have been published. It constitutes 0.2-1.5% of colorectal cancers [36,49]. In a review of 38 patients with colorectal SCC, the mean age was 57.6 years, with an almost equal male to female ratio [49]. The majority (63.2%) of patients had lymph node metastases and 39.5% had liver metastasis. Locations of colorectal SCC are in the anorectum – 47.4%, cecum – 18.4%, ascending colon – 18.4%, sigmoid colon – 7.9% and transverse colon – 7.9% [49]. Most patients were treated by resection only, with a median survival of 85.1 weeks. No specific risk factors for colorectal SCC were identified.

Molecular and histopathological characteristics

Morphologically, SCCGIT is identical to SCLC. Like its pulmonary counterpart, SCCGIT has solid architecture composed of round to fusiform cells with large nuclei and scant cytoplasm arranged in clusters, sheets and trabeculae separated by a delicate fibrovascular stroma [3]. The mitotic rate is high, averaging 40-50 mitoses per 10 high-power fields. The markers of high proliferative activity (Ki-67, MIB-1, PCNA) are present in abundance [12]. SCCGIT is often associated with tumour cells of invasive and non-invasive carcinomas specific to the site of origin.

SCCGIT have genetic and molecular alterations typical of both SCLC and non-small cell carcinoma of the site of origin. Much like its pulmonary counterpart, SCCGIT overexpresses markers of cellular proliferation (such as the proliferating cell nuclear antigen (PCNA), MIB-1 and Ki-67). Additionally, SCCGIT have abnormalities in p53 expression and regulation, and p16INK4A-CDK4/6-Rb pathway, the most common alteration being loss of Rb expression and p16INK4A mutations [12]. Like many other tumours of gastrointestinal origin, SCCGIT overexpresses markers of angiogenesis and metastasis, such as factor VIII-related antigen, VEGF (vascular endothelial growth factor), PDGF (platelet-derived endothelial cell growth factor) and KOC (K homology domain-containing protein overexpressed in cancer) [41]. The occurrence of SCCGIT with invasive and non-invasive "conventional" carcinomas, association with the same risk factors and common molecular characteristics of SCCGIT with non-small cell carcinomas, support the theory that SCCGIT arise from epithelial stem cells capable of divergent differentiation [3,12].

Clinical manifestations

SCCGIT is diagnosed at advanced stage in most cases; therefore, clinical manifestations of the disease are not limited to the site of the tumour, but also include systemic symptoms of disseminated disease, such as fatigue, anorexia and weight loss [3]. The most common symptoms of esophageal SCC are dysphagia, weight loss and chest pain [29,32]. Several paraneoplastic disorders documented in esophageal SCC include diarrhea, neutrophilia [31], hypercalcemia [11], inappropriate antidiuretic hormone secretion [29] and sensorimotor neuropathy [40].

The presenting symptoms of SCC of the stomach, bile ducts, gallbladder, pancreas, small intestine, large intestine and rectum are indistinguishable from the clinical features of conventional carcinomas. They follow an aggressive course with an early propensity for distant spread to regional lymph nodes and the liver [26,34,36,38].

Pretreatment evaluation and staging

A dual approach can be used for staging and pretreatment evaluation of SCCGIT. While the Tumor Node Metastasis (TNM) system was utilized by some [29,47], the more accepted staging system for SCCGIT is based on that introduced by the Veterans' Administration Lung Study Group (VALSG) for primary SCC of the lung. This system defines limited stage (LS) disease as a tumour mass localized to the organ of interest with or without regional lymph node metastasis that can be included within one radiation therapy treatment portal. Extensive stage (ES) disease is defined by the presence of tumour beyond this. The VALSG system has been utilized in some larger series of patients [2,14,18,23], and should be recommended for sites where radiation therapy is feasible.

The purpose of pretreatment evaluation is not only to define the extent of the disease, but also to exclude the presence of SCLC. The majority of published series reported the use of the bronchoscopy with random biopsies and/or bronchoalveolar lavage and/or endobronchial brushing [2,14,18,29,32,33]. The staging workup should always include chest and abdominopelvic computer tomography and bone scan. Brain imaging is recommended if neurological symptoms are present. Bone marrow biopsy is indicated if there are abnormal blood counts or findings on the peripheral smear, without other evidence of disseminated disease. The role of other imaging modalities, such as positron emission tomography, magnetic resonance imaging and scans with radiolabeled somatostatin analogs, has not been established for SCCGIT.

Treatment

Despite aggressive locoregional and systemic treatment including surgery, radiation therapy and systemic chemotherapy, none has dramatically changed the landscape of therapy for SCCGIT. The clinical course of these tumours is known to be aggressive in general, with early dissemination and frequent recurrence and the overall prognosis is very poor compared with the common types of gastrointestinal tumours. Due to the infrequency of SCCGIT, the dismal prognosis and lack of randomized trials, there is still no consensus with regard to treatment. The vast majority of information is derived from retrospective data, mainly series on SCC of the esophagus and case reports of patients with SCC of other sites of the GI tract. Because of the similarity in biology and clinical course of SCCGIT compared to SCLC, the treatment approach in these tumours resembles the management of SCLC.

Localized disease

Surgery

In the past, the treatment approach for localized disease has been surgery alone or surgery with the addition of adjuvant therapy [10]. Considering an aggressive course and early systemic spread, surgery as the sole treatment modality for SCCGIT is not recommended. Galanis *et al.* reported eight patients with SCCGIT treated by surgery alone. All patients (5 colorectal, 1 pancreas, 2 esophagus) succumbed to the disease with a median time to recurrence of five months for colon SCC and two months for esophageal SCC [14]. Most case reports of gastric, gallbladder, and intestinal (including rectum) SCC treated by surgery alone demonstrated dismal results [6,19,28,30,38,43,45,49]. In a review of 93 patients with LS esophageal SCC, local treatment without systemic treatment, whether surgery or radiotherapy, was a strong negative prognostic factor associated with a median survival of 5 months versus 20 months for patients who received local-plus-systemic treatment [4]. Therefore, surgery should be used as part of a multimodality treatment. The exact role of surgery here has not yet been defined. It was suggested by some that resection of the residual disease after preoperative chemo- or chemoradiotherapy could be of benefit. In the study reported by Medgyesy, of four patients with LS esophageal SCC treated by preoperative chemotherapy or chemoradiotherapy, three had residual disease at surgery. Two patients were free from the disease 10 and 57 months after surgery [29].

Adjuvant or neo-adjuvant platinum-based chemotherapy was thought to improve results of surgery but, in their analysis of the results of a series of 64 patients with SCCGIT, Brenner *et al.* found that chemotherapy in addition to local treatment had a minor role [2]. In this series of patients, of the four patients treated with chemotherapy alone and 12 with chemotherapy plus other local treatments, only three remained free of disease. To support this view, all nine patients reported by Wu *et al.* with LS SCC of the esophagus who were treated by adjuvant systemic chemotherapy and radiation therapy had local or distant failures [48].

Radiotherapy

Radiotherapy (RT) can provide acceptable local control for SCCGIT. SCCGIT is a radiosensitive tumour with common partial response but rare complete response [2,18]. The doses reported for definitive RT of esophageal SCC ranged from 44.4 Gy/22 fx to 61.6 Gy/33 fx [18,23,29]. Most patients with esophageal SCC treated by RT alone progressed after treatment, most often outside the irradiated field [14,18]. Galanis *et al.* reported 16 patients with extrapulmonary SCC who were treated by RT alone. All patients achieved temporary control but subsequently progressed: 13 outside the irradiated field and five within [14]. Additionally, six of seven patients with LS SCCGIT treated by RT alone from the Memorial Sloan Kettering Cancer Center (MSKCC) database had locoregional recurrence of their disease [2]. Therefore, RT should not be used as a single modality for the treatment of LS SCCGIT.

Chemotherapy

SCCGIT is a chemosensitive tumour with reported response rates as high as 90% [1,3,18]. Unlike SCLC, most responses were partial (about 15% complete responses), reflecting the frequent mixed histology of these tumours. The chemotherapy regimens used for SCCGIT were extrapolated from the treatments used for SCLC. Platinum derivatives and etoposide were the most frequently cited agents. The median duration of response ranged from 3 to 8.5 months. In spite of the high rates of response, most were short-lived. In a series of 13 patients treated at Massachusetts General Hospital, seven patients were treated with chemotherapy alone [18]. A variety of regimens was used, with most patients receiving combinations of cyclophosphamide, etoposide and cisplatin. While, five of six patients responded to chemotherapy with two complete responses, four patients died after five months and two died within 12 months. Based on this, chemotherapy as sole treatment for LS SCCGIT should be discouraged.

Combination treatment

A multimodality approach, utilizing local treatment (surgery or RT) and systemic chemotherapy has become the most accepted approach for the treatment of LS SCCGIT. In their review of 93 patients with LS esophageal SCC, Casas *et al.* reported a statistically significant difference in median survival in patients treated with local treatments only (RT or surgery) *vs.* patients who received local-plus-systemic treatments (5 months, n=50, *versus* 20 months, n=43; $p<0.0001$) [4]. No significant difference in survival for different types of local treatments was found in this review due to the few cases reported.

The M.D. Anderson Cancer Center series included six patients with LS esophageal SCC, of whom four were treated with a combined approach (two patients were treated with RT alone because of technical difficulties in delivering chemotherapy). Three of these four patients were treated by preoperative sequential or concomitant chemo-radiotherapy and one by preoperative chemotherapy. All but one received a cisplatin and etoposide regimen before and during their RT treatment. Radiation doses varied from 30 Gy/10 fx to 59.4 Gy/33 fx. Treatment complications were not reported. All surgical specimens contained residual disease, underlining the necessity of surgery after chemo-radiation. Of the four patients who underwent surgery, two were alive with no evidence of disease at 10 and 57 months after diagnosis. One patient developed multiple brain metastases five months after surgery and died 16 months after diagnosis. One patient died from postoperative complications [29].

In the MSKCC series of patients that included 14 patients with LS esophageal SCC, five of six long-term survivors were treated by induction chemotherapy followed by chemo-radiotherapy without surgery [23]. In this recent report, 11 patients were treated initially by at least two courses of platinum compounds (all but one received cisplatin) with etoposide or irinotecan and paclitaxel (one patient). One patient received alternating cycles of cisplatin/etoposide and cisplatin/doxorubicin/vincristine (the "CAV "regimen). Of these, four patients developed early progressive or metastatic disease during the treatment. Of the remaining seven patients, six were treated with concomitant chemo-radiotherapy that included a platinum compound and etoposide. The prescribed radiation doses were 50.4 Gy/28 fx, except for one patient who received 45 Gy/28 fx. Based on this, the management of SCCGIT should include a multimodality treatment.

Prophylactic cranial irradiation (PCI)

Although PCI is an established treatment in LS SCLC and ES SCLC that responds to chemotherapy [42], there is no data regarding this mode of treatment in SCCGIT. Some authors insist that the incidence of brain metastases is lower in SCCGIT than in SCLC and, therefore, do not recommend PCI for patients with SCCGIT [3,15]. Cicin *et al.* compared 54 cases of SCLC to 11 cases of extrapulmonary SCC [7]. In this study that included five patients with SCCGIT, brain metastasis at diagnosis was noted in 20% of patients with SCLC, while none of the patients with extrapulmonary SCC presented with brain metastasis, not even patients with ES SCCGIT. Subsequent brain metastases were observed in two patients (1 rectum, 1 gallbladder). Unfortunately, most series of patients did not report the incidence of brain metastasis on presentation or after treatment, complicating the conclusion on the usefulness of this treatment. On the other hand, in a very recent series of patients from MSKCC, one patient with LS esophageal SCC who achieved complete response after initial chemotherapy was treated with PCI [23].

Extensive disease

Patients with ES SCCGIT had much poorer prognoses than those with SCC at other locations. As in SCLC, SCCGIT responds well to platinum-based chemotherapy but the responses are typically short-lived [17,32]. Nevertheless, chemotherapy improves survival in patients with ES SCCGIT. As demonstrated by Casas *et al.* in a review of 95 patients with ES esophageal SCC, the only independent prognostic variable in both univariate and multivariate analysis was treatment or lack of treatment [4]. The median survival reported for patients who were not treated (n=30) with chemotherapy was only one month, while the median survival of patients who were treated (n=65) was five months. Whether or not chemotherapy improves survival of patients with SCC in other sites of the gastrointestinal tract is unknown, but many authors have reported favourable responses to cisplatin-based, adriamycin-based and irinotecan-based chemotherapy [9,13,14,21,49]. The latter combination was especially recommended for intestinal SCC, because of frequent cases of mixed SCC-adenocarcinoma [3,37]. The average number of treatment cycles reported was 4 (range, 3-6) [22,39,44], but this does not imply that four is the recommended number of treatment cycles. Until proven otherwise, patients should be treated until progression of the disease. Anecdotal reports have limited information on other regimens, but none were compared with the commonly used platinum-based chemotherapy. Matsui and colleagues reported treatment of gastric SCC with regimens used for gastric adenocarcinoma treatment based on tegafur and uracil or on fluorouracil and mitomycin [28]. 5-Fluorouracil or lomustine-based regimens were also used, but no responses were observed [14].

Radiation therapy is very effective as palliative therapy for achieving symptom control for metastatic SCCGIT, especially for painful bone metastasis, spinal cord compression syndrome and brain metastases. Moreover, RT can be used for palliation of dysphagia, gastric outlet obstruction, jaundice and intestinal obstruction. There are no recommended doses but, as mentioned earlier, the dose should be extrapolated from SCLC.

References

1. Bennouna J, Bardet E, Deguiral P, Douillard JY (2000) Small cell carcinoma of the esophagus: analysis of 10 cases and review of the published data. Am J Clin Oncol 23: 455-9
2. **Brenner B, Shah MA, Gonen M *et al.* (2004) Small-cell carcinoma of the gastrointestinal tract: a retrospective study of 64 cases. Br J Cancer 90: 1720-6**
3. Brenner B, Tang LH, Shia J *et al.* (2007) Small cell carcinomas of the gastrointestinal tract: clinicopathological features and treatment approach. Semin Oncol 34: 43-50
4. **Casas F, Ferrer F, Farrús B *et al.* (1997) Primary small cell carcinoma of the esophagus: a review of the literature with emphasis on therapy and prognosis. Cancer 80: 1366-72**
5. Chetty R, Clark SP, Pitson GA (1993) Primary small cell carcinoma of the pancreas. Pathology 25: 240-2
6. Chuang SS, Lin CN, Chu CH, Chen FF (1999) Small cell carcinoma of the gallbladder: report of two cases. Pathol Oncol Res 5: 235-8
7. Cicin I, Karagol H, Uzunoglu S *et al.* (2007) Extrapulmonary small-cell carcinoma compared with small-cell lung carcinoma: a retrospective single-center study. Cancer 110: 1068-1076.
8. Cioppa T, Marrelli D, Neri A *et al.* (2007) A case of small-cell gastric carcinoma with an adenocarcinoma component and hepatic metastases: treatment with systemic and intra-hepatic chemotherapy. Eur J Cancer Care 16: 453-7
9. Debois JM, De Vriendt P, Charles K (1998) Small cell carcinoma of the gallbladder. Acta Chir Belg 98: 110-2
10. Eimoto T, Hayakawa H (1980) Oat cell carcinoma of the stomach. Path Res Pract 168: 229-36
11. Fereidooni F, Horvath E, Kovacs K (2003) Humoral hypercalcemia of malignancy due to bipartite squamous cell/small cell carcinoma of the esophagus immunoreactive for parathyroid hormone related protein. Dis Esophagus 16: 335-8
12. Frazier SR, Kaplan PA, Loy TS (2007) The pathology of extrapulmonary small cell carcinoma. Semin Oncol 34: 30-8
13. Fujii H, Aotake T, Horiuchi T *et al.* (2001) Small cell carcinoma of the gallbladder: a case report and review of 53 cases in the literature. Hepatogastroenterology 48: 1588-93

3

14. Galanis E, Frytak S, Lloyd RV (1997) Extrapulmonary small cell carcinoma. Cancer 79: 1729-36
15. Haider K, Shahid RK, Finch D *et al.* (2006) Extrapulmonary small cell cancer: a Canadian province's experience. Cancer 107: 2262-9
16. Ho KJ, Herrera GA, Jones JM, Alexander CB (1984) Small cell carcinoma of the esophagus: evidence for a unified histogenesis. Hum Pathol 15: 460-8
17. Hoff PM, Pazdur R (1999) Small cell carcinoma of the gastrointestinal tract,. In Reghavan DBM. Johnson DH, Meropol NJ *et al.* Textbook of uncommon cancers (ed. 2) NJ Wiley &Sons, 463-7
18. **Huncharek M, Muscat J (1995) Small cell carcinoma of the esophagus: the Massachusetts General Hospital Experience, 1978-1993. Chest 107: 179-81**
19. Ihtiyar E, Algin C, Isiksoy S, Ates E (2005) Small cell carcinoma of rectum: a case report. World J Gastroenterol 11: 3156-8
20. Jun SR, Lee JM, Han JK, Choi BI (2006) High-grade neuroendocrine carcinomas of the gallbladder and bile duct: report of four cases with pathological correlation. J Comput Assist Tomogr 30: 604-9
21. Kaiho T, Tanaka T, Tsuchiya S *et al.* (2005) A case of small cell carcinoma of the common bile duct. Hepatogastroenterology 52: 363-7
22. Kim JH, Lee SH, Park J *et al.* (2004) Extrapulmonary small-cell carcinoma: a single-institution experience. Jpn J Clin Oncol 34: 250-4
23. **Ku GY, Minsky BD, Rusch VW *et al.* (2008) Small-cell carcinoma of the esophagus and gastroesophageal junction: review of the Memorial Sloan-Kettering experience. Ann Oncol 19: 533-7**
24. Kuraoka K, Taniyama K, Fujitaka T *et al.* (2003) Small cell carcinoma of the extrahepatic bile duct: case report and immunohistochemical analysis. Pathol Int 53: 887-91
25. Law SY, Fok M, Lam KY *et al.* (1994) Small cell carcinoma of the esophagus. Cancer 73: 2894-9
26. Maitra A, Tascilar M, Hruban RH *et al.* (2001) Small cell carcinoma of the gallbladder: a clinicopathologic, immunohistochemical, and molecular pathology study of 12 cases. Am J Surg Pathol 25: 595-601
27. Matsui K, Jin XM, Kitagawa M, Miwa A (1998) Clinicopathologic features of neuroendocrine carcinomas of the stomach: appraisal of small cell and large cell variants. Arch Pathol Lab Med 122: 1010-7
28. Matsui T, Kataoka M, Sugita Y *et al.* (1997) A case of small cell carcinoma of the stomach. Hepatogastroenterology 44: 156-60
29. **Medgyesy DC, Wolff RA, Putnam JB, Ajani JA (2008) Small cell carcinoma of the esophagus the University of Texas M. D. Anderson Cancer Center experience and literature review. Cancer 88: 262-7**
30. Miyaji M, Ogoshi K, Nakamura K *et al.* (1999) Small mucosal carcinoma of the stomach with para-aortic lymph node metastasis: a case report and review of the literature. Eur J Gastroenterol Hepatol 11: 343-6
31. Nagashima R, Mabe K, Takahashi T (1999) Esophageal small cell carcinoma with ectopic production of parathyroid hormone-related protein (PTHrp), secretin, and granulocyte colony-stimulating factor (G-CSF). Dig Dis Sci 44: 1312-6
32. **Nichols GL, Kelsen DP (1989) Small cell carcinoma of the esophagus. The Memorial Hospital experience 1970 to 1987. Cancer 64: 1531-3**
33. Nishimaki T, Suzuki T, Nakagawa S *et al.* (1997) Tumor spread and outcome of treatment in primary esophageal small cell carcinoma. J Surg Oncol 64: 130-4
34. O'Byrne KJ, Cherukuri AK, Khan MI *et al.* (1997) Extrapulmonary small cell gastric carcinoma: A case report and review of literature. Acta Oncol 36: 78-80
35. Ordóñez NG, Cleary KR, Mackay B (1997) Small cell undifferentiated carcinoma of the pancreas. Ultrastruct Pathol 21: 467-74
36. Saclarides TJ, Szeluga D, Staren ED (1994) Neuroendocrine cancers of the colon and rectum. Results of a ten-year experience. Dis Colon Rectum 37: 635-42
37. Sairenji T, Fujii Y, Eriguchi M (2001) A case of esophageal small-cell carcinoma responding to chemotherapy with CTP-11. Gan To Kagaku Ryoho 28: 1283-6
38. Sarsfield P, Anthony PP (1990) Small cell undifferentiated ("neuroendocrine") carcinoma of the colon. Histopathology 16: 357-63
39. Sengoz M, Abacioglu U, Salepci T *et al.* (2003) Extrapulmonary small cell carcinoma: multimodality treatment results. Tumori 89: 274-7

40. Shimoda T, Koizumi W, Tanabe S *et al.* (2006) Small-cell carcinoma of the esophagus associated with a paraneoplastic neurological syndrome: a case report documenting a complete response. Jpn J Clin Oncol 36: 109-12
41. Simon R, Bourne PA, Yang Q *et al.* (2007) Extrapulmonary small cell carcinomas express K homology domain containing protein overexpressed in cancer, but carcinoid tumors do not. Hum Pathol 38: 1178-83
42. Slotman B, Faivre-Finn C, Kramer G *et al.* (2007) Prophylactic cranial irradiation in extensive small-cell lung cancer. N Engl J Med 357: 664-72
43. Sonoda Y, Yamaguchi K, Nagai E *et al.* (2003) Small cell carcinoma of the cystic duct: a case report. J Gastrointest Surg 7: 631-4
44. Soto DE, Eisbruch A (2007) Limited-stage extrapulmonary small cell carcinoma: outcomes after modern chemotherapy and radiotherapy. Cancer J 13: 243-6
45. Sugawara G, Yamaguchi A, Isogai M *et al.* (2004) Small cell neuroendocrine carcinoma of the ampulla of Vater with foci of squamous differentiation: a case report. J Hepatobiliary Pancreat Surg 11: 56-60
46. Takubo K, Nakamura K, Sawabe M *et al.* (1999) Primary undifferentiated small cell carcinoma of the esophagus. Hum Pathol 30: 216-21
47. Vrouvas J, Ash DV (1995) Extrapulmonary small cell cancer. Clin Oncol 7: 377-81
48. Wu Z, Ma JY, Yang JJ *et al.* (2004) Primary small cell carcinoma of esophagus: report of 9 cases and review of literature. World J Gastroenterol 10: 3680-2
49. Yasui O, Tsukamoto F, Kudo K (2006) Small cell undifferentiated carcinoma of the ascending colon with rapid enlargement after resection: report of a case and review of the literature. Tohoku J Exp Med 209: 361-7
50. Zamboni G, Franzin G, Bonetti F *et al.* (1990) Small-cell neuroendocrine carcinoma of the ampullary region. A clinicopathologic, immunohistochemical, and ultrastructural study of three cases. Am J Surg Pathol 14: 703-13

Anorectal melanoma

4

S. Vieillot and D. Azria

Five Essential Points

1. *Anorectal melanoma has a poor prognosis, with an overall 5-year survival rate between 10 and 20%, and a median survival of 12-18 months.*
2. *Prognostic factors are similar to those for cutaneous melanoma: depth of parietal infiltration and stage of the disease.*
3. *Conservative surgery is recommended if technically possible with safe excision margins to improve local control. Overall survival is not modified by the surgical technique.*
4. *Adjuvant radiotherapy following conservative surgery leads to a local control similar or even superior to that obtain with an APR.*
5. *There is no recommendation for the treatment of metastatic anorectal melanoma.*

Introduction

Anorectal melanoma (ARM) is a rare tumour representing only 0.5 to 1% of anorectal tumours [10,30] and 1 to 2% of melanomas [39]. At the level of the digestive tract, the anorectum region is the first site for the development of melanoma. Since the first description by Moore [24] in 1857, only a few cases have been reported in literature. Due to the rarity of this disease, it is impossible to carry out prospective studies. Therefore, management of ARM is not well defined due to the fact that only data on retrospective studies, with very few patients, studied over a long period of time – sometimes decades – are available. A review of these retrospective series has been carried out so as to determine the best therapeutic strategy and to formulate recommendations.

Clinical diagnosis and extended evaluation

Patients have a median age of 60-65 years at diagnosis with the male/female ratio predominantly female (1:1.2) [10,14,34]. Prognosis is poor, with an overall 5-year survival rate estimated at between 10 and 20%, the median survival time being 12-18 months [14,34]. Symptoms are not specific at diagnosis: most often these are rectal haemorrhage more or less associated with a sensation of an anorectal mass [14,34]. To some degree, reports also mention pain, transit disturbances, anal pruritus or the discovery of an inguinal adenopathy. The time lag between appearance of symptoms and diagnosis is long (4 to 5 months) [13,34] and this is probably responsible for the severity of this disease even if it is difficult to prove that an earlier diagnosis may change the prognosis.

In more than half of the cases, on proctologic examination ARM manifests itself as an ulcero-vegetative tumour or a polypoid and pediculate lesion [23]. The characteristic blackish colour of a melanoma is present in 50% of cases.

Endoscopic ultrasonography is recommended on the locoregional extension to evaluate the extent of parietal invasion and perirectal lymph node invasion [9]. Table 1 presents a summary of this classification.

A thoracoabdopelvic tomodensitometry is indicated for the extended evaluation. In fact, very often one is faced with disease that is already metastatic at time of diagnosis (26-38% according to the series) [13,34]. ARM presents a significant haematogenous effusion. The usual metastatic sites include the lungs, liver, pelvic lymph nodes followed by the bone and peritoneum [34,40].

Following evaluation, ARM may be classified into three stages: (I) localized N0M0, (II) localized N+M0 and (III) metastatic. It is also important to evaluate the thickness of the parietal infiltration.

Table 1 – Endoscopic classification according to Bullard [9].

T1: sub-mucosal invasion
T2: sphincter/muscle invasion
T3: perianal /perirectal fat invasion
T4: invasion of adjacent organs

Prognostic factors

Knowledge of prognostic factors will improve therapeutic outcome in ARM. However, it is difficult to define them from such small retrospective series. Nevertheless, some factors, similar to those of cutaneous melanomas, stand out. The latter are well defined in the literature and are used to determine therapeutic strategy. Balch *et al.* have shown, on analysis of 17 600 patients suffering from a cutaneous melanoma, that for localised stages, parietal infiltration and ulceration were correlated to survival [3].

Wanebo *et al.* have revealed a correlation between thickness of parietal infiltration and disease-free survival (DFS) in ARM. In their series, the three long survivors (10 years) had a depth of parietal infiltration of less than 1.7 mm while the 23 patients having a tumour of more than 2 mm are all dead or alive with disease [39]. However, it is to be noted that Brady reported, in a subsequent analysis, on two long-term survivors, from the same institution, showing depths of 2.5 mm and 6 mm [7]. Other authors have also described long-term survivors having a parietal infiltration of more than 20 mm. [6]

Another more recent series finds this same prognostic factor to be significant, with a 5-year DFS of 19% *vs* 66% ($p = 0.04$) for tumours of more than 4 mm [4]. In the same analysis, the lymph node status also appears to be of prognostic significance with a 5-year DFS of 45% for patients with non-involved lymph nodes *vs* 0% when they are invaded.

Goldman *et al.* found size, while Slingluff *et al.* found tumour stage ($p = 0.005$) to be significant [16,32].

Finally, Dubé *et al.* have shown, in a univariate analysis that there is a poor prognosis in the presence of the following factors: stages II ($p = 0.001$) and III ($p = 0.011$), positive margins ($p = 0.003$) and tumour thickness > 20 mm ($p = 0.013$) [15].

With a certain similarity in relation to cutaneous melanomas, it is thus observed that depth of parietal infiltration and stage of the disease emerge as prognostic factors.

Pathology

ARM is a proliferation of fusiform or round cells. But it is an entity that shows great morphological variability. Distinction from other tumours (undifferentiated carcinomas, high grade sarcomas, GIST, lymphomas) is sometimes difficult, the more so when it concerns an amelanotic form (20% of cases). Immunohistochemistry enables a differentiation between ARM and other tumours. The proteins used are the same as for cutaneous melanomas: S100, HMB45, MelanA, Vimentin, Tyrosinase, which have been confirmed in several analyses [6,12,17].

Treatment

Surgery

For a long time, the standard therapy for localised stage I and II ARM has consisted of complete surgical resection only, with systemic treatment being reserved for metastatic patients. The surgical technique, nevertheless, has remained controversial, the older series favouring a heavy surgical approach with or without clearance, justified by the significant benefit in terms of local control and for some authors, even a tendency towards disease-free survival [7,32,39].

The more recent series favour a local transanal resection (TAR), allowing the preservation of the sphincter even though there is no benefit in overall survival [9,34,40]. In fact, these series confirm an improvement in local control through an abdominoperitoneal resection (APR) in the order of 70% *vs* 35% for TAR, but overall survival is not modified by the surgical technique and remains poor, at around 15-20% at 5 years. In addition, isolated relapses without metastatic disease are rare.

Table 2 shows results in terms of overall survival, disease-free survival and relapses in retrospective series with more than 10 patients since 1990 [5,7,9,16,19,21,27,28,30,32,34,40].

Table 2 – Treatment outcome after surgery.

Study	Year	Collection period	No. patients	OS at 5 years %	OS at 5 years %		DFS at 5 years %		LR % (number)		RR %		DR %	
					APA	TAR	APA	TAR	APA	TAR	APA	TAR	APA	TAR
Ross [28]	1990	-	32	3	19.5 m	18.9 m	0	8	(4/14)	58 (7/12)	-	-	-	-
Goldman [16]	1990	1970-1984	49	4	12 m	13 m	7	6	27 (4/15)	50 (9/18	-	-	-	-
Slingluff [32]	1990	1974-1990	24 (17 stage I)	8	34 m	33.4 m	0	0	50 (3/6) #	100 (7/7) #	-	-	-	-
Konstadoulakis [19]	1995	1975-1991	15 (13 M0)	9	25%	0	-	-	22 (2/9)"	50 (3/6)"	-	-	-	-
Brady [7]	1995	1929-1993	71	17	-	-	27	5	8	8	27	8	-	-
Luna-Perez [21]	1996	1980-1996	15 (7 stage I)	0	-	-			83 (5/6)	100 (1/1)	-	-	-	-
Roumen [30]	1996	-	34	-	25*	30*			5 (1/18)	75 (12/16)	-	-	-	-
Thibault [34]	1997	1939-1993	50 (37 M0)	22 / 30 M0	-	-	19	18	81 (21/26)	91 (10/11)	-	-	-	-
Bullard [9]	2003	1988-2002	5	33 to 2 years	25	4	29		50	18	25	27	75	36
Weyandt [40]	2003	1992-2001	19 (13 M0)	ns	-	-			0 (0/5)	62.5 (5/8)	-	-	-	-
Pessaux [27]	2004	1977-2002	40	17 (17 months)	30	19	14		22 (2/9)	48 (10/21)	-	-	-	-
Belli [5]	2008	1975-2006	40 (17 M0)	18.5	18.5	18.5	15.4	20.8	0	45.8	15.4	16.7	69.2	33.3

OS: overall survival, DFS: disease-free survival, LR: local relapse, RR: regional relapse, DR: distance relapse
APA: abdomino-perineal amputation, TAR: transanal resection
* to 7 years
# locoregional relapse
" includes metastatic patients

The fact that APR is associated with a better local control without impact on survival or the manifestation of metastases, suggests that systemic disease is already present at diagnosis. It is then difficult to justify such a mutilating surgical approach, except if the volume and tumour extension renders the conservative surgery impossible – the more so when the prognosis is poor. Two recent series have reported non-significantly different locoregional or distance relapse rates in spite of the surgical technique (Belli *et al.*: local relapse (LR) to 5 years 15.4% *vs* 16.7%, p = 0.98 and distance relapse (DR) 69.2% *vs* 33.3%, p = 0.1; Bullard *et al.*: 25 *vs* 27 and 75 *vs* 36) [5,9].

Therefore a conservative surgery is justified when it is technically possible with safe excision margins. Rossetti *et al.* noted the existence of intraparietal metastases up to 2 cm from the primary tumour that justifies margins of 1 to 2 cm during conservative surgery [29]. Nowadays, an APR cannot be justified only because of the achievement of safe margins that cannot be obtained with a conservative approach.

An APR is also not justified even if it allows the excision of the pelvic lymph nodes. The presence of such diseased lymph nodes, whether they are resected or not, gives an almost zero survival at 5 years [15]. It is the sign of systemic disease, leading inevitably to death of the patient, whether or not clearance is carried out. A palliative therapeutic lymph node dissection may be proposed, but this will not have any impact on the prognosis.

Lumboaortic, pelvic or inguinal prophylactic lymphadenectomy have not shown any gain in terms of survival but increased the risk of morbidity [11,38].

Prophylactic clearance does not therefore have any therapeutic role but it may have a prognostic impact. However, at present no treatment is available which can modify the prognosis with regard to lymph node status, contrary to other pathologies such as for the breast and this approach seems to be useless at present. The sentinel lymph node technique, which is well defined in the management of cutaneous melanomas, has been studied far less in ARM. The literature only reports some rare cases which do not allow conclusions to be drawn. This technique remains to be investigated [22,31,35].

Adjuvant treatment

Adjuvant treatment after conservative surgery has been suggested as being responsible for additional toxicity. Furthermore, local relapse does not impact overall survival. Bullard *et al.* have emphasized the potential importance of such a treatment in their series [9]: two patients presented an isolated regional metastatic relapse and were given a surgical clearance with an adjuvant treatment. During the following 5 years, they were free from local relapse or development of metastases.

Radiotherapy

Ballo *et al.* confirmed the benefits of adjuvant radiotherapy after surgery [4]. From 1989 to 2000, 23 patients with ARM benefited from TAR followed by adjuvant radiotherapy (hypofractionated: 30 Gy in 5 fractions for 2.5 weeks). Nine patients were also given systemic treatment (chemotherapy n = 4, immunotherapy n = 2 or both n = 3). The 5-year overall survival, relapse-free survival and metastasis-free survival were 31%, 37% and 35% respectively. The 5-year local and regional lymph node control rates were 74% and 84% respectively. They are similar to those obtained after APR. Univariate analyses have revealed that patients whose radiotherapy fields included the primary tumour as well as the drainage sites, had a higher 5-year local control rate (81% *vs* 0%, $p < 0.001$). Five patients presented a local relapse and three presented a regional relapse. These two relapses concerned radiotherapy treatments that included the primary tumour site only. It may be noted that the two relapses were located on the border line. Toxicity after radiotherapy was quite acceptable with a 5-year survival without complications of 71%.

Bujko *et al.* also noted the importance of adjuvant radiotherapy that includes the drainage sites so as to eradicate occult lymph node disease, often present even at localized stages [8].

Moozar *et al.* also reported a series of 14 patients, of whom 7 had surgery with adjuvant radiotherapy at different stages of their disease. Although the difference was not significant, overall survival was 12 months for patients having undergone a surgical excision versus 16.5 months for those who benefited from adjuvant radiotherapy [25].

Adjuvant radiotherapy following conservative surgery, can lead to a local control similar or even superior to that obtain with an APR only, given that the fields are not only focused on the primary tumour but also on drainage sites.

Chemotherapy and immunotherapy

Terada *et al.* observed an ARM case treated by APR with chemotherapy and a post-operative immunotherapy consisting of dacarbazine, nimustine hydrochloride, vincristine sulphate and interferon-beta. No relapse was recorded within the following 2 years [33]. Apart from reports on isolated and anecdotal cases, such as the one reported by Bullard *et al.* [9], the literature does not provide any data concerning adjuvant systemic treatment of ARM. The widely disappointing information on cutaneous melanomas can only be transposed. The 2003 French "Standards, Options and Recommendations" did not support the indication for chemotherapy or an adjuvant vaccination. Interferon-alpha has a marketing authorisation in France for melanomas of "initial poor prognosis" but is only considered as an option, given the controversial results obtained on overall survival [35]. The efficacy of chemotherapy and immunotherapy as adjuvant treatments has yet to be proven.

Neo-adjuvant treatment

The literature does not provide sufficient data to justify the implementation of a neo-adjuvant treatment by radiotherapy or chemotherapy. Although Uner *et al.* reported, with a time lapse of 30 months, a case of a stenosing ARM, free from local relapse or metastases, treated by a discharge colostomy followed by pre-operative radiotherapy followed by local surgery [37], the rare reports on patients having received a neo-adjuvant treatment for ARM concern essentially those having initially benefited from radiotherapy or radiochemotherapy for an undifferentiated carcinoma. Due to the absence of a definitive diagnosis, pathological verification was carried out, revealing a diagnosis of anorectal melanoma. [25]

Treatment of metastatic disease

Over the past two decades, biochemotherapy (BCT) has been widely studied in cutaneous metastatic melanomas [1]. With the chemotherapy (cisplatine, vinblastine and dacarbazine) and immunotherapy (Interleukin-2 IL2 and Interferon IFN) combination response rates in the order of 50% can be obtained, of which 10% to 20% are complete responses. The median survival time is around 11-12 months. In metastatic ARM, no randomised studies have been carried out and only data on retrospective series with very few participants, using similar treatments as for cutaneous melanomas, is available. Ulmer *et al.* have reported a metastatic ARM case treated with intra-tumour interferon-beta and systemic chemotherapy with dacarbazine. The patient obtained a complete regression of the primary tumour with a partial regression of metastases [36].

Koskal *et al.* observed a case of metastatic ARM of the liver treated by APR followed by chemotherapy and sub-cutaneous postoperative immunotherapy (intraportal cisplatin, interferon-alpha and interleukin-2). A complete regression of hepatic metastases was seen [20].

The largest published series is that of the MDACC team [18] concerning patients with metastatic ARM between 1991 and 2001. All patients received a BCT treatment and the results agreed with those obtained for cutaneous melanomas: 44% (8 patients) overall response, of which 11% (2 patients) had a complete response with a median survival time of 12.2 months.

However, this treatment has a significant toxicity, with 95% of patients presenting grade 3 or higher toxicity in the last phase III trial published on metastatic cutaneous melanomas [2]. Moreover, this trial confirmed that BCT treatment brought an increase in the response rate and progression-free survival, but without any impact on overall survival. This treatment is no longer recommended for metastatic cutaneous melanomas due to the complexity in administering the treatment and its toxicity. It is therefore difficult to define recommendations for the treatment of metastatic anorectal melanomas. BCT produces results, but at the price of a significant toxicity. It is important that the biology of these tumours is studied so that adapted therapies can be developed.

Conclusion

Surgery (TAR with clear margins) is the mainstay of treatment. This approach gives less morbidity and it enables preservation of the rectum while overall survival is unaltered. APR remains a valid alternative when clear surgical margins are impossible with a conservative procedure, when there is local relapse and in the case of palliative treatment for symptoms which cannot be controlled by other means. In the absence of an effective systemic treatment, the presence of lymph node invasion (pre- or per-operative) renders APR useless and clearance is only proposed as a palliative treatment. The presence of metastases – apart from those giving rise to uncontrollable symptoms – are a contra-indication for APR.

Giving adjuvant radiotherapy to the primary tumour including drainage sites results in a high local control, at least as good as with non-conservative surgery and without any doubt, gives a better quality of life. It should be an integral part of the management strategy in case of limited options.

However, this disease has a high metastatic potential and systemic treatment with biochemotherapy, even although it is not yet indicated as an adjuvant treatment due to the absence of proof of efficacy, should in fact be carried out in a metastatic situation, even if the relevant modalities are not well defined (chemotherapy alone?, in association with immunotherapy?, what type of treatment for second or third line therapy?).

Recommendations are presented in Table 3. Poor prognosis is attributable to the inherent characteristics of the disease and to late diagnosis and these two factors may probably be linked. Progress remains to be made in the early screening and diagnosis of these tumours as well as in the understanding of the biological mechanism involved, so as to provide a basis on which to propose adapted therapies.

Table 3 – Guidelines (adapted from Weyandt [40]).

N0 M0	Thickness	< 1 mm : 1- 4 mm: > 4 mm:	TAR 1 cm margin otherwise resumption or adjuvant RT TAR 2 cm margin otherwise resumption or adjuvant RT APR or TAR and adjuvant RT
N+M0	TAR + clearance and adjuvant RT		
M+	No systematic surgery, in presence of symptoms only Systemic treatment: immunotherapy, chemotherapy		

References

1. Atkins MB (2006) Cytokine-based therapy and biochemotherapy for advanced melanoma. Clin Cancer Res 12: 2353s-2358s
2. Atkins MB, Hsu J, Lee S *et al.* (2008) Phase III trial comparing concurrent biochemotherapy with cisplatin, vinblastine, dacarbazine, interleukin-2, and interferon alfa-2b with cisplatin, vinblastin, and dacarbazine alone in patients with metastatic malignant melanoma (E3695): a trial coordinated by the eastern cooperative oncology group. J Clin Oncol 26: 5748-54
3. Balch CM, Soong SJ, Gershenwald JE *et al.* (2001) Prognostic factors analysis of 17,600 melanoma patients: validation of the American Joint Committee on Cancer melanoma staging system. J Clin Oncol 19: 3622-34
4. **Ballo MT, Gershenwald JE, Zagars GK *et al.* (2002) Sphincter-sparing local excision and adjuvant radiation for anal-rectal melanoma. J Clin Oncol 20: 4555-8**
5. Belli F, Gallino GF, Vullo SL *et al.* (2008) Melanoma of the anorectal region. The experience of the national cancer institute of Milano.J Cancer Surg ESJO x: 1-6
6. Ben-Izhak O, Levy R, Weill S *et al.* (1997) Anorectal malignant melanoma: A clinicopathologic study, including Immunohistochemistry and DNA Flow Cytometry. Cancer 79: 18-25
7. **Brady MS, Kavolius JP, Quan SHQ (1995) Anorectal melanoma: a 64 year experience at Memorial Sloan-kettrering Cancer center (review). Dis Colon Rectum 38: 146-51**
8. Bujko K, Nowacki MP, Liszka-Dalecki P (1998) Radiation therapy for anorectal melanoma. A report of three cases. Acta Oncologica 37: 497-9
9. Bullard KM, Tuttle TM, Rothenberg DA *et al.* (2003) Surgical therapy for anorectal melanoma.J Am Coll Surg 196: 206-11
10. Cagir B, Whiteford MH, Topham A *et al.* (1999) Changing epidemiology of anorectal melanoma. Dis Colon Rectum 42: 1203-8
11. Chiu YS, Unni KK, Beart RW Jr (1980) Malignant melanoma of the anorectum. Dis Colon Rectum 23: 122-4
12. Chute DJ, Cousar JB, Mills SE (2006) Anorectal malignant melanoma : morphologic and immunohistochemical features. Am J Clin Pathol 126: 93-100
13. Cooper PH, Mills SE, Allen MS (1982) Malignant melanoma of the anus. Dis Colon Rectum 25: 693-703
14. Droesch JT, Flum DR, Mann GN (2005) Wide local excision or abdominoperineal resection as the initial treatment for anorectal melanoma? The American Journal of Surgery 189: 446-9
15. Dube P, Elias D, Bonvalot S (1997) Melanome primitive anorectal. J Chir 134: 3-8
16. Goldman S, Glimelius B, Pahlman L (1990) Anorectal malignant melanoma in Sweden: report of 49 patients. Dis Colon Rectum 33: 874-7
17. Hussein MR (2008) Extracutaneous malignant melanomas. Cancer Invest 26: 516-34
18. Kim KB, Sanguino AM, Hodges C *et al.* (2004) Biochemotherapy in patients with metastatic anorectal mucosal melanoma. Cancer 100: 1478-83
19. Konstadoulakis MM, Ricaniadis N, Walsh D, Karakousis CP (1995) Malignant melanoma of the anorectal region. J Surg Oncol 58: 118-20

4

20. Koskal N *et al.* (2000) Complete remission of the liver metastases of anorectal melanoma with regional chemotherapy: a case report. Hepatogastroenterology 47: 612-4
21. Luna-Perez P, Rodriguez DF, Macouzet JG (1996) Anorectal malignant melanoma. Surg Oncol 5: 165-8
22. Mariolis-Sapsakos T, Malamitsi J, Yakoumakis E, Orfanos F (2008) Is sentinel node mapping useful in anorectal melanoma? Hell J Nucl Med 11: 39-42
23. Melhouff MM, El Amrani N, Mathieu-Daud H, Dubois JB (1995) Les mélanomes malins anorectaux. A propos de 5 cas : revue de la littérature. Ann Gastroenterol Hepatol 3: 209-12
24. Moore WD (1857) Recurrent melanosis of the rectum after previous removal from the verge of the anus in a man aged 65. Lancet 1: 290-4
25. Moozar KL, Wong S, Couture J (2003) Anorectal malignant melanoma: treatment with surgery or radiation therapy, or both.Can J Surg 46: 345-9
26. Negrier S, Saiag P, Guillot B *et al.* (2005) Recommandations pour la pratique clinique: Standards, options et recommendations 2005 pour la prise en charge des patients adultes atteints d'un melanoma cutané M0. Ann Dermatol Venereol 132: 10s43-51
27. Pessaux P, Pocard M, Elias D *et al.* (2004) Surgical management of primary anorectal melanoma. Brit J Surg91: 1183-7
28. Ross M, Pezzi C, Pezzi T *et al.* (1990) Patterns of failure in anorectal melanoma: a guide to surgical therapy. Arch Surg 125: 316-6
29. Rossetti C, Koukouras D, Eboli M *et al.* (1997) Primary anorectal melanomas: an institutional experience. J Exp Clin Cancer Res 16: 81-5
30. Roumen RMH (1996) Anorectal melanoma in the Netherlands: a report of 63 patients. Eur J Surg Oncol 22: 598-601
31. Sanli Y, Turkmen C, Kurul S *et al.* (2006) Sentinel lymph node biopsy for the staging of anal melanoma:report of two cases. Ann Nucl Med 20: 629-31
32. Slingluff CL Jr, Vollmer RT, Seigler HF (1990) Anorectal melanoma: clinical characteristics and results of surgical management in twenty-four patients. Surgery 107: 1-9
33. Terada R, Ito S, Kobayashi M *et al.* (2002) Anorectal melanoma: successful treatment by surgical excision and combination chemoimmunotherapy. Hepatogastroenterology 49: 1545-8
34. **Thibault C, Sagar P, Nivatvongs S *et al.* (1997) Anorectal melanoma an incurable disease? Dis Colon Rectum 40: 661-8**
35. Tien HY, McMasters KM, Edwardes MJ, Chao C (2002) Sentinel lymph node metastasis in anal melanoma: a case report. Int J Gastrointest Cancer 32: 53-6
36. Ulmer A (2002) Successful palliation of stenosing anorectal melanoma by intratumoral injections with natural interferon-beta.Melanoma Res 12: 395-8
37. Uner A, Mentes BB, Egehan I, Duursun A (2003) Neoadjuvant radiotherapy in anorectal malignant melanoma. Int J Clin Prat 57: 65-7
38. Urist MM, Maddox WA, Kennedy JE, Balch CM (1983) Patient risk factors and surgical morbidity after regional lymphadenectomy in 204 patients. Cancer 51: 2151-6
39. **Wanebo HJ, Woodruff JM, Farr GH, Quan SH (1981) Anorectal melanoma. Cancer 47: 1891-900**
40. **Weyandt GH, Eggert AO, Houf M *et al.* (2003) Anorectal melanoma: surgical management guidelines according to tumour thickness. Br J Cancer 89: 2019-22**

Primary adenocarcinoma of the anal canal

5

Y. Belkacémi, P. Rouanet and M. Jafari

Five Essential Points

1. *Adenocarcinoma of the anal canal can be separated into three main categories:*
   . Tumours arising from the mucosal surface
   . Tumours arising from anal glands (AGC)
   . Tumours arising along fistulous tracts
2. *The loss of expression of p63 and CK5/6 in AGC compared with normal anal gland mucosa and its negativity for CDX2 compared with colorectal carcinoma could comprise an immunostaining panel that may be helpful for pathologic subclassification.*
3. *Age, gender, T stage, N stage, tumour differentiation and treatment modality are suggested to be prognostic factors.*
4. *The eradication of primary tumour occurs more often in patients who have received more than 54 Gy. Combined chemotherapy should be based on drugs such as fluoropyrimidines, platinum salts or mitomycin.*
5. *Abdomino-perineal resection should no longer be considered to be the primary treatment option. It could be reserved for salvage treatment of those tumours not responding to primary radio-chemotherapy, and for treatment of recurrent disease.*

Introduction

Anal tumours represent 5% of all anorectal malignancies [5]. Adenocarcinoma of the anal canal is considered as very rare and more aggressive than epidermoid cancers. It is thought to arise from the stratified columnar epithelium lining the anal glands, which have their openings in the transitional zone of the canal and extend into the submucosa to penetrate the internal sphincter [12, 25, 34]. Current adenocarcinoma management is controversial and experience with this disease remains largely anecdotal or is based on very small series. For some authors, primary abdomino-perineal resection should be considered as "the gold standard" [1, 4, 17, 34]. For others, combined radiochemotherapy, which has been widely reported to be very effective in epidermoid cancers of the anal canal, should be adopted as a possible treatment in certain patients with adenocarcinoma histology [18, 19, 22, 30, 31].

To address some of these uncertainties and to discuss the best management of this malignancy, this chapter presents an overview of past research, recent developments and ongoing controversies from pathology to treatment strategy in adenocarcinoma of the anal canal.

Pathogenesis

Squamous cell carcinomas represent almost 85% of all anal canal tumours, whereas adenocarcinoma rates reported in the literature range from 5 to 19% [4, 19]. Thus, our understanding of the pathogenesis and management of squamous cell carcinoma of the anal canal is better documented than that of adenocarcinoma.

The anatomic definitions of anal tumours vary considerably in the literature, which has led to confusion regarding diagnosis and treatment. In general, two clinical entities exist: tumours of the anal canal and those of the anal margin. The anal canal is lined by squamous mucosa which is present between the anal verge and the pectinate line. The latter represents the border between the more distal squamous mucosa and a transitional area of squamous and non-squamous mucosa. Tumours arising within the anal canal distal to the pectinate line are most often keratinizing squamous-cell carcinoma, whereas those arising within the transitional mucosa above the pectinate line are mostly non-keratinizing squamous-cell carcinoma.

The pathogenesis of anal canal adenocarcinoma is not completely clear. For over thirty years, numerous factors such as local chronic inflammation, pre-existing fistula and Crohn's disease have been reported to be associated with the development of anal canal carcinoma [9, 20]. More recently, the human papillomavirus, which is sexually transmitted, has also been incriminated in epidermoid anal cancer pathogenesis [13, 31]. An excellent review of anatomical features, histological findings and predisposing factors can be found in papers by Ryan *et al.* [30, 31].

Adenocarcinoma of the anal canal can be separated into three main categories:

- Tumours arising from the mucosal surface,
- Tumours arising from anal glands and
- Tumours arising along fistulous tracts.

The identification of mucins is a key element in the diagnosis of adenocarcinoma. Historically, it is difficult to differentiate subclassification of extramucosal adenocarcinoma from anal gland carcinoma (AGC). The definitive criterion for the diagnosis of AGC is the demonstration of continuity of the tumour with normal anal glands. However, in a significant proportion of cases, a direct relation of the tumour to anal glands cannot be established because of obliteration of the point of origin, removal of the primary tumour site, associated inflammatory change, or the vagaries of sampling. Recently, it has been suggested that the loss of expression of p63 and CK5/6 in AGC, compared with normal anal gland mucosa and its negativity for CDX2 compared with colorectal carcinoma, could comprise an immunostaining panel that may be helpful in the diagnosis of AGC [21].

Prognostic factors

In adenocarcinoma of the anal canal the low number of patients in published series does not permit any consistent analysis for local or distant prognosis. Thus, the parameters reported for squamous cell carcinoma are generally considered as the basis for decision making in adenocarcinoma without consistent data, the latter obtained largely from anecdotal experience or from very small series.

Tumour size and tumour mobility are important prognostic factors for patients with squamous cell cancer of the anal canal. Mobile lesions of no more than 2 cm in diameter can be cured in approximately 80% of cases, whereas survival rates are no higher than 50% when tumour size exceeds 5 cm [35]. In addition, the probability of nodal involvement is directly related to tumour size [8, 26, 32, 35]. To date, limited data are available with regard to prognostic factors of anal canal adenocarcinoma. In the study of the Rare Cancer Network (RCN) (www.rarecancer.net) in which 82 cases of adenocarcinomas were studied [6], four independent prognostic factors were identified: T stage, N stage, tumour differentiation and treatment modality. Among these factors, which have also been reported for squamous cell carcinoma, tumour length (> 4 *versus* ≤ 4 cm) which influenced survival rates in univariate analyses, was not identified as an independent factor in the multivariate model for adenocarcinoma. Moreover, neither tumour width nor tumour circumference were found to be a prognostic factor. Conversely, tumour grade, which is an independent prognostic factor in squamous cell carcinoma [38], was also identified for adenocarcinoma in the RCN study [6].

In the RCN report, other parameters such as age and gender were not found to be prognostic factors for adenocarcinoma. With regard to gender, a female predominance is generally observed in squamous cell carcinomas [19, 33, 37, 38,]. Myerson *et al.* [23] reported in addition to early tumour stage and epidermoid histology, the significant favourable impact of female gender on survival. In adenocarcinoma, we observed a slight male predominance [6] as in other reports [1,4,18,23,33] but gender has never been reported to be a prognostic factor.

Age in anal cancer patients is highly variable with a peak incidence observed during the seventh decade of life. The age of patients reported in both adenocarcinoma and squamous cell carcinoma ranges between 25 and 94 years old [4, 8, 14, 19, 24, 37, 38]. This is not generally reported to be a prognostic factor but it could be a restrictive factor for the use of standard chemotherapy (CT) doses in addition to loco-regional radiotherapy.

Treatment strategy

Combined modalities

The management of squamous cell carcinoma of the anal canal, which is better documented than that of adenocarcinoma, has undergone profound changes over the last 30 years. Several studies demonstrated that combined treatment provides results equivalent to surgery with the advantage of preserving sphincter function. Some other reports confirmed these results, and for many years, the only obvious benefit from chemoradiation protocols was in sphincter function preservation; without any impact on survival. Thus, radiochemotherapy was advocated as the treatment of choice for these anal canal carcinomas. In their review, Ryan *et al.* concluded that squamous cell carcinomas could be cured with radiochemotherapy without APR, and approximately one half of the patients with local recurrence after combined treatment would be successfully treated with salvage surgery either using APR or more recently with the trans-anal techniques [30].

Because of its rarity and apparent heterogeneity, anal canal adenocarcinoma has been less frequently studied and optimal therapeutic strategies less defined. To date, various available therapeutic options have been discussed but neither comparative nor analytical epidemiological studies have been conducted that might help to resolve this issue.

In contrast with squamous cell carcinoma, chemoradiation was not recognized early on as a primary treatment modality in adenocarcinoma of the anal canal. Until the nineties, most authors recommended radical surgery as the treatment of choice [1, 7, 9]. However, this has been associated with a poorer prognosis than in squamous cell carcinoma with 5-year survival rates ranging between 17% and 42%. In the RCN study, we observed overall survival rates of 21% and 29% at 5 years in the two surgical groups [6].

When considering advanced anal canal tumours, patients with an adenocarcinoma also have a poorer prognosis than those with a squamous cell carcinoma, with survival rates not reaching more than 5% [1, 5, 10, 18, 29]. This may be due partly to the widespread use of combined radiochemotherapy as the principle treatment for squamous cell carcinoma as compared to adenocarcinoma. In the National Cancer Database Report, the majority of patients with squamous cell carcinoma were managed principally with combined treatment whereas 3/4 of those with adenocarcinoma underwent surgery [23]. In small surgical series of adenocarcinomas treated with APR or local excision, the number of patients surviving at long term remains very low [4, 17], with a crude 5-year survival of 4.8% [17].

Over the last 10 years, some small retrospective adenocarcinoma series have reported radiochemotherapy to be an interesting primary treatment option [1, 18, 19, 22, 34]. In a large study of 192 anal canal cancers, Klas *et al.* [19] identified 36 patients with adenocarcinoma. Twenty-two (61%) of them were managed with surgery alone (6 APR and 16 local excisions) and 14 (39%) with surgery followed by chemoradiation. The 5-year survival and local recurrence rates were 63% and 21% respectively. Table 1 shows the results of small series of adenocarinoma treated with combined radiochemotherapy.

About 50% of patients unresponsive to radiation (or chemoradiation) can be cured by APR [2, 19, 27]. This conclusion has been drawn from a study by Abel *et al.* [1] which included 38 adenocarcinomas treated with radiation and/or CT as an adjunct to surgery or as the prime modality. In this series, APR was ultimately required in 75% of patients. However, single or bimodality therapies may not be sufficient for locally and regionally advanced T3, T4 and N2 tumour control. The prognosis of advanced adenocarcinomas is very poor, with 5-year survival rates about 5% [1, 5, 10, 18, 29]. In the RCN study, the 5-year survival was 9% for T4 tumours and 13% for N2 disease. Klas *et al.* [19] observed better results in their series of 36 patients. The authors attributed their good results to the use of chemoradiation either preoperatively or postoperatively. Indeed, to improve our results in advanced tumours, trimodality therapy could be considered as an interesting alternative.

In the RCN report, analyses were performed according to 3 treatment modalities. The combined radiochemotherapy group did better than the other two surgical groups. Moreover, the combined radiochemotherapy modality was a favourable independent prognostic factor in the multivariate analysis [6].

Table 1 – Results of combined radiochemotherapy.

Authors	n	N of pts CRT-CT	Median FU (years)	LRR
Klas *et al.* [19]	36	39%	–	21%
Tarazi *et al.* [34]	7	100%	–	14%
Longo *et al.* [22]	7	–	5.1	CRT-CT > APR
Joon *et al.* [18]	15	40%	6.6	0%
Belkacémi *et al.* [6]	82	38%	4.7	35%

Abbreviations: CRT-CT: combined radiochemotherapy; FU: follow-up; LRR: local recurrence rate; APR: abdominoperineal resection.

Radiation therapy modality

In terms of radiation therapy, the total dose required for anal cancer sterilization has been the subject of debate. Retrospective studies have suggested that permanent eradication of primary tumour occurred more often in patients who had received a dose over 54 Gy of external beam radiation therapy [11, 16]. This dose-effect relationship has also been noted at lower dose ranges. Klas *et al.* [19] found an improved survival in patients who had received more than 45 Gy compared with those who had received less than 35 Gy ($p < 0.05$). In the RCN study, there was no influence of total dose on tumour control and survival. As compared to rectal adenocarcinomas, the total dose should be in excess of 45 Gy, at least in the preoperative setting. For example, in cT2 distal rectal adenocarcinomas, a total dose of 50.4 Gy cannot result in more than 15% of complete response in patients who refuse the required APR. With this dose, the rate of local failure in the 78% of patients who underwent a sphincter-sparing operation was 10% [28].

On the other hand, nodal dose should also be assessed. The inguinal dose may be different according to the lymph node involvement and treatment modality. In the study by Joon *et al.* [18], the total dose delivered to inguinal nodes in patients with T3 and T4 tumours treated with concurrent radiochemotherapy, was 54 Gy and 45 Gy respectively, in patients with or without nodal involvement. When radiotherapy was used alone, the doses were increased to 60 Gy and 50 Gy, respectively. In the RCN study, 78% of the patients had no initial inguinal lymph node involvement. The majority of them (84%) received prophylactic radiotherapy at a dose of 38-50 Gy. In the combined therapy group, the inguinal prophylactic dose in the 77% of patients who had no lymph node involvement was 44 Gy. Two patients classified as N2 received 66 Gy. Thus, these data suggest that the total dose should be adapted to the nodes status. However, in the context of primary combined radiochemotherapy modality, the impact of inguinal prophylactic irradiation on regional control and survival is still not clear.

Systemic therapy

In a radiochemotherapy study using 5-fluorouracil associated with mitomycin or carboplatin for epidermoid cancer, acute toxicity was acceptable, although a high number of patients exhibited chronic treatment-related symptoms [15, 38]. In the RCN adenocarcinoma study, we also observed a slightly higher late toxicity in the combined group as compared to the surgical group but the difference was not statistically significant [6]. In the study by Joon *et al.* [18], mitomycin was administered as a bolus of 10 mg/m^2 (day 1) and 5-fluorouracil at a dose of 1,000 mg/m^2 in a continuous infusion (day 1 to 4 and 29 to 32). The results were better in the combined therapy group but 2/4 patients developed major toxicity and required dose modifications of the chemotherapy.

Because of the small number of patients in the reported series of anal canal adenocarcinoma, the optimal CT combination is unknown. For epidermoid carcinomas, CT protocols have been more extensively investigated using combined 5-fluorouracil-mitomycin and radiotherapy compared to radiotherapy alone. The combined schedule resulted in fewer local failures, in a lower likelihood of recurrence and in a lesser probability of subsequent colostomy due to persistent disease, however with similar 3-year survival.

The role of CT in the prevention of distant metastases in anal canal cancers is unclear. In the combined modality groups, the rate of metastasis varies between 5.5% and 17% [3, 19, 36, 38]. However in adenocarcinoma, Joon *et al.* (18) did not observe any distant failures in the 6 patients treated with combined

5

radiochemotherapy after a median follow-up of 6.6 years. The lung and liver are recognized to be the most frequent sites of distant metastases from anal canal cancers. Shindo (33) reported lung and liver metastases in 13% of epidermoid cancers and in 18% of adenocarcinomas. In the RCN study, 17 patients (20%) developed metastases. The most frequent sites were the lung and liver [6].

References

1. Abel ME, Chiu YSG, Russel TR *et al.* (1993) Adenocarcinoma of the anal glands: results of a survey. Dis Colon Rectum 36: 383-7
2. Allal AS, Laurencet FM, Reymond MA *et al.* (1999) Effectiveness of surgical salvage therapy for patients with locally uncontrolled anal carcinoma after sphincter-conserving treatment. Cancer 86: 405-9
3. Bartelink H, Roelofsen F, Eschwege F *et al.* (1997) Concomitant radiotherapy and chemotherapy is superior to radiotherapy alone in the treatment of locally advanced anal cancer: results of a phase III randomized trial of the European Organization for Research and Treatment of Cancer Radiotherapy and Gastrointestinal Cooperative groups. J Clin Oncol 15: 2042-9
4. Basik M, Rodriguez-Bigas MA, Penetrante R *et al.* (1995) Prognostic and recurrence patterns of anal adenocarcinoma. Am J Surg 169: 233-7
5. Beahars OH, Wilson SM (1976) Carcinoma of the anus. Ann Surg 184: 422-8
6. **Belkacémi Y, Berger C, Poortmans P *et al.* (2003) Primary adenocarcinoma of the anal canal management: a retrospective multicenter study from the Rare Cancer Network. Int J Radiat Oncol Biol Phys 56: 1274-83**
7. Berg HK (1990) Adenocarcinoma of the anal canal. Md Med J 39: 675-8
8. Boman BM, Moertel CG, O'Connell MJ *et al.* (1984) Carcinoma of the anal canal: a clinical and pathological study of 188 cases. Cancer 54: 114-25
9. Buchwalter JA, Jurayj MN (1957) Relationship of chronic anorectal disease to carcinoma. Arch Surg 75: 352-61
10. Cabrera A, Tsukada Y, Pickeren JW (1966) Adenocarcinoma of the anal canal and perineal tissues. Ann Surg 164: 152-6
11. Cummings BJ, Kane TJ, O'Sullivan B *et al.* (1991) Epidermoid anal cancer: treatment by radiation alone or by radiation and 5-fluorouracil with or without mitomycin C. Int J Radiat Oncol Biol Phys 21: 1115-25
12. Fenger C, Morson BC (1989) Anal duct carcinoma. Dis Colon Rectum 32: 355-7
13. Frisch M, Glimelius B, van den Brule AJ *et al.* (1997) Sexually transmitted infection as a cause of anal cancer. N Engl J Med 337: 1350-8
14. Frost DB, Richards PC, Montagne ED *et al.* (1984) Epidermoid cancer of the anorectum. Cancer 53: 1285-93
15. Gabriele AM, Rovea P, Solo B *et al.* (1997) Radiation therapy and chemotherapy in the conservative treatment of carcinoma of the anal canal: survival and late morbidity in a series of 25 patients. Anticancer Res 17: 653-6
16. Hughes LL, Rich TA, Delclos L *et al.* (1989) Radiotherapy for anal cancer: experience from 1979-1987. Int J Radiat Oncol Biol Phys 17: 1153-60
17. Jensen SL, Shokouh-Amiri MH, Hagen K (1988) Adenocarcinoma of the anal ducts: a series of 21 cases. Dis Colon Rectum 31: 268-72
18. **Joon DL, Chao MW, Ngan SY *et al.* (1999) Primary adenocarcinoma of the anus: a retrospective analysis. Int J Radiat Oncol Biol Phys 45: 1199-205**
19. Klas JV, Rothenberger DA, Wong WD *et al.* (1999) Malignant tumors of the anal canal: the spectrum of disease, treatment, and outcomes. Cancer 85: 1686-93
20. Kline RJ, Spencer RJ, Harrisson Jr RG (1964) Carcinoma associated with fistula-in-ano. Arch Surg 89: 989-94
21. **Lisovsky M, Patel K, Cymes K *et al.* (2007) Immunophenotypic characterization of anal gland carcinoma: loss of p63 and cytokeratin 5/6. Arch Pathol Lab Med 131: 1304-11**
22. Longo WE, Vernava AM III, Warde TP *et al.* (1995) Rare anal canal cancers in the US veteran: patterns of disease and results of treatment. Am J Surg 61: 495-500
23. Myerson RJ, Karnell LH, Menk HR (1997) The National Cancer Database Report on carcinoma of the anus. Cancer 80: 805-15
24. O'Brien PH, Jenrette JM, Wallace KM *et al.* (1982) Epidermoid carcinoma of the anus. Surg Gynecol Obstet 155: 745-51

25. Parks AG (1970) Mucin secreting adenocarcinoma of anal gland origin. Br J Surg 57: 434-6
26. Pintor MP, Northover JM, Nicholls RJ (1989) Squamous cell carcinoma of the anus at one hospital from 1948 to 1984. Br J Surg 76: 806-10
27. Procard M, Tiret E, Nugent K *et al.* (1988) Results of salvage abdominoperineal resection for anal cancer after radiotherapy. Dis Colon Rectum 41: 1488-93
28. Renegan R, Paty P, Wong WD *et al.* (2005) Distal cT2N0 rectal Cancer: is there an alternative to abdominoperineal resection? J Clin Oncol 23: 4905-12
29. Rich TA, Ajani JA, Morrisson WH *et al.* (1993) Chemoradiation therapy for anal canal: radiation plus continuous infusion of 5-fluorouracil with or without cisplatin. Radiother Oncol 27: 209-15
30. Ryan DP, Compton CC, Mayer RJ (2000) Carcinoma of the anal canal. N Engl J Med 342: 792-800
31. Ryan DP, Mayer RJ (2000) Anal carcinoma: histology, staging, epidemiology, treatment. Curr Opin Oncol 12: 345-52
32. Schlienger M, Krzisch C, Pène F *et al.* (1989) Epidermoid carcinoma of the anal canal treatment results and prognostic variables in a series of 242 cases. Int J Radiat Oncol Biol Phys 17: 1141-51
33. Shindo K (1981) Epidermoid carcinoma compared with adenocarcinoma of the anal canal. Aust N Z J Surg 51: 426-9
34. Tarazi R, Nelson RL (1994) Anal adenocarcinoma:a comprehensive review. Sem Surg Oncol 10: 235-40
35. Touboul E, Schlienger M, Buffat L *et al.* (1995) Conservative versus non conservative treatment of epidermoid carcinoma of the anal canal for tumors longer or equal to 5 centimeters. A retrospective comparison. Cancer 75: 786-93
36. UKCCCR Anal Cancer Trial Working Party (1996) Epidermoid anal cancer: results from UKCCCR randomized trial of radiotherapy alone versus radiotherapy, 5-fluorouracil and mitomycin. Lancet 348: 1049-54
37. Valentini V, Montello G, Leone MV *et al.* (1997) Organ preservation in carcinoma of the anal canal. Rays 22: 447-53
38. Wagner JP, Mahe MA, Romestaing P *et al.* (1994) Radiation therapy in the conservative treatment of carcinoma of the anal canal. Int J Radiat Oncol Biol Phys 29: 17-23
39. Zaren HA, Delone FX, Lerner HJ (1983) Carcinoma of the anal gland: case report and review of the literature. J Surg Oncol 13: 250-4

Anal margin tumours

6

M. Schlienger and E. Touboul

Five Essential Points

1. *Prevention of anal margin cancers by repeated search and treatment of benign loco-regional lesions, in particular in patients at risk of immunodeficiency.*
2. *After positive biopsy, loco-regional and general evaluation including HIV status before any treatment.*
3. *TNM classification permits the choice of a conservative treatment:*
   - *T1 and small T2 N0 (<3 cm) excision with 1 cm margin; careful local and nodal follow-up;*
   - *T2 N0 (3 to 5 cm) pelvic RT + elective inguinal RT;*
   - *T3 – T4 N0-N1 (>5 cm): pelvic + inguinal RT + CT.*
4. *Careful prolonged follow-up permits an appropriate salvage of local or loco-regional failures.*
5. *Treatment of HIV-positive patients: 2 mandatory contemporary treatments:*
   - *Treatment of AM tumour according to TNM stage and*
   - *Treatment of immunodeficiency (favorable factor: CD4 count >200 mm^3)*

Introduction

Cancers of the anal margin (AM) are cutaneous cancers (peri-anal skin cancers) occurring on the peri-anal area outside the anal verge. This funnel-shaped skin area is defined by a circle measuring 10 cm in diameter centred on the anal orifice. For some authors, the lower part of the anal canal, a non-keratinizing squamous epithelium area below the pectinate line, is part of the anal margin. Frequently AM tumours are included in series on "anal or anal canal" cancers (AC). In the prospective trial of the UKCCCR 1997 [25] on "anal cancers", comparing radiotherapy (RT) alone *vs* RT + chemotherapy, 134 (23 %) of 587 cases were AM tumours; unfortunately, their results were not separated from the anal canal group.

AM tumours represent about 15 % of tumours of anal region, therefore they are considered as rare tumours and 80 to 85 % are epidermoid epitheliomas. For several years, an increase in their frequency has been noticed as they are being found in young or middle aged homosexual men who are frequently HIV positive.

Changes of management over time of anal margin carcinomas

Treatment modalities have evolved over the last forty years. In the sixties, small tumours (T1 < 2 cm and small T2 < 3 cm) had a local conservative excision. Larger tumours, (T2 > 3 cm, T3 and T4) had an abdomino-perineal resection (APR) and RT was used as palliative or salvage treatment.

During the early seventies, the possibility of local cure of AC tumours by conservative treatment with external RT and or brachytherapy was assessed. Subsequently, concomitant chemotherapy (CT) was combined with RT by Nigro [14] with 5FU and Mitomycin, initially as a preoperative (APR) irradiation for larger AC tumours. The encouraging results led Papillon [16] and Cummings [5] to use this protocol to treat AC tumours conservatively as well as large AM lesions. At the present time, the same conservative principles are the basis of AM epidermoïd carcinoma treatment, while APR has become salvage treatment.

Results of treatment

Tables 1 and 2 summarize 5 surgical series with 203 patients and 7 RT series with 193 patients.

Five surgical series (1963-1989) (Table 1)

a) T1 and T2 N0 AM tumours treated by local excision (n = 134): according to Jensen [12], given the high rate of late local recurrences, frequent life-long examinations are necessary. Further local excision can be successfully performed (7 survivors/8 patients in the Greenhall series) [10]. In the surgical series, there was no evaluation of sphincter function nor of post-operative late complications.
b) T3 and T4 N0-N1 tumours treated by APR (n = 54): the number of APR as first treatment was 52 cases (n = 4 to 18; median 10). LC was recorded in one series 63% [10]. There was no evaluation of complications.

Table 1 – Anal margin epidermoid carcinoma: five surgical series 1963-1989.

	n	T1+T2 T3-T4	Excision	APR	Local control	Nodal Failure in N0	5-year survival
Dillard 1963 [8]	23	?	10	10 50%	?	?	Excis: 30% APR: 90%
Schraut 1983 [22]	16	9 T1..	11	4 31%	9/11 82%	?	4/5= 67% /10y
Greenhall 1985 [10]	48	31/42 74% 11	31	11 23%	Ex: 18/31 58 % APR: 7/11	4	Ex: 20/31 64 % APR: 7/11 63%
Jensen 1988 [12]	76	?	43	9 12%	25/43 59%	5	85 % 5 y 63 % 10y
Pinnapinto 1989 [19]	73 (10 inoperable)	55 18	55 66 %	18 22%	57 %	?	Ex: 27/41 65% APR: 4/11 36%

Seven radiation therapy series: 1986-2005 (Table 2)

a) Three series had RT alone [7, 18, 24] including 50 T1-T2 (71%) and 20 T3-T4. They represented the early attempts to cure an AM tumour conservatively with external irradiation alone.

b) Four series [2, 5, 9, 16] had RT and Nigro-type CT: the introduction by Nigro [14] in 1975 of the combination of RT and CT (5FU + Mitomycin C) brought an improvement in the results of RT as a conservative treatment of AC tumours. The use of the same protocol for AM tumours by Cummings [5] and Papillon [15] gave improvements in local control and survival for advanced AM cases. Later, some authors, such as Bieri [2] and Grabenbauer [9], used the combination RT+CT for small lesions.

Preservation of anal sphincter function

As we have seen above, anal sphincter function was not evaluated after local excision. In the radiation-treated group there was an overall (T1 to T4) evaluation of preservation of function in cured patients: 67% for Bieri [2] and 82% of cured patients for Touboul [24]. Peiffert [18] reported a preservation rate of 89% for cured patients, but stressed the fact that anatomical preservation was not a guarantee for normal anal function.

Table 2 – Anal margin epidermoid carcinoma: 7 radiotherapy series (1986-2005).

	T1 T2 T3-T4	N+ N0	Exci- sion	Perineal +\- boost	RT+ Pelvis	Brachy.	RT+ CT	RT Ing N0	Compli- cations Grade 3-4	LC initial LC Salvage	Nodal failure In N0	5-Year survival	Sphincter preservation
Cummings 1986 (5) 29 pts	13 45% 16	4 14%	0	11 38%	0	1 boost	18 62%	0	3/11 1 colost	T1T2=:13/13... T3T4=:9/16 RT: 9/11 RT+CT: 15/17	2/4	F-up: 1-5y median 7Y	4 fibrosis 1 colostomye Good in cured
Cutuli 1988 (7) 21 pts	11 52% 10 48 %	3N+ 18 17%	?	20 95%	0	1	0	9 60 Co	3/21 14%	48% 62%	3/18 T2T3 Loc+T	63% T1-T2 40% T3T4	9/10: 90% Cured pts
Papillon 1992 (16) 57 pts	48 84% 9 16 %	15 26%	3+7	36 63 %	0	8	14/36 39%	2	3/57 7%	88% 98%	9 16 %	Crude 59% 100%T1 61% T2 12% T3	No loc fail for RT+ +CT
Touboul 1995 (24) 17 pts	15 88% 2 12%	2/17 12%	9 53%	10/17 59%	7	1	0	10/17 59%	2 12%	86.5% 13/15	1/13 8%	86.2 %	Overall 73.5% 11/15 Cured pts 82 % 9/11
Peiffert 1997 (18) 32 pts	24 75% 8 25%	6/26 19%	6/32 19%	1 3	11 5	12 exclusive	1	0 2/26 N0 recur	8/31 7 Gr3	Overall 77% salvage 93.5%	2/26 8%	Ov 56% Spec 69% N0: 100% N1: 40%	84% overall Cured pts 89%
Bieri 2001 (2) 24pts	18 74% 6 26%	4 17%	 3	16	14 Split	5	14/24 58% Nigro	17/24 71%	15/21 71%	69.5%/5y Salvage 1 exci. 4 APR	0	Overall 56% Specific 69.5%	Overall 16/24 67%
Grabenbauer 2005 (9) 14 pts	5 T2 9 T3-T4 36%	7 50%	0	0	14/14 gap	?	14/14 100%	6/14	1 grade 4)	Salvage 9/14	?	4/14 alive 54%	?

Nodal outcome in N0 patients (inguinal)

a) Surgical series (Table 1): Jensen [12] reported 5/76 (6.5%) inguinal node failure while Greenhall [10] reported 4/48 (8%).

b) RT series (1986-2005) (Table 2):
After perineal or pelvic irradiation alone, the rate of inguinal node failure was 8%, 15% and 17% according to the series [18, 24, 7].
After perineal irradiation +/- CT, Cummings [5] had no nodal evolution in 25 N0 patients but an unknown number of N0 had CT and Papillon [16] had nodal evolution in 9/43 N0 (21%) patients.
After elective inguinal irradiation + CT, Bieri [2] had no failure in 20 N0 patients while Grabenbauer [9] had no failure in 6 N0 patients in a series of 14 T2-T3, T4 patients.

In summary, there was about 7 to 15% nodal metachronous evolution in the absence of elective irradiation with or without concomitant CT.

Complications

The five surgical series [8, 10, 12, 19, 22] did not report any treatment-related complications after excision or APR. In the seven RT series, the LENT-SOMA grading system [21] was used for scoring late complications after 1995; grade 3 to 5 complications were reported (Table 2). In the two last series [2, 9] the late complication rate increased as a result of a more careful follow-up. Cutaneous, GI tract and hematologic toxicity with the combination of RT + Nigro CT has led to the move from mitomycin C to cisplatin [3] especially in HIV patients [17].

To conclude the survey of these rare tumour series, extended over long periods, one can underline several methodological difficulties which hamper the studies:

- the classification of anal region tumours in the margin or anal canal tumours can be difficult as stressed by Greenhall [10];
- partial data and lack of the required data for a meaningful study;
- division into subgroups as a function of the TNM classification [23];
- the inhomogeneity of treatment, which has been underlined by Greenhall [10] in the following words: "some tumours of his series having had APR might well have been treated satisfactorily by local excision".

Moreover, the use of new treatments for a part of a series [5, 16] introduces new parameters and the need to take into account new subgroups. However, in spite of these "methodological" difficulties, the literature shows that the outcome of these tumours has improved since the use of conservative treatments. The local excision of T1 tumours (T1 > 3cm T2) is a conservative surgical treatment even if a postoperative irradiation is necessary due to incomplete removal. All sizes of lesions (including T1 after biopsy) can be treated conservatively with RT (small tumours) or with combined RT/CT (larger tumours): APR represents the salvage treatment of both AM and AC tumours.

Current epidemiology

There are two groups of patients; the first group has the well-known characteristics of the "old series" [2, 5, 7, 9, 16, 18, 24]. The second group has been increasing over the last 10 to 15 years. It is composed of homosexual patients, mostly young or middle aged men with T3-T4 "anal" tumours (28 %) and HIV positivity. They represent a new clinical and therapeutic entity [1, 3, 11, 13, 17, 20, 26].

Clinical features

All loco-regional abnormality must be clinically investigated. In small lesions, one can distinguish AM from AC tumours. In advanced cases, it could be difficult to determine the origin of the tumour, i.e. AC lesion extending to the AM or AM lesions extending to the AC.

However, at the present time the treatment of advanced cases of AM or AC are similar. Size, circumference extension, distance between the lesion and the anal verge must be evaluated. Precisely oriented sketches and photography are a part of the initial work-up as well as anal digital examination and palpation of inguinal areas. Biopsy can then be performed. Deep loco-regional extension is investigated using endo-anorectal endoscopy and ultrasound. Distant spread is checked with the usual means: chest x-ray, CT scans or abdominal and pelvic ultrasound. The usual biologic tests are necessary, the most important being HIV and immunological status.

In women, a gynecological examination is mandatory to look for condylomatous lesions of the vulvo-vaginal region and cervix dysplasia. Biopsy of the tumour and cytology of abnormal nodes must be performed.

When excision is performed, the quality of removal should be checked to evaluate whether RT is necessary. The lesion should be classified according the TNM classification (23).

According to the HIV status, treatment should be planned as described below.

Treatment of non-HIV-positive patients

Tumours < 3 cm (T1< 2 cm and T2 < 3 cm)

Excision with a 1cm margin (occasionally associated with a skin graft for young patients with lesions distant to the anal verge). Post surgery RT or CT are not required. After biopsy, or in case of doubt about the quality of excision, perineal irradiation including a security margin is mandatory.

Tumours from 3 to 5 cm

Before the use of combined treatment, external beam RT alone, delivering 60 to 65 Gy in 7 to 8 weeks using x-ray and electrons, was able to cure a number of patients [7, 18, 24]. After 45 Gy, the field was usually coned down and a split course was frequently given [2, 9, 16, 24]. In some chosen cases, a boost was given with brachytherapy using low dose rate 192-iridium for lesions involving the lower part of the anal canal [18]. Large experience of the technique and perfect knowledge of the topography (the size of initial and residual lesion) is mandatory when considering treatment of these tumours.

Locally advanced lesions

T3 and T4 lesions have the same treatment as the homologous lesions of the anal canal, i.e. conservative curative combination of RT + CT (5 FU + mitomycin or cisplatin or other combinations). Mitomycin and cisplatin have been tested [4].

The RT box technique, used for large AC tumours allows treatment of primary AM tumours and inguinal areas (45 Gy for elective irradiation of these areas).

Inguinal regions : Positive nodes

Extensive nodal surgery, a factor for chronic edema of lower limbs, must be avoided. Irradiation is delivered using the box technique or to separate inguinal fields (with electrons) combined with perineal irradiation.

It seems that for T1-T2 < 3 cm elective RT is not necessary, provided a careful follow-up is possible. For T2 (3 to 5 cm) inguinal irradiation is a security, given the rarity of local post- irradiation changes. For T3 T4 N0 tumours, bilateral inguinal RT is mandatory. Previous results [5-16] have shown in N0 cases the absence of nodal secondary evolution after CT in T1-T2 N0 tumours.

Treatment of HIV-positive patients

At the present time, the majority of papers on anal malignancies in HIV-positive patients report series of anal region tumours, AM tumours not being specifically discussed [1, 3, 11, 13, 17, 20, 26]. The main reason is the use of the same treatments for the two sites because the goal is identical, i.e. conservation of anal function in a group of HIV-positive patients. In this last category, another contemporary treatment addressing the immunodeficiency is fundamental. In this short paper, we have mentioned some of them but, as mentioned above, anal margin tumours are not always distinguished. The therapeutic problem is to use in HIV-positive patients the RT + CT protocols which have proved their efficacy and acceptable tolerance in HIV-negative patients with AM tumours.

Local tumour excision could be applied for lesions ≤2cm, provided a very careful periodical follow-up is possible. For lesions between 2 and 5 cm, perineal RT combined with CT (5 FU + mitomycin or cisplatin) should be given. Elective inguinal RT in N0 patients is justified by combining it with CT, taking into account the known negative evolution of AC tumours in HIV patients [2, 3, 11, 17, 26].

A comparison between a series of 20 AC tumours in HIV-positive patients and a similar series of tumours in HIV-negative patients has shown that they had varying stages as there were more N+ and more organ deficiencies [26]. Clinical experience has shown that combined treatment can give rise to major toxicity in AM tumours, similar to toxicity described for AC lesions in HIV-positive patients. Toxicity is the reason for reduction of CT and of RT doses and for prolongation or interruption of treatment, eventually giving poorer results.

Several authors have stressed the importance of initial CD4 count to estimate prognosis. The outcome is a function of CD4 count (> or < $200/mm^3$). In a series of 17 patients [11] with CD4 count > $200/mm^3$, a high local control was reported (7/8) as well as acceptable toxicity. A similar experience [3] has been reported in 11 patients (local control, 9/11).

However, a high mortality rate was reported [20] in a series of 14 AC tumours, related to HIV, i.e. 40 % at one year. The same negative evolution has recently been described in a series of 23 patients [17]. All authors stressed the fact that vigorous anti-retroviral therapy, started before cancer treatment, may decrease toxicity and improve survival as advocated for AC epidermoïd carcinomas [15]. A cooperative phase II protocol of RT combined with cisplatin, 5 FU and cetuximab in HIV patients with AC or AM cancers has recently been initiated by the NCI [13].

Prevention of anal margin cancers

As recommended for AC tumours, PNH-related condylomatous lesions and *in situ* cancers of the ano-genital region should be periodically searched for and treated, while the HIV status must be checked [1]. The value of anti-PNH vaccination has not yet been assessed.

Conclusion

AM epidermoïd carcinomas are rare tumours, often reported in the literature with anal or anal region malignancies. Treatment in HIV-negative patients is similar to the treatment of AC tumours except for T1 and small T2, where conservative excision (and careful follow-up) is recommended. For larger tumours, perineal or pelvic irradiation can be used in combination with the Nigro-type CT. At the present time, the number of AM tumours has increased in a specific population of young or middle-aged homosexual men who are frequently HIV positive.

For HIV-positive patients, according to the literature, the same general approach should be used but potentially more toxicity and poorer results must be anticipated if the CD4 count is <200 mm3. Because of HIV disease, survival is short in spite of the high rate of local control obtained with the currently used combined protocols and in spite of the improvements in the treatment of immunodeficiency. New research programs with new drug combinations have been initiated.

References

1. Bauer P, Etienney I (2002) Therapeutiques du cancer épidermoïde de l'anus: particularité chez les sujets infectés par le VIH. Gastroenterol Clin Biol 26: 147-9
2. Bieri S, Allal AS, Kurtz JM (2001) Sphincter conserving treatment of carcinomas of the anal margin. Acta Oncol 40: 29-33
3. Cleator S, Fife K, Nelson M *et al.* (2000) Treatment of HIV associated invasive anal cancer with combined chemoradiation. Eur J Cancer 36: 754-8
4. Créhange G, Bosset M, Lorchel F (2006) Combining Cisplatin and mitomycin with radiotherapy in anal carcinoma. Dis Colon Rectum 50: 43-9
5. Cummings BJ, Keane TJ, Hawkins NV *et al.* (1986) Treatment of peri-anal carcinoma by radiation plus chemotherapy (RTCT). Int J Radiat Oncol Biol Phys 12 (suppl 1): 152
6. **Cummings BJ, Brierley JD, Anal c and Tanal. Chapter 55, In: Principles and Practice of Radiation Oncology. Ca Perez, LW Brady, EC Halperin, RK Schmidt-Ulrich (eds.) Lippincott Williams & Wilkins. Philadelphia 4th Edition 2004;1630-48**
7. Cutuli B, Fenton J, Labib A *et al.* (1988) Anal margin carcinoma: 21 cases treated at Institut Curie by exclusive conservative radiotherapy. Radiother Oncol 11: 1-6
8. Dillard BM, Spratt JS, Ackerman LV *et al.* (1963) Epidermoid cancer of anal margin and canal. Review of 79 cases. Arch Surg 86: 100-5

6

9. **Grabenbauer CG, Kessler H, Matzel KE (2005) Tumor site predicts outcome after radiochemotherapy in squamous cell carcinoma of the anal region: long term results in 101 patients. Dis Colon Rectum 48: 1742-51**
10. Greenall MJ, Quan SHQ, Stearns MW *et al.* (1985) Epidermoid cancer of the anal margin. Pathologic features, treatment, and clinical results. Am J Surg 149: 95-101
11. Hoffman R, Welton ML, Klencke B *et al.* (1999) The significance of pre-treatment CD4 count on the outcome and treatment tolerance of HIV-positive patients with anal cancer. Int J Radiat Oncol Biol Phys 44: 127-31
12. Jensen SL, Hagen K, Harling H *et al.* (1988) Long term prognosis after radical treatment for squamous-cell carcinoma of the anal canal and anal margin. Dis Colon Rectum 31: 273-8
13. NCI (2007) Cisplatin, fluorouracil, cetuximab and radiation therapy in treating patients with HIV and Stage I, Stage II or Stage III anal cancer. Clinical Trials.gov.NCT 00324415
14. Nigro N, Vaitkevicius VK, Considine BJ (1974) Combined therapy for cancer of the anal canal. A preliminary report. Dis Colon Rectum 17: 354
15. Papillon J, Renard L, Pipard G (1985) Le cancer de la marge de l'anus. J Eur Radiother 6: 23-34
16. Papillon J, Chassard JL (1992) Respective roles of radiotherapy and surgery in the management of epidermoid carcinoma of the anal margin. Series of 57 patients. Dis Colon Rectum 35: 422-9
17. Parthasarathy A, Glaubiger DL, Grant KM (2006) Treatment of anal carcinoma in HIV positive males. A single institution experience. Int J Radiat Oncol Biol Phys 3 suppl: 2139
18. **Peiffert D, Bey P, Pernot M *et al.* (1997) Conservative treatment by irradiation of epidermoid carcinomas of the anal margin. Int J Radiat Oncol Biol Phys 39: 57-66**
19. Pinna Pintor M, Northover JMA, Nicholls RJ (1989) Squamous-cell carcinoma of the anus, 1948 to 1984. Br J Surg 76: 806-10
20. Place RJ, Gregorcyk SG, Huber PL *et al.* (2001) Outcome analysis of HIV positive patients with anal squamous cell carcinoma. Dis Colon Rectum 44: 506-12
21. RTOG/EORTC (1995) Late effects working group.LENT SOMA tables. Radiother Oncol 35: 19-60
22. Schraut WH, Wang C, Dawson PJ *et al.* (1983) Depth of invasion, location, and size of cancer of the anus dictate operative treatment. Cancer 51: 1291-6
23. Sobin LH,Wittekind CH (eds) (1997) TNM classification of malignant tumors. UICC 5th edit New York AJ Wiley 70-3
24. **Touboul E, Schlienger M, Buffat L *et al.* (1995) Epidermoid carcinoma of the anal margin: 17 cases treated with curative-intent radiation therapy. Radiother Oncol 34: 195-202**
25. UKCCCR (1996) Anal cancer trial working party: Epidermoid anal cancer: results from the UKCCCR randomized trial of radiotherapy alone versus radiotherapy, fluorouracil and mitomycin. Lancet 348: 1049-54
26. Vatra B, Sobhani I, Aparicio T *et al.* (2002) Charactéristiques cliniques, thérapeutiques et pronostiques des carcinomes épidermoides du canal anal chez les malades VIH positifs. Gastroenterol Clin Biol 26: 150-6

Uncommon hepatobiliary tumours

7

M. Hübner, N. Halkic and N. Demartines

Five Essential Points

1. *Rare malignant liver tumours of the adult are a very heterogeneous group of malignancies, especially with regard to epidemiology, aetiology, histology and prognosis.*
2. *Common features of this group are a nonspecific presentation with abdominal pain and a hepatic mass. Diagnosis is commonly established only after surgery.*
3. *Overall, surgical R0 resection is the mainstay of therapy, often combined with chemotherapy, especially in primary hepatic lymphoma.*
4. *Liver transplant is a very good indication for patients with unresectable epithelioid haemangioendothelioma, even in the presence of metastatic disease.*
5. *Patients with rare liver tumours also profit from the rapid progress in the multimodality treatment of frequent liver tumours in high volume centres. Current treatment algorithms will surely be redefined, and new strategies will result in improved outcome.*

Introduction

A large amount of data is available on hepatocellular carcinoma, cholangiocarcinoma, and liver metastases of colorectal or neuroendocrine origin. During the last decade, a multidisciplinary diagnostic and therapeutic approach has led to a considerable improvement in outcome, especially in high volume centres. Based on a large body of evidence, comprehensive treatment algorithms have recently been defined for these frequent entities [1, 5, 27]. The therapeutic backbone remains surgical resection or liver transplant. This has been complemented by interventional radiology, local ablation and innovative chemotherapy [1, 5, 20, 27]. However, only very little is known about the treatment of rare liver tumours, and this chapter will focus entirely on these neglected rare malignancies. Because of their rarity, no large prospective series are available. Prognostic factors and the optimal treatment still need to be defined. We will review the available data on these "orphans", including rare epithelial and non-epithelial tumours, primary hepatic lymphoma as well as the veritable curiosities such as solitary fibrous tumour or carcinosarcoma. While treatment strategies are nowadays available for metastases from breast cancer, melanoma, and gastric cancer, rarities such as liver tumours of unknown origin constitute diagnostic and therapeutic challenges and have to be treated on a case-by-case basis [4, 5, 17, 19, 28, 32].

In this chapter, we aim to introduce the classification of liver tumours, to describe the epidemiology and characteristics of the relevant rare adult liver tumours and review available treatment options and their outcome for each malignancy.

7

Rare malignant liver tumours of the adult

Each tumour type will be discussed below. No details on surgical or interventional techniques are given, as these are no different from established algorithms for common liver tumours [1, 5, 27]. A two-phrase summary rounds off each paragraph, giving typical features and the recommended treatment strategy. Tables 2 and 3 give a synopsis with all essential facts for each entity described.

Classification

Table 1 shows a modified World Health Organization (WHO) classification of hepatobiliary tumours [10], excluding all benign and metastatic liver tumours (right column). In a second step, frequent malignancies and those affecting primarily children were eliminated. The remainder (in bold type) was selected for critical review of the literature.

Epithelial tumours

Epithelial malignancies evolve from hepatocytes or bile duct epithelium. This group features, among others, the common primary liver tumours, hepatocellular and cholangiocarcinoma.

Bile duct cystadenocarcinoma

Definition

Cystadenocarcinomas are malignant tumours which evolve from biliary epithelium [6, 10]. The cystic lesions are different from tumours arising from a congenital

Table 1 – Classification of liver tumours with emphasis on rare adult primaries [10].

	Malignant	Benign
Epithelial	Hepatocellular carcinoma* Cholangiocarcinoma* **Cystadenocarcinoma** **cHCC-CC** Hepatoblastoma§ Undifferentiated carcinoma§	Hepatocellular adenoma Focal nodular hyperplasia Bile duct adenoma Cystadenoma Biliary papillomatosis
Non-epithelial	**Epitelhioid haemangioendothelioma** **Angiosarcoma** Embryonal sarcoma§ Rhabdomyosarcoma§	Angiomyolipoma Lymphangioma Haemangioma Infantile haemangioendothelioma
Miscellaneous	Solitary fibrous tumour Teratoma§ Yolk sac tumour§ **Carcinosarcoma** Rhabdoid tumour§ **Primary hepatic lymphoma**	**Metastases** Breast cancer Melanoma Gastric cancer Unknown primary origin Others

This comprehensive overview of liver tumours has been adapted to the subject of this chapter, some entities might therefore not be included [10]. Benign and secondary tumours (right column), frequent malignancies (*) and mostly infantile tumours (§) have been excluded from this table. The remaining tumours (in **bold** type) have been selected for discussion in this review.
cHCC-CC: combined hepatocellular and cholangiocarcinoma.

Table 2 – Rare adult primary liver tumours: epidemiology and characteristics.

	Epidemiology	Etiology/Risk factors	Clinics/Diagnosis	Pathology
Cystadenocarcinoma	< 5% of all cystic liver lesions (+ cystadenoma) Onset around 50-60 years M/f ratio 1:1	Etiology largely unknown Evolving usually from cystadenoma	Abdominal pain, palpable mass Combination of US, CT, MRI FNA: atypical cells, mucus, CEA, CA 19-9	Multilocular cystic lesions (3-30 cm) Solid thickening with papillary projections
cHCC-CC	0.4-14% of all primary liver tumours Onset around 6th decade M > f	Association with viral hepatitis, cirrhosis (comparable to HCC)	Non-specific symptoms, 40% asymptomatic Tumour markers: CA 19-9 57%, AFP 82% Biopsies not advocated (bleeding and seeding)	Both components (> 10%) proven by immunostaining; mean size 7 cm 2 types: „transition tumour“ > „collision ...“
EHE	Incidence < 1/106 Mean age at onset 42 years M/f ratio 2:3	Unclear etiology No predisposing factors identified	Abdominal pain, weakness, weight loss Liver function tests frequently elevated Tumour markers usually normal	Multifocal, ill-defined (0,5-12 cm) tumours Preservation of portal structures F VIII-related antigen, CD 31/34 (> 90%)
Angiosarcoma	0.5-2% of all primary liver tumours Prevalence 0.14-0.25/106, 200 new cases/year Onset around 6-7th decade, m/f ratio 3:1	Thorotrast, arsenic, vinyl chloride, steroids (42%), cirrhosis (20%) Pathogenesis: oxidative damage?	Weakness, abdominal pain, weight loss Acute abdomen due to tumour rupture (15%) Imaging unspecific, cave biopsies (bleeding)	Grayish spongy fibrous masses (up to 5 cm) Hemorrhage, infarction, necrosis Destruction of hepatic architecture, CD31/34
PHL	0.016% of all non-Hodgkin's lymphomas B-cell: 5th decade, m/f ratio 2.3:1 T-cell: mean age 20 years, m/f ratio 5:1	Association with AIDS and chronic liver disease (10%)	Abdominal pain, weight loss, fever LDH (50%), liver function tests (70%) and beta-2-microglobulin (90%), imaging + biopsy	Solitary > multiple tumours, rarely diffuse preservation of the acinar landmarks B-cell/ CD20, CD79a
SFT	About 40 cases in the literature 6th decade of life; female > male	Unknown etiology Not linked to viral hepatitis/cirrhosis	Abdominal pain, palpable mass Diagnosis by histopathology (specimen)	gray-with firm tumours (2-45 cm) capsule (90%); CD34, Vimentin, Desmin
Carcinosarcoma	About 20 cases in the literature, median onset around 60 years; m/f ratio 1:1	Unknown etiology	Abdominal pain, weight loss Diagnosis only after surgical resection	Intimate mixture (> 30%) of carcinomatous and sarcomatous component; size 5-14 cm

Abbreviations in order of appearance: cHCC-CC: combined hepatocellular and cholangiocarcinoma; EHE: Epithelioid haemangioendothelioma; PHL: Primary hepatic lymphoma; SFT: Solitary fibrous tumour; m/f ratio: male-to-female ratio; US: Ultrasonography; CT: Computed tomography; MRI: Magnetic resonance imaging; FNA: Fine needle aspiration, CEA- , CA 19-9: Carbohydrate antigen 19-9; HCC: Hepatocellular carcinoma; AFP: Alpha-fetoprotein; CD: cluster of differentiation; AIDS: Acquired immune deficiency syndrome; LDH: Lactate dehydrogenase.

Table 3 – Rare adult primary liver tumours: treatment options, predictors, prognosis.

	Surgical treatment options	Chemotherapy/Other	Metases/Prognostic predictors	Outcome/Prognosis
Cystadenocarcinoma	R0 resection	experimental	Frequent metastases: LN, lungs, pleura, peritoneum	5 year disease-free -87% (after R0 resection) Outcome worse in men
cHCC-CC	R0 resection + hilar lymphadenectomy	Interventional radiology (TACE, RF); palliative chemotherpy?	LN metastases (44%): predictive of poor survival LN metasases/neurovascular invasion 72%): -> high recurrence rate	5 years disease-specific -50% (after R0 resection)
EHE	R0 resection (but 90% unresectable) Liver transplantation Tumour debulking contraindicated	Interventional radiology (TACE, RF); chemotherapy, anti-angiogenics (anti-VEGF antibodies, rapamycine)	Synchroneous metastases (40%): Lungs, peritoneum, LN, bone, spleen High cellularity, vascular invasion: poor prognosis	5 years overall 40% range: 55-83% liver transplanatation, 75% R0 resection, 30% chemotherapy, 5% best palliative
Angiosarcoma	R0 resection Liver transplantation contraindicated	Chemoresistant; no improvement in survival by other strategies	Distant metastases (20-60%): Lung, bone, spleen, adrenal gland	Median overall survival 5-6 months 2 years survival 3%
PHL	Resection (or liver transplantation) <u>in combination</u> with chemotherapy	Early and aggressive chemotherapy, new antibodies; radiotherapy ineffective	Prognosis depending largely on histological type and grade: nodular > diffuse, B-cell > T-cell	Unpredictable: Median overall survival 15 months (range: 3-124)
SFT	Only therapy: R0 resection-	Experimental	Unknown	6 months overall 100%
Carcinosarcoma	Only therapy: R0 resection-	Experimental	Unknown	Rarely alive 6 months after surgery

Abbreviations in order of appearance: cHCC-CC: combined hepatocellular and cholangiocarcinoma; EHE: Epithelioid haemangioendothelioma; PHL: Primary hepatic lymphoma; SFT: Solitary fibrous tumour; LN: Lymph node; TACE: Transarterial chemoembolisation, RF: Radiofrequency; anti-VEGF: anti-Vascular endothelial growth factor.

cystic malformation or intrahepatic lithiasis. They are lined by epithelium with papillary infoldings that may be mucus-secreting or, less frequently, serous [10].

Epidemiology

Cystadenocarcinoma arises generally in a pre-existing biliary cystadenoma, but aetiology remains unclear. Cystadenoma and cystadenocarcinoma together represent only 5% of all solitary liver cysts [6, 14, 30]. While cystadenoma is more frequent in women, cystadenocarcinoma has an equal sex distribution. Onset is around 50-60 years [5, 6, 10, 14, 30].

Clinical presentation and diagnosis

Symptomatic patients present usually with abdominal pain or a palpable mass. Elevation of CA 19-9 is infrequent. [5, 6, 10, 30]. Preoperative distinction between cystadenoma and cystadenocarcinoma is virtually impossible. However, benign lesions can mostly be excluded based on radiological findings and fine needle aspirations (FNA). Cystadenocarcinoma appears on CT and MRI as a multifocal cystic tumour with tiny papillary folds within the cystic wall [5, 6, 10]. FNA often contains atypical cells, mucinous material, and elevated levels of CEA and CA 19-9 [6].

Pathological features

The multifocal cystic lesions (3-30 cm) are filled with clear mucinous, bile-stained, or blood-tinged fluid [5, 6, 10, 14, 30]. Malignant change typically involves parts of the cyst lining that consists of tall columnar cells with nuclear atypia and mitoses. Areas of solid thickening, large papillary projections and invasion of the adjacent parenchyma are clues to malignancy differentiating this tumour from cystadenoma. Cystadenocarcinoma presents mostly as a well-differentiated tubulopapillary or tubular adenocarcinoma [5, 10].

Prognosis and treatment

Cystadenocarcinoma is usually a well-defined tumour permitting complete resection with a 5-year disease-free survival of up to 87% [5, 10, 14, 30]. Tumours behave more aggressively in men [5, 10, 30]. Patients with unresectable tumours, due to intrahepatic spread or metastatic disease (regional lymph nodes, lungs, pleura, or peritoneum), carry a bad prognosis that seems to be only slightly better than for patients with cholangiocarcinoma [5, 10].

Cystadenocarcinoma presents as a multilocular adenocarcinoma arising from intrahepatic bile ducts. Preoperative diagnosis is difficult, but complete resection offers a good prognosis.

Combined hepatocellular and cholangiocarcinoma (cHCC-CC)

Definition

cHCC-CC shows features of both hepatocellular and cholangiocarcinoma. Unequivocal elements of both entities are closely combined in a variable distribution. While the so-called "transition" type shows intermixed patterns, "collision tumours" consist of separate areas of hepatocellular and cholangiocarcinoma [5, 9, 10, 13, 26]. The hypothesis of a distinct entity is supported by the same multiple allelic losses in both tumour components, suggestive of divergent differentiation from a single clone [5, 10].

Epidemiology

Depending on the classification and the region, cHCC-CC represents up to 14% of all primary hepatic malignancies [5, 10, 13, 26]. It occurs more frequently in patients with viral hepatitis or cirrhosis [5, 13, 26]. Geographic, age and sex distribution follow largely that of hepatocellular carcinoma with onset in the 6th decade and a male preponderance [5, 10, 13, 26].

Clinical presentation and diagnosis

Clinical presentation is non specific, and 40% of patients are asymptomatic [5, 13, 26]. Elevated CA 19-9 and AFP levels are frequent (57 and 82%, respectively) in cHCC-CC [5, 10, 13, 26]. As for cholangiocarcinoma, preoperative diagnosis is difficult, and even combined imaging modalities are inaccurate concerning diagnosis and staging [13, 26]. Preoperative biopsies are completely unreliable and should be avoided [5, 26].

Pathological features

Macroscopic appearance is similar to hepatocellular carcinoma; presence of bile and mucus is typical for the combined tumour. Mean tumour size at diagnosis is about 7 cm [26]. Clear identification of a significant amount (> 10%) of both components by immunostaining is mandatory for diagnosis [5, 10, 26]. Transitional-type tumours are more frequent than collision-type tumours, and the predominant component can be either hepatocellular or cholangiocarcinoma [26]. Vascular invasion (72%) and nodular metastases (44%) are frequent and depend largely on the size and the predominating component of the primary tumour [26]. Metastases feature either hepatocellular or a mixed pattern of differentiation [5, 10].

Prognosis and treatment

Generally, treatment and prognosis depend on the major component, and on the underlying disease [13, 26]. cHCC-CC shows higher frequency of nodal and distant metastases, and carries a worse prognosis compared to hepatocellular carcinoma. Nodal spread is the only predictor of poor survival [5, 10, 13, 26]. Curative resection should, therefore, include hilar lymph node dissection. Five-year disease-specific survival after curative resection can be over 50%, and is comparable to hepatocellular carcinoma [13, 26]. Neurovascular infiltration and lymphonodal metastases are predictors of a high recurrence rate [26]. Local recurrence is very frequent, and occurs usually in the first two years after resection. While multidisciplinary treatment can still achieve a median survival of about one year, patients treated with palliative care only die after 4 months [13, 26]. The role of liver transplant, interventional techniques, chemotherapy, and/or radiotherapy remains unclear [13].

cHCC-CC is a distinct entity with components of both, hepatocellular and cholangiocarcinoma. While aetiology is rather similar to hepatocellular carcinoma, prognosis and treatment options are similar to those for cholangiocarcinoma.

Non-epithelial tumours

Primary hepatic sarcomas are rare tumours of vascular origin that represent approximately 10% of hepatic sarcomas and only 0.1-2% of all hepatic malignancies [5, 12, 25, 31]. They are slightly more common in children [5, 25]. There is no aetiological link to pre-existing liver disease [5].

Epithelioid haemangioendothelioma

Definition

Epithelioid haemangioendothelioma (EHE) is a rare primary sarcoma with a variable malignant potential. It originates from endothelial cells and is characterized by epithelioid or spindle cells growing along preformed vessels, or forming new vessels [5, 10].

Epidemiology

EHE occurs at a mean age of 42 years (range: 12-86) with a male-to-female ratio of 2:3. Incidence is less than $1/10^6$, and aetiology remains unclear [5, 10, 19, 22].

Clinical presentation and diagnosis

Symptomatic patients (80%) present usually with abdominal pain, weakness, weight loss or hepatosplenomegaly. Jaundice and liver failure are rare [5, 10, 18, 19, 22, 31]. Elevation of alkaline phosphatase (42-69%), gamma-glutamyl transpeptidase (45%), bilirubine (20-25%) or transaminases (25-40%) is frequent, while tumour markers tend to be normal [18, 19, 22]. EHE appears on CT typically hypodense with an irregular outline, focal calcifications (20%) and hypervascularised areas within the tumour after intravenous contrast. The early type shows a nodular "peripheral pattern", while the later confluent type appears diffuse and with infiltration of the large vessels [5, 10, 19, 22].

Pathological features

EHE appears in the form of bilobar, multifocal, ill-defined fibrous masses (0,5-12 cm) [5, 18, 22]. Nests of pleiomorphic tumour cells grow typically along sinusoids or vessels and often invade Glisson's capsule. The hepatic acinar landmarks are preserved despite extensive infiltration [5, 10, 18, 19, 22]. Diagnosis is based on the absence of epithelial differentiation and detection of the vascular marker factor VIII-related antigen (91-100%), as well as the endothelial markers CD 31 and 34 (86 and 94%, respectively) [5, 10, 18, 19, 22]. High tumour cellularity and vascular invasion carry a bad prognosis [5, 10, 18, 19].

Prognosis and treatment

EHE has a variable and unpredictable natural course. Due to slow progression, prognosis is relatively good compared to other liver malignancies. Five-year overall survival is around 40%, ranging from 5% (no treatment) up to around 75% following curative liver resection [5, 10, 19, 22, 31]. About 40% of the patients have synchronous metastases in lungs, peritoneum, lymph nodes bones or spleen [5, 10, 18, 19, 22]. Furthermore, most patients have large multifocal tumours in both lobes, rendering a curative resection possible in only 10% of the patients [5, 19, 22]. Debulking procedures are strongly discouraged as tumours behave more aggressively after palliative resection due to stimulated angiogenesis [18, 22]. Given the slow progression and the relatively good prognosis of EHE, liver transplant has been evaluated for unresectable EHE with encouraging 5-year survival rates of 55-83% [5, 19, 22]. Liver transplant (and resection) is a valuable option in patients with metastases which, in contrast to most other tumours, tend to remain stable under immunosuppression [22]. Chemotherapy, radiotherapy, and/or interventional strategies have only moderate impact on tumour progression with a 5-year survival of 30% [5, 10, 19, 22, 29]. The value of antiangiogenic agents (rapamycin, anti-vascular endothelial growth factor antibodies) remains to be assessed [18, 19].

EHE is a slowly growing sarcoma characterized by preservation of a lobular architecture. The prognosis after liver resection or transplant is rather good.

Angiosarcoma

Definition

Angiosarcoma is a highly malignant tumour of vascular origin. It is composed of spindle and pleiomorphic cells that line or invade the lumina of sinusoids and small veins [10].

Epidemiology

Angiosarcoma is the most common primary sarcoma of the liver that accounts for up to 2% of all primary liver malignancies. Prevalence is around 0.14-0.25/million with about 200 new cases per year, worldwide [5, 10, 19]. Compared to EHE, incidence is later in life (6-7th decade) with a male-to-female ratio of 3:1 [5, 10, 19]. Twenty percent of the affected patients have concomitant liver cirrhosis and 25-42% of all cases have been linked to exposure to vinyl-chloride monomer, thorotrast, arsenic compounds, anabolic steroids or other chemical agents [5, 8, 10, 19]. Oxidative damage might play a role in pathogenesis, as mutations in K-ras-2 gene have been found in 29% of the sporadic and in 40% of the thorotrast-associated cases [5, 10].

Clinical presentation and diagnosis

Patients are usually symptomatic and present with weakness, abdominal pain, weight loss and nausea [5, 19, 31]. Hepatosplenomegaly, ascites and jaundice are frequent findings [5, 19]. Thrombocytopenia and acute abdominal crisis because of tumour rupture are typical complications (15%) in advanced stage. Imaging is rather non-specific and percutaneous biopsies are contraindicated due to high risk of bleeding (ca. 5% mortality) [5, 10].

Pathological features

The typical grey-white spongy masses (up to 5 cm) affect the entire organ and extend along preformed vascular channels. Consecutive liver-cell atrophy finally results in cavities, containing tumour debris or clotted blood and in areas of hemorrhage, infarction and necrosis. Thorotrast deposits are associated with considerable periportal and subcapsular fibrosis. CD31 and CD34 are highly sensitive but not specific for angiosarcoma. Distinction from EHE is made on the basis of destruction of the hepatic architecture and a higher degree of cytological atypia. Metastatic sarcoma can be excluded only on clinical grounds [5, 10, 19].

Prognosis and treatment

Angiosarcoma is a very aggressive and chemoresistant disease with poor prognosis. Distant metastases are present in 20-60% of cases, mostly in lung, bone, spleen and the adrenal glands [5, 10, 19]. The median survival from diagnosis is as low as 5-6 months, with a 2-year overall survival of only 3% [5, 8, 10, 31]. Curative resection is the only possible cure that is rarely achievable due to the rapid growth and ill-defined lesions. Liver transplant was abandoned because of high recurrence rate and a median survival of only 7 months [11, 19]. Systemic chemotherapy does not improve survival in unresectable patients [5, 29].

Angiosarcomas are aetiologically linked to environmental toxins, and characterised histologically by disruption of the hepatic architecture. Curative resection is the only therapy that is rarely possible and still associated with a dismal prognosis.

Primary hepatic lymphoma

Definition

Primary hepatic lymphoma (PHL) is defined as extranodal lymphoma that has its primary clinical presentation in the liver. While distant spread can occur, the main disease is localized in the liver and therapy is usually directed at this site [5, 10, 19].

Epidemiology

Secondary liver involvement is frequent in haematogenous malignancies, and ranges from 30% in multiple myeloma up to 80-100% in chronic leukaemia. On the contrary, PHL is very rare and accounts for only about 0.016% of all cases of non-Hodgkin's lymphomas [23]. Usually, PHL presents in the form of large B-cell lymphomas in males (2.3:1) in their 5th decade of life [5, 10, 23]. T-cell lymphomas are very rare, very aggressive and occur very early (mean age, 20 years, male-to-female ratio, 5:1). There is an aetiologic association with AIDS and chronic liver disease (10%) [5, 10, 19, 23].

Clinical presentation and diagnosis

Typical symptoms include abdominal pain, weight loss, fever and hepatosplenomegaly [5, 7, 10, 23]. Radiologically, PHL can easily be taken for hepatocellular carcinoma, cholangiocarcinoma or metastases. Diffuse lymphoma infiltration can mimic hepatic inflammation. PET-CT can add valuable information concerning extrahepatic involvement [2, 21, 23]. Typical laboratory findings include very high serum lactate dehydrogenase levels (50%), abnormal liver function tests (70%) and/or an elevated beta-2-microglobulin (90%, prognostic value) [5, 7, 10, 23]. Diagnosis is usually confirmed by biopsy [5, 19].

Pathological features

PHL usually presents as solitary (55-60%) or multiple tumours (35-40%), rarely with diffuse infiltration [5, 7, 10, 23]. The monomorphic medium-sized cells infiltrate portal triads and the adjacent parenchyma, either as destructive tumour nodules or in a more diffuse fashion with preservation of the acinar landmarks [23]. Conversely, metastatic lymphoma shows a diffuse infiltrate pattern. The B-cell type expresses CD20 and CD79a. [5, 10].

Prognosis and treatment: PHL carries a poor prognosis but the individual course is very unpredictable (survival range: 3-124 months), depending mainly on histological type and grade [5, 23]. The nodular type has a better prognosis than the diffuse type and B-cell type compares favourably with T-cell lymphomas [5, 10, 19, 23]. Early and aggressive chemotherapy, including targeted antibodies, remains the mainstay of therapy with a median survival of about 15 months [19, 23]. Surgical resection followed by systemic chemotherapy is the mainstay of treatment, while chemotherapy alone or combined with radiotherapy can be used in inoperable patients [5, 10, 19, 23].

PHL presents as a solitary or multilocular tumour of large B-cells with no relevant extrahepatic manifestation that can be linked to immunosuppression or chronic liver disease. Aggressive chemotherapy therapy should be combined with surgical resection.

Miscellaneous

These true "orphans" comprise a heterogeneous collection of very rare tumours that are only reported in from of case reports. Epidemiology, treatment and prognosis are controversial.

Solitary fibrous tumour

Definition

Solitary fibrous tumour (SFT) is a semi malignant tumour of mesenchymal origin that combines different features. Some authors refer to them as sarcomas, and classification does not yet seem to be clearly defined [3, 5, 10, 15, 25, 31].

Epidemiology

SFT occurs usually in the pleura. Hepatic SFT is very rare with only about 40 cases described in the literature [3, 15, 24]. Etiology is almost unknown with no association to viral hepatitis or cirrhosis. SFT appears in the 6th decade with a slight female preponderance [3, 10].

Clinical presentation and diagnosis

Clinical presentation is non specific with abdominal pain or a palpable mass [3]. Lesions vary considerably in size (2-45 cm), and can appear in either lobe, sometimes as pedunculated tumours [3, 10]. Radiological imaging does not contribute to diagnosis. Tumour markers or other laboratory tests tend to be negative [3].

Pathological features

SFT is characterised by greyish-white firm nodules which are sharply demarcated and surrounded by a well-defined capsule (90%) [3]. They contain areas with alternating cellular and relatively acellular areas. Large tumour size and necrosis, associated with pleiomorphic atypical cells and a high mitotic rate are features of malignant potential [3]. Positive immunostaining for CD34, vimentin and desmin is rather specific for SFT [3, 10, 15].

Prognosis and treatment

Diagnosis is usually established by histopathology after resection. R0 resection provides a relatively favourable prognosis with a 6 month survival of 100%. Very little is known about additional treatment options [3, 5, 25, 31].

Solitary fibrous tumour is a very rare tumour of variable size. The well-defined tumours are usually eligible for curative resection with a good prognosis.

Carcinosarcoma

Definition

Hepatic carcinosarcoma contains both sarcomatous and carcinomatous elements. Some authors prefer therefore the term "malignant mixed tumour" [10, 16].

Epidemiology

Approximately 20 cases of this extremely rare tumour are reported in the literature [16, 25, 31]. Males and females are equally affected and median onset is around 55-

67 years [16, 31]. Aetiology and risk factors are unknown but incidence might be largely underestimated and actually account for up to 6% of all primary malignancies [16].

Clinical presentation and diagnosis

Based on case reports, patients present typically with unspecific symptoms, such as abdominal pain and weight loss [16].

Pathology features

Carcinosarcomas are rather large tumours (5-14 cm) that contain areas of hemorrhage and necrosis [16]. Carcinomatous (hepatocellular or cholangiocellular) and sarcomatous components are closely mixed, and usually account for at least 30% of the neoplasm in each case [10, 16]. While the carcinomatous part is mainly conventional hepatocellular carcinoma, sarcomatous components are highly variable [16]. Differentiation from true sarcomas might be very difficult, and necessitates specimens of sufficient size [5, 31].

Prognosis and treatment

Diagnosis is usually made only after surgical resection, which is the only promising treatment option. Despite R0 resection, patients are rarely alive six months after surgery [16, 25, 31].

Carcinosarcomas are very rare tumours, mixed of sarcomatous and carcinomatous components. Surgical resection delivers occasionally satisfactory outcome, but prognosis is generally poor.

References

1. **Blumgart LH, Belghiti J, Jarnagin WR *et al.* (2007) Surgery of the Liver, Biliary Tract, and Pancreas. Saunders Elsevier, Philadelphia**
2. Chan WK, Tse EW, Fan YS *et al.* (2008) Positron emission tomography/computed tomography in the diagnosis of multifocal primary hepatic lymphoma. J Clin Oncol 26: 5479-80
3. Changku J, Shaohua S, Zhicheng Z *et al.* (2006) Solitary fibrous tumor of the liver: retrospective study of reported cases. Cancer Invest 24: 132-5
4. Choi EA, Abdalla EK (2007) Patient selection and outcome of hepatectomy for non-colorectal non-neuroendocrine liver metastases. Surg Oncol Clin N Am 16: 557-77.
5. **Clavien PA, Fong Y, Lyerly HK *et al.* (2004) Malignant Liver Tumors: Current and Emerging Therapies. Jones and Bartlett Publishers International, London**
6. Del Poggio P, Buonocore M (2008) Cystic tumors of the liver: a practical approach. World J Gastroenterol 14: 3616-20
7. Emile JF, Azoulay D, Gornet JM *et al.* (2001) Primary non-Hodgkin's lymphomas of the liver with nodular and diffuse infiltration patterns have different prognoses. Ann Oncol 12: 1005-10
8. Forbes A, Portmann B, Johnson P *et al.* (1987) Hepatic sarcomas in adults: a review of 25 cases. Gut 28: 668-74
9. Goodman ZD, Ishak KG, Langloss JM *et al.* (1985) Combined hepatocellular-cholangiocarcinoma. A histologic and immunohistochemical study. Cancer 55: 124-135.
10. **Hamilton SR, Aaltonen LA (2000) Pathology and Genetics of Tumours of the Digestive System. In: Kleihues P, Sobin LH (eds) World Health Organization Classification of Tumours. IARC Press, Lyon, France**
11. Husted TL, Neff G, Thomas MJ *et al.* (2006) Liver transplantation for primary or metastatic sarcoma to the liver. Am J Transplant 6: 392-7
12. Japan LCSGo (1990) Primary liver cancer in Japan. Clinicopathologic features and results of surgical treatment. Ann Surg 211: 277-87

7

13. Kassahun WT, Hauss J (2008) Management of combined hepatocellular and cholangiocarcinoma. Int J Clin Pract 62: 1271-8
14. Kim HG (2006) [Biliary cystic neoplasm: biliary cystadenoma and biliary cystadenocarcinoma]. Korean J Gastroenterol 47: 5-14
15. Korkolis DP, Apostolaki K, Aggeli C *et al.* (2008) Solitary fibrous tumor of the liver expressing CD34 and vimentin: A case report. World J Gastroenterol 14: 6261-4
16. Lao XM, Chen DY, Zhang YQ *et al.* (2007) Primary carcinosarcoma of the liver: clinicopathologic features of 5 cases and a review of the literature. Am J Surg Pathol 31: 817-26
17. Lazaridis G, Pentheroudakis G, Fountzilas G *et al.* (2008) Liver metastases from cancer of unknown primary (CUPL): a retrospective analysis of presentation, management and prognosis in 49 patients and systematic review of the literature. Cancer Treat Rev 34: 693-700
18. Lerut JP, Orlando G, Adam R *et al.* (2007) The place of liver transplantation in the treatment of hepatic epitheloid hemangioendothelioma: report of the European liver transplant registry. Ann Surg 246: 949-57; discussion 957
19. **Lerut JP, Weber M, Orlando G *et al.* (2007) Vascular and rare liver tumors: a good indication for liver transplantation? J Hepatol 47: 466-75**
20. Llovet JM, Ricci S, Mazzaferro V *et al.* (2008) Sorafenib in advanced hepatocellular carcinoma. N Engl J Med 359: 378-90
21. McCormack L, Hany TI, Hubner M *et al.* (2006) How useful is PET/CT imaging in the management of post-transplant lymphoproliferative disease after liver transplantation? Am J Transplant 6: 1731-6
22. **Mehrabi A, Kashfi A, Fonouni H *et al.* (2006) Primary malignant hepatic epithelioid hemangioendothelioma: a comprehensive review of the literature with emphasis on the surgical therapy. Cancer 107: 2108-21**
23. Noronha V, Shafi NQ, Obando JA *et al.* (2005) Primary non-Hodgkin's lymphoma of the liver. Crit Rev Oncol Hematol 53: 199-207
24. Perini MV, Herman P, D'Albuquerque LA *et al.* (2008) Solitary fibrous tumor of the liver: report of a rare case and review of the literature. Int J Surg 6: 396-9
25. Poggio JL, Nagorney DM, Nascimento AG *et al.* (2000) Surgical treatment of adult primary hepatic sarcoma. Br J Surg 87: 1500-5
26. Portolani N, Baiocchi GL, Coniglio A, et al. (2008) Intrahepatic cholangiocarcinoma and combined hepatocellular-cholangiocarcinoma: a Western experience. Ann Surg Oncol 15: 1880-90
27. Poston G, Blumgart L (2003) Surgical Management of Hepatobiliary and Pancreatic Disorders. Martin Dunitz, a member of the Taylor & Francis Group, London
28. Reddy SK, Barbas AS, Marroquin CE *et al.* (2007) Resection of noncolorectal nonneuroendocrine liver metastases: a comparative analysis. J Am Coll Surg 204: 372-82
29. Steward WP (1997) Chemotherapy for metastatic soft tissue sarcomas. Cancer Treat Res 91: 157-72
30. Vogt DP, Henderson JM, Chmielewski E (2005) Cystadenoma and cystadenocarcinoma of the liver: a single center experience. J Am Coll Surg 200: 727-33
31. Weitz J, Klimstra DS, Cymes K *et al.* (2007) Management of primary liver sarcomas. Cancer 109: 1391-6
32. Yedibela S, Gohl J, Graz V *et al.* (2005) Changes in indication and results after resection of hepatic metastases from noncolorectal primary tumors: a single-institutional review. Ann Surg Oncol 12: 778-85

Unusual pancreatic tumours

8

T.V.F. Nguyen and A.-C. Dupont-Gossart

Five Essential Points

1. *In case of well-differentiated pancreatic endocrine tumours, a multi-disciplinary approach is recommended. Current therapy allows good control of the hormonal and clinical symptoms and a combination of different therapeutic options offers better long term survival.*
2. *Poorly-differentiated metastatic pancreatic endocrine tumours are chemosensitive but their prognosis remains unfavourable.*
3. *Significant progress has been made in the management of liver metastases, with the use of technically advanced surgical procedures, including extensive resections, and local ablation techniques, such as radiofrequency, allowing either curative treatment or symptom control in palliative situations.*
4. *For cystic pancreatic tumours (CPT), surgical resection is indicated for most symptomatic lesions and in patients for whom the surgical risk is low. Management in patients without symptoms has not been accurately defined yet because there is no reliable test that can accurately distinguish between benign and potential malignant CPT or predict the risk of progression to invasive cancer.*
5. *Pancreatic metastasis can occur very late, particularly in case of renal cell carcinoma emphasizing the importance of prolonged follow-up. Surgical treatment should be attempted whenever curative resection is possible.*

Introduction

As pancreatic neoplasms include a large variety of tumours, we limit this review to those tumours whose treatment can lead to relatively good outcome. The therapeutic strategy in such cases remains controversial. In this chapter, we review the current management of endocrine tumours, cystic tumours and metastases to the pancreas.

Pancreatic endocrine tumours

General features

Pancreatic endocrine tumours (PET) are rare epithelial tumours that can be benign or malignant, and represent less than 10% of all pancreatic tumours [30]. These tumours express neuroendocrine markers such as synaptophysin and chromogranin

A, and produce different hormones : gastrin, insulin, glucagon, somatostatin, vasoactive intestinal polypeptide, growth hormone-releasing factor and adrenocorticotropic hormone. PET are classified as functioning and nonfunctioning tumours, depending on the presence or absence of clinical syndromes and hormonal secretion. The incidence of PET is low: 0.2 to 0.4 per 100,000 persons per year [40]. In decreasing order of frequency, there are gastrinoma, insulinoma, glucagonoma, vipoma, somatostatinoma and tumours with inappropriate hormone secretion (GH-RH, ACTH, neurotensin). PET are generally sporadic but may be associated with Multiple Endocrine Neoplasia type 1 (MEN-1), which encompass about 25% gastrinoma and 5% insulinoma. Tumour evolution is usually slow, even in the presence of metastases, which are diagnosed in about 60% of cases [30]. Management of PET depends on whether or not the tumour is functioning, on the presence or absence of metastases, on the histological differentiation and on whether or not there is association with MEN-1. Considerable therapeutic progress has been made in recent years and several therapeutic options are currently available, including curative or palliative surgery, local treatment with hepatic artery chemo-embolization or radiofrequency ablation, systemic treatment with somatostatin analogs, interferon, chemotherapy and targeted radionuclide therapy. However, the indications and outcomes of the various therapeutic options are poorly defined, due to the low incidence of the disease, and due to the absence of prospective randomized studies which include both patients with pancreatic and digestive endocrine tumours. Therefore, the therapeutic strategy must be decided by a multidisciplinary team for each patient on a case-by-case basis. The various treatment options, as well as their respective indications and outcomes, are detailed here.

Surgery

Surgery represents the only potentially curative treatment, and the feasibility of surgical resection should always be assessed. Technical resection of the primary tumour depends on the symptomatology, as well as the size, localization in the pancreas and distance from the Wirsung canal. If no metastatic disease is present, surgery consists of enucleation for sporadic small benign tumours, such as insulinoma, which are considered as benign in 90% of cases (provided histopathology demonstrates complete excision and benign features). In other cases, surgery consists of a left pancreatectomy with or without splenectomy, median pancreatectomy, Kausch-Whipple pancreatoduodenectomy, or even total pancreatectomy in selected cases. The morbidity of these surgical resections is about 30% for enucleation and segmentary pancreatectomy and can reach 50% in case of pancreatoduodenectomy [37]. These operations are also performed in localized disease arising from other functioning, as well as non-functioning tumours. When PET are associated with MEN-1, primary lesions are often multiple. Sub-total left pancreatectomy is performed in this context, with a recurrence rate of less than 10% in the case of insulinoma associated with MEN-1 [36]. In patients with gastrinoma associated with MEN-1, surgery is controversial, as data suggest a recurrence rate of 100% at 10 years in surgically-treated patients [34]. In palliative situations, surgery is indicated for well-differentiated disease in order to control the hormonal syndrome (through a debulking surgery) [29] or to treat local complications (jaundice, bleeding by duodenal invasion, segmentary portal hypertension).

Liver surgery

At the time of diagnosis, half of all patients present hepatic metastases. Liver surgery with curative intent is possible in only about 10 % of patients [40].

Resection of hepatic metastases from well-differentiated endocrine tumours can provide significant symptomatic benefit in patients with functioning tumours and may improve overall survival, regardless of the clinical syndrome [29, 39]. Five-year survival in patients with resected liver metastases is about 70% [13, 43], compared to 40% for non-resected cases [28]. Hepatic resection depends on the number and localization of lesions and the proportion of remaining healthy liver. Surgical techniques include metastasectomy, minor (≤ 3 Couinaud segments) or major hepatectomy, either or not associated with preoperative portal vein embolization or local therapy, such as radiofrequency [13]. Concomitant surgery of the primary tumour and metastases is possible, but a mortality rate of 5% has been reported in cases of large pancreatic tumour removal [13] and morbidity is between 30% and 45% [13, 43].

Liver transplant

Liver transplant (LT) is a possible therapeutic option for patients with non-resectable limited hepatic metastases of well-differentiated PET. Indications for LT are controversial, because cure is not likely to occur, with a poor disease-free survival of less than 25% at 5 years, while overall 5-year survival is about 50% [25, 26]. Some patients with surgically unresectable tumours and uncontrollable symptoms, in whom all other therapies (chemotherapy, interferon therapy, somatostatin analogues or intrahepatic chemotherapy) have been unsuccessful, may benefit from transplantation for palliation. Recommendations are based on a limited level of evidence (retrospective, non-meta-analysis data; multivariate analysis). LT may be reserved for young patients (under 50 years of age), in whom the primary tumour was previously removed, with characteristics that appeared to be good prognostic markers in a large retrospective analysis with 103 patients [25]. In a recent retrospective study, assessing 85 patients treated with liver transplant (41 with a duodenopancreatic endocrine tumour), the association of PET and hepatomegaly were unfavourable prognostic factors, with a 5 year survival rate of 12%. In the absence of hepatomegaly, this rate increased to 66%. [26].

Somatostatin analogs

Few prospective studies including both PET and other digestive endocrine tumours have demonstrated the efficacy of somatostatin analog treatment, notably with the use of prolonged release somatostatin analogs. In PET, somatostatin analog treatments allow tumour stabilization in about 50% of patients, with a median time ranging from 9.5 to 25 months [11, 45]. Objective response is exceptional.

Local treatments

Hepatic arterial chemoembolization

Liver metastases of endocrine tumours are often hypervascular. Arterial embolization of the hepatic artery induces ischaemia of the tumour cells, thereby reducing their hormone output and causing liquefaction. Ischaemia of tumour cells also increases their sensitivity to chemotherapeutic substances such as doxorubicin or streptozotocin. Contra-indications for chemoembolization include complete portal vein obstruction, liver insufficiency and biliary reconstruction. Response rate is about 50% in PET, with control of clinical symptoms of between 60 and 80% of cases [10, 38, 41].

Radiofrequency ablation

This is a relatively new therapeutic approach reserved for patients with localized or residual disease and possibly as a complement to surgery. Lesion destruction can be performed percutaneously or laparoscopically with one or more electrode tips producing hyperthermia at around 60 degrees. The main limitations for radiofrequency ablation are: tumour size less than 35 mm, number of metastases less than 5 and lesions located near large vessels. Response rates of between 87 and 96% have been described with a response duration of up to 25 months [2, 18].

Chemotherapy

Chemotherapy may be used for inoperable or metastatic disease. Treatment regimens are determined according to histological differentiation and tumour course. In progressive and well-differentiated PET, the combination of doxorubicin and streptozotocin is the most effective chemotherapy, yielding long-term objective response rates ranging from 33 to 69% [14, 32]. The combination is effective in both functioning and non-functioning tumours. However, this regimen is not suitable for some patients because of doxorubicin-induced toxicity, notably heart failure. A combination of streptozotocin and 5-fluorouracil should be used in patients with contraindications to doxorubicin.

Poorly differentiated PET frequently respond to treatment with etoposide plus cisplatin. Even with high chemosensitivity with response rates between 40 and 60%, median survival does not exceed 18 months [31].

Interferon

Few data are available about interferon therapy in PET. A review of literature from 380 patients with both PET and digestive endocrine tumours, reported an objective response rate of 11% and stable disease rate of 35% [35]. About 15 to 20% of patients have progressive clinical or biochemical disease.

Targeted therapy

Numerous receptors in signal transduction seem to be involved in the growth of endocrine tumours (VEGFR, EGFR, IGFR1, PDGFR, PI3K, AKT and mTOR). Interesting results were found with Sunitinib (a small molecule kinase inhibitor with activity against a number of tyrosine kinase receptors, including notably VEGFR and PDGFR) and RAD001, an oral inhibitor of mTOR, in advanced and pre-treated PET. A phase II study evaluating sunitinib in 66 pre-treated PET showed a disease control rate of 85% (objective response: 16.7%, stable disease: 68%). Median time to tumour progression was 7.7 months and the one-year survival rate was 81% [22]. RAD001 (everolimus) was assessed in a phase II study, alone (arm A: 115 patients) or associated with intra-muscular octreotide (arm B: 45 patients) in progressing PET after chemotherapy [54]. Clinical benefit was considerable and of long duration: 76.5% for RAD001 alone and 82.2% for combined RAD001 and octreotide. Median progression-free survival was 9.3 months with RAD001 and 12.9 months with both RAD001 and octreotide [54]. Median global survival was not reached after 18 months of follow-up. Phase III studies are still ongoing [54].

Targeted radionuclide therapy

The treatment principle is to give radionuclide therapy when there is abnormally increased uptake of the corresponding imaging agent. Somatosatin analogues coupled to radionuclides emitting beta-radiation, such as ^{90}Y or ^{177}Lu, give encouraging results in terms of tumour shrinkage. Kwekkeboom *et al* evaluated the treatment with a radiolabeled somatostatin analog octreotate in 131 patients with gastroenteropancreatic tumour including 33 non-functioning PET, 8 gastrinomas and 2 insulinomas [23]. The response rate was as follows:

1. non functioning PET: complete response (CR) 9%, partial response (PR) 22%, minor response (MR) 22% and stable disease (SD) 34%, respectively;
2. gastrinoma: PR 63%, MR 25% and SD 12%, respectively;
3. insulinoma: PR 50% [23].

Serious side-effects were rare. Pre-treatment with amino-acid infusion reduced tubular octreotide binding and minimised renal damage. Targeted radionuclide therapy is not currently available in daily routine practice and its role in the therapeutic armamentarium remains to be defined. It could be a useful palliative option for symptomatic patients with inoperable or metastatic tumours, progressive under chemotherapy, or who have received a maximum cumulative dose of anthracyclines, and with tumours that present an uptake of In111-pentaoctreotide (Octreoscan) scintigraphy.

Therapeutic management

According to histological differentiation and disease stage, we recommend the following therapeutic strategy (Fig. 1). In case of well-differentiated PET, curative surgery of primary tumour and metastases should be proposed for patients with a good performance status. If disease is not resectable, tumour progression and symptoms should determine the therapeutic choice. Observation is recommended for stable disease without symptoms. In case of stable disease with symptoms, somatostatin analogs should be proposed. If symptoms are not controlled, then chemo-embolization, chemotherapy, local destructive therapy or debulking surgery should be proposed. In case of progressive disease, chemo-embolization should be preferred for predominant liver disease, or systemic chemotherapy for extra-hepatic metastatic disease. Targeted radionuclide therapy and targeted therapies may be discussed in case of progression under chemotherapy or chemotherapy toxicity.

In case of poorly-differentiated PET, after curative surgery, adjuvant treatment is not recommended. In case of advanced disease, chemotherapy should be proposed. Surgery is ineffective in advanced disease.

Cystic tumours

Epidemiology, pathology and natural history

The World Health Organization (WHO) classification describes three levels of malignancy for cystic pancreatic tumours (CPT): benign, borderline and malignant tumours [19] and this definition was updated by Kosmahl *et al.* in 2004 [21].

CPT represent only 10 to 15% of cystic pancreatic lesions. Pseudocysts (following acute or chronic pancreatitis) constitute the main differential diagnosis, comprising more than 70% of all cystic lesions within the pancreas. The incidence of CPT is estimated at 1/5000. We focus here on borderline and malignant cystic tumours.

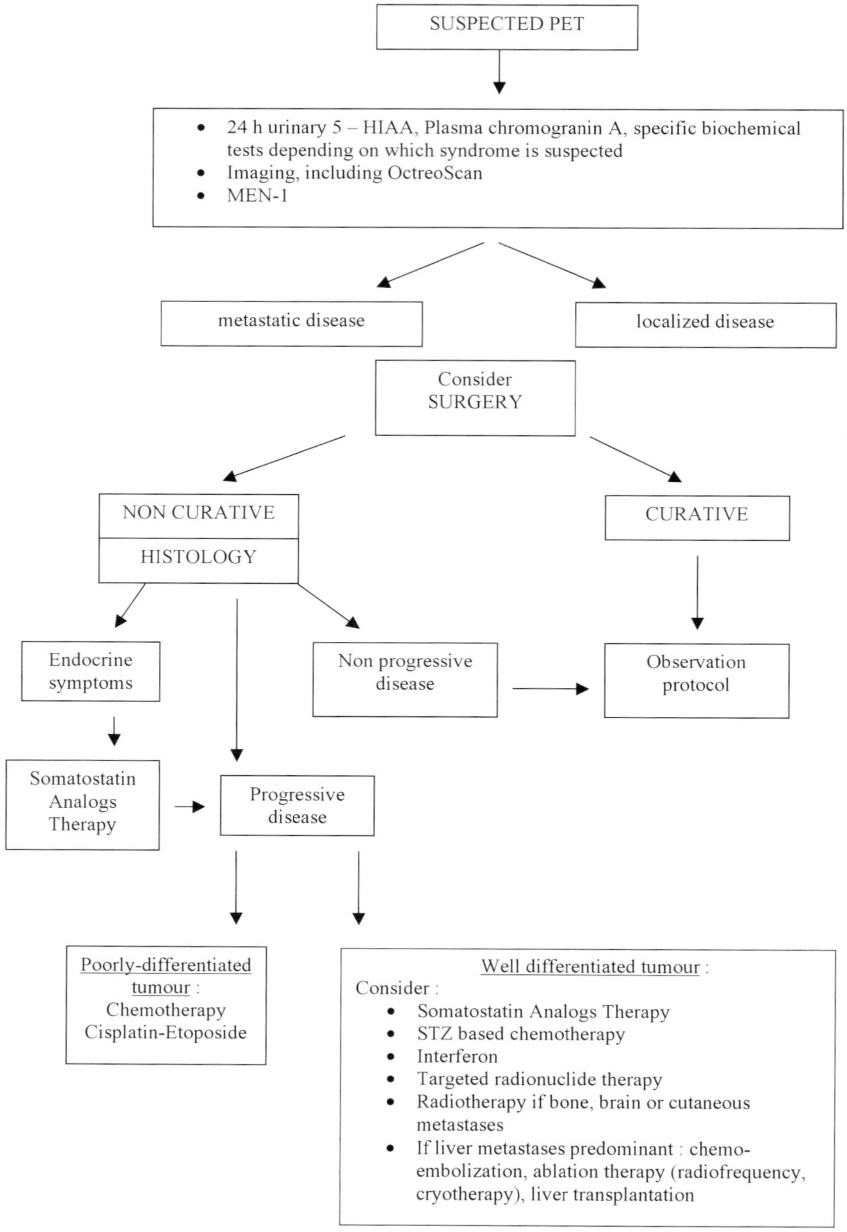

Fig. 1. Algorithm for the management of pancreatic endocrine tumours (PET).

Serous cystadenoma

Serous cystic neoplasm represent 32% of CPT [24]. They occur mainly in women (70-80% of cases). They are usually benign and slow-growing tumours. The risk of malignant transformation is exceptional, estimated to be less than 3% [48]. The classic form is a unique tumour composed of numerous microcysts whose size varies from a few millimetres to less than 2 cm, with a spongy and honeycombed pattern and lined with glycogen-rich cells. A variant is the serous macrocystic adenoma, a feature that can make difficult the distinction from mucinous cystadenomas. The presence of a central scar is a diagnostic feature, but is only observed in about 20% of cases.

Mucinous cystic tumour

These are the most frequent cystic pancreatic tumours: among CPT, the prevalence is 28% for mucinous cystadenoma and 15% for mucinous cystadenocarcinoma. They are found mainly in middle aged women and more frequently developed in the body and tail of the pancreas [24]. In macroscopic pathology, there are few macrocysts (diameter: 1-30 cm) with internal segmentation and clear fluid. Their key feature is a dense mesenchymal ovarian-like stroma and absence of any connection with the ductal system. The uncommon finding of peripheral eggshell calcifications is specific for a mucinous cystic tumour and highly predictive for the development of cancer [8, 49]. Despite some controversy, the coexistence of mucinous cystadenoma and cystadenocarcinoma, heralds slow malignant transformation from mucinous cystadenoma to cystadenocarcinoma. In addition, Singh *et al.* showed evidence of a molecular progression towards malignancy by mutations of the KRAS oncogene [44].

Intraductal papillary mucinous tumours

Their histological definition is an uncommon proliferation of the epithelium of a pancreatic duct. They represent 5% of CPT and preferentially occur in the 6th and 7th decades of life with an equal distribution between men and women. The principal localization is the head of pancreas in 70% of cases, but in 10% of cases, an invasion of the whole gland is found. Distended ducts displaying profuse papillary fronds and filled with mucus and/or solid vegetations are characteristic of these tumours. They are divided into 2 anatomical sub-types: (1) those confined to secondary ducts (side-branch type) and (2) those involving the main pancreatic duct (main-duct type); or a combination of both. Predictive morphologic criteria of a malignant transformation are main duct or mixed types, obstruction of a pancreatic biliary duct, main duct diameter of more than 10 to 15 mm, a side-branch duct diameter of more than 30 to 40 mm and presence of mural nodules of more than 3 mm [3]. Histologically, such tumours display marked differences with a well-differentiated intestinal sub-type and a pancreato-biliary sub-type, which is associated with a poorer survival [44, 49].

Solid pseudo papillary tumours

These tumours represent less than 5% of CPT and occur in young adults (median age of 26), more frequently in non-Caucasian people [7]. The sex ratio for women is 95%. They are borderline malignant tumours characterized by a low grade potential for the development of invasive cancer. However, in the absence of curative treatment, locoregional involvement and distant metastasis can occur [5, 50]. The classic morphology is a solid mass of large size (mean diameter of 9 cm, [7]) characterized by mixed features, necrosis and haemorrhage.

Diagnosis

Imaging

Most patients with a pancreatic cystic lesion do not have any symptoms, except for those with intraductal papillary mucinous tumours, which are diagnosed in 40% of cases following an acute episode of pancreatitis. Such tumours are often discovered incidentally due to the wide use of radiological imaging. Endoscopic ultrasonography (EUS) and CT scan are the most effective techniques. EUS can show millimetric structures such as vegetations, thickened walls or small microcysts [4]. In association with a retrograde cholangiopancreatography, characteristic findings of mucinous-filled defects, ductal dilatation and papillary projections can be visualized [17]. Diagnosis of CPT was possible in 92-96% of cases in a Japanese study [20], but these excellent results were not replicated in more recent studies [5], underlining the problem of interobserver agreement [1]. CT allows the characterization of cystic tumours using the following criteria: peripheral calcifications of the cyst wall, central scar, segmentation, mural nodules, hypervascularisation, or other findings in favour of acute or chronic pancreatitis. In order to simplify decision-making with regard to management, Sahani *et al.* has proposed an image-based classification resulting in four subtypes: unilocular cyst, microcystic lesions, macrocystic lesions and cysts with solid component [42]. Magnetic resonance imaging (MRI) has the advantage of a better sensitivity to show fluid inside microcystic lesions. Furthermore, MRI performed with a cholangiopancreatography can determine the presence of a connection between the duct and the cystic tumour and the extent of an intraductal papillary mucinous tumour toward the main pancreatic duct. However, the ability of these imaging techniques to accurately detect borderline or malignant disease remains questionable [9]. PET scan may be helpful to resolve this difficult question by offering an accurate discrimination between malignant and benign cystic lesions, as reported in a recent study [47].

Cytology and biochemical assessment

Cytologic examination and assessment of tumour markers and presence of amylase in the cyst fluid are currently performed by EUS, which is the safest technique for guiding fine needle aspiration of cystic lesions. Reports on the accuracy of cytological analysis vary from a specificity of only 40% up to more than 90% [51, 52]. Mucin and fluid viscosity may be used to characterize mucinous tumours, which tend to have high mucin content and subsequently a higher viscosity [27]. Amylase-rich fluid is an indicator of communication between a cyst and the ductal system and is therefore commonly found in pseudo-cyst and intraductal papillary mucinous tumours, but with higher levels in pseudo-cysts. Different cut-off levels of tumour markers such as carcinoembryonic antigen (CEA) and CA 19-9 have been evaluated in the diagnosis of malignant or premalignant cystic lesions: although they are not sensitive, if raised, they appear to be highly specific. A pooled analysis of 450 patients showed that cut-off values of less than 5 ng/ml for CEA and less than 37 ng/ml for CA 19-9, strongly suggest a serous cystadenoma or a pseudocyst and a cut-off value of less than 250 U/l for amylase would exclude a pseudocyst [51].

Treatment

The decrease in morbidity and mortality associated with pancreatic resections has led to the increasing use of surgery for the pre-emptive treatment of premalignant cystic lesions. Furthermore, the appropriate pancreatic segment where the cystic lesion is located should be resected (distal, proximal or middle pancreatectomy). Splenectomy is rarely done and performed only in case of suspicion of invasive cancer of the pancreatic tail. However, in intraductal papillary mucinous tumours, because of their longitudinal extent along ducts, resection margins must be carefully examined intraoperatively, leading to total pancreatectomy in 15% of patients [46].

In patients at high risk of surgical resection, EUS-assisted ethanol ablation therapy of CPT can be considered: for macrocyst lesions measuring between 1 and 5 cm, ethanol lavage has shown good results in terms of cyst resolution or epithelial ablation, as reported by Brugge *et al.* in a study of 25 patients [6].

Management

The management of CPT has not yet been standardized. In symptomatic patients (biliary duct obstruction, acute pancreatitis...), with a low surgical risk and for whom cystic tumours show a substantial risk of degeneration, surgical resection is the most appropriate treatment. However, evaluation and management in patients without any symptoms, for whom cystic tumours were discovered incidentally, are poorly defined. Several treatment algorithms have been proposed based on observational studies [12, 16, 49, 53]. High resolution CT and/or MRI should be performed initially. In the absence of obvious criteria for malignant disease, EUS can provide further precise morphologic features of the lesion and an opportunity to perform aspiration of the fluid or a biopsy of the cyst wall in order to diagnose potentially malignant disease. Patients who have characteristic features of main duct or mixed intraductal papillary mucinous neoplasm or cyst with solid component or peripheral calcification should be proposed for surgery. Patients with unilocular cyst, which is not characteristic of pseudocyst or macrocysts, should undergo EUS with cyst fluid analysis (cytology, viscosity, amylase, CEA and

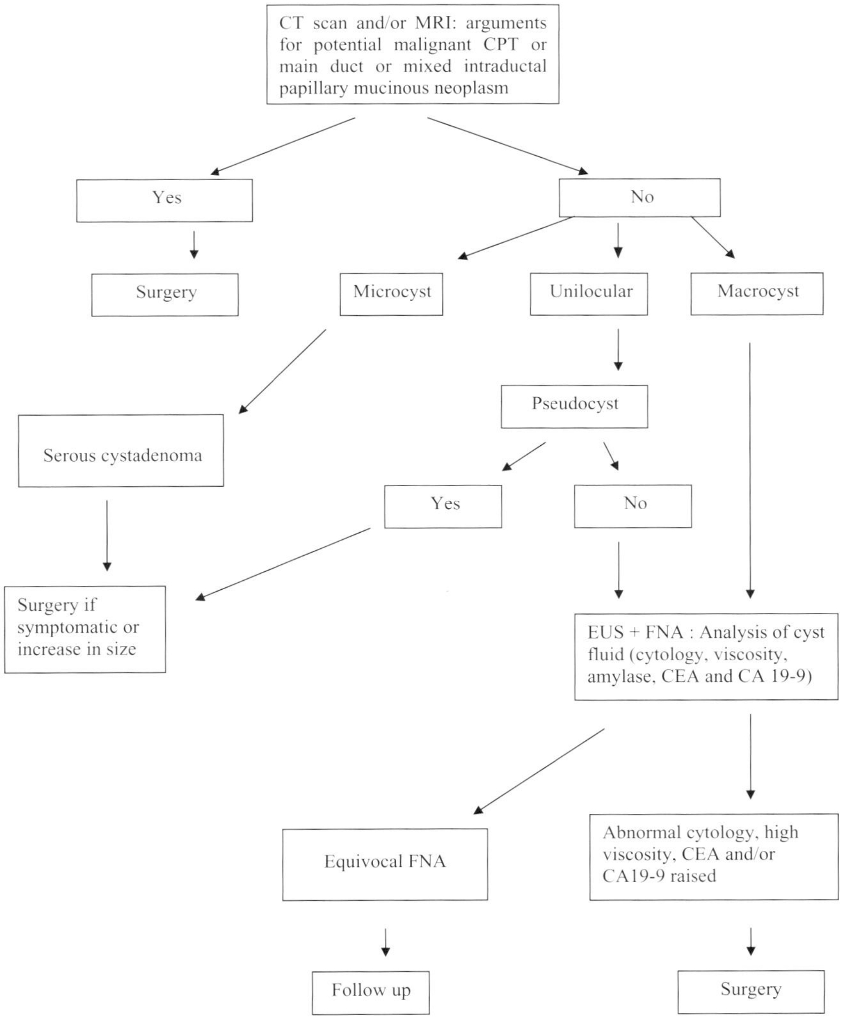

Fig. 2. Algorithm for the management of CPT incidentally discovered.

CA 19-9). In addition, rate of growth and life expectancy are important variables to consider in the perspective of non-operative management, although the exact modalities of follow-up have not yet been well-defined. Our recommendations for the management of CPT are summarized in Figure 2.

Pancreatic metastases

Metastasis of other cancers to the pancreas are usually incidental findings in patients with known metastatic disease, but solitary metastases have been reported: Faure *et al.* found that 3% of all pancreatic resections performed for malignant disease concern pancreatic metastases of renal-cell carcinoma [15]. Most pancreatic metastases develop from primary kidney, lung, breast, colon tumours and melanoma. These lesions are rarely symptomatic and are discovered coincidently during regular surveillance. Distinguishing a metastatic lesion from a primary tumour or a locoregional invasion of gastrointestinal tumour is not an easy diagnosis, even for the pathologist. If a CT scan shows a well-delineated and highly vascular mass, this is more in favour of a metastasis than of a primary pancreatic cancer, which tends to be relatively hypovascular. This must still be distinguished from a primary neuroendocrine tumour, which is also hypervascular. The most reliable method for diagnosis remains a tumour biopsy, which is best obtained with endoscopic ultrasound and fine needle aspiration. Treatment modalities depend on the type of primary tumour and the localization of other metastases. In the medical literature, the two main prognostic factors are the primary localization and resectability. The longest survival reported has always concerned patients who underwent surgery for a primary renal cancer with long disease-free interval and curative resection for the pancreatic metastasis: a 5-year survival of 31% has been reported for patients treated by surgery for a solitary metastasis due to renal cell carcinoma [15]. In these cases, radiotherapy, chemotherapy or immunotherapy should be discussed whenever surgery is not feasible [33].

This finding underscores the importance of regular prolonged surveillance, particularly after treatment of renal cell carcinoma.

References

1. Ahmad NA, Kochman ML, Brensinger C *et al.* (2003) Interobserver agreement among endosonographers for the diagnosis of neoplastic versus non-neoplastic pancreatic cystic lesions. Gastrointest Endosc 58: 59-64
2. Berber E, Flesher N, Siperstein AE (2002) Laparoscopic radiofrequency ablation of neuroendocrine liver metastases. World J Surg 26: 985-90
3. Bernard P, Scoazec JY, Joubert M *et al.* (2002) Intraductal papillary-mucinous tumors of the pancreas: predictive criteria of malignancy according to pathological examination of 53 cases. Arch Surg 137: 1274-8
4. Brandwein SL, Farrell JJ *et al.* (2001) Detection and tumor staging of malignancy in cystic, intraductal and solid tumors of the pancreas by EUS. Gastrointest Endosc 53: 722-7
5. Brugge WR, Lauwers GY, Sahani D *et al.* (2004) Cystic neoplasms of the pancreas. N Engl J Med 351: 1218-26
6. Brugge WR (2008) Management and outcomes of pancreatic cystic lesions. Digestive and Liver Disease 40: 854-9
7. Buetow PC, Buck JL, Pantongrag-Brown L *et al.* (1996) Solid and papillary epithelial neoplasm of the pancreas: imaging-pathologic correlation on 56 cases. Radiology 199: 707-11

8. Campbell F, Azadeh B (2008) Cystic neoplasms of the exocrine pancreas. Histopathology 52: 539-41
9. Curry CA, Eng J, Horton KM, et al (2000) CT of primary cystic pancreatic neoplasms: can CT be used for patient triage and treatment? Am J Roentgenol 175: 99-103
10. Dominguez S, Denys A, Madeira I *et al.* (2000) Hepatic arterial chemoembolization with streptozotocin in patients with metastatic digestive endocrine tumours. Eur J Gastroenterol Hepatol 12: 151-7
11. Ducreux M, Ruszniewski P, Chayvialle JA *et al.* (2000) The antitumoral effect of the long-acting somatostatin analog lanreotide in neuroendocrine tumors. Am J Gastroenterol 95: 3276-81
12. **Edirimanne S, Connor SJ (2008) Incidental pancreatic cystic lesions. World J Surg 32: 2028-37**
13. **Elias D, Lasser P, Ducreux M *et al.* (2003) Liver resection (and associated extrahepatic resections) for metastatic well-differentiated endocrine tumors: a 15-year single center prospective study. Surgery 133: 375-82**
14. Eriksson B, Skogseid B, Lundqvist G *et al.* (1990) Medical treatment and long-term survival in a prospective study of 84 patients with endocrine pancreatic tumors. Cancer 65: 1883-90
15. Faure JP, Tuech JJ (2001) Pancreatic metastasis of renal cell carcinoma : presentation treatment and survival. J Urol 165: 20-2
16. Goh BK, Tan YM, Chung YF *et al.* (2007) Pancreatic cyst : a proposed management algorithm based on current evidence. Am J Surg 193: 749-55
17. Hara T, Yamaguchi T, Ishihara T *et al.* (2002) Diagnosis and patient management of intraductal papillary-mucinous tumor of the pancreas by using peroral pancreatoscopy and intraductal ultrasonography. Gastroenterology 122: 34-43
18. Hellman P, Ladjevardi S, Skogseid B *et al.* (2002) Radiofrequency tissue ablation using cooled tip for liver metastases of endocrine tumors. World J Surg 26: 1052-6
19. Kloppel GS, Solcia E, Longnecker DS *et al.* (1996) Histological Typing of Tumors of the Exocrine Pancreas. World Health Organization. International Histological Classification of Tumours. 2nd ed. Berlin, Heidelberg, New York: Springer, pp.15-21
20. Koito K, Namieno T, Nagakawa T *et al.* (1997) Solitary cystic tumor of the pancreas: EUS-pathologic correlation. Gastrointest Endosc 45: 268-76
21. Kosmahl M, Pauser U, Peters K *et al.* (2004) Cystic neoplasms of the pancreas and tumor-like lesions with cystic features: a review of 418 cases and a classification proposal. Virchows Arch 445: 168-78
22. Kulke MH, Lenz HJ, Meropol NJ *et al.* (2008) Activity of sunitinib in patients with advanced neuroendocrine tumors. J Clin Oncol 26: 3403-10
23. Kwekkeboom DJ, Teunissen JJ, Bakker WH *et al.* (2005) Radiolabeled somatostatin analog [177Lu-DOTA0,Tyr3]octreotate in patients with endocrine gastroenteropancreatic tumors. J Clin Oncol 23: 2754-62
24. Le Borgne J, de Calan L, Partensky C (1999) Cystadenomas and cystadenocarcinomas of the pancreas: a multiinstitutional retrospective study of 398 cases. French Surgical Association. Ann Surg 230: 152-61
25. Lehnert T (1998) Liver transplantation for metastatic neuroendocrine carcinoma: an analysis of 103 patients. Transplantation 66: 1307-12
26. **Le Treut YP, Grégoire E, Belghiti J *et al.* (2008) Predictors of long-term survival after liver transplantation for metastatic endocrine tumors: an 85-case French multicentric report. Am J Transplant 8: 1205-13**
27. Linder JD, Geenen JE, Catalano MF (2006) Cystic fluid analysis obtained by EUS-guided FNA in the evaluation of discrete cystic neoplasms of the pancreas. Gastrointest Endosc 64: 697-702
28. Madeira I,T erris B, Voss M *et al.* (1998) Prognostic factors in patients with endocrine tumours of the duodenopancreatic area. Gut 43: 422-7
29. McEntee GP, Nagorney DM, Kvols LK *et al.* (1990) Cytoreductive hepatic surgery for neuroendocrine tumors. Surgery 108: 1091-6
30 Mignon M, Cadiot G, Aparicio T (2005) Tumeurs endocrines pancréatiques : Diagnostic clinique et biologique. In : Traité de pancréatologie clinique. Lévy P, Rusniewski P, Sauvanet A Eds. Flammarion Médecine-Sciences, pp. 289-300
31. Moertel CG, Kvols LK, O'Connell MJ *et al.* (1991) Treatment of neuroendocrine carcinomas with combined etoposide and cisplatin. Evidence of major therapeutic activity in the anaplastic variants of these neoplasms. Cancer 68: 227-32

32. Moertel CG, Lefkopoulo M, Lipsitz S *et al.* (1992) Streptozocin-doxorubicin, streptozocin-fluorouracil or chlorozotocin in the treatment of advanced islet-cell carcinoma. N Engl J Med 326: 519-23
33. Moussa A, Mitry E, Hammel P *et al.* (2004) Pancreatic metastases a multicentric study of 22 patients. Gastroenterol Clin Biol 28: 872-6
34. Norton JA, Fraker DL, Alexander HR *et al.* (1999) Surgery to cure the Zollinger-Ellison syndrome. N Engl J Med 341: 635-44
35. Oberg K (2000) Interferon in the management of neuroendocrine GEP-tumors: a review. Digestion 62 Suppl 1: 92-7
36. O'Riordain DS, O'Brien T, van Heerden JA *et al.* (1994) Surgical management of insulinoma associated with multiple endocrine neoplasia type I. World J Surg. 18: 488-93; Discussion 493-4
37. Phan GQ, Yeo CJ, Hruban RH *et al.* (1998) Surgical experience with pancreatic and peripancreatic neuroendocrine tumors: review of 125 patients. J Gastrointest Surg 2: 472-82
38. Perry LJ, Stuart K, Stokes KR *et al.* (1994) Hepatic arterial chemoembolization for metastatic neuroendocrine tumors. Surgery 116: 1111-6; Discussion 1116-7
39. Que FG, Nagorney DM, Batts KP *et al.* (1995) Hepatic resection for metastatic neuroendocrine carcinomas. Am J Surg 169: 36-42; Discussion 42-33
40. Ramage JK, Davies AH, Ardill J *et al.* (2005) Guidelines for the management of gastroenteropancreatic neuroendocrine (including carcinoid) tumours.Gut. 54: iv1-16
41. Ruszniewski P, Rougier P, Roche A *et al.* (1993) Hepatic arterial chemoembolization in patients with liver metastases of endocrine tumors. A prospective phase II study in 24 patients. Cancer 71: 2624-30
42. **Sahani DV, Kadavigere R, Saokar A (2005) Cystic pancreatic lesions: a simple imaging based classification system for guiding management. Radiographics 25: 1471-84**
43. Sarmiento JM, Que FG, Grant CS *et al.* (2002) Concurrent resections of pancreatic islet cell cancers with synchronous hepatic metastases: outcomes of an aggressive approach. Surgery 132: 976-82; Discussion 982-3
44. Singh M, Maitra A (2007) Precursor lesions of pancreatic cancer: molecular pathology and clinical implications. Pancreatology 7: 9-19
45. Shojamanesh H, Gibril F, Louie A *et al.* (2002) Prospective study of the antitumor efficacy of long-term octreotide treatment in patients with progressive metastatic gastrinoma. Cancer 94: 33143
46. Sohn TA, Yeo CJ, Cameron JL *et al.* (2004) Intraductal papillary mucinous neoplasms of the pancreas: an updated experience. Ann Surg 239: 788-97; Discussion 797-9
47. Sperti C, Pasquali C, Decet G *et al.* (2005) F-18-fluorodeoxyglucose positron emission tomography in differentiating malignant from benign pancreatic cysts: a prospective study. J Gastrointest Surg 9: 22-8
48. Strobel O, Z'Graggen K, Schmitz-Winnenthal FH *et al.* (2003) Risk of malignancy in serous cystic neoplasms of the pancreas. Digestion 68: 24-33
49. Tanaka M, Chari S, Adsay V *et al.* (2006) International consensus guidelines for management of intraductal papillary mucinous neoplasms of the pancreas. Pancreatology 6: 17-32
50. Tipton SG, Smyrk TC, Saar MG (2006) Malignant potential of solid pseudopapillary neoplasm of the pancreas. Br J Surg 93: 733-7
51. **Van der Waaij LA, van Dulleman HM, Porte RJ (2005) Cyst fluid analysis in the differential diagnosis of pancreatic cystic lesions: a pooled analysis. Gastrointest Endosc 62: 383-9**
52. Volmar KE, Vollmer RT, Jowell PS (2005) Pancreatic FNA in 1000 cases: a comparison of imaging modalities. Gastrointest Endosc 61: 85461
53. Walsh RM, Vogt DP, Henderson JM *et al.* (2008) Management of suspected pancreatic cystic neoplasms based on cyst size. Surgery 144: 677-85
54. Yao Y, Lombard-Bohas C *et al.* (2008) A phase II trial of daily oral RAD001 (everolimus) in patients with metastatic pancreatic neuroendocrine tumors (NET) after failure of cytotoxic chemotherapy. Ann Oncol 19: abstr 508PD

Section 4
Genitourinary tumours

Rare tumours of the renal pelvis and ureter

1

M. Ozsahin and A. Zouhair

Five Essential Points

1. *Translational-cell carcinoma (TCC) is the most common upper urinary tract tumour.*
2. *Heavy cigarette smoking or chronic use of laxatives or non-steroidal anti-inflammatory drugs is associated with increased risk of TCC of the upper urinary tract.*
3. *Hematuria is the main symptom.*
4. *Open or laparascopic surgery in the mainstay of treatment.*
5. *The place of adjuvant chemo- and/or radiotherapy is not proven.*

Introduction

Primary transitional-cell carcinoma (TCC) of the renal pelvis or ureter is a relatively rare disease. It accounts for less than 1% of genitourinary neoplasms, and 5-7% of all urinary tract tumours [16]. Its incidence increases with age, the peak of diagnosis being in the sixth and the seventh decades of life [22]. Male gender has an increased incidence [16, 22]. It arises from the lining surface epithelium [25]. Adverse prognostic factors are high grade pathology and/or advanced stage. Most available data are from retrospective studies and surgery is the mainstay of the treatment. Chemotherapy and/or radiation therapy as adjuvant or primary treatment for selected patients can be used; however, prospective studies are needed to confirm their use.

Etiology and Pathology

The etiology of primary TCC of the renal pelvis or ureter is similar to that reported for TCC of the bladder [29]. Heavy cigarette smoking and chronic use of laxatives or non-steroidal anti-inflammatory drugs such as phenacetin are reported to have a strong association with this cancer [14, 30]. Occupational exposure to organic chemicals has been associated with higher risk of developing upper urinary tract urethelial cancers in workers in the chemical, petrochemical, or plastics industries [14]. The surface epithelium of the urinary tract exposed to potential carcinogens may develop a "field cancerization" resulting in synchronous or metachronous involvement of multifocal areas [15]. Endemic nephropathies, such as Balkan nephropathy, an indolent inflammatory process occurring in the Balkan countries, or nephropathy from China secondary to the ingestion of Chinese herbs containing *Aristolochia fangchi*, which is used for weight reduction, are associated with the development of TCC of the renal pelvis or ureter [26, 31]. Environmental factors such as radon inhalation and minerals in the drinking water are reported to increase the risk of TCC of the renal pelvis or ureter [14]. Genetic factors such as Lynch syndrome are also reported to increase the risk of cancers of the upper urinary tract [20, 27].

The most common type of renal pelvis and ureter cancers is TCC [15]. Squamous-cell carcinomas, adenocarcinomas, or sarcomas are uncommon [18]. Morphologically, TCC of the renal pelvis and ureter, like the bladder TCC, can be papillary or solid, and associated with carcinoma *in situ*. The prognosis of TCC is better than other histological subtypes [13].

Clinical presentation

Macroscopic or microscopic hematuria is present in 75-90% of the patients. Flank pain, occurring in 20-40% of the patients, secondary to obstructive tumour mass, can mimic an uretheral calculus [3]. Urinary symptoms (dysuria, pollakiuria, etc) may occur in 25-50% of the patients [3, 13]. Physical examination is generally normal, with the exception of a palpable flank mass in less than 10% of the patients.

Staging and diagnostic work-up

TCC of the renal pelvis or ureter can spread locally by direct extension to adjacent anatomical structures, or can be disseminated by lymphatic or hematogenous pathways [8]. Urine cytology, intravenous pyelography, and/or ureteroscopy are used to detect the primary tumour. Routine staging includes chest radiograph and/or thoraco-abdominal CT combined with assessment of hepatic, renal and hematologic chemistry. Radionuclide bone scan is also recommended to exclude bone metastases. The UICC (Union International Contre le Cancer) staging system classifies this disease according to tumour (T), nodes (N) and metastases (M) (Table 1) [32].

Treatment of non metastatic disease

The treatment of renal pelvis and ureter tumours is open or laparoscopic surgery varying from conservative to more extensive surgical procedures, *i.e.* radical nephroureterectomy including the removal of the contents of Gerota's fascia with the ipsilateral ureter and a cuff of bladder at its distal extent [12]. The entire ipsilateral ureter should be removed as 20-50% of the patients with residual ureteral stumps develop tumours within the stump [10, 28]. Following surgery, locoregional failure is reported in 9 to 15% of patients with low grade and low stage disease and in 30 to 50% of those with high grade and advanced disease [9, 24].

In bladder cancer, an organ-preserving approach using combined chemo- and radiotherapy has been used successfully [33]. The same approach can also be applied in upper urinary tract tumours if surgery is not possible.

Table 1 – Definition of TNM staging for tumours of renal pelvis and ureter [32].

Primary Tumour (T)	
TX	Primary tumour cannot be assessed
T0	No evidence of primary tumour
Ta	Papillary noninvasive carcinoma
Tis	Carcinoma *in situ*
T1	Tumour invades subepithelial connective tissue
T2	Tumour invades the muscularis
T3	For renal pelvis only: tumour invades beyond muscularis into peripelvic fat or the renal parenchyma For ureter only: tumour invades beyond muscularis into periureteric fat
T4	Tumour invades adjacent organs, or through the kidney into the perinephric fat
*Regional Lymph Nodes (N)**	
NX	Regional lymph nodes cannot be assessed
NO	No regional lymph node metastasis
N1	Metastasis in a single lymph node, 2 cm or less in greatest dimension
N2	Metastasis in a single lymph node, more than 2 cm but not more than 5 cm in greatest dimension; or multiple lymph nodes, none more than 5 cm in greatest dimension
N3	Metastasis in a lymph node more than 5 cm in greatest dimension
Distant Metastasis (M)	
MX	Distant metastasis cannot be assessed
MO	No distant metastasis
MI	Distant metastasis

* Note: laterality does not affect the N classification.

Despite aggressive primary surgery, locoregional failure remains high. Adjuvant radiation therapy has been advocated by some authors [1, 3, 5, 6, 33] but its benefit is unclear. Some studies suggest no benefit from adjuvant radiotherapy, but data from clinical experience are limited without any conclusive results from prospective studies [21, 28]. Data from the literature are summarized in Table 2. Generally speaking, in patients with adverse factors, such as high grade or stage, close or positive surgical margins or positive lymph nodes, postoperative radiotherapy may be considered. The role of adjuvant chemotherapy is also unproven. Recent retrospective results show that using modern cytotoxic agents combined with radiotherapy or used alone seem to be associated with a better outcome [2, 11, 17, 23]. In this setting, prospective studies are warranted in large collaborative groups.

Table 2 – Postoperative radiotherapy in urothelial renal pelvis and/or ureter tumours: data from the literature.

Author [ref]	N	Dose (Gy)	Residual tumour after surgery	Results
Babaian [14]	8	18.25-59	8 out of 8	Control: 4 of 8; local control: 7 of 8
Brookland [6]	9	40-60	4 of 9	Control: 5 of 9; local control: 8 of 9
	11	-	1 of 11	Control: 3 of 11; local control 8 of 11
Brady [5]	2	40-50	2 of 2	Control: 1 of 2
Cozad [10]	10	37.4-56	3 of 10	Local control: 9 of 10
Czito [11]	31	46.9	5 of 31	Control: 15 of 31; local control: 23 of 31
Maulard-Durdux [21]	26	45	?	Local control: 21 of 26
Ozsahin [28]	45	20-66	15 of 45	Local control: 33 of 45
	81	-	18 of 81	Local control: 51 of 81

The 5-year overall survival of TCC of the upper urinary tract according to the data from the National Cancer Institute SEER program [25] is 95% in *in situ* tumours, 89% in localized disease, 63% in node positive patients and 17% in metastatic disease.

Treatment of advanced disease

Many treatment options exist for management of advanced or metastatic disease including surgery, radiation therapy and/or chemotherapy, depending on the performance status of the patient and his/her comorbidities. Urothelial cancers are reported to be responsive to cisplatin-based chemotherapy regimens [19]. Taxanes and/or gemcitabine have also been used in this setting [4, 7].

Conclusion

In patients with TCC of the renal pelvis and/or ureter, radical surgery should be carried out whenever possible. Locoregional failure remains high. With the introduction of more sophisticated treatment planning, conformal techniques and intensity modulation, the role of postoperative radiation therapy remains to be reassessed. Adjuvant chemotherapy using novel drugs and/or targeted agents should also be evaluated prospectively.

References

1. Babaian RJ, Johnson DE, Chan RC (1980) Combination nephroureterectomy and postoperative radiotherapy for infiltrative uroteral carcinoma. Int J Radiat Oncol Biol Phys 6: 1229-32
2. Bamias A, Deliveliotis C, Fountzilas G *et al.* (2004) Adjuvant chemotherapy with paclitaxel and carboplatin in patients with advanced carcinoma of the upper urinary tract: a study by the Hellenic Cooperative Oncology Group. J Clin Oncol 22: 2150-4
3. Batata MA, Whitemore WF, Hilaris BS *et al.* (1975) Primary carcinoma of the ureter: a prognostic study. Cancer 35: 1626-32
4. Bellmunt J, Guillem V, Paz-Ares L *et al.* (2000) Phase I-II study of paclitaxel, cisplatin, and gemcitabine in advanced transitional-cell carcinoma of the urothelium. J Clin Oncol 18: 3247-55
5. Brady LW, Gislason GJ, Faust DS *et al.* (1968) Radiation therapy: a valuable adjunct in the management of carcinoma of the ureter. JAMA 206: 2871-4
6. Brookland RK, Richter MP (1985) The postoperative irradiation of transitional cell carcinoma of the renal pelvis and ureter. J Urol 133: 952-5
7. Burch PA, Richardson RL, Cha SS *et al.* (2000) Phase II study of paclitaxel and cisplatin for advanced urothelial cancer. J Urol 164: 1538-42
8. **Buskirk SJ, Wong WW, Haddock MG *et al.* (2007) Kidney and ureteral carcinoma. In: Gunderson LL, Tepper JE (Eds.): Clinical Radiation Oncology, 2nd Ed. Philadelphia, Churchill Livingstone pp. 1287-1306**
9. Charbit L, Gendroau MC, Mee S *et al.* (1991) Tumors of the upper urinary tract: 10 years of experience. J Urol 146: 1243-6
10. Cozad SC, Smalley SR, Austenfeld M *et al.* (1995) Transitional cell carcinoma of the renal pelvis or ureter: patterns of failure. Urology 46: 796-800
11. **Czito B, Zietman A, Kaufman D *et al.* (2004) Adjuvant radiotherapy with and without concurrent chemotherapy for locally advanced transitional cell carcinoma of the renal pelvis and ureter. J Urol 172: 1271-5**

12. Freiha FS (1994) Renal, renal pelvis and ureteral tumours: should retroperitoneal nodes be treated? Front Radiat Ther Oncol 28: 155-63
13. Holmang S, Lele SM, Johansson SL (2007) Squamous cell carcinoma of the renal pelvis and ureter: incidence, symptoms, treatment, and outcome. J Urol 178: 51-6
14. Jensen OM, Knudsen JB, McLaughlin JK *et al.* (1988) The Copenhagen case-control study of renal pelvis and ureter cancer: role of smoking and occupational exposures. Int J Cancer 41: 557-61
15. Johansson S, Angervall L, Bengtsson U *et al.* (1976) A clinicopathologic and prognostic study of epithelial tumors of the renal pelvis. Cancer 37: 1376-83
16. Kirkali Z, Tuzel E (2003) Translitional cell carcinoma of the ureter and renal pelvis. Crit Rev Oncol Hematol 47: 155-69
17. Kwak C, Lee SE, Jeong IG *et al.* (2006) Adjuvant systemic chemotherapy in the treatment of patients with invasive translitional cell carcinoma of the upper urinary tract. Urology 68: 53-7
18. Li MK, Chung WL (1987) Squamous cell carcinoma of the renal pelvis. J Urol 138: 269-71
19. Loehler PJ Sr, Einhorn LH, Elson PJ *et al.* (1992) A randomized comparison of cisplatin alone or in combination with methotrexate, vinblastine, and doxorubicin in patients with metastatic urothelial carcinoma: a cooperative group study. J Clin Oncol 10: 1066-73
20. Lynch HT, Ens JA, Lynch JF (1990) The Lynch syndrome II and urological malignancies. J Urol 143: 24-8
21. Maulard-Durdux C, Dufour B, Hennequin C *et al.* (1996) Postoperative radiation therapy in 26 patients with invasive transitional cell carcinoma of the upper urinary tract: no impact on survival? J Urol 155: 115-7
22. Mellemgaard A, Carstensen B, Norgaard N *et al.* (1993) Trends in the incidence of cancer of the kidney, pelvis, ureter and bladder in Denmark 1943-88. Scand J Urol Nephrol 27: 327-32
23. Michael M, Tannock IF, Czaykowski PM *et al.* (1998) Adjuvant chemotherapy for high-risk urothelial transitional cell carcinoma: the Pricesss Margaret Hospital experience. Br J Urol 82: 366-72
24. Miyao N, Masumori N, Takahashi A *et al.* (1998) Lymph node metastasis in patients with carcinomas of the renal pelvis and ureter. Eur Urol 33: 180-5
25. Munoz JJ, Ellison LM (2000) Upper tract urothelial neoplasms: incidence and survival during the last 2 decades. J Urol 164: 1523-5
26. Nortier JL, Martinez MC, Schmeiser HH *et al.* (2000) Urothelial carcinoma associated with the use of a Chinese herb (Aristolochia fangchi). New Engl J Med 342: 1686-92
27. Orphali SL, Shols GW, Hagewood J *et al.* (1986) Familial translational cell carcinoma of renal pelvis and upper ureter. Urology 27: 394-6
28. Ozsahin M, Zouhair A, Villa S *et al.* (1999) Prognostic factors in urothelial renal pelvis and ureter tumours: a multicentre Rare Cancer Network study. Eur J Cancer 35: 738-43
29. Parkin DM, Pisani P, Ferlay J (1993) Estimates of the world-wide incidence of 18 major cancers in 1985. Int J Cancer 54: 594-606
30. Pommer W, Bronder E, Klimpel A *et al.* (1999) Urothelial cancer at different tumour sites: role of smoking and habitual intake of analgesics, and laxatives. Results of the Berlin Urothelial Cancer Study. Nephrol Dial Transplant 14: 2892-7
31. Sattler TA, Dimitrov T, Hall PW (1977) Relation between endemic (Balkan) nephropathy and urinary-tract tumours. Lancet 1: 278-80
32. Sobin LH, Wittekind C (2002) TNM Classification of Malignant Tumours. 6th Ed. New York, Wiley-Liss
33. Zouhair A, Ozsahin M, Schneider D *et al.* (2001) Invasive bladder carcinoma: a pilot study of conservative treatment with accelerated radiotherapy and concomitant cisplatin. Int J Cancer 96: 350-5

Rare tumours of the urethra

F.Ö. Dinçbaş

2

Five Essential Points

1. *Squamous cell carcinoma is the most common urethra tumour.*
2. *Chronic irritation and inflammation, sexually transmitted disease, human papillomavirus is associated with increased risk of squamous cell carcinoma.*
3. *Bleeding, perineal pain, urinary frequency, dysuria, decreased flow and urinary obstruction are the common symptoms.*
4. *Prognosis depends upon the tumour localization. Distal tumours do better than the proximal tumours. Surgery forms the mainstay for treatment of carcinoma of the urethra. Superficial tumours may be treated with TUR and fulguration. Tumours invading the corpus spongiosum and localized to the distal half of the penis are best treated with a partial or total penile amputation in male patients, while aggressive treatment such as anterior pelvic exenteration is often needed in female patients.*
5. *The role of both adjuvant chemo- and/or radiotherapy is not proven. Neoadjuvant chemotherapy may be used for locally advanced tumours. Adjuvant treatment of cases with rare tumours should be treated according to the general rules of the treatment of these histologies in the other part of the body.*

Introduction

Urethral tumours are rare both in men and women and are usually seen in the sixth decade of life; however 10% of them are reported in men younger than 40 years [9]. The most frequent histology is squamous cell carcinoma [34]. There is no racial predisposition. Local invasion and lymph node metastases are seen at the early phase of the disease. In retrospective series, most of the patients were diagnosed in advanced stage and 46% of them were understaged at presentation [13,16]. Multidisciplinary treatment schedules with surgery, radiation therapy and chemotherapy are used to treat these tumours, although it is not easy to confirm definite treatment schedules as these tumours are so uncommon. Also, as etiology, histology and presentation is different in the two sexes, it is appropriate to consider the treatment and prognosis separately. *Suggest: Etiology, histology and presentation is different in the two sexes and treatment and prognosis should be considered separately.*

Male Urethra Tumours

Primary tumours of the urethra are very rare and make up less than 1% of genitourinary tumours in males [16]. The etiologic factors for male urethral cancer are chronic infection or inflammation, chronic foreign body (catheter etc.), sexually transmitted disease and human papillomavirus (HPV) [62,67]. Current reports show that there is increased incidence of urethra tumours, which might be related with some exogenous factors such as arsenic exposure and dietary habits [16,60].

The most common symptom is bleeding, perineal pain, urinary frequency, dysuria, decreased flow and urinary obstruction [9]. The common localization of urethral tumours is bulbomembranous urethra (60%), the penile urethra (30%) and the prostatic urethra (10%) respectively [14]. Tumours with a bulbomembranous urethra location have a worse prognosis, compared to those localized in other parts of the urethra [4,9]. Involved inguinal nodes are found in approximately 20% of patients with urethral cancer at presentation [59]. They may invade the vascular spaces of the corpus spongiosum. Bulbomembranous urethral cancer may invade the prostate, perineum, and scrotum. They may metastasize to the regional lymph nodes, which are superficial and deep inguinal, external iliac, obturator, and hypogastric nodes. Hematogenous metastasis is rare and seen usually in advanced disease [59].

Pathology

The most common histology is squamous cell with an incidence of approximately 80%. The other common histologies are transitional cell carcinoma (15%) and adenocarcinomas or undifferentiated tumours (5%) [59]. The histology differs according to the location of the tumour. Most of the carcinomas of the prostatic urethra are transitional cell and adenocarcinoma, while squamous carcinomas are common in the penile urethra [16]. Squamous cell carcinoma has a locally infiltrative pattern and is seen more in men than in women. Adenocarcinomas of the urethra tend to be in the prostatic urethra and are likely to arise from the surface mucosa or from periurethral glands. Malignant transformation of the glandular elements of urethritis cystica might be responsible for mucinous adenocarcinoma of the urethra [67]. Increased numbers of bulbomembronous adenocarcinoma are reported in South Taiwan, related to arsenic exposure in drinking water [60]. This has the same prognosis as the other histologies [59].

Diagnostic work-up and Staging

Diagnostic work-up consists of physical examination, blood and urine analysis, cystoscopy and urethroscopy, urethrogram, abdominopelvic CT, chest radiography; occasionally lymphangiography is required.

There are several staging systems for carcinoma of the urethra. The most commonly used staging is the UICC (Union International Contre le Cancer) staging system which classifies this disease according to tumour (T), nodes (N), and metastases (M) [52] (Table 1).

Table 1 – UICC TNM staging of Urethra (male and female).

Ta.	Noninvasive papillary, polypoid, or verrucous carcinoma
Tis.	Carcinoma *in situ*
T1.	Tumour invades subepithelial connective tissue
T2.	Tumour invades any of the following: corpus spongiosum, prostate, periurethral muscle
T3.	Tumour invades any of the following: corpus cavernosum, beyond prostatic capsule, anterior vagina, bladder neck
T4.	Tumour invades other adjacent organs
Transitional cell carcinoma of prostate (prostatic urethra)	
Tis pu.	Carcinoma in situ, involvement of prostatic urethra
Tis pd.	Carcinoma in situ, involvement of prostatic ducts
T1.	Tumour invades subepithelial connective tissue
T2.	Tumour invades any of the following: prostatic stroma, corpus spongiosum, periurethral muscle
T3.	Tumour invades any of the following: corpus cavernosum, beyond prostatic capsule, bladder neck (extraprostatic extension)
T4.	Tumour invades other adjacent organs (invasion of bladder)
N - Regional Lymph Nodes	
NX.	Regional lymph nodes cannot be assessed
N0.	No regional lymph node metastasis
N1.	Metastasis in a single lymph node 2 cm or less in greatest dimension
N2.	Metastasis in a single lymph node more than 2 cm in greatest dimension, or multiple lymph nodes
M - Distant Metastasis	
MX.	Distant metastasis cannot be assessed
M0.	No distant metastasis
M1.	Distant metastasis

Treatment

Tumours of the distal urethra are diagnosed earlier than the proximal, bulbomembranous urethral tumours. Surgery is the primary treatment modality for treatment of male urethral tumours [11,14]. Transurethral resection and fulguration can be used for superficial tumours [11]. Invasive tumours (T2, T3) are best treated with radical surgery. Partial or total penectomy with radical cystoprostatectomy are performed according to the localization of the tumour [11,40]. Partial penectomy can be done for those patients with tumour in the distal urethra, without invasion of the corpus spongiosum or corpora cavernosum and have 2 cm of clear tumour margins. There are few reports of penis-sparing surgery [7]. Advanced tumours require total penectomy. Advanced proximal and prostatic urethra tumours can be managed by radical cystoprostatectomy and total urethrectomy with urinary diversion [14]. Pelvic and inguinal lymph node dissection is indicated if there is palpable adenopathy. Five-year survival rates after lymphadenectomy are reported at between 12-66% [59]. In the Dalbagni *et al.* series, most of the patients were treated with surgery; the local control rate was 51%, and the 5-year overall survival was 42% [9]. Survival was better in the patients with anterior lesions (69%), compared to those with posterior lesions (26%) [9].

Radiation therapy is used for selected patients with early-stage lesions of the anterior urethra who refuse surgery. However, the results of treatment with only radiotherapy are not good [34]. External-beam radiotherapy of 50 to 60 Gy was delivered during 6 weeks. The radiotherapy results are comparable with surgery for distal urethral tumours [47]. Preoperative radiotherapy is used for advanced disease, in order to decrease locoregional recurrence. The locoregional control rate was 29% for those patients [27].

Multimodality treatment with combined chemo-radiation with surgical excision for locally advanced urethral carcinomas has been reported by Baskin *et al.* with a disease-free survival rate of 60% [3]. Other series supported the efficacy of multimodality treatment both for male and female squamous cell carcinomas of the urethra [24,33,53]. Adjuvant radiotherapy (45Gy) and concurrent chemotherapy with 5-fluorouracil (5FU) and Mitomycin C has been proposed for patients with bulbomembranous infiltration in order to preserve the penis [43]. Neoadjuvant chemotherapy with methotrexate, vinblastine, doxorubicin, and cisplatin followed by surgery or irradiation is preferred for advanced carcinoma of the prostatic urethra with TCC [15,52]. The results with neoadjuvant chemotherapy or chemoradiotherapy followed by surgery results seem to be better than surgery only in disease-free and overall survival for high stage urethral tumours [15].

Carcinoma of the Female Urethra

Urethral tumours are 4 times more frequent in women than in men. The peak incidence is in the sixth decade [14]. They are common in Caucasian women when compared with non-whites.

Chronic inflammation, irritation, proliferative lesions, HPV are the risk factors. Urethral bleeding, palpable mass or induration, urinary discharge, dysuria, urinary frequency are the common symptoms [59].

Anterior urethral lymphatics drain into the superficial and deep inguinal nodes, while the posterior urethra drains into the external iliac, hypogastric, and obturator lymph nodes. At presentation, one third of patients has inguinal lymph node involvement and one fifth has pelvic lymph node metastases [14].

Pathology

The common histology is squamous cell carcinomas (60%) for female urethral tumours; however the incidence is lower than in men [14]. Transitional cell carcinoma (20%), adenocarcinoma (10%), undifferentiated tumours (8%), and melanoma (2%) are the other less frequent tumours [14]. Clear-cell carcinoma is a rarely seen tumour of the female urethra.

Diagnostic work-up and Staging

Pelvic examination under anesthesia, cystourethroscopy with biopsy, CT or MRI of the pelvis and abdomen, and chest x-ray are used for staging of female urethral carcinoma.

UICC TNM staging has been adapted to female urethral cancer [54].

Treatment

Treatment is based on the stage at the time of initial presentation. Thus, most of the distal urethral tumours have a better prognosis than the proximal urethral tumours [59]. Local excision is used for low-stage carcinoma of the distal urethra. Proximal urethra tumours are more aggressive than distal tumours. Radical surgery such as anterior pelvic exenteration, that is defined as en bloc total urethrectomy, cystectomy with pelvic lymphadenectomy, hysterectomy with salpingectomy, and removal of the anterior wall of the vagina, is often performed. Resection of the symphysis pubis and ramus inferior is required when there is involvement of the pubic symphysis [27]. Occasionally, resection of the pubic symphysis and inferior rami are needed when there is bone invasion. Anterior exenteration is another option for locally advanced disease; however, the survival rates are very low [59]. Dalbagni *et al.*, reported the 5-year disease-specific survival as 46%, with 89% survival for low-stage tumours compared with 33% for high-stage disease [10].

Radiation therapy can be used in patients with low-stage urethral carcinoma. It can be applied by brachytherapy alone or combined with external-beam radiation. Definitive brachytherapy doses are 50-60 Gy for sole therapy, and 20-25 Gy after pelvic irradiation for combined radiotherapy. Proximal urethral tumours with bladder neck invasion and bulky tumours are treated by combined external beam and brachytherapy [29]. Brachytherapy seems to decrease the risk of local recurrence [37]. Survival rates are reported as 55% in patients treated with radiotherapy plus surgery and 34% in those treated with radiation alone. However aggressive treatment may result in a high complication rate [19,42].

Neoadjuvant chemotherapy and preoperative radiation therapy, followed by surgery, is also recommended for advanced female urethral carcinoma. In advanced disease, MVAC chemotherapy for transitional-cell carcinomas and mitomycin C plus 5-FU for squamous cell carcinoma and preoperative radiation, followed by surgery is preferred in some centres [53]. Local control rates seem to be higher for the patients treated by combined treatment schedules [10]. However, the prognosis for women with carcinoma of the urethra is poor.

Other Rare Tumours, Diagnosis,Treatment

Clear cell adenocarcinoma (CCA)

CCA of the urinary tract is very rare, 39 cases being reported in the English-language literature to date [56]. They are seen in the bladder rather than the urethra [38,56]. CCA of the urethra is more common among women than men and 56% of cases has association with urethral diverticulum [44]. Young and Scully first introduced the term ‘clear cell tumours’ for these tumours in 1985 [68]. The histogenesis of these tumours in the bladder and urethra is still unclear. They were originally categorized as “mesonephric adenocarcinoma”, although there is no clear evidence for this origin [68]. In contrast, the latest data have shown that they have a similar staining pattern as non-mullerian tumours and tissues, including urothelial carcinoma [44,56]. There is limited information about the prognosis and therapeutic recommendations of clear cell carcinoma. Extensive surgical resection was the primary treatment choice in most of the reported cases [44]. There is some experience in adjuvant radiotherapy or chemotherapy with the patients who had clear cell carcinoma of the bladder; however, the number of cases is insufficient to justify conclusions on the optimal treatment [17,30].

Melanomas of the urethra

Malignant melanoma is a rare disease in the genitourinary tract and the incidence is 1% of all melanomas and 4% of all urethral tumours [20,26]. Urethra and penis are the common localisation in the genitourinary tract [2,51]. It is seen 3 times more frequently in women than men [45,60]. The distal urethra is the common location [20]. More than 160 patients have been reported in English language literature [55]. Secondary melanomas, metastatic from the glans penis or labia are reported more frequently than primary melanomas of the urethra. The symptoms are similar to the other tumours of urethra: melanuria, dysuria, hematuria, palpable mass are the most common symptoms. Average duration from the onset of symptoms to diagnosis is quite long [20]. Malignant melanoma should be kept in mind if the histopathology is other than transititional cell carcinoma for urethral tumours. Malignant melanoma has microscopic variability and can resemble other histologies [26]. Therefore, immunohistochemistry analysis must be performed. HMB-45 and S-100 protein are positive in the tumour cells [26,46]. Primary malignant melanoma of the urethra is an aggressive tumour and the prognosis is poor, most of the patients dying within 3 years with distant metastasis [12,20,50]. Treatment schedules differ according to the localization and the extent of invasion. While this is an uncommon histology, there are no defined guidelines for treatment. However surgery is the primary treatment: tumour excision with partial urethrectomy, partial amputation with a 2-cm margin, total urethrectomy being performed in early stage tumours where radical surgery, cystouretherectomy, vaginectomy, vulvectomy and lymph node dissection with or without radiotherapy are preferred for the treatment of invasive tumours [12,45]. IFN-α is an immunotherapy which can be applied as an adjuvant treatment. There is little evidence with regard to the efficacy of adjuvant chemotherapy and immunotherapy in the treatment of urethral melanoma [61,66]. Primary or postoperative radiotherapy are used in some series [29,45]. The local recurrence rate is high in partial surgeries and most of the patients died within 2 years.

Neuroendocrine tumours (NET) of the urethra, carcinoid tumour and small cell carcinoma of urethra

NETs comprise a wide spectrum of cells classified from carcinoid tumours to small cell carcinomas [63]. They are thought to arise from the differentiation of the pluripotent stem cells of the urethral epithelium. Neuroblastoma, a small-cell variant of osteosarcoma, Merkel cell tumour and metastatic small-cell should be considered for differential diagnosis [1]. Carcinoid tumours are described in the urogenital tract, such as bladder, prostate and urethra [41]. In 1975, Sylora *et al.* first reported the carcinoid tumour of the urethra [57]. Carcinoid tumours are small polypoid nodules, of sizes varying from 3 to 8 mm. To our knowledge, four cases each of carcinoid tumour and primary NET for penile urethra have been reported in the literature [1,6,25,41]. There seems to be a male tendency for NETs of the urethra. Immunohistochemically, neuron specific-enolase and chromagranin, synaptophysin and cytokeratin staining were positive in the tumour cells [41].

Optimal management is unclear due to the small number of cases. Definitive surgery, including penectomy + prostavesiculectomy, penectomy + cystoprostatectomy + supravesical diversion with pelvic lymphadenectomy is the main treatment. Disease-free survival rates of longer than 2 years have been reported for the 4 patients, except for one who died in the 16th month with regional and visceral metastases [41]. It seems there is no adjuvant role for radiotherapy or chemotherapy in the treatment of carcinoid tumours, however close follow-up is recommended. For the patients with large-cell neuroendocrine or small-cell carcinoma of the urethra, combined modalities with adjuvant chemo- and radiotherapy can be recommended considering the successful results from the pulmonary NETs treated in the same way [1].

Hematologic neoplasms of the urethra

Non-Hodgkin lymphoma and mucosa associated lymphoma (MALT)

Primary urethral lymphoma cases have been reported. Non-Hodgkin's lymphoma (NHL) of the genitourinary tract as primary disease is rare [8]. The most common site is the bladder, followed by the prostate and very rarely in the urethra. Vaginal spotting, dysuria, urinary outflow obstruction are the common symptoms [48]. Most of them are seen in the sixth and seventh decade of life. To our knowledge, there are 15 female cases of malignant lymphoma of the urethra and 5 male cases reported in the literature [8,22,23,48]. Diagnostic work up should be performed for staging. Treatment guidelines for NHL in other sites are recommended. After transurethral resection, adjuvant multi-agent chemotherapy or external or intracavitary radiotherapy can be applied, according to the histology and stage of the disease. One-year survival is reported as 91% for local stage and 35% for disseminated stage cases [48,49]. There are 14 cases reported as marginal zone of B-cell MALT lymphoma of the urethra [21,36]. External radiotherapy can be applied after transurethral biopsy of the mass [31].

Extramedullary plasmacytomas

Extramedullary plasmacytomas are usually seen in the respiratory tract, lymph nodes and spleen [64]. Urinary tract plasmacytomas including bladder and kidney are seen rarely; to our knowledge only 7 cases have been reported in the English-language literature [18,28,35,39]. The papillary lesions are located in the urethra. Lambda light chain proteins have been found in the pathologic specimens and are produced by plasma cells. Bone marrow biopsy, Bence-Jones proteinuria and other tests have to be performed in order to distinguish from multiple myeloma [64]. The patients were succesfully treated by transurethral resection, transurethral resection plus radiotherapy and radiotherapy only, as plasmacytoma cells are radiosensitive [18,32,35].

Other rare histologies

There are only single cases of granulocytic sarcoma, granular cell tumour and lymphoepithelioma-like carcinoma of the urethra reported in the literature to our knowledge [5,58,65].

Conclusion

In conclusion, tumours of the urethra are very rare. Treatment alternatives are considered according to the location and extent of invasion of the tumour. Treatment schedules are generally similar for all histologies, except for hematologic malignancies. Surgical resection varying from transurethral resection to urethro-cystoprostatectomy and pelvic exenteration is the standard treatment. Adjuvant treatment with radiotherapy and chemotherapy can be added, according to the stage and histology of the tumour.

Références

1. Altintas S, Blockx N, Huirzing M *et al.* (2007) Small-cell carcinoma of the penile urethra: a case report and a short review of the literature. Annals Oncol 18: 801-9
2. Arai K, Joko M, Kagebayashi Y *et al.* (1993) Primary malignant melanoma of the female urethra:a case report. Jpn J Clin Oncol 23(1): 74-7
3. Baskin L, Turzan C (1992) Carcinoma of the male urethra: Management of locally advanced disease with combined chemotherapy, radiotherapy, and penile-preserving surgery. Urology 39: 21-5
4. Catto JW, Yates DR, Rehman I *et al.* (1984) Behavior of urothelial carcinoma with respect to anatomical location. J Urol 177(5): 1715-20
5. Chatin BA, Manning JT, Ordonez NG (1984) Hematologic neoplazms with initial manifestations in lower urinary tract. Urology 23(1): 35-42
6. Chen KTK (2001) Primary carcinoid tumor of the urethra. J Urol 166: 1831-2
7. Christopher N, Arya M, Brown RS *et al.* (2002) Penile preservation in squamous cell carcinoma of the bulbomembranous urethra. BJU Int 89(4): 464-5
8. Curry NS, Chung CJ, Potts W, Bissada N (2993) Isolated lymphoma of genitourinary tract and adrenals. Urology 41(5): 494-8
9. **Dalbagni G, Zhang ZF, Lacombe L, Herr HW (1999) Male urethral carcinoma: analysis of treatment outcome. Urology 53(6): 1126-32**
10. **Dalbagni G, Zhang ZF, Lacombe L, Herr HW (1998) Female urethral carcinoma: an analysis of treatment outcome and a plea for a standardized management strategy. Br J Urol 82(6): 835-41**
11. Davis JW, Schellhammer PF, Schlossberg SM (1999) Conservative surgical therapy for penile and urethral carcinoma. Urology 53: 386
12. **DiMarco DS, DiMarco CS, Zincke H *et al.* (2004) Outcome of surgical treatment for primary malignant melanoma of the female urethra. J Urol 171(2 Pt 1): 765-7**
13. Dinney CP, Johnson DE, Swanson DA *et al.* (1994) Therapy and prognosis for male anterior urethral carcinoma:an update. Urology 43: 506-14
14. **Flanigan C (2005) Urethral Cancer. In: Richie JP, D'Amico A (Eds.). Urologic Oncology, 1st Ed. Philadelphia, Elsevier Saunders, pp. 675-685**
15. Gheiler EL, Tefilli MV, Tiguert R *et al.* (1998) Management of primary urethral cancer. Urology 52: 487-93
16. Gillitzer R, Hampel C, Wiesner C *et al.* (2008) Single-instution experience with primary tumours of the male urethra. BJU International 101(8): 964-8
17. Gögüs C, Baltacı S, Orhan D, Yaman O (2003) Clear cell adenocarcinoma of the male urethra. Int J Urol 10(6): 348-9

18. Gokce O, Acar O, Tunc M *et al.* (1998) Primary urethral plasmacytoma: a case report and literature review. Kaohsiung J Med Sci 24(5): 274-7
19. Grigsby PW (1998) Carcinoma of the urethra in women. Int J Radiat Oncol Biol Phys 41(3): 535-41
20. Gupta R, Bhatti SS, Dinda AK, Singh MK (2007) Primary melonoma of the urethra: a rare neoplasm of the urinary tract. Int Urol Nephrol 39: 833-6
21. Hara M, Stake M, Ogino H *et al.* (2002) Primary ureteral mucosa-associated lymphoid tissue (MALT) lymphoma-patological and radiological findings. Radiat Med 20(1): 41-4
22. Hatcher PA, Wilson DD (1997) Primary lymphoma of the male urethra. Urology 49(1): 142-4
23. Inuzuka S, Koga S, Imanishi D *et al.* (2003) Primary malignant lymphoma of the female urethra. Anticancer Res 23: 2925-7
24. Johnson D, Kessler J, Ferrigni R *et al.* (1989) Low dose combined chemotherapy/radiotherapy in the management of locally advanced urethral squamous cell carcinoma. J Urol 141: 615
25. Katayama M, Hara A, Hirose Y *et al.* (2003) Carcinoid tumor in the female urethal orifice; rare case report and a review of the literature. Pathol Int 53(2): 102-5
26. Katz EE, Suzue K, Willie M *et al.* (2005) Primary malignant melanoma of the urethra. Urology 65: 389-2005
27. Klein FA, Whitmore WF, Herr HW *et al.* (1983) Inferior pubic rami resection with en bloc radical excision for invasive proximal urethral carcinoma. Cancer 51: 1238-42
28. Kraus-Tiefenbacher U, Gutwein S, Höpner U *et al.* (2004) Plasmacytoma of the urethra. Onkologie 27(2): 166-8
29. Kuettel MR Parda DS, Harter KW *et al.* (1997) Treatment of female urethral carcinoma in medically inoperable patients using external beam irradiation and high dose rate intracavitary brachytherapy. J Urol 157: 849-60
30. Kurosaka S, Irie A, Mizoguchi H *et al.* (2005) Advanced clear-cell adenocarcinoma of the bladder successfully treated by radical surgery with adjuvant chemoradiotherapy. Int J Clin Oncol 10(5): 362-5
31. Kurtman C, Andrieu MN, Baltaci S *et al.* (2001) Conformal radiotherapy in primary non-Hodgkin's lymphoma of the male urethra. Int Urol Nephrol 33(3): 537-9
32. Lemos N, Melo CR, Soares IC *et al.* (2000) Plasmacytoma of the urethra treated by excisional biopsy. Scand J Urol Nephrol 34(1): 75-6
33. Licht MR, Klein EA, Bukowski R *et al.* (1995) Combination radiation and chemotherapy for the treatment of squamous cell carcinoma of the male and female urethra. J Urol 153: 1918
34. Mansur DB, Chao C (2008) Penis and male urethra. In: Halperin EC, Perez CA, Brady WB (Eds.) Principles and Practice of Radiation Oncology, 5th Ed. Philadelphia, Lippincot Williams & Wilkins, pp. 1519-1531
35. Mark JA, Pais VM, Chong FK (1990) Plasmacytoma of the urethra treated with transurethral resection and radiotherapy. J Urol 143(5): 1010-1
36. Masuda A, Tsujii T, Kojima M *et al.* (2002) Primary mucosa-associated lymphoid tissue (MALT) lymphoma arising from the male urethra. A case report and review of the literature. Pathol Res Pract 198(8): 571-5
37. Milosevic MF, Warde PR, Banerjee D *et al.* (2000) Urethral carcinoma in women: results of treatment with primary radiotherapy. Radiother Oncol 56: 29-35
38. Miller J, Karnes RJ (2008) Primary clear cell adenocarcinoma of the proximal female urethra: a case report and review of the literature. Clin Genitourin Cancer 6(2): 131-3
39. Mordkin RM, Skinner DG, Levine AM (1996) Long-term disease-free survival after plasmacytoma of the urethra: a case report and review of the literature. Urology 48(1): 149-50
40. Mostofi FK, Davis CJ, Sesterhenn IA (1992) Carcinoma of the male and female urethra. Urol Clin North Am 19: 347-58
41. Murali R, Kneale K, Lalak N, Delprado W (2006) Carcinoid tumors of the urinary tract and prostate. Arch Pathol Lab Med 130: 1693-706
42. Narayan P, Konety B (1992) Surgical treatment of female urethral carcinoma. Urol Clin North Am 19: 373-82 Review

2

43. Oberfield RA, Zinman LN, Leibenhaut M *et al.* (1996) Management of invasive squamous cell carcinoma of the bulbomembranous male urethra with coordinated chemo-radiotherapy and genital preservation. Br J Urol 78: 573-8
44. Oliva E, Amin MB, Jimenez R, Young RH (2002) Clear cell carcinoma of the urinary bladder:a report and comparison of four tumors of mullerian origin and nine of probable urethelial origin with discussion of histogenesis and diagnostic problems. Am J Surg Pathol 26: 190-7
45. Oliva E, Quinn TR, Amin MB *et al.* (2000) Primary malignant melanoma of the urethra:a clinicopathologic analysis of 15 case. Am J Surg Pathol 24(6): 785-96
46. Radhi JM (1997) Urethral malignant melanoma closely mimicking urothelial carcinoma. J Clin Pathol 50: 250-62
47. Raghavaiah NV (1978) Radiotherapy in the treatment of carcinoma of the male urethra. Cancer 41: 1313-6
48. Rajan N, Allman D, Scaglia B *et al.* (1995) Non-Hodgkin's lymphoma of the male urethra. J Urol 153(6): 1916-7
49. Richter LA, Hegde P, Taylor JA 3rd (2007) Primary non-Hodgkin's B-cell lymphoma of the male urethra presenting as stricture disease. Urology 70(5): 1008.e11-2
50. Rikaniadis N, Konstadoulakis MM, Tsibloulis B et al. (1998) Long term survival of a female patient with primary malignant melanoma of the urethra. Eur J Surg Oncol 24(6): 607-8
51. Sanchez–Ortiz R, Huang SF, Tamboli P *et al.* (2005) Melanoma of the penis, scrotum and male urethra: a 40 year single institution experience. J Urol 173(6): 1958-65
52. Scher HI, Yagoda A, Herr HW *et al.* (1998) Neoadjuvant M-VAC (methotrexate, vinblastine, doxorubicin and cisplatin) for extravesical urinary tract tumors. J Urol 139: 475
53. Shah A, Kalra J, Silber L *et al.* (1985) Squamous cell cancer of the female urethra: Successful treatment with chemoradiotherapy. Urology 25(3): 284-6
54. Sobin LH and Wittekind Ch (eds.) (2002) In: International Union Against Cancer TNM Classification of Malignant Tumours, 6th edition New York, Wiley-Liss
55. Sugiyama EV, Chan KJ, Kapp DS (2008) Management of melanomas of the female genital tract. Curr Opin Oncol 20: 565-9
56. Sun K, Huan Y, Unger PD (2008) Clear cell adenocarcinoma of urinary bladder and urethra:another urinary tract lesion immunoreactive for P504S. Arch Pathol Lab Med 132(9): 1417-22
57. Sylora HO, Diamond HM, Kaufman M *et al.* (1975) Primary carcinoid tumor of the urethra. J Urol 114(1): 150-3
58. Tamas E, Matthew EN, Schoenberg M, Epstein J (2007) Lymphoepithelioma-like carcinoma of the urinary tract: a clinicopathological study of pure and mixed cases. Modern Pathol 20: 828-34
59. **Trabulsi EJ, Gomella LG (2009) Cancer of Urethra And Penis. In: DeVita VT, Theodore SL, Rosenberg SA (Eds.), Cancer, Principles & Practice of Oncology, 8th Ed. Philadelphia, Lippincot Williams & Wilkins, pp. 1452-1462**
60. Tsai Y-S, Yang W-H, Tong Y-C *et al.* (2005) Experience with primary urethral carcinoma from the blackfoot disease-endemic area of South Taiwan: increased frequency of bulbomembranous adenocarcinoma? Urol Int 74: 229-34
61. Watanabe J, Yamamato S, Souma T *et al.* (2000) Primary malignant melanoma of the male urethra. Int J Urol 7: 351-3
62. Wiener JS, Liu ET, Walther PJ (1992) Oncogenic human papillomavirus type 16 is associated with squamous cell cancer of the male urethra. Cancer Res 52: 5018
63. Wick MR (2000) Neuroendocrine neoplasia:current concepts. Am J Clin Pathol 113: 331-5
64. Witjes JA, de Vries JDM, Schaafsma HE *et al.* (1991) Extramedullary plasmacytoma of the urethra: A case report. J Urol 145: 826-8
65. Yokoyama H, Kontani K, Komiyama I *et al.* (2007) Granular cell tumor of the urethra. Int J Urol 14: 461-2
66. Yoshizawa T, Kawata N, Katsuhiko S *et al.* (2007) Primary Malignant Melanoma of the Female Urethra. Urology 70: 13-6
67. Yvgenia R, Ben BM, Sibi J, Koren R (2005) Mucinous adenocarcinoma of posterior urethra. Report of a case. Path Res Pract 201(2): 137-40
68. Young D, Bilello S, Gomelsky A (2007) Squamous cell carcinoma in situ in a female urethral diverticulum. South Med J 100(5): 537-9

Uncommon bladder cancers

C. Durdux and O. Mir

3

Four Essential Points

1. *Close follow-up is mandatory in patients presenting with chronic inflammatory bladder process (chronic catheterization, bladder exstrophy,...), prolonged cyclophosphamide therapy or previous pelvic radiation therapy, given the likelihood of neoplastic transformation.*
2. *Irrespective of the histological subtype (except for lymhomas), optimal treatment is based on radical cystectomy (+/- pelvic lymphadenectomy), with negative resection margins.*
3. *Recommended treatment of lymphomas is based on radiation therapy and chemotherapy.*
4. *Chemotherapy must be added to local treatment for small cell carcinomas and carcinosarcomas.*

Introduction

Non-urothelial neoplasm of the bladder is rare in western countries and accounts for less than 5% of all vesical tumours combined. The histological types include adenocarcinoma (incidence rate, 0.5-2%), non-bilharzial squamous cell carcinoma (SCC, 3-7%), carcinoïds and small cell carcinoma (0.5%), sarcomas (< 0.1%), paraganglioma (< 0.1%), melanoma (< 0.1%) and lymphomas (< 0.1%). Apart from these, bladder location of metastasis has been described in a few studies. Most of these non-transitional cell tumours will not be encountered within a lifetime of practicing oncology, but when they do occur, they present a diagnostic and therapeutic challenge. We propose to review the main data concerning the etiology, diagnosis and optimal management of adult uncommon bladder cancer. Pediatric bladder tumours and urachus carcinomas will not be discussed here.

Adenocarcinoma

Pure adenocarcinoma of the bladder is the third most frequent type of bladder cancer after transitional cell and squamous cell cancers [71]. Tumours appear ulcerative, papillary or nodular, with a predilection for the trigone or the bladder dome. Multiple tumours are present in approximately 50% of cases [18]. It occurs more frequently in areas of endemic schistosomiasis, in males in the sixth decade [6]. Moreover, it is the most common tumour arising in patients with bladder exstrophy (4% life-time risk), after a long period of catheterization [58] or during chronic inflammatory process such as endometriosis. Symptoms are not specific (hematuria, dysuria). The histological patterns may be glandular, not otherwise specified, colonic (enteric type), papillary or mucinous. No grading system has been uniformly accepted. Immunohistochemical assessment with PSA antibody allows the differentiation of primary bladder carcinoma – which appears as negative – from prostate adenocarcinoma with bladder extension. Signet cell carcinoma is a rare variant of adenocarcinoma, with approximately 70 cases reported in the literature, including bladder and urachus locations [21]. It occurs more often in males and is characterized by a thick bladder wall with loss of contractility, evolving to the linitis plastica in a third of cases. The natural history of these tumours is silent asymptomatic local progression, leading to a late diagnosis with unresectable disease. Another rare variant of adenocarcinoma is clear cell or mesonephric carcinoma, mostly described in the female urethra [74].

Most patients with localized adenocarcinoma of the bladder have been treated by radical cystectomy with bilateral lymphadenectomy. Partial cystectomy could be proposed for monocentric lesions located on the mobile bladder wall. Andestrom *et al.* reported a 54% 5-year survival in a series of 15 patients treated by partial cystectomy [6]. The addition of pre-operative irradiation did not improve survival. For unresectable tumours, there are a few studies of tumour response to radiotherapy. Intra-arterial 5-Fluorouracil infusion has been shown to be effective in advanced stages [25], with an objective response in five of eight patients in Logothetis's series [36]. Bavendam *et al.* suggests that evaluation of a CMV regimen could be worthwhile [8]. The 5-year survival rates of patients with bladder adenocarcinomas are poor, ranging between 11% and 55% according to stage [22, 27, 34, 42, 57, 71]. The largest series with 185 patients, reported by El Mekresh *et al.*, mentioned a 55% 5-year survival rate but has exclusively included adenocarcinomas associated with schitosomiasis which may account for a more favourable prognosis [18].

Non-bilharzial squamous cell carcinoma

Pure SCC of the bladder must be distinguished from transitional cell cancer with common partial squamous differentiation. Pure SCC is an epithelial neoplasm that exclusively displays squamous aspects with squamous pearls, keratohyaline granules and intercellular bridges. The literature reports male and black race predominance with occurrence in sixth decade. Risk factors are chronic bacterial urinary tract infections, chronic irritative factors such as vesical calculi, indwelling catheters for paraplegic patients or intermittent self-cathetherization for exstrophy, cigarette smoking, medication (cyclophosphamide, intravesical BCG) [32, 62, 66]. Human papilloma viruses do not play a significant role in carcinogenesis of SCC [38]. Abnormalities on chromosomes 3, 8, 10, 13 and 17 have been detected. Studies on uropakin II gene expression, correlated to the differentiation of urothelium, found significant differences between transitional carcinoma and SCC [20]

Further, verrucous carcinoma is an extremely rare variant of SCC (3-4%) characterized by a gross exophytic tumour with slow growth rate, low incidence of lymph node and distant metastasis and almost always associated with schistosomal cystitis [17] or condyloma acuminata [28].

Symptoms of SCC at diagnosis are not specific (hematuria, dysuria) but urinary tract infection is generally present (30 to 93% of patients in Johnson's series) [31]. Most of the tumours present as a solitary locally advanced disease in the trigone or lateral walls, with extension beyond the bladder wall in 75% of cases [55]. Distant metastasis are infrequent (8-10%) [72]. For resectable tumours, treatment is based on partial or radical cystectomy with bilateral pelvic lymph node dissection. In this group, 5-year survival ranged from 34% to 50% according to stage [31, 48, 50, 55, 65]. In the study by Nishiyama *et al.*, 5-year survival after cystectomy did not differ between transitional cell carcinoma (68%) and SCC (60.8%); in multivariate analysis, histological feature did not appear as an independent prognostic factor [43]. Pre-operative radiotherapy (40 to 50 Gy in 4-5 weeks) could protect against pelvic recurrence [31, 64]. For located unresectable tumours, exclusive radiotherapy has been proposed with poor results from 5% to 18% 5-five-year survival. Radiotherapy remains controversial for verrucous forms with possible anaplastic transformation [15]. In all these series, the number of included patients was small and did not exceed 35. Standard chemotherapy regimens such as M-VAC or CMV appear to have limited impact on the disease due to the relative chemoresistance of SCC [35]. No objective response to neoadjuvant M-VAC was seen [61]. Novel agents such as taxanes, or gemcitabine have not yet been evaluated in this particular histological pattern of bladder cancer.

Carcinoïds and small cell carcinoma

Primarily small cell or neuroendocrine carcinoma of the bladder is an uncommon entity of bladder tumours with around 300 reported cases and a 0.5% incidence of all primary bladder malignancies [12]. The sex ratio is 3:1 for men. Only 5 cases of carcinoïds (benign or malignant) have been described in the literature. In the same way, large cell neuroendocrine carcinoma is extremely rare [9]. The largest series concern small cell carcinoma. Small cell bladder cancer originates from the totipotent stem cells present in the submucosa of the bladder [56]. Microscopically, small cell carcinoma looks like lung form, composed of uniform oat cells with scant cytoplasm, hyperchromatic nuclei, necrosis and frequent mitotic figures. Additional immunohistochemical staining for chromogranin A and synaptophysin confirm the neuroendocrin origin. MIB-1 proliferation index (Ki 67) is often greater than 80%. C-kit and E-GFR expression is found in more than 25% of patients, opening new ways of treatment [68]. Small cell bladder cancer could be pure or associated to transitional cell cancer, adenocarcinoma or SCC [1, 10], with similar endoscopic aspect. Hematuria and metastasis (lymph nodes, liver, bone, lung, brain) are present at diagnosis in 90% and 67% of cases respectively [63]. Paraneoplastic syndrome is rare (hypercalcemia). Reports on patients with small cell bladder cancer suggest that it behaves similarly to small cell lung cancer. Local treatments alone yield poor results but systemic chemotherapy by etoposide-cisplatin provides survival improvement [13, 45]. In Sved's series, 7 patients who underwent cystectomy alone died between 1 to 25 months after surgery. Adding chemotherapy, 13 to 18 patients were alive at a mean of 27 months [63]. Similar results with systemic etoposide-cisplatin in a neoadjuvant and/or adjuvant setting have been published by Walther *et al.* [67]. For Siefter-Radtke who reported MD Anderson Cancer Center's experience of 25 patients treated by cystectomy with or without postoperative chemotherapy, 5-year-survival has been dramatically improved with neoadjuvant chemotherapy (78% with neoadjuvant regimen *versus* and 26% when surgery was performed first) [57]. The role of radiotherapy appears controversial. Chemoradiation seemed to be successful in localized stages as reported by Lohrisch [37] but results reported by Sved were poor with a mean survival < 8 months [63].

Sarcomas

All histological subtypes have been described among primary sarcomas of the urinary bladder, but leiomyosarcomas and angiosarcomas appear as the more frequent [49]. Rhabdomyosarcomas of the bladder, mainly occur in children and are exceptional in adults. The pathologic diagnosis relies on the same morphological and immunohistochemical features as other soft-tissue sarcomas, and no specific imaging characteristics have been identified to date. The most common sites of distant metastases are the lungs, bone, brain, and liver [59]. Optimal treatment includes surgery with negative margins [59] and chemotherapy based on the most active agents in soft-tissue sarcomas (namely doxorubicin and ifosfamide). The role of radiotherapy in the adjuvant setting still needs to be defined.

Angiosarcoma

Angiosarcomas mostly occur in middle-aged and elderly men (mean age of 65 years, sex ratio 8 male: 1 female) [19, 54, 70]. Twenty-four cases of bladder angiosarcoma have been reported [19, 54, 70], including 8 cases occurring after radiation therapy. Gross hematuria is the most common presentation, with bulky tumour (mean size: 7 cm) located in the trigone and/or dome. Overall survival was poor, with 5-year survival rates close to 35%. Longer-term survival has been demonstrated in patients who have had a multimodal approach to treatment, which combines radical surgery with chemotherapy and radiotherapy.

Leiomyosarcoma

Up to 80 cases of primary bladder leiomyosarcoma have been reported in the last 10 years [16, 39, 51], with a mean age of 62 years and a sex ratio of 3 male: 1 female. Eight cases occurred in patients previously treated with cyclophosphamide [4]. The most common symptoms at presentation were gross hematuria (80% of patients), pollakiuria (25%), and dysuria (20%). The Memorial Sloan Kettering Cancer Center disease stage system is a significant predictor of survival of patients with bladder leiomyosarcoma ($p = 0.018$) [51]. Radical cystectomy is the standard therapy for locally invasive disease with a 5-year disease-specific survival rate close to 60%. Literature supports the benefit of peri-operative chemotherapy. In this way, Sawhney *et al.* [53] reported near-complete pathologic response to neoadjuvant chemotherapy with gemcitabine and docetaxel.

Carcinosarcomas

Sarcomatoid carcinoma and carcinosarcoma of the bladder contain epithelial and mesenchymal elements. From Perret's review, primary heterologous carcinosarcoma of the urinary bladder predominantly occurred in elderly men, most often at advanced stage and rapidly became lethal [47]. Some heterologous carcinosarcomas should be regarded as a variant of sarcomatoid carcinoma (metaplastic carcinoma) with prominent heterologous differentiation. Loss of heterozygosis has been described on chromosomal arms 9p, 9q, 8p, and 8q [24]. Regarding overall prognosis, patients with carcinosarcoma (HR 2.00, 95% CI 1.65-2.41) are at higher risk of death compared to those with urothelial carcinoma [73]. One complete pathologic response was described after neoadjuvant chemoradiotherapy. Other reported cases received doxorubicin-based chemotherapy [29, 47].

Paraganglioma

This tumour probably arises from embryonic nests of chromaffin cells in the detrusor sympathic plexus (neural crest). It is termed pheochromocytoma (PC) if hormonally active. It represents 0.06% of bladder tumours and 10% of extra-adrenal PC, slightly more common in women and in the fifth decade, malignant in 10% of cases, generally as sporadic form, sometimes associated with Recklinghausen neurofibromatosis [69]. Symptoms at presentation are non specific (hematuria) but micturitional attacks with hypertension, headache, blurred vision, diaphoresis, resulting from catecholamine release are present in 50% of cases with elevated serum and urinary levels of catecholamines. For diagnosis, cystoscopy should be performed after adrenergic blockade under surgical conditions and biopsy should be avoided. It generally shows a solitary submucosal or intramural nodule. Nuclear scanning with MIBG is the imaging of choice for diagnosis with high sensitivity (77-90%) and specificity (95-100%) [33] and PET-scan could also be useful [30]. The standard treatment of PC is partial cystectomy with pelvic node dissection with the same precautions taken as for any other PC with adrenergic blockade. The ipsilateral hypogastric vein should be temporarily occluded before tumour manipulation to avoid paroxysmal hypertensive episodes [2, 52].

Melanoma

Melanoma of the bladder (MMB) is most commonly a metastatic location of a cutaneous melanoma. But rare cases of primary MMB or of the female urethra have been reported [23, 26]. The histogenesis of these tumours is unclear, possibly related to a neural crest origin. Symptoms are not specific. Cystoscopy reveals a darkly pigmented exophytic bladder lesion. Histologically, MMB resembles other melanoma with large malignant cells arranged in nests with variable amounts of pigment [12]. Immunochemistry with HMB-45 and S100 protein is positive. Few cases of amelanotic malignant melanoma of female urethra have been described [41]. Radical cystectomy and bilateral lymphadenectomy are recommended for localized MMB. Adjuvant treatment has not been evaluated [60].

Lymphomas

Most frequently, bladder lymphoma reflects widespread metastatic hematologic disease. However about 90 cases of primary lymphomas of the bladder have been reported [3]. The majority are non-Hodgkin lymphoma (NHL) of B-cell type, in which 14% were follicular lymphomas [44]. Primary extranodal marginal zone lymphomas of mucosa associated lymphoid tissue (MALT type) have also been described and were associated with an excellent prognosis [11]. An important female preponderance was found (sex ratio, 1 male: 6.5 females) with a 64 year median-age and frequent chronic cystitis history. In contrast to most other primary bladder tumours, treatment consists of local radiotherapy which achieves remission in a high percentage of patients [3].

Others

Cyclophosphamide-induced bladder cancer

Cyclophosphamide-induced bladder cancers generally present as transitional cell carcinomas, although sarcomas (mostly leiomyosarcomas) have been described. They can occur after more than one year of oral cyclophosphamide treatment, with a 7-9 fold relative risk, proportional to the cumulative dose of cyclophosphamide (beyond 20 g) and with a median interval from treatment to cancer diagnosis of 7 years [5]. Acrolein, one of the cyclophosphamide metabolites, is recognized as the main carcinogenic agent for the bladder, but the immunosuppressive effect of cyclophosphamide may also play a role in carcinogenesis [5]. Thus, bladder assessment should be recommended for patients receiving continued cyclophosphamide treatment.

Metastasis to the urinary bladder (BM)

Secondary bladder tumours can be classified according to their origins [14]:

- metastatic cells (MC) reaching the bladder by contiguous invasion from an adjacent cancer (prostate, colon, rectum or cervix uteri);
- MC from upper urinary tract carcinomas ("drop metastases"), which should be considered as multifocal carcinoma;
- MC reaching the bladder by hematogenous route or by lymphatic spread, discussed here.

The most common primary tumours (80% of cases) are stomach and lung cancer in men, and stomach, colon and breast in women [40]. Bladder metastases (BM) are usually part of a widespread process, with frequent ureteral and lymph node involvement [14]. Nevertheless, several cases of solitary BM have been reported [7]. BM usually occurs several years after the treatment of the primary (7 months-14 years) [14]. Although MC generally infiltrate the muscularis, less than 50% of BM are symptomatic [46]. When BM are symptomatic, dysuria, hematuria and pollakiuria should prompt a cystoscopy and biopsy. The subsequent management depends on the primary tumour [14].

References

1. Abbas F, Civantos F, Benedetto P, Soloway MS (1995) Small cell carcinoma of the bladder and prostate. Urology 46(5): 617-30
2. **Abol-Enein H, Kava BR, Carmack AJ (2007) Nonurothelial cancer of the bladder. Urology 69(1 Suppl): 93-104**
3. Al-Maghrabi J, Kamel-Reid S, Jewett M *et al.* (2001) Primary low-grade B-cell lymphoma of mucosa-associated lymphoid tissue type arising in the urinary bladder: report of 4 cases with molecular genetic analysis. Arch Pathol Lab Med 125(3): 332-6
4. Al-Zahrani AA, Kamal BA, Eldarawani HM, Hashim TM (2006) Leiomyosarcoma of the bladder in a 16-year-old girl with a history of cyclophosphamide therapy for bilateral retinoblastoma during infancy. Saudi Med J 27(4): 531-3
5. Alexandre J, Lévy V, Hunault M *et al.* (1996) Bladder neoplasms and cyclophosphamide. Apropos pf 3 cases and review of the literature. Bull Cancer 83(11): 945-50
6. Anderström C, Johansson SL, von Schultz L (1983) Primary adenocarcinoma of the urinary bladder. A clinicopathologic and prognostic study. Cancer 52(7): 1273-80

7. Bardales RH, Pitman MB, Stanley MW *et al.* (1998) Urine cytology of primary and secondary urinary bladder adenocarcinoma. Cancer 84(6): 335-43
8. Bavendam TG, Kramolowsky EV, Mitros FA (1989) Invasive adenocarcinoma of bladder response to cisplatinum, methotrexate, and vinblastine chemotherapy. Urology 33(1): 53-6
9. Bertaccini A, Marchiori D, Cricca A *et al.* (2008) Neuroendocrine carcinoma of the urinary bladder: case report and review of the literature. Anticancer Res 28(2B): 1369-72
10. Cheng L, Pan CX, Yang XJ *et al.* (2004) Small cell carcinoma of the urinary bladder: a clinicopathologic analysis of 64 patients. Cancer 101(5): 957-62
11. Cohen DD, Lamarre C, Lamarre L, Saad F (2002) Primary low-grade B-cell lymphoma of the urinary bladder: case report and literature review. Can J Urol 9(6): 1694-7
12. **Dahm P, Gschwend JE (2003) Malignant non-urothelial neoplasms of the urinary bladder: a review. Eur Urol 44(6): 672-81**
13. Davis MP, Murthy MS, Simon J *et al.* (1989) Successful management of small cell carcinoma of the bladder with cisplatin and etoposide. J Urol 142(3): 817
14. Debois JM (2002) TxNxM1, The anatomy and clinics of metastatic cancer. In: 1st ed. Boston: Kluwer; Chapter 4, Metastases to the urogenital system; pp. 106-28
15. Demian SD, Bushkin FL, Echevarria RA (1973) Perineural invasion and anaplastic transformation of verrucous carcinoma. Cancer 32(2): 395-401
16. Dotan ZA, Tal R, Golijanin D *et al.* (2006) Adult genitourinary sarcoma: the 25-year Memorial Sloan-Kettering experience. J Urol 176(5): 2033-8
17. El-Bolkainy MN, Mokhtar NM, Ghoneim MA, Hussein MH (1981) The impact of schistosomiasis on the pathology of bladder carcinoma. Cancer 48(12): 2643-8
18. El-Mekresh MM, el-Baz MA, Abol-Enein H, Ghoneim MA (1998) Primary adenocarcinoma of the urinary bladder: a report of 185 cases. Br J Urol 82(2): 206-12
19. Engel JD, Kuzel TM, Moceanu MC *et al.* (1998) Angiosarcoma of the bladder: a review. Urology 52(5): 778-84
20. Fadl-Elmula I, Gorunova L, Lundgren R *et al.* (1998) Chromosomal abnormalities in two bladder carcinomas with secondary squamous cell differentiation. Cancer Genet Cytogenet 102(2): 125-30
21. Fiter L, Gimeno F, Martin L, Gómez Tejeda L (1993) Signet-ring cell adenocarcinoma of bladder. Urology 41(1): 30-3
22. Grignon DJ, Ro JY, Ayala AG *et al.* (1991) Primary adenocarcinoma of the urinary bladder. A clinicopathologic analysis of 72 cases. Cancer. 1991 Apr 15;67(8): 2165-72
23. Gupta R, Bhatti SS, Dinda AK, Singh MK. Primary melanoma of the urethra: a rare neoplasm of the urinary tract. Int Urol Nephrol 39(3): 833-6
24. Halachmi S, DeMarzo AM, Chow NH *et al.* (2000) Genetic alterations in urinary bladder carcinosarcoma: evidence of a common clonal origin. Eur Urol 37(3): 350-7
25. Hatch TR, Fuchs EF (1989) Intra-arterial infusion of 5-fluorouracil for recurrent adenocarcinoma of bladder. Urology 33(4): 311-2
26. Helpap B (2001) Nonepithelial neoplasms of the urinary bladder. Virchows Arch 439(4): 497-503
27. Henly DR, Farrow GM, Zincke H (1993) Urachal cancer: role of conservative surgery. Urology 42(6): 635-9
28. Horner SA, Fisher HA, Barada JH *et al.* (1991) Verrucous carcinoma of the bladder. J Urol 145(6): 1261-3
29. Hoshi S, Sasaki M, Muto A *et al.* (2007) Case of carcinosarcoma of urinary bladder obtained a pathologically complete response by neoadjuvant chemoradiotherapy. Int J Urol 14(1): 79-81
30. Hwang JJ, Uchio EM, Patel SV *et al.* (2003) Diagnostic localization of malignant bladder pheochromocytoma using 6-18F fluorodopamine positron emission tomography. J Urol 169(1): 274-5
31. Johnson DE, Schoenwald MB, Ayala AG, Miller LS (1976) Squamous cell carcinoma of the bladder. J Urol 115(5): 542-4
32. Kantor AF, Hartge P, Hoover RN, Fraumeni JF Jr (1988) Epidemiological characteristics of squamous cell carcinoma and adenocarcinoma of the bladder. Cancer Res 48(13): 3853-5
33. Klingler HC, Klingler PJ, Martin JK Jr *et al.* (2001) Pheochromocytoma. Urology 57(6): 1025-32

34. Kramer SA, Bredael J, Croker BP *et al.* (1979) Primary non-urachal adenocarcinoma of the bladder. J Urol 121(3): 278-81
35. Loehrer PJ Sr (1992) Chemoradiotherapy in locally advanced bladder carcinoma. Semin Oncol 19(4 Suppl 11): 92-5
36. Logothetis CJ, Samuels ML, Ogden S (1985) Chemotherapy for adenocarcinomas of bladder and urachal origin: 5-fluorouracil, doxorubicin, and mitomycin-C. Urology 26(3): 252-5
37. Lohrisch C, Murray N, Pickles T, Sullivan L (1999) Small cell carcinoma of the bladder: long term outcome with integrated chemoradiation. Cancer 86(11): 2346-52
38. Maloney KE, Wiener JS, Walther PJ (1994) Oncogenic human papillomaviruses are rarely associated with squamous cell carcinoma of the bladder: evaluation by differential polymerase chain reaction. J Urol 151(2): 360-4
39. Martin SA, Sears DL, Sebo TJ *et al.* (2002) Smooth muscle neoplasms of the urinary bladder: a clinicopathologic comparison of leiomyoma and leiomyosarcoma. Am J Surg Pathol 26(3): 292-300
40. Melicow MM (1974) Tumors of the bladder: a multifaceted problem. J Urol 112: 467-78
41. Nakamoto T, Inoue Y, Ueki T *et al.* (2007) Primary amelanotic malignant melanoma of the female urethra. Int J Urol 14(2): 153-5
42. Nakanishi K, Kawai T, Suzuki M, Torikata C (1996) Prognostic factors in urachal adenocarcinoma. A study in 41 specimens of DNA status, proliferating cell-nuclear antigen immunostaining, and argyrophilic nucleolar-organizer region counts. Hum Pathol 27(3): 240-7
43. Nishiyama H, Habuchi T, Watanabe J *et al.* (2004) Clinical outcome of a large-scale multi-institutional retrospective study for locally advanced bladder cancer: a survey including 1,131 patients treated during 1990-2000 in Japan. Eur Urol 45(2): 176-81
44. Ohsawa M, Aozasa K, Horiuchi K, Kanamaru A (1993) Malignant lymphoma of bladder. Report of three cases and review of the literature. Cancer 72(6): 1969-74
45. Pan CX, Zhang H, Lara PN Jr, Cheng L (2006) Small-cell carcinoma of the urinary bladder: diagnosis and management. Expert Rev Anticancer Ther 6(12): 1707-13
46. Perez-Mesa C, Pickren JW, Woodruff MN, Mohallatee A (1965) Metastatic carcinoma of the urinary bladder from primary tumors in the mammary gland of female patients. Surg Gynecol Obstet 121(4): 813-8
47. Perret L, Chaubert P, Hessler D, Guillou L (1998) Primary heterologous carcinosarcoma (metaplastic carcinoma) of the urinary bladder: a clinicopathologic, immunohistochemical, and ultrastructural analysis of eight cases and a review of the literature. Cancer 82(8): 1535-49
48. Prempree T, Amornmarn R (1984) Radiation management of squamous cell carcinoma of the bladder. Acta Radiol Oncol 23(1): 37-42
49. Raghavan D (2006) Textbook of uncommon cancer. 3rd ed. New York: John Wiley & Sons; 857 p
50. Richie JP, Waisman J, Skinner DG, Dretler SP (1976) Squamous carcinoma of the bladder: treatment by radical cystectomy. J Urol 115(6): 670-2
51. Rosser CJ, Slaton JW, Izawa JI *et al.* (2003) Clinical presentation and outcome of high-grade urinary bladder leiomyosarcoma in adults. Urology 61(6): 1151-5
52. Samaan NA, Hickey RC, Shutts PE (1988) Diagnosis, localization, and management of pheochromocytoma. Pitfalls and follow-up in 41 patients. Cancer 62(11): 2451-60
53. Sawhney R, Curry N, Burks T, Chaudhary UB (2007) Locally advanced leiomyosarcoma of the urinary bladder: near-complete pathologic response to neoadjuvant gemcitabine and docetaxel. Anticancer Drugs 18(6): 745-7
54. Seethala RR, Gomez JA, Vakar-Lopez F (2006) Primary angiosarcoma of the bladder. Arch Pathol Lab Med 130(10): 1543-7
55. Serretta V, Pomara G, Piazza F, Gange E (2000) Pure squamous cell carcinoma of the bladder in western countries. Report on 19 consecutive cases. Eur Urol 37(1): 85-9
56. Shahab N (2007) Extrapulmonary small cell carcinoma of the bladder. Semin Oncol 34(1): 15-21
57. Siefker-Radtke AO, Gee J, Shen Y *et al.* (2003) Multimodality management of urachal carcinoma: the M. D. Anderson Cancer Center experience. J Urol 169(4): 1295-8
58. Smeulders N, Woodhouse CR (2001) Neoplasia in adult exstrophy patients. BJU Int 87(7): 623-8

59. **Spiess PE, Kassouf W, Steinberg JR *et al.* (2007). Review of the M.D. Anderson experience in the treatment of bladder sarcoma. Urol Oncol 25(1): 38-45**
60. **Sternberg CN, Swanson DA. (1997). Non-transitional cell bladder cancer. Principles and practice of genitourinary Oncology. Lippincott-Raven, Philadelphia**
61. Sternberg CN, Yagoda A, Scher HI *et al.* (1985) Preliminary results of M-VAC (methotrexate, vinblastine, doxorubicin and cisplatin) for transitional cell carcinoma of the urothelium. J Urol 133(3): 403-7
62. Stonehill WH, Goldman HB, Dmochowski RR (1997) The use of urine cytology for diagnosing bladder cancer in spinal cord injured patients. J Urol 157(6): 2112-4
63. Sved P, Gomez P, Manoharan M *et al.* (2004) Small cell carcinoma of the bladder. BJU Int 94(1): 12-7
64. Swanson DA, Liles A, Zagars GK (1990) Preoperative irradiation and radical cystectomy for stages T2 and T3 squamous cell carcinoma of the bladder. J Urol 143(1): 37-40
65. Utz DC, Schmitz SE, Fugelso PD, Farrow GM (1973) Proceedings: A clinicopathologic evaluation of partial cystectomy for carcinoma of the urinary bladder. Cancer 32(5): 1075-7
66. Wall RL, Clausen KP (1975) Carcinoma of the urinary bladder in patients receiving cyclophosphamide. N Engl J Med 293(6): 271-3
67. Walther PJ (2002) Adjuvant/neoadjuvant etoposide/cisplatin and cystectomy for management of invasive small cell carcinoma. J. Urol 167 (4): 285 [Abstract 1124]
68. Wang X, MacLennan GT, Lopez-Beltran A, Cheng L (2007) Small cell carcinoma of the urinary bladder-histogenesis, genetics, diagnosis, biomarkers, treatment, and prognosis. Appl Immunohistochem Mol Morphol 15(1): 8-18
69. Whalen RK, Althausen AF, Daniels GH (1992) Extra-adrenal pheochromocytoma. J Urol 147(1): 1-10
70. Williams S, Romaguera R, Kava B (2008) Angiosarcoma of the bladder: case report and review of the literature. ScientificWorld Journal 8: 508-11
71. Wilson TG, Pritchett TR, Lieskovsky G *et al.* (1991) Primary adenocarcinoma of bladder. Urology 38(3): 223-6
72. Wishnow KI, Dmochowski R (1988) Pelvic recurrence after radical cystectomy without preoperative radiation. J Urol 140(1): 42-3
73. Wright JL, Black PC, Brown GA *et al.* (2007) Differences in survival among patients with sarcomatoid carcinoma, carcinosarcoma and urothelial carcinoma of the bladder. J Urol 178(6): 2302-6
74. Young RH, Scully RE (1985) Clear cell adenocarcinoma of the bladder and urethra. A report of three cases and review of the literature. Am J Surg Pathol 9(11): 816-26

Neuroendocrine small cell carcinoma of the prostate: A brief review of pathology, clinical characteristics and treatment guidelines

4

M.E. Stein and A. Kuten

Five Essential Points

1. *SCPca is a rare entity.*
2. *SCPca is very aggressive, even in early disease.*
3. *There is no surveillance policy, even in early stages, unlike the usual adenocarcinoma of the prostate.*
4. *Surgical treatment should be considered in very early disease.*
5. *Combined modality treatment (cisplatin-based chemotherapy, mainly VP-16) and pelvic + prostatic region boost radiation therapy is the preferred mode in the majority of cases.*

Introduction

Extrapulmonary small cell carcinoma (EP-SCC) has been increasingly recognized as a clinico-pathologic entity with biologic behaviour and prognosis distinct from pulmonary small cell carcinoma (P-SCC). The first report of EP-SCC was published by Duguid *et al.* [14] in 1930. Since then, EP-SCC has been observed in almost every non-pulmonary site with an overall incidence of 0.1-0.4% [41]. Due to the rarity of these tumours, exact treatment guidelines are still lacking.

Small cell carcinoma of the prostate (SCPca), also known as neuroendocrine SCPca, was first described by Wenk *et al.* in 1977 [43]. Since then, the incidence of this entity has been estimated at less than 2% of *de novo* prostatic malignancies [32]. These tumours are considered to be highly aggressive, with a median survival of 5-10 months. Clinical features which might lead to a suspicion of SCPca include a rapidly growing local/pelvic mass, unresponsiveness to hormonal therapy, visceral metastases at presentation, and a disproportionately low prostate-specific antigen (PSA) level in the setting of advanced/metastatic disease [12, 32]. A thorough literature search was done to gather as much information as possible concerning the rare entity of SCPca.

Etiology

In recent years, much evidence has emerged that neuroendocrine (NE) cells which are present in the normal and pathological prostate have a central role in regulating growth differentiation and homeostasis of the normal and malignant prostate [12, 20]. Neuroendocrine differentiation of the prostate appears to be associated with poor prognosis, tumour progression and an androgen-independent state, for which there is currently no successful therapy [12, 20, 32, 38].

These neuroendocrine cells are the main components of SCPca, and they tend to differentiate or de-differentiate into neuroendocrine carcinoma, which is also known as small cell neuroendocrine carcinoma, undifferentiated carcinoma, pure small cell carcinoma, or anaplastic carcinoma of the prostate [1, 20].

Some authors [1, 10, 12, 32] consider SCPca to be a de-differentiation of the typical adenocarcinoma of the prostate, arising in the course of disease progression and representing an aggressive and terminal phase . Other authors [25, 26] suggest that SCPca is derived from argentaffin or argirophyllic cells present in the prostate or from multipotential epithelial cells with diverse differentiation possibilities. Regardless of its cellular origin, it is always necessary to confirm (clinically, biochemically and radiologically) that it is a primary prostatic neoplasm and not a metastasis of a pre-existing pulmonary tumour.

Prostatic neuroendocrine cells have regulatory functions, being a part of the widely-distributed amino precursor and decarboxylation (APUD) system. APUD cells produce and release regulatory peptides such as serotonin, the chromogranin family (chromogranin A, chromogranin B and secretogranin); peptides of the calcitonin family; the parathormone (PTH)-related protein; thyroid stimulating hormone (TSH) and human chorio-gonadotropin (HCG)-like peptides; glucagon, bombesin-like peptides, somatostatin, carcino embryonic antigen (CEA), and neuron specific enolase (NSE) [1, 11, 34]. However, even the detection of ectopic hormone production is infrequently combined with typical paraneoplastic clinical manifestations by SCPca.

All SCC, including SCPca, show the same microscopic, immunohistochemical and ultrastructural features. Histopathological diagnosis of SCPca is achieved through an ultrastructural study which reveals the presence of dense neurosecretory granules in the cytoplasm *via* light microscopy with silver stains and through specific immunohistochemical staining [18]. Immunohistochemical examination of the neoplastic tissue is mandatory for the correct diagnosis of SCPca. It is generally accepted that the presence of a positive reaction for chromogranin A, synapthophysin and NSE constitutes sufficient evidence of neuroendocrine differentiation [13, 15, 44]. Chromogranin A is much more specific than NSE and seems to be the best marker of SCPca in blood and tissue, with its serum value used to show the progression of therapy resistance in prostate carcinomas [13, 15].

Neuroendocrine SCPca also exhibits intense staining of vascular endothelial growth factor (VEGF) [18]. Correlation has been found between the total numbers of the tumour marker chromogranin A positive cells and the total amount of VEGF-containing NE-cells in individual tumours. A subset of these cells may secrete transforming growth factor alpha (TGF-A), and the presence of these angiogenic factors may be used in diagnosis, follow-up, estimation of prognosis, and for targeting specific molecular sites. Their presence shows a more aggressive phenotype [2, 21-23].

Pathology

The histological examination of SCPca is undistinguishable from P-SCC. Differential diagnosis should be between SCPca and poorly differentiated adenocarcinoma of the prostate. In addition to the pure form of SCPca, we can find adenocarcinoma mixed with features of SCPca progressing to pure SCPca, adenocarcinoma progressing to mixed adenocarcinoma and SCPca, along with mixed SCPca and adenocarcinoma on presentation [41]. The proportion of the small cell component may range from a small focus of the tumour burden to the predominant histology. Mitotic activity and necrosis are generally prominent.

Small cell carcinoma of the prostate shows ultrastructural evidence of both primitive epithelial and neuroendocrine differentiation. Tumour cells show scant cytoplasmic organelles and sparse neurosecretory granules. The immunophenotype of SCPca supports both epithelial and primitive neuroendocrine differentiation [38, 41]. It shows immunoreactivity with common neuroendocrine markers such as NSE, neurofilaments, synaptophysin, leu 7, epithelial membrane antigen (EMA), leukocyte common antigen (LCA) and chromogranin A (most specific marker) [44], and is almost always negative for PSA. Small cell carcinoma of the prostate shows a high proliferative rate, as demonstrated by immunohistochemical staining for MIB-1 and through flow-cytometric studies of S-phase fraction [9, 18, 25].

The differential diagnosis includes metastatic PSCC, other neuroendocrine tumours, various round blue cell tumours, metastatic melanoma, lymphoma and poorly differentiated carcinoma. Differential diagnostic measures include morphologic light microscopic features, immunostaining and the introduction of tumour-specific markers. Clinical presentation and radiological findings are also important in distinguishing SCPca and metastatic PSCC (normal basic radiograph and computed tomography scan of the chest and normal sputum cytology or negative bronchoscopy).

Clinical presentation

The most typical age at diagnosis is 61 to 70 years. Some authors [31, 32] suggest a range from 24 to 90 years. Male to female ratio is 1:1. The most common presenting symptoms are bladder outlet obstructive syndrome, either due to a massive prostatic tumour mass alone or with periprostatic and/or pelvic lymphadenopathy. Additional local symptoms include pelvic or abdominal/para-aortic lymphadenopathy), pain, hematochezia or hematuria [19, 31, 32]. Metastatic disease is also common at the time of diagnosis of SCPca and includes massive hepatic involvement with hepatic failure, ascites, pleural effusion, edema, lung and bone metastases and spinal cord compression with neurological symptoms. Brain metastases are rare at presentation. Hydronephrosis and/or renal failure is also a frequent finding at diagnosis [31, 32]. In rapidly developing disease, patients exhibit systemic signs like anorexia, weight loss, diarrhoea, weakness and malaise. Hypercalcemia in connection with extensive lytic bone lesions and deep venous thromboses due to hypercoagulability or venous compression have also been described [7, 27, 31].

Paraneoplastic syndromes [6, 19, 24, 32, 42, 43] have also been described. The most common are Cushing's syndrome, PTH-like hormone secretion with hypercalcemia, glucagon and thyroid stimulating hormone (TSH) secretion and the syndrome of inappropriate anti-diuretic hormone secretion. Neurological symptoms as a part of a paraneoplastic syndrome include peripheral neuropathy, limbic encephalitis and Eaton-Lambert syndrome (myasthenia gravis).

Diagnosis

On digital rectal examination, the prostate could be normal, could show localized palpable nodularity, or could be diffusely firm or irregular with multiple nodules (extracapsular extension) [32]. These findings are unlikely to be distinguishable from typical prostatic adenocarcinoma or benign enlargement of the prostate. In advanced disease, the physician may observe jaundice, cachexia, and ascites or diffuse lymphadenopathy [31, 32, 42].

Laboratory findings are non-specific. Erythrocyte sedimentation rate (ESR), alkaline phosphatase and lactate dehydrogenase (LDH) levels may be elevated in widespread disease. Anemia of chronic disease may also be a part of the clinical picture [16, 32].

Serum and tissue chromogranin A and NSE have been identified as markers of the neuroendocrine differentiation. Their levels can correlate with the degree of aggressiveness and the tumour burden [13, 15]. Even prostate-non-specific serum tumour markers such as CEA and cancer antigen 19-9 are often elevated in SCPca. PSA elevation, ranging mainly between 4 to 10 ng/ml, is generally noted in about 30% of SCPca patients and can suggest discordant involvement with PSA-producing typical adenocarcinoma and possible responsiveness to hormonal treatment, but it does not correlate with tumour burden [6, 25, 32]. In patients with a high disease volume, low serum PSA, poorly differentiated disease and poor or insufficient response to hormonal treatment, SCPca should be considered.

Staging

The tumour-node-metastasis (TNM) staging for prostate cancer has been used, and Galanis *et al.* [18] used a two stage system as for pulmonary SCC. Limited disease was defined as tumour localized to organ of origin and the locoregional lymph nodes that can be encompassed within one radiation therapy treatment portal. Any evidence of disease beyond that was classified as extensive disease.

Measures necessary for staging include trans-rectal ultrasound (TRUS), which may identify abnormalities of the prostate and involved periprostatic lymph nodes which can be used to direct needle biopsies. Additional local staging and metastatic evaluation can be accomplished with bone scan, computed tomography (CT) scan or Magnetic Resonance Imaging (MRI) [3, 28, 32]. Somatostatin, a tetradecapeptide neuroendocrine hormone of hypothalamic origin, through receptors on normal and malignant prostate cells, has a strong affinity to prostate tumours with a role in the control of prostate growth and function. Radiolabeled somatostatin analogs that bind to somatostatin receptors are increasingly used to visualize primary neuroendocrine small cell carcinoma and metastases scintigraphically [1]. Indium-11-octreoscan can be used to evaluate metastatic bone disease especially [36].

Brink *et al.* [8] and Fricke *et al.* [17] demonstrated that {18}-fluoro-2-deoxy-D-glucose positron emission tomography (FDG-PET) in small cell neuroendocrine lung carcinoma and in prostate cancer is potentially useful for correct initial staging and can demonstrate exactly true "stage migration", thereby affecting patient management. It is also useful in monitoring of patients with small cell neuroendocrine carcinoma and may be superior to bone scan in detecting bone metastases.

Treatment

Due to the rarity of SCPca, the dismal prognosis and the lack of large, randomized trials, there is still no consensus regarding fixed guidelines for the treatment of SCPca. All our results are based on case reports and very few comparative studies. Most authors [30, 32, 33, 35, 38] use cisplatin-based chemotherapy (mainly with VP-16 (etoposide)) and radiation therapy, either with curative intent or for palliation of local symptoms or symptomatic visceral metastases (painful metastatic bone disease; metastatic hepatomegaly). Unlike very early adenocarcinoma of the prostate, surveillance policy alone is not recommended even for incidentally detected SCPca.

Radical prostatectomy has been curative in selected patients with small-burdened or incidentally diagnosed prostatic SCC, in most cases when co-existing with typical prostatic adenocarcinoma [7, 32]. Transurethral resection of the prostate (TURP) can relieve obstructive symptoms but is not curative. All these patients should be treated with at least 4-6 cycles of cisplatin-based chemotherapy. The role of adjuvant radiation therapy following radical prostatectomy is still controversial. In localized disease, it should be considered according to the pathological (positive surgical margins) or clinical (symptomatic local disease, extracapsular extension) staging.

Response rate is variable. Complete remission is very rare. Papandreou *et al.* [33] summarized their phase II study based on 38 SCPca patients treated with at least four courses of doxorubicin/etoposide/cisplatin. All assessable patients presented with locally advanced disease, incurable with radiotherapy or surgery, and/or visceral metastases. Twenty-two (61%) patients achieved partial remission and 8% stable disease. The overall best responses were demonstrated by bone scan and reduction of pain. The median time-to-progression and overall survival were 5.8 months and 10.5 months, respectively. Toxicity was higher in this patient population and the chemotherapy regimen failed to improve outcome over other studies [30, 35].

The responsiveness of EP-SCC and SCPca to chemotherapy has led to experiments aiming to improve outcome, such as maintenance therapy, the use of alternating non-cross resistant regimens, administration of consolidation therapy, the use of high-dose chemotherapy and autologous stem cell rescue. While all these approaches consistently failed to improve outcome, they showed increased toxicity [32].

The role of hormonal treatment in SCPca is controversial [27]. In patients with mixed histologies, hormonal treatment by orchiectomy or luteinizing hormone releasing hormone (LHRH) analogs, such as Zoladex or Lucrin, should be used according to stage and prognostic factors and the guidelines used for typical adenocarcinoma. Due to the lack of clear evidence based on large comparative studies and long-term follow-up, treatment decisions are often based on empirical considerations and physician's decision alone. In any case, hormonal treatment should not be used as the sole therapy in SCPca.

Radiation therapy is very effective in the palliative treatment of symptomatic metastatic SCPca, especially painful bony secondaries and spinal cord compression. Patients with brain metastases should be treated with chemotherapy and radiation therapy to the whole brain with various dose schedules ranging between 40 Gy in 20 fractions to 30 Gy in 10 fractions [9, 32, 36, 39]. As in metastatic and chemosensitive PSCC and germ cell tumour, clinical and radiological regression of brain metastases as well as marked symptomatic relief can be demonstrated, most probably due to disruption and penetration through the blood-brain-barrier. Due to the rarity of brain relapse following failure of treatment, there is no necessity for prophylactic whole brain irradiation [5].

Somatostatin receptors have been identified in normal and malignant prostate cells and somatostatin analogs have been shown to exert antiproliferative action in these cells, substantially decreasing the proteins secreted by these cells. Practically, following octreoscan positivity for metastatic SCPca, somatostatin analogs and their radionuclide derivatives might exert palliative effect in symptomatic metastatic SCPca [20, 36, 40]. Also, the neuroendocrine cell product Bombesin, whose

4

antagonists have been shown to have very strong mitogenic activity, can inhibit growth and invasiveness of malignant prostate cells and are currently being tested against small cell neuroendocrine carcinomas [20].

The role of adjuvant radiation therapy for early or localized disease (with or without periprostatic or pelvic lymphadenopathy) following chemotherapy is still unclear and controversial, as are exact guidelines concerning daily fractions, total dose and the boundaries of the irradiation volume. The administration schedule for radiation therapy before, after or concomitantly with chemotherapy is also unclear. Most physicians prefer to adopt the guidelines used in PSCC, limited disease (irradiation of the primary tumour and involved/potentially involved lymph nodes), albeit without prophylactic whole brain irradiation. Asmis *et al.* [5] and Spiess *et al.* [35] believe that surgical resection with or without radiation therapy combined with chemotherapy should be considered as treatment strategy in local/early SCPCa. This modality may provide better local control and potential survival benefit.

Small cell carcinoma of the prostate has been found to respond to some innovative therapeutic approaches, targeted molecules such as membrane glycolipids and glycoproteins, receptor tyrosine kinases and neuropeptides and their receptors [29]. New agents include small molecule inhibitors directed at membrane receptor tyrosine kinases, such as C-IHT (imatinib mesylate) and the recombinant humanized monoclonal antibodies bevacizumab directed at the vascular endothelial growth factor (VEGF) which is present massively in SCPca cells and is responsible for tumour angiogenesis [21, 29].

For adjuvant therapy after radical surgery, a minimum of four cycles of chemotherapy should be given. Following TURP, or in the presence of adverse pathologic features after radical prostatectomy, radiation therapy should follow chemotherapy. Due to the rarity of SCPCa, no exact guidelines for total dose and boundaries of irradiation volume could be given. Due to the propensity for local and pelvic lymph node relapse, the volume in early, potentially curative disease should include the pelvic lymph nodes with a dose of 40-50 Gy and the prostate up to 72 Gy [4, 30, 32].

Stein *et al.* [37] summarized retrospectively, within the framework of the Rare Cancer Network study, 30 patients from 7 medical centres (including Rambam Medical Centre) suffering from SCPca either in an early/localized or in an advanced/metastatic stage. Patients were treated with cisplatin-based chemotherapy (with VP-16 +/- other agents) and pelvic radiotherapy aiming at local control. Even although various chemotherapy regimes, different radiotherapy schedules and doses were used, the following conclusions could be drawn:

1. Even in localized stage, SCPca is a very aggressive disease with a poor prognosis.
2. Despite initial responses, the common cisplatin based chemotherapy plus radiotherapy failed to improve outcome markedly.
3. The optimal radiation schedule and dose for achieving local control is still unknown. The experience favours a total dose of nearly 70 Gy to the prostate region.
4. Prophylactic cranial irradiation is unnecessary.

Prognosis

The prognosis for SCPca patients is very poor. Adverse factors include advanced stage, high amount of neuroendocrine differentiation, total lack of hormone responsiveness, presence of paraneoplastic syndrome while, according to the large retrospective study of Spiess *et al.* [35], high serum LDH level and low albumin level at the time of diagnosis is predictive of inferior disease-free survival.

Median survival is measured in months and long-term survivors are rare. Patients diagnosed with early adenocarcinoma and incidental finding of small cell neuroendocrine tumour should be offered the option of radical prostatectomy and adjuvant chemotherapy. The best remissions and survival can be achieved in early disease patients treated with at least 4-6 courses of cisplatin-based chemotherapy and radical radiation therapy. Metastatic disease occurs early in the course of disease. Initial response to chemotherapy is shown but relapse is unavoidable. The presence of the paraneoplastic syndrome may be a poor prognostic factor.

Conclusions

The rarity of SCPCa precludes therapeutic prospective randomized trials. Generally, these tumours with their neuroendocrine differentiation are considered high-grade and are associated with both local and distant symptoms at the time of presentation. Various radio-chemotherapy schedules have not improved tumour control and survival of patients. Further research may lead to advances in the understanding of neuroendocrine differentiation and the development of novel agents, targeting the SCPCa on the molecular level.

References

1. Abrahamsson PA (1999) Neuroendocrine differentiation in prostatic carcinoma. Prostate 39:135-48
2. Adlakha H, Bostwick DG (1994) Paneth cell-like change in prostatic adenocarcinoma represents neuroendocrine differentiation: report of 30 cases. Hum Pathol 25: 135-9
3. Adshead F, De Graeff A, Mansi JL *et al.* (1991) Small cell carcinoma of the prostate: implications for management. Br J Urol 67: 217-8
4. Anker CJ, Dechet C, Isaac JC *et al.* (2008) Small-cell carcinoma of the prostate. J Clin Oncol 26:1168-71
5. Asmis TR, Reaume MN, Dahrouge S *et al.* (2006) Genitourinary small cell carcinoma: a retrospective review of treatment and survival patterns at The Ottawa Hospital Regional Cancer Center. BJU Int 97: 711-5
6. Baird AD, Cornford PA, Helliwell T *et al.* (2002) Small cell prostate cancer with anti-Hu positive peripheral neuropathy. J Urol 168: 192
7. Bolton DM, Chiu ST, Clarke S *et al.* (1994) Primary small cell carcinoma of the prostate: unusual modes of presentation. Aust N Z J Surg 64: 91-4
8. Brink I, Schumacher T, Mix M *et al.* (2004) Impact of [18F] FDG-PET on the primary staging of small-cell lung cancer. Eur J Nucl Med Mol Imaging 31:1614-20
9. Clegg N, Ferguson C, True LD *et al.* (2003) Molecular characterization of prostatic small-cell neuroendocrine carcinoma. Prostate 55: 55-64
10. Cohen RJ, Glezerson G, Haffejee Z (1992) Prostate-specific antigen and prostate-specific acid phosphatase in neuroendocrine cells of prostate cancer. Arch Pathol Lab Med 116: 65-6
11. Di Sant'Agnese PA (1992) Neuroendocrine differentiation in carcinoma of the prostate. Diagnostic, prognostic, and therapeutic implications. Cancer 70: 254-68
12. Di Sant'Agnese PA, Cockett AT (1994) The prostatic endocrine-paracrine (neuroendocrine) regulatory system and neuroendocrine differentiation in prostatic carcinoma: a review and future directions in basic research. J Urol 152: 1927-31
13. Di Sant'Agnese PA, de Mesy Jensen KL (1987) Neuroendocrine differentiation in prostatic carcinoma. Hum Pathol 18: 849-56
14. Duguid J, Kennedy R (1930) Oat cell tumors of the mediastinal glands. J Pathol Bacteriol 33: 93-9

4

15. Fernandes RC, Matsushita MM, Mauad T *et al.* (2001) Prostate carcinoma with neuroendocrine differentiation: case report and literature review. Rev Hosp Clin Fac Med Sao Paulo 56: 153-8
16. Freedy RM, Miller KD Jr (1990) Small-cell carcinoma of the prostate: metastases to the brain as shown by CT and MR with pathologic correlation. AJNR Am J Neuroradiol 11: 947-8
17. Fricke E, Machtens S, Hofmann M *et al.* (2003) Positron emission tomography with 11C-acetate and 18F-FDG in prostate cancer patients. Eur J Nucl Med Mol Imaging 30: 607-11
18. Galanis E, Frytak S, Lloyd RV (1997) Extrapulmonary small cell carcinoma. Cancer 79: 1729-36
19. Ghandur-Mnaymneh L, Satterfield S, Block NL (1986) Small cell carcinoma of the prostate gland with inappropriate antidiuretic hormone secretion: morphological, immunohistochemical and clinical expressions. J Urol 135: 1263-6
20. Hansson J, Abrahamsson PA (2001) Neuroendocrine pathogenesis in adenocarcinoma of the prostate. Ann Oncol 12: S145-52
21. Harper ME, Glynne-Jones E, Goddard L *et al.* (1996) Vascular endothelial growth factor (VEGF) expression in prostatic tumours and its relationship to neuroendocrine cells. Br J Cancer 74: 910-6
22. Harper ME, Goddard L, Glynne-Jones E *et al.* (1993) An immunocytochemical analysis of TGF alpha expression in benign and malignant prostatic tumors. Prostate 23: 9-23
23. Harper ME, Goddard L, Glynne-Jones E *et al.* (1995) Epidermal growth factor receptor expression by northern analysis and immunohistochemistry in benign and malignant prostatic tumours. Eur J Cancer 31A: 1492-7
24. Haukaas SA, Halvorsen OJ, Nygaard SJ *et al.* 1999) Cushing's syndrome in prostate cancer. An aggressive course of prostatic malignancy. Urol Int 63: 126-9
25. Helpap B, Kollermann J (1999) Undifferentiated carcinoma of the prostate with small cell features: immunohistochemical subtyping and reflections on histogenesis. Virchows Arch 434: 385-91
26. López Cubillana P, Martínez Barba E, Prieto A (2001) Oat-cell carcinoma of the prostate. Diagnosis, prognosis and therapeutic implications. Urol Int 67: 209-12
27. Moore SR, Reinberg Y, Zhang G (1992) Small cell carcinoma of prostate: effectiveness of hormonal versus chemotherapy. Urology 39: 411-6
28. Munechika H, Kitanosono T, Gokan T *et al.* (1995) Small cell carcinoma of the prostate: CT and MRI findings. Radiat Med 13: 137-42
29. Murray N, Salgia R, Fossella FV (2004) Targeted molecules in small cell lung cancer. Semin Oncol 31: 106-11
30. Oesterling JE, Hauzeur CG, Farrow GM (1992) Small cell anaplastic carcinoma of the prostate: a clinical, pathological and immunohistological study of 27 patients. J Urol 147: 804-7
31. Okada H, Gotoh A, Ogawa T *et al.* (1996) Two cases of small cell carcinoma of the prostate. Scand J Urol Nephrol 30: 503-8
32. Palmgren JS, Karavadia SS, Wakefield MR (2007) Unusual and underappreciated: small cell carcinoma of the prostate. Semin Oncol 34: 22-9
33. Papandreou CN, Daliani DD, Thall PF *et al.* (2002) Results of a phase II study with doxorubicin, etoposide, and cisplatin in patients with fully characterized small-cell carcinoma of the prostate. J Clin Oncol 20: 3072-80
34. Pearse A (1969) The cytochemistry and ultrastructure of polypeptide hormone-producing cells of the APUD series and the embryologic, physiologic and pathologic implications of the concept. J Histochem Cytochem 17: 303-13
35. Spiess PE, Pettaway CA, Vakar-Lopez F *et al.* (2007) Treatment outcomes of small cell carcinoma of the prostate: a single-center study. Cancer 110: 1729-37
36. Spieth ME, Lin YG, Nguyen TT (2002) Diagnosing and treating small-cell carcinomas of prostatic origin. Clin Nucl Med 27: 11-7
37. Stein ME, Bernstein Z, Ufuc A *et al.* (2008) Small cell (neuroendocrine) carcinoma of the prostate: Etiology, diagnosis, prognosis and therapeutic implications. A retrospective study of 30 patients from the Rare Cancer Network. Am J Med Sci 336: 478-88
38. Tetu B, Ro JY, Ayala AG *et al.* (1987) Small cell carcinoma of the prostate. Part I. A clinicopathologic study of 20 cases. Cancer 59: 1803-19
39. Tremont-Lukats IW, Bobustuc G, Lagos GK *et al.* (2003) Brain metastasis from prostate carcinoma: The M.D. Anderson Cancer Center experience. Cancer 98: 363-8

40. Tzannou IA, Karapanagiotou EM, Charpidou A *et al.* (2007) The use of radiolabeled somatostatin analog scintigraphy in the staging of small cell lung cancer patients. Am J Clin Oncol 30: 503-6
41. van der Heijden HF, Heijdra YF (2005) Extrapulmonary small cell carcinoma. South Med J 98: 345-9
42. Venkatesh PK, Motwani B, Sherman N *et al.* (2004) Metastatic pure small-cell carcinoma of prostate. Am J Med Sci 328: 286-9
43. Wenk RE, Bhagavan BS, Levy R *et al.* (1977) Ectopic ACTH, prostatic oat cell carcinoma, and marked hypernatremia. Cancer 40: 773-8
44. Yao JL, Madeb R, Bourne P *et al.* (2006) Small cell carcinoma of the prostate: an immunohistochemical study. Am J Surg Pathol 30: 705-12

Uncommon tumours of the testis

I. Alexandre, E. Horn and F. Selle

5

Five Essential Points

1. *Orchidectomy, as for "usual" testicular neoplasia is the first line of therapy. Sparing surgery is an option in some specific cases.*
2. *Lymph node dissection is required for many histological subtypes of rare tumour of the testicle.*
3. *Usual tumour markers are negative*
4. *If chemotherapy is required, it is rarely "standard chemotherapy" used for usual subtypes such as BEP (bleomycin, etoposide, cisplatin) or EP (etoposide, cisplatin). It is often chosen based on tumour histology, as for other localizations of the same histology*
5. *Long-term follow up is recommended as late recurrence can occur up to fifteen years on.*

Introduction

Testicular neoplasms are rare pathologies that occur most frequently in the young adult with an incidence of 3:100,000 men per year and account for 1-2% of all neoplasms.

For the most common forms of testicular neoplasms, the maximum age of incidence occurs between 15 and 35 years with a good prognosis, 90% of patients being cured.

Diagnosis of rare testicular tumours is made in similar fashion to that of more widespread tumours of the testis: self-palpation of the nodule and swelling or heaviness of the testis. Occasionally, a tumour may be discovered by pain in the testis or other symptoms related to extended disease. Less frequently, an examination for infertility may uncover a rare testicular tumour.

Definitive histology is usually determined after orchidectomy [13].

Germ Cell Tumours

Germ cell tumours represent 90-95% of testicular tumours and can be of three types: seminomatous (30-40%), non-seminomatous (60-70%) and mixed tumours. They are not described here and treatment is well-defined [13].

Non germ cell tumours

They account for less than 10% of adult testicular tumours and more than 30% of childhood testicular tumours. These tumours are usually composed of a single cellular type. Long-term follow-up is always recommended since long-term recurrence has been reported [14].

5

Leydig cell tumours

Leydig cell tumours represent 1 to 3% of testicular tumours and are bilateral in less than 10% of cases. They may be seen in patients with Klinefelter's syndrome or cryptorchidism. The adult form usually occurs between 30 and 60 years of age and may present with gynecomastia or loss of libido [37]. In about 50% of cases, testicular nodules are seen following ultrasound imaging for infertility or gynecomastia evaluation, as small, solid and well-defined peripheral tumours. Magnetic Resonance Imaging (MRI) is also helpful [10]. About 20% of cases present during childhood and diagnosis is made due to precocious puberty [34]. Serum levels of estrogen, estradiol or testosterone can be elevated while low serum gonadotropin is often associated with this tumour while αFP, hCG and LDH are normal [37].

Histologically, polygonal Reinke's crystals figure prominently and are observed in 30-40% of cases. Fatty vacuoles and lipofuscin pigment are observed in 15% of cases [14]. Mutations in gene coding for fumarate hydratase and the luteinizing hormone/choriogonadotropin receptor have been found [10].

Prognosis is usually good. However, tumours may be malignant with metastases in about 10% of cases, particularly in the elderly. In 20% of cases, metastases are synchronous; 40% of metastases occur within 2 years [37]. Size, necrosis, aneuploidy, amplified MIB-1 and mitotic activity may be suggestive of more aggressive tumours. Benign Leydig cell tumours are diploid with less significant MIB-1 [14] expression.

Patients undergo orchidectomy and retroperitoneal lymph node dissection (RLND) for malignant forms. In these cases, radiotherapy and chemotherapy are ineffective with high mortality. In benign cases, orchidectomy is sufficient. Sparing surgery may be chosen for small malignant tumours [37].

Sertoli cell tumours

Sertoli cell tumours account for 1% of testicular tumours and are a heterogeneous group with only 20% of cases being malignant. Median age at diagnosis is 45 years with patients presenting with a slow-growing testicular mass. Gynecomastia may be associated with primary malignant forms of the tumour. Serum estradiol is elevated in 5% of cases [28].

Histologically, cells are eosinophilic and may be vacuolated. Charcot-Bottcher crystals may also be present [14]. Malignant forms are poorly differentiated with necrosis, vascular invasion and a high mitotic index. However, features of Leydig cell tumours may persist. The most frequently observed cytogenetic abnormality is a gain on the X chromosome [28].

For patients with metastatic Sertoli cell tumours, RLND, chemotherapy and radiotherapy are performed [20].

Large-cell calcifying Sertoli cell tumour (LCCSCT) is a rare subtype with fewer than 50 reported cases. Tumours are often multiple, bilateral (40%), benign, occurring primarily in adolescents. A single patient, the oldest at 44 years of age, presented with a malignant tumour. Endocrine signs such as gynecomastia, sexual precocity or adrenal cortex nodular hyperplasia were present, while serum markers were normal [7].

Associations between LCCSCT and dysplastic syndromes have been reported such as the Carney complex (characterized by cardiac myxoma, endocrine overactivity, schwannomas and spotty skin pigmentation) [12], Peutz-Jeghers syndrome (an autosomal dominant disease characterized by intestinal hamartomatous polyps, mucocutaneous melanocytic macules and higher risk of colon, stomach or pancreatic cancers) [41] or androgen insensitivity syndrome. Sporadic onset of LCCSCT accounts for 60% of cases [14].

Ultrasound imaging shows specific features including multiple tumour sites and large calcifications. Histologically, tumours are composed of large Sertoli cells with eosinophilic and sometimes vacuolated cytoplasm. Tumour cells are arranged in nodules with focal calcifications. Radical orchidectomy is standard treatment for LCCSCT. Treatment of the bilateral form in young adults includes either a bilateral radical orchidectomy or enucleation of the less affected testis preceded by sperm storage and followed by close monitoring [7].

Sclerosing Sertoli cell tumour (SSCT): Fewer than 15 cases of SSCT have been reported with the first case described in 1991. Median age at diagnosis is about 35 years without a single prepubertal case reported. Tumours are painless, unilateral, small in size and fail to produce hormones. Except for one reported case, these tumours have a low malignancy potential.

Histologically, tumours are composed of small neoplastic tubules delimited by extensive sclerotic stroma. Treatment consists of orchidectomy with option of sparing surgery [31].

Sertoli cell tumour, not otherwise specified: Median age of occurrence is approximately 45 years. Malignant tumours may be misdiagnosed as seminomas. Reported cases of unilateral tumours lack defining clinical features. Seven percent of patients present metastases at diagnosis.

Necrosis, a high mitotic rate, vascular invasion and a size greater than 5 cm suggest the malignant form of this tumour type. Moreover, tumours with seminoma-like features appear to be more malignant and tend to metastasize [20].

Granulosa cell tumours

Granulosa cell tumours derive from epithelial cells of the spermatic cord and are classified as either juvenile or adult type. The juvenile type is one of the most frequent congenital testicular neoplasms, usually occurring in children under the age of 1 year [4].

Only 23 cases of adult type have been reported with 5 being metastatic [2]. Tumours often present as a painless testicular mass that grows slowly for months or years. Due to abnormal hormonal secretions such as estrogen, gynecomastia is associated in 25% of cases [9]. Classical serum markers are normal but serum level of inhibin and Müllerian-inhibiting hormone may be elevated as in the ovarian type [14]. Predictive factors for metastasis include hemorrhage, necrosis, size greater than 7 cm and presence of vascular or lymphatic invasion. The juvenile type usually occurs within the first 6 months of life and is generally benign [20].

Histological criteria for granulosa tumours are similar to the ovarian type. Microfollicles, Call-Exner bodies and "coffee bean" nuclei are typical histological patterns [9].

In reported cases, adjuvant treatment for the localized tumour was not performed. One patient with metastases in the retroperitoneal lymph nodes underwent a radical orchidectomy followed by RLND and radiotherapy. He remained disease-free 14 years following diagnosis [25].

Tumours of the thecoma/fibroma group

These tumours are slow growing and occur between 30 and 40 years of age. Fewer than 30 cases have been reported. There are no signs of abnormal hormonal secretion and serum markers are normal. In reported cases, there have been no recurrences or metastatic progressions. Histologically, these tumours are similar to the ovarian type with fusiform cells and several small blood vessels. Surgery is the treatment of choice [14].

Gonadoblastoma

Gonadoblastoma is a rare tumour seen only in dysgenetic gonads with ambiguous genitalia and Turner syndrome with Y chromosome material. Frequency in these patients is about 30%.

Development of gonadoblastoma is associated with a specific part of the Y chromosome: the gonadoblastoma locus on the Y chromosome or the GBY region. This region contains the gene encoding TSPY (testis-specific protein on the Y chromosome), which has an oncogenic function. Gonadoblastoma is a precursor lesion for tumours of the dysgenetic gonad. It has the potential to progress to invasive dysgerminoma but also to embryonal carcinoma, teratoma, yolk sac tumour or choriocarcinoma. Histologically, tumours are composed of large germ cells identical to those of seminoma, small cells identical to immature Sertoli or granulosa cells and calcifications. Gonadoblastoma expresses TSPY, PIAP, and c-kit. Preventive treatment consists of early gonadectomy and gender assignment. This controversial treatment results in definitive infertility and necessitates hormone replacement therapy. Some physicians propose a conservative treatment. For example, Cools *et al.* proposed initial bilateral biopsies in order to predict neoplastic evolution if undifferentiated gonadal tissue is found [26, 35].

Neuroendocrine tumours (carcinoid tumours)

Primary testicular carcinoid tumours represent less than 1% of testicular neoplasms. Primary tumours constitute the majority of reported cases and 20-25% are coupled with teratomas. The latter have a worse prognosis than a carcinoid tumour alone [36]. Median age of diagnosis is 45 years although diagnosis may range between 10-83 years. In few cases (1-3%), a carcinoid syndrome may be associated with a large testicular mass. It is often linked to the highly malignant type and often related to liver metastases. Carcinoid syndrome may disappear after orchidectomy for localized tumour [33].

Immunohistochemical test results are positive for chromogranin, serotonin, neuron specific enolase and a moderate level of cytokeratin. Primary tumours and metastases cannot be differentiated histologically. Other sites for primary tumours must be excluded [27].

If the tumour is at a localized stage, orchidectomy must be performed. Roughly 10% of tumours will metastasize and chemotherapy is then necessary including a combination of platinum and etoposide, sometimes octreotide as well as radiotherapy for metastatic lymph nodes [36]. Patients with primary carcinoid tumour and teratoma should undergo RLND. In addition to CT scan and octreotide scintography, serum serotonin and urinary 5-hydroxyindoleacetic acid (5-HIAA) may be used as valuable markers in patient follow-up [33]. Because of late recurrences at up to 10 years or more, long-term follow-up is needed [27].

Ovarian-type surface epithelial tumours

Ovarian-type surface epithelial tumours are very rare and are histologically similar to ovarian epithelial tumours. Serum marker CA125 may be elevated and help during follow-up.

Serous tumours arise frequently from the tunica vaginalis (TV). It is the most common of all ovarian-type carcinomas. Roughly half of them are borderline cystadenoma while the other half are cystadenocarcinomas. They may arise from the regressed Müllerian duct system [8].

Histologically, they present features identical to ovarian tumours: papillary serous carcinoma with psammoma bodies presenting over time. Cystic lesions are usually serous tumours of borderline malignancy. Differential diagnosis of a serous tumour from mesothelioma may be difficult although immunohistochemistry can help in this. The tumours are negative for mesothelioma markers such as calretinin or N-cadherin and positive for ovarian epithelial tumour markers such as epithelial membrane antigen (EMA) or CA125 [16].

Following classical surgical removal of the testis and RLND, additional platinum-based chemotherapy is performed (carboplatin plus paclitaxel) [29].

Mucinous tumours may emerge in the testis and paratestis [1]. The median age of occurrence is 64 years. Mucinous tumours are well-demarcated masses and appear as multiple-cavity cystic tumours on ultrasound imaging. They may arise from any part of the mature cystic monodermal or multidermal teratoma (dermoid cyst) with malignant transformation [5].

Histologically, they present a mixture of mucinous and epithelial cells and can exhibit intestinal or endometrial differentiations. Cystic tumours contain a gelatinous substance that may sometimes be ossified. Most tumours are either benign or borderline. In the case of cystadenocarcinoma, spread to the peritoneum may occur causing carcinomatosis.

Treatment consists of orchidectomy for all cases and additional platinum-based chemotherapy only for the malignant type. However, malignant type has high mortality rates regardless of additional treatment [1].

Brenner tumours: Only five cases have been published. Tumours show the histological features of ovarian Brenner tumours: a nest of transitional cells associated with non-keratinized squamous and transitional carcinomas. Both poor prognosis and benign evolution have been reported. Patients underwent radical orchidectomy alone [14, 40].

Only two cases of clear cell adenocarcinoma have been reported: one arising from the TV and one from the parenchyma, both highly malignant [32, 40]. Renal or prostate cancer must be excluded [15].

Sarcomas

Fewer than 30 cases have been reported with a highly variable age of occurrence [39, 6]. Clinical and radiological differences that could reveal diagnosis before surgery were absent. Histological subtypes found, from most to least common, included leiomyosarcoma, rhabdomyosarcoma and spindle-cell sarcoma, fibrosarcoma, osteosarcomas, chondrosarcomas and finally, liposarcomas. Sarcomas may emerge from an existing teratoma. This fact is important because of the associated poor prognosis [14]. A single case of testicular leiomyosarcoma occurring after radiotherapy as a relapse of an acute lymphoblastic leukemia has been reported. Histologically, diagnosis is made in difficult cases with the help of immunohistochemistry: presence of a germ cell tumour is excluded by the expression of vimentin or cytokeratin [39, 6].

The specificity of each subtype and the management of non-metastatic sarcomas has been reported as follows:

- Leiomyosarcomas were treated by orchidectomy. In one case, RLND was performed which were negative. No adjuvant chemotherapy was given [39].

- Rhabdomyosarcomas are more frequent in paratesticular tissue. Intratesticular tumours are sometimes associated with either mature or immature teratoma. They have poor prognosis due to high grade chemoresistant tumours. RLND is required [23, 24].
- Spindle-cell sarcomas have poor chemosensitivity and radiosensitivity. RLND should be performed [6].
- Osteo- and chondrosarcomas are very rare with only seven cases of each reported. In all cases, patients were older than 50 years. Ultrasound can aid diagnosis with imaging of focal calcifications. Their origin is unclear but malignant transformation of a teratoma is possible. Orchidectomy alone and long-term follow-up is recommended [11, 22].
- Liposarcomas generally develop in paratesticular tissue (spermatic cord) and account for 20% of non-metastatic sarcomas. Patients are generally older than 50 years. Regardless of tumour origin, treatment consists of an orchidectomy and occasionally a wide excision of the hemiscrotum. RLND is controversial. Myxoid and well-differentiated tumours are usually localized whereas round-cell tumours are heterogeneously spread and highly malignant. Local relapse is frequent and sometimes delayed. For metastatic disease, chemotherapy using schemes used in the treatment of other sarcomas with the same histology, was given. For some subtypes such as liposarcoma, surgery may be proposed for metastases [38].

Adenocarcinoma of the rete testis

This is a very rare tumour of unknown origin occurring in adults over the age of 40 years. Clinical symptoms include a scrotal mass sometimes associated with hydrocele and occasionally, epididymitis. An inguinal hernia may sometimes hide symptoms. Nodules may spread to the scrotal and perineal skin. About 20% of patients has symptomatic metastatic disease while 30% has asymptomatic disease, almost all disease being in the lymph nodes or lungs. Histological criteria are: absence of histologically similar extrascrotal primary tumour, tumour centered on the testicular hilum, histological transition from the unaltered rete testis, solid growth pattern and absence of another testicular neoplasm.

In reported cases, treatments include orchidectomy with or without RLND followed by chemotherapy and/or radiotherapy with little response when metastatic. One-year overall survival is approximately 60% [14, 3].

Mesothelioma

Mesothelioma can occur in the testis, as the TV is part of the reflected peritoneum. Fewer than 100 cases have been reported. Malignant mesothelioma and mesothelioma of the TV are linked to asbestos exposure, between 30 and 40% of reported cases of the latter having had a history of exposure [21, 30]. Other possible risk factors include radiotherapy, radiation exposure and viral infections [18]. Median age of incidence is between 55 and 75 years. Patients often present with an enlargement of the scrotum over several months with hydrocele [17]. Tumour markers are absent. The majority of cases are diagnosed intraoperatively with hemorrhagic hydrocele or a papillary or fibrotic aspect of the TV. Treatment consists primarily of surgery with inguinal orchidectomy and additional lymphadenectomy of retroperitoneal or iliac nodes. These are positive in roughly two-thirds of the cases. Organ-sparing surgery carries the risk of local reccurrence, linked to metastatic development. Adjuvant radiotherapy may be performed for patients with local mesothelioma after surgery with clear margins. The majority of recurrences occur within the 2 years following diagnosis. For disseminated disease, chemotherapy (doxorubicin and cyclophosphamide in most reported cases) failed to produce complete remission, while short remissions were obtained with radiotherapy.

Mesothelioma has a poor prognosis with a median survival at 2 years of 60%. Prognostic factors include age over 60 years and primary metastatic disease [30]. Some late recurrences after a period of 15 years have been reported [17].

Conclusion

Testicular tumours are rare and heterogeneous tumours that must be identified and classified for appropriate treatment. For some, preoperative or intra-operative identification can be done which may avoid radical surgery. Germ cell tumours should be excluded when establishing a diagnosis.

Because of the small number of each type, definitive recommendations for management cannot be provided. For most testicular tumours, radical orchidectomy is sufficient treatment and is sometimes completed with RLND for lymphatic spread or when there are signs of possible lymph node metastases. Chemotherapy and/or radiotherapy are rarely needed in adjuvant strategies. When necessary, equivalent treatment schemes to those used for more usual histological types, can be used. Regardless of the tumour type, long-term follow-up is recommended.

To improve management of these rare tumours, case registration could be informative as large series are lacking. Several trials on the use of targeted therapy (HDAC inhibitors) and immunotherapy (interleukin-12) vaccinotherapy (ras peptide cancer vaccine) are ongoing. We await data on sunitinib and germ cell tumour as well as bevacizumab for which very few cases have been reported in the literature. High dose chemotherapy has also been combined with bevacizumab in a published case report [19].

Acknowledgement

We acknowledge the valued collaboration of Maxime Japkowicz, Joseph Gligorov, Stéphane Provent and Jean-Pierre Lotz of the University Pierre et Marie Curie, Hopital Tenon, Paris, France.

References

1. Al-Qahtani M, Morris B, Dawood S *et al.* (2007) Malignant mesothelioma of the tunica vaginalis. Can J Urol 14(2): 3514-7
2. Anderson GA(1995) Sclerosing sertoli cell tumor of the testis. A distinct histological subtype. J Urol 154(5): 1756-8
3. Banfield GK, Brookstein R (1995) Rhabdomyosarcoma arising in teratoma of the testis. J R Army Med Corps 141(3): 167-8
4. Brown B, Ram A, Clayton P *et al.* (2007) Conservative management of bilateral Sertoli cell tumors of the testicle in association with the Carney complex: a case report. J Pediatr Surg 42(9): E13-5
5. Caccamo D, Socias M, Truchet C (1991) Malignant Brenner tumor of the testis and epididymis. Arch Pathol Lab Med 115(5): 524-7
6. Canales BK, Lukasewycz SJ, Manovel JC *et al.* (2005) Postradiotherapy intratesticular leiomyosarcoma. Urology 66: 657.e19-20
7. Chang B, Borer JG, Tan PE *et al.* (1998) Large-cell calcifying Sertoli cell tumor of the testis: case report and review of the literature. Urology 52: 520-23

5

8. Cheville JC. (1999) Classification and pathology of testicular germ cell and sex cord-stromal tumors. Urol Clin North Am 26: 595-609
9. Cools M, Stoop H, Kersemaekers AMF *et al.* (2006) Gonadoblastoma arising in undifferentiated gonadal tissue within dysgenetic gonads. J Clin Endocrinol Metab 91(6): 2404-13
10. Ditonno P, Lucarelli G, Battaglia M *et al.* (2007) Testicular granulosa cell tumor of adult type: a new case and a review of the literature. Urol Oncol. 25(4): 322-5
11. Dupré F, Zachar D, Choquenet C *et al.* (2001) Paratesticular serous papillary carcinoma: a case report. Ann Pathol 21: 63-6
12. Fernandez GC, Tardaguila F, Rivas C *et al.* (2004) MRI in the diagnosis of testicular Leydig cell tumour. B J Radiol 77: 521-4
13. **Guarch R, Rivas A, Puras A (2005) Papillary serous carcinoma of ovarian type of the testis with borderline differentiation. Histopathology 46: 588-90**
14. Haines IE, Schwarz MA, Westmore DD *et al.* (1985) Rhabdomyosarcoma in a patient treated for metastatic germ cell tumour of the testis containing teratoma – a case report. Aust N Z J Surg 55(2): 141-3
15. Hayashi T, Iida S, Taguchi J *et al.* (2001) Primary carcinoid of the testis associated with carcinoid syndrome. Int. J. Urol 8(9): 522-4
16. **Hisano M, Souza FM, Malheiros DM *et al.* (2006) Granulosa cell tumor of the adult testis: report of a case and review of the literature. Clinics 61(1): 77-8**
17. Hodzic J, Golka K, Schulze H (2004) Primary testicular carcinoid. Med Sci Monit 10(8): 46-8
18. Humphrey PA (1997) Clear cell neoplasms of the urinary tract and male reproductive system. Semin Diagn Pathol 14(4): 240-52
19. Jones MA, Young RH, Scully RE (1995) Malignant mesothelioma of the tunica vaginalis. A clinicopathologic analysis of 11 cases with review of the literature. Am J Surg Pathol Jul 19(7): 815-25
20. Kirschner-Hermanns R, Füzesi L, Sohn M (1994) [Therapy of primary testicular chondrosarcoma]. Urologe A 33(6): 517-20
21. Krege S, Beyer J, Souchon R *et al.* (2008) European consensus conference on diagnosis and treatment of germ cell cancer: a report of the second meeting of the European Germ Cell Consensus group (EGCCCG). Eur Urol 53(3): 478-513
22. Lachkar A, Sibert L, Gobet F *et al.* (2000) A rare tumour: spermatic cord liposarcoma. Prog Urol 10(6): 1228-31
23. Markou A, Vale J, Vadgama B *et al.* (2002) Testicular leydig cell tumor presenting as primary infertility. Hormones 1(4): 251-4
24. Matoska J, Ondrus D, Talerman A (1992) Malignant granulosa cell tumor of the testis associated with gynecomastia and long survival. Cancer 69(7): 1769-72
25. Nistal M, Revestido R, Paniagua R (1992) Bilateral mucinous cystadenocarcinoma of the testis and epididymis. Arch Pathol Lab Med 116(12): 1360-3
26. Niewenhuis JC, Wolf MC, Kass EJ (1994) Bilateral asynchronous Sertoli cell tumor in a boy with the Peutz-Jeghers syndrome. J Urol 152(4): 1246-8
27. Pectasides D, Glotsos J, Bountouroglou NG *et al.* (2002) Primary carcinoid of the testis with metastases. Case report and review of the literature. J Buon 7(2): 153-6
28. Peterson JT, Greenberg SD, Buffler PA (1984) Non-asbestos-related malignant mesothelioma. Cancer 54: 951-60
29. Plas E, Riedl CR, Pflüger H (1998) Malignant mesothelioma of the tunica vaginalis testis, review of the literature and assessment of prognostic parameters. Cancer 83: 2437-46
30. Schoeneich G, Oehlmann U, Gustmann C *et al.* (2005) Primary intratesticular sarcoma of the testis: a rare manifestation of testicular cancer. Scand J Urol Nephrol 39(3): 249-50
31. **Sesterhenn IA, Cheville J, Woodward PJ *et al.* (2004) Sex cord/gonadal stromal tumours. In: Eble JN, Sauter G, Epstein JI, Sesterhenn IA (eds) Pathology and genetics. Tumours of the urinary system and male genital organs. IARC, Lyon, pp 250-8**
32. Skailes GE, Menasce L, Banerjee SS et al. (1998) Adenocarcinoma of the rete testis. Clin Oncol 10: 401-3
33. Su MT, Lee IW, Kuo PL (2006) Presence of TSPY transcript and absence of transcripts of other Y chromosomal genes in a case of microscopic gonadoblastoma. Gynecol Oncol 103(1): 357-60
34. **Talerman A, Roth LM (2007) Recent advances in the pathology and classification of gonadal neoplasms composed of germ cells and sex cord derivatives. Int J Gynecol Pathol Jul 26(3): 313-21. Review**

35. Tazi H, Karmouni T, Ouali M (2006) Osteosarcoma of the testis. Int J Urol 13(3): 323-4
36. Tulunay O, Gögüfl C, Baltaci S *et al.* (2004) Clear cell adenocarcinoma of the tunica vaginalis of the testis with an adjacent uterus-like tissue. Pathol Int 54(8): 641-7
37. Ulbright TM, Young RH (2003) Primary mucinous tumors of the testis and paratestis: a report of nine cases. Am J Surg Pathol 27(9): 1221-8
38. Vaughn DJ, Rizzo TA, Malkowicz SB (2005) Chemosentivity of malignant ovarian-type surface epithelial tumor of testis. Urology 66: 658.e7-9
39. Verdorfer A, Höllrigl A, Strasser U *et al.* (2007) Molecular-cytogenetic characterisation of sex cord stromal tumours: CGH analysis in sertoli cell tumours of the testis. Virchows Arch 450: 425-31
40. Voigt W, Kegel T, Maher G *et al.* (2006) Bevacizumab plus high-dose ifosfamide, etoposide and carboplatin (HD-ICE) as third-line salvage chemotherapy induced an unexpected dramatic response in highly platinum refractory germ-cell cancer. Ann Oncol Mar 17(3): 531-3
41. Young RH, Scully RE (1986) Testicular and paratesticular tumors and tumor-like lesions of ovarian common epithelial and müllerian types. A report of four cases and review of the literature. Am J Clin Pathol 86(2): 146-52

Primary testicular lymphoma

6

A. Zouhair, R.O. Mirimanoff and M. Ozsahin

Five Essential Points

1. *Primary testicular lymphoma (PTL) is a rare disease accounting for 1% of non-Hodgkin's lymphomas.*
2. *PTL occurs in older patients. It is a lethal disease.*
3. *For early stage, the treatment consists of orchidectomy followed by chemotherapy and prophylactic scrotal RT with/or without iliac and paraortic lymph node RT.*
4. *For advanced stage, CT is the treatment of choice while the place of scrotal RT can be discussed.*
5. *Both in early or advanced disease, intrathecal CT is warranted to prevent CNS relapse.*

Introduction

Primary extranodal lymphoma of the testis is a lethal disease, second only to primary brain lymphoma; median survival is 12 to 24 months. It accounts for approximately 1% of non-Hodgkin's lymphomas, 4% of all extranodal non-Hodgkin's lymphomas, 5% of all testicular malignancies, with an estimated incidence of 0.26/100'000 per year [6,21]. Primary testicular lymphoma (PTL) is essentially an intermediate or high-grade lymphoma, and diffuse large-cell type is the most common one [4]. In contrast to other testicular malignancies, PTL occurs mostly in patients older than 50 years of age [9]. After adequate locoregional and systemic treatment, the central nervous system (CNS) remains the most frequent site of recurrence (up to 30%). Therefore, prophylactic intrathecal (IT) chemotherapy (CT) combined with systemic treatment has been introduced to improve outcome [17]. We review in this chapter some data concerning pathology, staging, prognosis, and finally treatment options for different stages of PTL.

Pathology, staging and prognosis

As for all situations with any suspected tumour in the testes, the primary option remains inguinal orchidectomy for diagnosis and treatment. Orchidectomy is important because it removes the tumour located in the so-called "sanctuary site" with good local control and provides important information on grade and pathology subtype [13]. Histologically, 80-90% of primary testicular lymphomas are diffuse large-cell type with B-cell immunophenotype [11]. Complete initial staging work-up is the same as for all other non-Hodgkin's lymphomas. Cerebrospinal fluid (CSF) examination for malignant cells is recommended due to the high incidence of CNS relapse. Recently, PET or PET-CT is widely used in initial lymphoma staging but few data are available on primary testicular lymphoma [15]. The majority of patients with PTL present stage I or II disease according to Ann-Arbor staging [18]. PTL, like other aggressive extranodal non Hodgkin's lymphomas, shows a tendency to spread and relapse at several extranodal sites including the CNS, contralateral testis, Waldeyer's ring, skin, pleura, lung, or soft tissues [5]. The prognosis of PTL is poor even in early stage despite the combination of orchidectomy followed by anthracyclin-based chemotherapy, radiation therapy and CNS prophylaxis. The majority of patients fail within the first two years following treatment, and mainly in the CNS [2,7].

Treatment options

Given the rarity of PTL, its treatment has not been standardized. Up to now, no prospective trial has been published. Available data are reported by some single institutions and/or by international collaborative groups active in rare diseases [20,22]. The management of PTL depends on stage either at initial diagnosis or after relapse following an adequate initial treatment.

Treatment of early stage I-II

The universally accepted treatment modality for stage I and II aggressive nodal lymphoma is either chemotherapy (cyclophosphamide, doxorubicin, vincristin, prednison; CHOP) combined with rituximab or chemotherapy (CT) followed by radiation therapy (RT) [10,12]. However, an optimal treatment approach has not been defined for extranodal lymphomas. Also no randomized studies have been performed to evaluate the superiority of combined modality treatment to RT or CT alone, especially in testicular lymphoma, where there is an increased incidence of relapse (50-80%) following orchidectomy and RT without chemotherapy [14]. Regarding these results and the patterns of failure, the use of systemic CT combined with prophylactic intrathecal CT has become an important part of the management of early disease. Connors *et al.* [1], in their study of 15 patients with stage IE and IIE disease, administered (following orchidectomy) a doxorubicin-based CT with testicular RT, and observed 93% actuarial relapse-free survival. However, in a retrospective study by Fonseca *et al.* [5] including 62 patients, no beneficial effect of combined treatment compared to single modality was observed. In their study, only 10 patients, including 3 with stage I disease, received combined modality treatment. Moreover, only 4 patients received intrathecal-CT, and 2 of these already had leptomeningeal involvement at diagnosis. It is, therefore, difficult to draw a conclusion about the inefficacy of combined treatment. Zouhair *et al.* evaluated the outcome of a series of 36 patients in a multicentre Rare Cancer Network study [20]. Most patients (80%) had CHOP-CT combined with intrathecal-CT in 17 patients (47%). Testicular RT was delivered to the scrotum alone in 12 patients, or also to the iliac and para-aortic lymph nodes in 8. No relapse was observed in the irradiated volumes. The majority of relapses (12 out of 14) were observed in extranodal sites. Eight patients (22%) had CNS relapse. The 5-year overall, lymphoma-specific, and disease-free survival were 47%, 66%, and 43% respectively. In a series of 34 patients with localized disease registered in the British National Lymphoma Investigation, Crellin *et al.* [2] found that CHOP-CT was insufficient to prevent CNS relapse. In a Danish trial, 24 out of 39 patients with early stage managed by orchidectomy and doxorubicin-based CT had a relapse rate of 15.4%, while for patients not treated with adjuvant CT, the relapse rate was 63.6% [11]. The median relapse-free (28 vs. 14 months) and overall survival (43 vs. 17% at 2 and 5 years) were in favour of adjuvant CT. Data from MD Anderson Cancer Center have shown that despite doxorubicin-based adjuvant CT in 22 patients, CNS and/or contralateral testis were involved in all relapsing patients. These patients did not receive any prophylactic medication [18]. Tondini *et al.* [17] have reported the treatment in 16 out of 29 patients with localized disease with the same CT regimen as in the MD Anderson study but completed with prophylactic RT to regional lymph nodes in 85% of patients. After a median follow-up of 7 years, one-third of patients are alive. In a retrospective study from several French cancer centres, patients were divided into 3 groups (orchidectomy alone, orchidectomy + RT, and orchidectomy + RT + CT) without any CNS prophylaxis [7]. Thirty-two out of 84 patients relapsed mainly in the CNS. There was no significant difference in terms of overall, disease-specific or disease-free survival between the three groups. Zucca *et al.* [22] reported a large retrospective international survey in 373 patients with PTL mainly at stage I-II. The median age at diagnosis was 66 years. Anthracyclin-based CT was administered to 68% of patients, and prophylactic intrathecal CT was given to 18%. Prophylactic scrotal RT was administered in 36% of the patients. Median overall survival was 4.8 years, and median progression-free survival was 4 years. The survival curves showed no clear evidence of a substantial proportion of cured patients. Combination of CT with an anthracyclin-based regimen improved the outcome especially when 6 cycles or more were given. Patients receiving at least 30 Gy locoregional RT had a significantly longer overall survival. Darby *et al.*, from UK, reported the outcome of 30 PTL patients with early stage [3]. Eleven patients (37%) had orchidectomy alone, 12 (40%) orchidectomy + adjuvant CT, and 4 patients orchidectomy + CT + RT. A complete remission was observed in 84%. Twelve patients (40%) relapsed after a median follow-up of 73 months. The majority of relapses occurred in the lymph nodes (58%). One relapse in CNS, one in bone, one in skin and 2 in the contralateral testis were observed. The authors suggest that a combined modality approach is more effective (orchidectomy + CT+RT). A prospective trial conducted by the GOELAMS (Groupe Ouest Est d'Etude des Leucemies Aigues et Maladies du Sang) in stage I-IIE primary non-Hodgkin's lymphoma of 494 patients, analysed the outcome in a subgroup of 16 patients with PTL [8]. All patients received 3 cycles of anthracyclin-based CT followed by regional RT on inguinal, iliac and para-aortic lymph nodes. Prophylactic intrathecal CT was given in all patients. Relapses occurred in extranodal sites in 4, in abdominal lymph nodes in 1, in CNS in 1 and in the contralateral testis in one patient. After a median follow-up of 73.5 months, the probability of disease-free and overall survival were 70% and 65%, respectively. They concluded that their good results were attributed to the use of regional RT and CNS prophylaxis.

In conclusion, patients with stage IE should be managed with anthracyclin-based chemotherapy and scrotal RT. Furthermore, in stage IIE some authors propose, following CT, scrotal RT combined with nodal RT to the pelvic and/or para-aortic lymph nodes [16]. However, CNS prophylaxis with intrathecal CT is warranted to prevent the high incidence of CNS relapse.

Treatment of advanced stage III-IV

The treatment of choice for advanced disease in PTL is standard anthracyclin-based chemotherapy plus rituximab. Despite a higher rate of relapse in the contralateral testis (in up to 50% of patients), prophylactic scrotal irradiation is recommended by some authors [18], while others propose RT only for symptomatic patients, or in case of bulky disease [19]. Prophylactic intrathecal-CT to prevent CNS relapse (which occurs in about 50% of patients) is also considered in patients achieving complete remission [11]. Some authors propose adding high-dose methotrexate in young patients but this has not been proven. Many authors reported that intrathecal-CT did not appear to alter the CNS relapse pattern [5,18,20]. A median survival of less than 6 months is reported, confirming the dismal outcome of this entity. High-dose CT supported by autologous stem-cell rescue remains an investigational option.

Treatment of relapse or refractory disease

Treatment of relapse or refractory disease after initial treatment is unknown [19]. No prospective trial results are available in the literature. The decision to treat depends on many factors (age, performance status, previous treatment, etc). PTL is predominantly a disease of older men with multiple co-morbidities and short life expectancy. Palliative supportive care should be given in these situations. However, young patients can be managed by an aggressive approach.

Conclusion

Given the lack of randomized data in this rare disease, treatment options are based only on data available from retrospective studies but few of these include large number of patients. The prognosis remains very poor despite combined CT and RT following orchidectomy. Treatment of relapses at extranodal sites, contralateral testis and/or CNS needs to be further investigated using new molecular approaches and/or more aggressive management.

References

1. **Connors JM, Klimo P, Voss N *et al.* (1988) Testicular lymphoma: Improved outcome with early brief chemotherapy. J Clin Oncol 6: 776-81**
2. Crellin AM, Hudson BV, Bennett MH *et al.* (1993) Non-Hodgkin's lymphoma of the testis. Radiother Oncol 27: 99-106
3. Darby S, Hancock BW (2005) Localised non-Hodgkin's lymphoma of the testis: the Sheffield lymphoma group experience. Int J Oncol 26: 1093-9
4. Eskey CJ, Whitman GJ, Chew FS (1997) Malignant lymphoma of the testis. Am J Roentgenol 169: 822
5. **Fonseca R, Habermann TM, Colgan JP *et al.* (2000) Testicular lymphoma is associated with a high incidence of extranodal recurrence. Cancer 88: 154-61**
6. Gospodarowicz MK, Sutcliffe SB, Brown TC *et al.* (1987) Patterns of disease in localized extranodal lymphomas. J Clin Oncol 5: 875-80
7. Lagrange JL, Ramaioli A, Theodore CH *et al.* (2001) Non-Hodgkin's lymphoma of the testis: a retrospective study of 84 patients treated in the French anticancer centers. Ann Oncol 12: 1313-9

8. Linassier C, Desablens B, Lefrancq T *et al.* (2002) Stage I-IIE primary non-Hodgkin's lymphoma of the testis:results of a prospective trial by the GOELAMS study group. Clin Lymphoma 3: 167-72
9. Lobo FD, Bansal R, Naik R *et al.* (1998) Primary testicular lymphoma. J Indian Med Assoc 96: 193-4
10. Miller TP, Dahlberg S, Cassady R *et al.* (1993) Chemotherapy alone compared with chemotherapy plus radiotherapy for localized intermediate- and high-grade non-Hodgkin's lymphoma. N Eng J Med 329: 21-6
11. Moller MB, d'Amore F, Christensen BE (1994) Testicular lymphoma: A population-based study of incidence, clinicopathological correlations and prognosis. The Danish Lymphoma Study Group, LYFO. Eur J Cancer 30: 1760-4
12. Reyes F, Lepage E, Ganem G *et al.* (2005) ACVBP versus CHOP plus radiotherapy for localized aggressive lymphoma. N Eng J Med 352: 1197-205
13. Salem YH, Miller HC (1994) Lymphoma of genitourinary tract. J Urol 151: 1162-70
14. Shahab N, Doll DC (1999) Testicular lymphoma. Semin Oncol 26: 259-69
15. Spaepen K, Stroobants S, Dupont P *et al.* (2001) Prognostic value of positron emission tomography (PET) with fluorine-18 fluorodeoxyglucose (18FFDG-PET) after first line chemotherapy in non-Hodgkin's lymphoma: is (18FFDG-PET) a valid alternative to conventional diagnostic methods: J Clin Oncol 19: 414-9
16. Tepperman BS, Gospodarowicz MK, Bush RS *et al.* (1982) Non-Hodgkin's lymphoma of the testis. Radiology 142: 203-8
17. Tondini C, Ferreri AJM, Siracusano L *et al.* (1999) Diffuse large-cell lymphoma of the testis. J Clin Oncol 17: 2854-8
18. **Touroutoglou N, Dimopoulos MA, Younes A *et al.* (1995) Non-Hodgkin's lymphoma of the testis. Testicular lymphoma: late relapses and poor outcome despite doxorubicin-based therapy. J Clin Oncol 13: 1361-7**
19. Vitolo U, Ferreri AJM, Zucca E (2008) Primary testicular lymphoma. Critical Reviews in Oncology/Hematology 65: 183-9
20. **Zouhair A, Weber D, Belkacémi Y *et al.* (2002) Outcome and patterns of failure in testicular lymphoma: A multicenter rare cancer network study. Int J Radiat Oncol Biol Phys 52: 652-6**
21. Zucca E, Roggero E, Bertoni F *et al.* (1997) Primary extranodal non-Hodgkin's lymphomas. Part 1:gastrointestinal, cutaneous and genitourinary lymphomas: Ann Oncol 8: 727-37
22. **Zucca E, Conconi A, Mughal TI *et al.* (2003) Patterns of outcome and prognostic factors in primary large-cell lymphoma of the testis in a survey by the international extranodal lymphoma study group. J Clin Oncol 21: 20-7**

Human chorionic gonadotropin-producing seminoma

7

R.-O. Mirimanoff and A. Zouhair

Five Essential Points

1. *HCG-producing seminoma (HCG+S) is an uncommon entity and belongs to the overall category of pure seminoma.*
2. *Clinical presentation, behaviour and work-up should be the same as for non-secreting seminoma (HCG-S).*
3. *HCG+S tumours are not more resistant to radiation therapy (RT) or chemotherapy (CXT) than HCG-S tumours.*
4. *RT remains an excellent option in stage I and IIa disease with chemotherapy as an alternative; overall prognosis is excellent.*
5. *Surveillance in early stage HCG+S is followed by a higher relapse rate than in early stage HCG-S.*

Introduction

Pure testicular seminoma is one of the most curable cancers, with overall cure rates and survivals of around 97% [19, 29]. However, the management and prognosis of human chorionic gonadotrophin (HCG)-secreting seminoma have been controversial for a long time. It has been said that this subcategory of seminoma carried a worse prognosis than that of non-secreting seminoma. The aim of this chapter is to review relevant aspects of this relatively uncommon subtype of testicular cancer and to demonstrate that the overall management and prognosis are the same as for those with non-HCG producing seminoma.

Incidence

Seminoma of the testicle accounts for approximately 1% of all male cancers [15] and represents about 50% of germ cell tumours in men (17). Patients with genuine pure seminoma can present with elevated HCG serum levels. This occurs, on average, between 8% and 40% of all seminomas, although recent studies have suggested higher proportions [13, 14, 23]. This wide range is likely to be due to several factors: 1) the various frequencies at which hormonal determinations were done in various institutions, 2) the sensitivity of the method for HCG or βHCG determination, 3) whether the measurements were done in plasma or in tumour tissue by immunoperoxidase, and 4) the differences in tumour stage between the various series [11, 14, 20, 24, 31]. For example, in one of the largest reports, out of 1169 records of patients with pure seminoma, 132 (or 11%) were found to be HCG positive. The β fraction of HCG (βHCG) is thought to be a more sensitive marker than HCG: in one study of 54 patients with pure seminoma, βHCG was positive in 83% and HCG in only 50% of the same patients [14].

Anatomy and Pathology

Seminoma arises from seminiferous tubular epithelium. It is thought to have always progressed from the well-known in situ stage or the intra-tubular germ cell neoplasia.

There are 3 main histologic subtypes of seminoma: the anaplastic, the classic and the rare spermatocytic type. Stage for stage, they appear to have an equivalent prognosis [26].

With regard to HCG-secreting seminoma, histological studies have shown by immunoperoxidase localisation that HCG is secreted by isolated syncithiotrophoblastic giant cells [2, 28]. It is not certain that all these giant cells are trophoblastic in origin, as various morphological forms of multinucleated cells can be found in pure seminoma, including the giant or "mulberry cell" and the Langerhans's giant cell [5]. The occurrence of positive immunohistochemical stain in surgical specimens ranges from 7 to 39% [31]. A particularly careful search for non-seminoma component should be done by the pathologist to rule out another non-seminomatous component of the testicular tumour.

Clinical presentation

Most seminomas present as a painless testicular mass. In a minority of patients metastases represent the first sign of disease with a palpable mass in the abdomen or head and neck. Except for the possible occurrence of gynecomastia in HCG-secreting seminoma, symptoms and signs are similar in both groups of patients. The frequency of gynecomastia is poorly or even not reported at all in most series, and is likely to be related to the HCG level. It is estimated to be about 10% of all HCG-positive cases. In one large report, 6% of all seminoma (i.e. positive and negative) presented with a gynecomastia [12].

Staging procedure

Staging procedures should be no different from those used in HCG-negative seminoma. Most experts will recommend a careful history and physical examination, testicular ultrasound, complete blood tests including tumour markers such as αFP, HCG, LDH and whole body CT scan [7, 21]. Contrary to HCG, elevated αFP is generally not to be found in pure seminoma and almost always indicates a different histological component of testicular tumours. In extremely rare instances, an "idiopathic" elevation of αFP was reported in pure seminoma [9]. Testicular biopsy should be avoided as it may cause disruption of lymphatic integrity and an increase in local recurrence rate [6]. A staging workup is dictated by the typical pattern of spread of seminoma to retroperitoneal lymph nodes with infrequent hematogenous spread, and this is similar in HCG secreting and non-secreting tumours [20, 32]. The 2000 TNM staging system is presented in table 1 and takes primarily into account the nodal status (size and number of lymph nodes), except for stage III.

Table 1 – 2002 TNM stage grouping of testicular cancer.

Stage	Definition
I	Any T stage, N0, M0
IIA	Any T stage, N1 (≤ 5 lymph nodes, ≤ 2 cm maximal diameter), M0
IIB	Any T stage, N2 (lymph nodes > 2 cm but ≤ 5 cm maximal diameter, M0
IIC	Any T stage N3 (lymph nodes > 5 cm maximal diameter), M0
III	Any T stage, any N stage, M1

Treatment

Surgery

Standard surgical management consists of a radical inguinal orchidectomy with high ligation of the spermatic cord. After surgery, elevated HCG levels should return to normal values in all cases of stage I [4, 24] whereas a persistently elevated value indicates a stage II or higher, with metastatic disease in lymph nodes or elsewhere [19]. In the latter situation, levels should return to normal after RT or chemotherapy [24].

Radiotherapy

Stage I

Radiotherapy has been the mainstay of treatment options after orchidectomy and remains a major option in Stage I. A review of 11 series has yielded a 97% survival rate [18]. It is generally accepted that a dose of 20-25 Gy to the para-aortic area is sufficient to achieve a high cure rate [7, 18, 21]. Older series have claimed that even with post-operative RT, HCG-positive seminomas carried a poorer prognosis but this was probably due to a bias in the stage distribution [7, 21]. Important series have now established that stage for stage, the prognosis remains excellent and comparable to this of non-secreting tumours. In 1993, we have published the first relatively large collection of HCG-positive seminoma treated by radiotherapy with 132 patients; 96 or 73% were stage I. Of these only one relapsed with a 5 yr relapse-free survival of 99% [20]. Interestingly, 7 of these stage I patients had a very high elevation of HCG, from 128 to 1,400 times the upper limit of normal value: all 7 patients were alive without recurrence [20]. The largest number of patients was reported from Germany in 1999: out of 726 evaluable patients, 378 had elevated HCG values [32]. In stage I, the cumulative relapse-free survival at 3 yrs was 94%, all patients receiving post-operative RT to infra-diaphragmatic nodes of 30 Gy [32]. These results were confirmed by smaller recent reports [4, 7].

Stage IIA

Generally, RT is still accepted as the standard for stage IIA. A review of 8 series has shown an overall survival rate of between 94% and 100% [18]. RT is delivered to para-aortic and ipsilateral iliac nodes, with doses between 23 and 30 Gy [18, 21]. Experience with HCG-positive seminoma is relatively limited in that stage. In our study, none of the 20 stage IIA patients relapsed after RT only (20). In the German series only one of the 42 patients with stage IIA recurred [32].

Stage IIB, IIC and Stage III

Current management for these tumours, regardless of HCG status, includes primary chemotherapy (*vide infra*) and the role of RT is now limited. Still, in our series, 2 of 7 patients with stage IIB and 3 of 8 patients with stage III relapsed, with a relapse-free survival of 65% at 5 yrs. All were treated initially with RT alone, and all received salvage therapy with chemotherapy, radiation therapy or both: 3 of 5 relapsing patients could be cured (20). In the German trial, patient with stage IIB were also generally treated with radiotherapy: of 38 patients, 8 or 21% relapsed [32]. In the same study, patients with stage IIC and III received primary chemotherapy (*vide infra*).

Chemotherapy

Stage I

Chemotherapy is now a new option for seminoma at any stage. A large randomized study has demonstrated that it was equivalent to radiotherapy in stage I [32]. Experience in HCG patients is still limited, but results of a series with 29 patients from Japan with various chemotherapy regimes yielded a 100% survival [25], and the results of the Spanish Germ Cell Cancer Cooperative Group study suggest that 2 courses of carboplatin in HCG negative and positive (34 pts) seminoma yielded also an excellent disease-free survival [1].

Stage IIA, IIB and IIC

As for stage I, there is a trend to treat any stage II with chemotherapy. This is especially true in stage IIB and beyond (= bulky disease) where radiotherapy alone is followed by a relapse rate of between 40 to 50%, even if many of the relapsing patients can be salvaged with chemotherapy [18]. So primary platin-based chemotherapy is now the standard for "bulky disease" seminoma, with cure rates of between 80 to 90% [3, 10, 16]. In the German experience with HCG-positive seminoma, the relapse rate after chemotherapy amongst 69 patients with stage IIC and III was only 9%, indicating a similar behaviour to that of the HCG negative seminoma [32].

Surveillance in Stage I

Post-orchidectomy surveillance is an accepted alternative to RT or chemotherapy in stage I seminoma as shown now in several large trials [8, 29, 30]. The relapse rate lies between 12 and 20% and most patients can be successfully salvaged. However, several risk factors such as tumour size, anaplastic type, necrosis and infiltration of the rete testis should be taken into account [1, 27, 30]. The Spanish report has shown that for patients managed with surveillance, a preoperative elevation of HCG adversely affected outcome in a multivariate analysis with a relapse rate of 20% *versus* 3.5 % in non-secreting seminoma [1]. Thus it seems appropriate to consider pre-operative HCG level along with the other prognostic factors in the overall recommendation to offer surveillance or not.

Prognostic factors

If we consider that the production of HCG is not an independent adverse prognostic factor, it is likely that all other prognostic factors are similar in both HCG-negative and HCG-positive seminoma. Some studies have shown a correlation between stage and the importance of HCG levels [13, 20, 32]. However, this is not a constant finding since in our study, 7 of 8 patients categorized as having a very high elevation (HCG values above 100 times the upper limit) were classified as stage I [20]. In the largest series of HCG-secreting seminoma, the following parameters were found to be significant for progressive disease: 1) T category; 2) infiltration of the tunica albuginea, epididymis and spermatic cord, 3) size 4) LDH levels, 5) presence of metastases, 6) stage I-IIc (32). Altogether, the overall prognosis of HCG-producing seminoma remains excellent (Table 2).

Table 2 – Series of HCG-producing seminoma.

Series	Year	Number of Patients	Treatment	Survival: All stages	Stage I	Stage II	Stage III	Mean or *median* follow up	Initial Chemo-therapy
Mirimanoff *et al.* (MGH) [19]	1985	10	RT	100%	3/3	6/6	1/1	*6 yrs*	
Mirimanoff *et al.* (RCN) [20]	1993	132	RT (± CXT)	94%	96/96	27/27	6/9	*4 yrs*	10/132
Suzuki *et al.* [25]	1998	29	CXT (± RT)	100%	NR	NR	NR	*6 yrs*	8/29
Weissbach *et al.* [32]	1999	378	RT (± CXT)	98%	NR	NR	NR	*36 mo*	NR
Bruns *et al.* [4]	2005	19	RT	100%	19/19	-	-	*6 yrs*	
Aparicio *et al.* [1]	2005	44	CXT or SRV	100%	44/44	-	-	*34 mo*	34/44

Abbreviations: RT radiotherapy; CXT chemotherapy; SRV surveillance; MGH data from Massachusetts General Hospital; RCN data from Rare Cancer Network; NR not reported.

Conclusions

HCG-producing seminoma is an uncommon subgroup of an uncommon tumour and is included in our definition of rare cancers. Its prevalence depends on many local institutional factors, but should be on average 20-30% and it is in part correlated to stage. Overall management including pre-therapeutic workup, staging and therapy should not be different from that for non-secreting seminoma, except perhaps as far as surveillance is concerned. This subgroup of seminoma is no more radio-resistant or chemo-resistant than other seminomas. Radiotherapy remains an excellent option in stage I and IIA whereas chemotherapy is an alternative in stage I and IIA and is standard in stage IIB and beyond. The prognostic factors are similar to those found in HCG-negative seminoma.

7

References

1. Aparicio J, Germà JR, García del Muro X *et al.* (2005) Risk-adapted management for patients with clinical stage I seminoma: the Second Spanish Germ Cell Cancer Cooperative Group study. J Clin Oncol 23: 8717-23
2. Bjurlin MA, August CZ, Weldon-Linne M (2007) Histologically pure stage I seminoma with an elevated beta-hCG of 4497 UI/l. Urology 70: 1007.e13-5
3. Bompas E, Fléchon A, Biron P *et al.* (2002) Management of advanced seminoma: retrospective study of 96 patients. Bull Cancer 89: 877-85
4. **Bruns F, Raub M, Schaefer U *et al.* (2005) No predictive value of beta-hCG in patients with stage I seminoma – results of a long-term follow-up study after adjuvant radiotherapy. Anticancer Res 25: 1543-6**
5. Butcher DN, Gregory WM, Gunter PA *et al.* (1985) The biological and clinical significance of HCG-containing cells in seminoma. Br J Cancer 51: 473-8
6. Capelouto CC, Clark PE, Ransil BJ *et al.* (1995) A review of scrotal violation in testicular cancer: is adjuvant local therapy necessary? J Urol 153: 981-5
7. **Coleman JM, Coleman RE, Turner AR *et al.* (1998) The management and clinical course of testicular seminoma: 15 years' experience at a single institution. Clin Oncol 10: 237-41**
8. Duchesne GM, Horwich A, Dearnaley DP *et al.* (1990) Orchidectomy alone for stage I seminoma of the testis. Cancer 65: 1115-8
9. Fléchon A, Droz JP (2001) Hereditary persistence of alfa-fetoprotein in testis disease. J Urol 165: 2004
10. Fosså SD, Stenning SP, Gerl A *et al.* (1999) Prognostic factors in patients progressing after cisplatin-based chemotherapy for malignant non-seminomatous germ cell tumours. Br J Cancer 80:1392-9
11. Hartmann M, Pottek T, Bussar-Maatz R *et al.* (1997) Elevated human chorionic gonadotropin concentrations in the testicular vein and in peripheral venous blood in seminoma patients. An analysis of various parameters. Eur Urol 31: 408-13
12. Hernes EH, Harstad K, Fosså S (1996) Changing incidence and delay in testicular seminoma in southern Norway (1981-1992). Eur Urol 30: 349-57
13. Hori K, Uematsu K, Yasoshima H *et al.* (1997) Testicular seminoma with human chorionic gonadotropin production. Pathol Int 47: 592-9
14. Hoshi S, Suzuki K, Ishidoya S *et al.* (2000) Significance of simultaneous determination of serum human chorionic gonadotropin (hCG) and hCG-beta in testicular tumor patients. Int J Urol 7: 218-23
15. Jemal A, Siegel R, Ward E *et al.* (2006) Cancer statistics, 2006. CA Cancer J Clin 56: 106-30
16. Mencel PJ, Motzer RJ, Mazumdar M *et al.* (1994) Advanced seminoma: treatment results, survival and prognostic factors in 142 patients. J Clin Oncol 12: 120-6
17. McGlynn KA, Devesa SS, Sigurdson AJ *et al.* (2003) Trends in the incidence of testicular germ cell tumors in the United States. Cancer 97: 63-70
18. Mirimanoff RO (2003) Radiotherapy of testicular seminoma: changes of the past 10 years. Cancer Radiother 7(suppl 1): 70s-77s
19. Mirimanoff RO, Shipley WU, Dosoretz DE *et al.* (1985) Pure seminoma of the testis: the results of radiation therapy in patients with elevated human chorionic gonadotropin titers. J Urol 134: 1124-6
20. **Mirimanoff RO, Sinzig M, Krüger M *et al.* (1993) Prognosis of human chorionic gonadotropin-producing seminoma treated by postoperative radiotherapy. Int J Radiat Oncol Biol Phys 27: 17-23**
21. Neill M, Warde P, Fleshner N (2007) Management of low-stage testicular seminoma. Urol Clin North Am 34: 127-36
22. **Oliver RT, Mason MD, Mead GM *et al.* (2005) Radiotherapy versus single-dose carbopatin in adjuvant treatment of stage I seminoma: a randomised trial. Lancet 366: 293-300**
23. Paus E, Fosså SD, Risberg T *et al.* (1987) The diagnostic value of human chorionic gonadotrophin in patients with testicular seminoma. Br J Urol 59: 572-7
24. Rüther U, Rothe B, Grunert K *et al.* (1994) Role of human chorionic gonadotropin in patients with pure seminoma. Eur Urol 26: 129-33
25. Suzuki K, Nakazato H, Kurokawa K *et al.* (1998) Treatment of stage I seminoma: should beta-HCG positive seminoma be treated aggressively? Int Urol Nephrol 30: 593-8

26. Ulbright TM (2004) Testicular and paraatesticular tumors. In: Mills SE, Greenson JK, Oberman HA (eds) Sternberg's diagnostic surgical pathology. 4th edn. Lippincott William & Wilkins, Philadelphia: p2168
27. Von der Maase H, Specht L, Jacobsen GK *et al.* (1993) Surveillance following orchidectomy for stage I seminoma of the testis. Eur J Cancer 29A: 1931-4
28. Von Hochstetter AR, Sigg C, Saremaslani P *et al.* (1985) The significance of giant cells in human testicular seminomas. A clinico-pathological study. Virchows Arch A Pathol Anat Histopathol 407: 309-22
29. Warde P, Gospodarowicz MK, Panzarella T *et al.* (1995) Stage I testicular seminoma: results of adjuvant irradiation and surveillance. J Clin Oncol 13: 2255-62
30. Warde P, Specht L, Horwich A *et al.* (2002) Prognostic factors for relapse in stage I seminoma managed by surveillance: a pooled analysis. J Clin Oncol 20: 4448-52
31. Weissbach L, Bussar-Maatz R (1993) HCG-positive seminoma. Eur Urol 23(S2): 29-32
32. Weissbach L, Bussar Maatz R, Löhrs U *et al.* (1999) Prognostic factors in seminoma with special respect to HCG: results of a prosptective multicentre study. Seminoma Study Group. Eur Urol 36: 601-8

Section 5
Gynecological tumours

Rare ovarian cancers

1

J. Gligorov, I. Ray-Coquard, P. Pautier, É. Pujade Lauraine, F. Selle, C. Lhommé, J.-P. Lotz, P. Morice and P. Duvillard

Five Essential Points

1. *Principles of treatment of rare ovarian cancers are dictated by the pathological report. The WHO ovarian tumours histological classification includes the 3 more common histological types, which are surface epithelial-stromal tumours, sex cord-stromal tumour and germ cell tumours..*
2. *Usually the general principles of surgical ovarian treatment have to be respected in cases of rare ovarian cancers.*
3. *Systemic treatment options are usually in agreement with the general strategy applied in a particular histological group of tumours. (Taxane-platinum combined therapy for rare surface epithelial-stromal tumours, BEP regimens for germ cell tumours)*
4. *Because some of those rare ovarian cancers arise in rather young women, fertility preservation is an important issue to discuss in localized tumours.*
5. *For optimal results it is important to treat patients according to existing guidelines or they should be oriented toward specialized centres with a specific interest for this type of tumour and adequate department of pathology.*

Introduction

Tumours of the ovary represent about 30% of all cancers of the female genital system. Ovarian cancer is the fifth leading cause of death from cancer in women and the leading cause of death from gynaecological cancer. The annual worldwide estimated incidence is about 200.000 new cases and the annual mortality rate is about 115.000 [9].

Ovarian tumours are classified according to histology, which dictates many aspects of clinical management. Ovarian cancer is staged by the FIGO staging system (similar to the AJCC system) and uses information theoretically obtained after surgery or complete body imaging. The WHO histological classification [10] (Table 1) includes the 3 more common histological types, which are:

- Surface epithelial-stromal tumours (or ovarian epithelial carcinoma), are the most common ovarian neoplasms. These include serous, mucinous and endometrioid tumours (these 3 categories accounting for 90% of ovarian cancers in North America and Western countries), but also more rare clear cell tumours, transitional cell tumours and squamous cell tumours. All these histological subtypes of surface epithelial-stromal tumours can be malignant, borderline or benign.
- Sex cord-stromal tumour, including estrogen-producing granulosa cell tumour and virilizing Sertoli-Leydig cell tumour or arrhenoblastoma, accounting for 5% to 10% of all ovarian cancers.

1

Table 1 – WHO classification of tumours of the ovary.

1. Surface epithelial-stromal tumours	1.1 Serous tumours: benign, borderline, malignant 1.2 Mucinous tumours, endocervical-like and intestinal-type: benign, borderline, malignant 1.3 Endometrioid tumours: benign, borderline, malignant, epithelial-stromal and stromal 1.4 Clear cell tumours: benign, borderline, malignant 1.5 Transitional cell tumours: Brenner tumour, Brenner tumour of borderline malignancy, malignant Brenner tumours, transitional cell carincoma (non-Brenner type) 1.6 Squamous cell tumours 1.7 Mixed epithelial tumours (specify components): benign, borderline, malignant 1.8 Undifferentiated carcinoma
2. Sex cord-stromal tumours	2.1 Granulosa-stromal cell tumours: granulosa cell tumours, thecoma-fibroma group 2.2 Sertoli-stromal cell tumours, androblastomas: well-differentiated, Sertoli-Leydig cell tumour of intermediate differentiation, Sertold-Leydig cell tumour poorly differentiated (sarcomatoid), retiform 2.3 Sex cord tumour with annular tubules 2.4 Gynandroblastoma 2.5 Unclassified or of mixed cell types 2.6 Steroid (lipid) cell tumours: stromal luteoma, Leydig cell tumours, unclassified
3. Germ cell tumours	3.1 Primitive germ cell tumours (dysgerminoma; yolk sac tumours; embryonal carcinoma; polyembryoma; non-gestational choriocarcinoma 3.2 Biphasic or triphasic teratoma (immature or mature) 3.3 Monodermal teratoma and somatic-type tumours associated with dermoid cysts
4. Germ cell sex cord-stromal tumour of non-gonadoblastoma type	4.1 Gonadoblastoma 4.2 Mixed germ cell-sex-cord-stromal tumour
5. Tumours of rete ovarii	5.1 Adenocarcinoma 5.2 Adenoma 5.3 Cystadenoma 5.4 Cystadenofibroma
6. Tumours of uncertain origin and miscellaneous tumours	Among these small cell carcinoma, hypercalcaemic type
7. Tumour-like conditions	Including luteoma of pregnancy
8. Lymphoid and haematopoietic tumours	
9. Secondary tumours	

– Germ cell tumours, accounting for approximately 30% of all ovarian tumours but usually only 5% of ovarian cancers as the vast majority of germ cell tumours are teratomas, most of these being benign. Germ cell tumours seem to be more frequent in some Asian countries including Japan.

More rare cancers are described in Table 1. In this chapter, we will focus more specifically on the treatment of germ cell cancers, sex cord-stromal cancers, more rare surface epithelial stromal tumours and other very rare and specific primary cancers excluding secondary tumours, lymphoid and hematopoietic tumours, tumour-like conditions and miscellaneous tumours not specific to the ovary.

It is important to stress that usually the general principles of ovarian treatment have to be respected in cases of rare ovarian cancers [1]. The main reason is because rare ovarian cancers are frequently diagnosed at the time of the initial surgery. Concerning strategy and systemic treatment options, these are usually in agreement with the general strategy applied in a particular histological group of tumours. For example, systemic treatment for rare surface epithelial-stromal tumours is mostly a taxane-platinum combined therapy while BEP regimens are given for germ cell tumours [2,3].

Rare surface epithelial-stromal tumours

Surface epithelial-stromal tumours are the most frequent ovarian cancers. Among these, even if serous, mucinous and endometrial carcinomas are frequent, it is important to emphasize that stage IA-B, grade 1 and 2 mucinous carcinomas have a particularly good prognosis.

Malignant müllerian mixed tumour (MMMT)

Also known as carcinosarcoma, malignant mesodermal mixed tumour or metaplastic carcinoma, MMMT is a highly aggressive neoplasm containing malignant epithelial and mesenchymal elements and a subgroup of endometrioid tumours. The incidence is low representing less than 1% of ovarian malignancies. There are no specific recommendations concerning the surgical treatment of this histological subtype. The 5-year survival rate is 78%, 63%, 24%, 6% according to FIGO stage I, II, III or IV respectively. Guidelines usually recommend the use of chemotherapy even for stage I disease. Adenosarcomas are biphasic tumours characterized by a proliferation of müllerian-type epithelium with a mesenchymal component. The most important treatment for adenosarcoma is surgery. Chemotherapy and radiation therapy may be applied, however no established guidelines exist.

Endometrial stromal and undifferentiated ovarian sarcoma (ESS)

Also a subcategory of endometrioid tumours, ESS is a monophasic sarcomatous tumour characterized by a diffuse proliferation of neoplastic cells similar to stromal cells of proliferative endometrium. The importance of an undifferentiated ovarian sarcoma component influences the prognosis of the disease. Treatment is classically surgical and some successful treatments of advanced disease with hormonal drugs (aromatase inhibitors, progestins) have been reported [7].

Clear cell adenocarcinoma (CCA)

CCA is a rare ovarian cancer (<5%) arising from endometriosis or from the surface epithelium. The differential diagnosis always includes germ cell tumours and particularly yolk sac tumour in which elevated serum alpha foeto proteins are always found. The 5-year survival rate is 69%, 55%, 14%, 4% according to FIGO stage I, II, III or IV respectively. Despite their aggressive clinical course, ACC are still treated similarly to the other surface epithelial-stromal cancers with platinum-taxane based combination chemotherapy after initial surgery.

Transitional cell carcinoma and Brenner tumour

This entity includes ovarian cancers composed of epithelial elements, histologically resembling urothelium and its neoplasm. The WHO histological classification clearly distinguishes benign Brenner tumours from borderline and malignant Brenner tumours (without invasive transitional epithelium) and transitional cell carcinomas (TCC) in which a malignant transitional cell tumour is not associated with a benign or borderline Brenner component. Transitional cell carcinoma is the pure or predominant element in 6% of ovarian carcinomas. Even if the 5-year survival rate is 35%, pure TCC are usually considered to be more chemosensitive.

1

Concerning Brenner tumours, only 5% are malignant and 80% of them are stage 1 at the time of the diagnosis and they have a better prognosis than stage matched transitional cell carcinomas.

Squamous cell carcinoma (SCC)

Most SCC are classified in the germ cell tumour category as they arise from dermoid cysts. Here are considered SCC composed of squamous epithelial cells that are not of germ cell origin. The incidence is very rare (<1%) and the prognosis is usually poor even if there is a very limited number of publications concerning the item [4].

Undifferentiated carcinoma (UC)

According to WHO criteria (primary ovarian carcinoma with no differentiation or only small foci of differentiation) UC represents 4-5% of ovarian cancers. More than 90% of the tumours are discovered in stages III and IV, the reason for the 5-year survival being worse than that of ovarian serous or transitional cell tumours.

Mixed epithelial tumours (MET)

MET are defined as a an epithelial ovarian tumour composed of an admixture of two or more of the five major cell types of surface epithelial-stromal tumours. The incidence is variable (0,5% - 4%) and usually due to variability in the histological definition. Concerning the prognosis, the dominant cell type generally dictates behaviour except for the serous component that always dictates the prognosis even if it is not the dominant cell type.

Borderline tumours

Borderline ovarian tumours are a subset of epithelial ovarian tumours without stromal invasion that have a very favourable prognosis. Even if in 15 to 40% of cases there is peritoneal implant, the diagnosis should be based on the primary ovarian tumour and extensive sampling is required to firmly establish the diagnosis. Borderline tumours comprise approximately 15% of all epithelial ovarian tumours. The mean age of occurrence is approximately 10 years younger than that in women with malignant ovarian cancer. Surgery is the usual treatment for borderline tumours. To date, no medical therapy after optimal surgery has been shown to clearly improve outcomes. Surgical staging is crucial and principles are the same as in invasive cancers. Because many women with borderline tumours are of child-bearing age, conserving fertility is a frequent challenge. There is no evidence that a conservative surgical approach – consisting of unilateral oophorectomy and removal of peritoneal implants – has an adverse effect on survival in patients with stage I borderline tumours. Even if the recurrence rate is higher after conservative surgery, effective surgery for recurrent disease leads to equivalent survival.

Sex cord-stromal cancers (SCSC)

Sex cord-stromal tumours account for about 8% of ovarian cancers. These include ovarian tumours composed of granulosa cells, Theca cells, Sertoli cells, Leydig cells and fibroblasts of stromal origins. Tumours usually secret steroid hormones explaining the clinical presence of androgen or estrogen and rarely, Cushings syndrome. General strategic considerations concerning the treatment of SCSC consist of initial surgery leading to diagnosis, staging and treatment (even in stage IV disease) with lack of interest concerning lymphadenectomy. In case of stage IA and IB disease no systematic adjuvant treatment with chemotherapy is given. In all other situations the chemotherapy regimen is usually PEB (Platinum, Etoposide, Bleomycin) for 3 to 4 cycles with potential value of paclitaxel carboplatin chemotherapy regimens. Secondary surgery is indicated in case of incomplete initial surgery.

Granulosa cell tumour Group (GCTP)

This group of tumours represents 2% of all ovarian tumours. Two major subtypes (adult and juvenile) are recognized. More than 95% of granulosa cell tumours are of adult type and are caracterized by the FOXL2 mutation. Nearly 90% of patients have stage I disease which remains the most important prognostic factor. The juvenile form is defined according to the age of the patient (< 30 years) at the time of diagnosis. In that case and because of the age criteria, small cell carcinoma associated with hypercalcemia, which also occurs in children and young women, could be a differential diagnosis.

Sertoli-Leydig cell tumour group (SLCTG)

SLCTG (also called arrhenoblastoma) accounts for less than 1% of ovarian neoplasms and intermediate and poorly differentiated forms are most common. Clinically one-third of patients are virilised and others may have estrogenic symptoms. A familial occurrence of SLCTG possibly associated with thyroid disease has been reported [10]. More than 95% of SLCTG are located in one ovary only. The great majority of the SLCTG tumours are benign, but approximately 20% of all SLCTG will relapse with, at that time, poor prognosis. The prognosis is good in well differentiated and stage I disease but the 5-year survival rate for poorly differentiated tumours is only 50%. Chemotherapy is proposed in case of presence of bad prognostic factors (advanced stage, poorly differentiated, presence of heterologous elements), but there is no consensus concerning the type. Usually a PEB regimen or a combination of anthracyclines and alkyklating agents is proposed.

Among SLCTG, Sertoli cell tumours are usually associated with Peutz-Jeghers syndrome. Tumours are frequently functional (most often estrogenic but sometimes androgenic). Typically benign, the aggressive forms are very rare.

Steroid cell tumours (SCT)

These are tumours composed of more than 90% of cells that resemble steroid hormone-secreting cells. One-third of these is malignant and their presence usually cause Cushing's syndrome. There is no standard defined systemic treatment due to the very low incidence (<0.5%) but they are usually treated as SLCTG.

Sex cord-stromal tumours of mixed or unclassified cell types

These are defined as exclusive sex cord-stromal tumours which are not granulosa, Sertoli-Leydig or steroid cell tumours. Among them gynandroblastoma is the more frequent histological type and is composed of Sertoli and granulosa cells (at least 10%) even if it is one of the rarest ovarian tumours. Androgenic symptoms are usual clinical features. Benign in the vast majority of the cases, endometrial hyperplasia is frequently present and must be screened. After surgery, chemotherapy is indicated only in case of relapse or advanced stage tumours.

Germ cell tumours (GCT)

Even if germ cell tumours account for 30% of primary ovarian tumours, the vast majority is benign and represented by mature cystic teratomas. The malignant germ cell tumours represent about 3% of all ovarian cancers in western countries but up to 20% in Asia. GCT are more frequent in the younger population (median age at presentation is about 18 years) explaining the challenge of conserving fertility, enhanced by the fact that those tumours are frequently diagnosed at an earlier stage (70% stage I), are usually very chemosensitive and can probably be cured by polychemotherapy only. Usually primitive malignant ovarian GCT are classified into dysgerminoma and non-dysgerminoma (yolk sac tumour, embryonal carcinoma, polyembryoma, non-gestational choriocarcinoma and mixed germ cell tumour). The distinction is important from a clinical and therapeutic point of view. The 5-year overall survival rate for dysgerminoma is close to 100% and only 75% for non-dysgerminoma primitive malignant ovarian GCT. Principles of treatment are dictated by the fact that GCT have a good prognosis, detected at an early stage, in a young population for whom fertility preservation is crucial and also that all the malignant GCT are chemosensitive to a PEB (Platinum, Etoposide, Bleomycin) regimen. Even if dysgerminomas are particularly radiosensitive, the risk of secondary infertility is important after radiation therapy, explaining why it is no longer frequently used in curative situations. Concerning surgery, even if unilateral oophorectomy is part of the diagnosis and treatment, neither bilateral oophorectomy nor hysterectomy or retroperitoneal lymph node dissection are systematically recommended. The general strategy is then after initial surgery, complementary treatment with 3 to 4 cycles of a PEB regimen.

Dysgerminoma

This tumour is identical to testicular seminoma. Dysgerminomas are very chemo and radiosensitive. Stage is the only prognostic factor. In cases of stage IA, there is no consensus concerning adjuvant systemic treatment after surgery. In case of no treatment the risk of relapse is close to 25% but the tumour is chemosensitive and those patients could be secondarily cured. For stage IB and more, 3 cycles of adjuvant PEB are usually indicated. Less toxic chemotherapy regimens such as PE or carboplatinum-etoposide could be proposed as in the treatment of seminomas

Non dysgerminoma primary ovarian malignant GCT

Yolk sac tumour

Malignant germ cell tumours in which there is differentiation into yolk sac structures, also formerly known as endodermal sinus tumours, comprise approximately 1% of ovarian malignancies. High levels of alpha-fetoprotein are present in the serum of most of the patients and can be used to monitor the response to the systemic PEB treatment.

Embryonal carcinoma

Very rare ovarian counterparts of the testicular homologue, ovarian embryonal carcinoma occurs almost exclusively in children and young women with an average age of 15 years. Elevated levels of beta-hCG may be present and are useful in monitoring the response to systemic PEB treatment.

Choriocarcinoma

Extremely rare as pure primary ovarian choriocarcinoma of germ cell origin (<1% of ovarian germ cell tumours), ovarian choriocarcinoma is seen more frequently as a component of a mixed germ cell tumour. High levels of beta-hCG are present in the serum of most of the patients and can be used to monitor the response to the systemic PEB treatment.

Other rare malignant tumours of the ovary

Small cell carcinoma of hypercalcemic type

Small cell carcinoma has the ultrastuctural features of an epithelial tumour but its precise lineage is uncertain. It is predominantly a tumour of young women with an average age of 24 years with some rare familial cases. About two thirds of patients have had hypercalcemia even if it is clinically asymptomatic in the great majority of the cases. Stage is the main prognostic factor with only 33% 5-year life expectancy for stage Ia disease and 6,5% for stages II to IV. Initially very chemosensitive, the tumour has become chemoresistant. Optimal surgery as in surface epithelial-stromal tumours is recommended but followed by an intensive chemotherapy regimen containing anthracyclines, cisplatinum, cyclophosphamide and vepeside.

Desmoplastic small round cell tumours (DSRCT)

Desmoplastic small round cell tumour is classified as a soft tissue sarcoma. It is an aggressive and rare tumour that primarily occurs as masses in the abdomen and could, in rare cases, develop from the ovary. DSRCT is associated with a unique chromosomal translocation (t11;22)(p13:q12), resulting in a EWS/WT1 transcript that is characteristic of this tumour. This transcript codes for a protein that acts as a transcriptional activator which fails to suppress tumour growth. The tumour is considered to be a childhood cancer that predominantly affects young adults. The prognosis for DSRCT remains poor with less than 20% of patients surviving beyond two to three years. Optimal surgery and intensive chemotherapy regimens including high dose chemotherapy programmes are under evaluation [5].

Conclusion

Non-epithelial malignant tumours of the ovary and rare surface-epithelial-stromal ovarian cancers are tumours whose natural history is not well known and for which prognostic factors still have to be defined; for these reasons all patients should be treated in specialized centres with a specific expertise in the treatment of this type

1

of tumour and with an expert department of pathology. Surgery, which remains a vital part of therapy, can rely on the efficacy of chemotherapy and must be aimed at preserving fertility. The effect of chemotherapy must be taken in account when deciding on a new intervention, which could be necessary in isolated cases. Indeed, recent studies report that apart from the tumour stage, the number of cases treated both in surgical and medical departments has prognostic significance [7].

International guidelines where available (http://www.nccn.org) or a dedicated website allowing physicians to ask for advice regarding the surgical and medical management of these patients through a discussion forum on the internet (http://www.sor-cancer.fr/) (http://www.arcagy.org/tmro/) are important for the improvement of care in those cancers.

The recently published francophone experience from the arcagy.org web forum discussion pannelists clearly demonstrate the importance of sharing experiences in management of rare ovarian cancers [6].

References

1. **Barakat RR, Markman M, Randall ME eds (2009) Principle and Practice of Gynecologic Oncology. 5th edition. Wolters Kluwer Health**
2. **Fletcher CDM ed (2001) Diagnostic Histopathology of tumours. 2nd edition. Churchill Livingston**
3. Guastalla JP, Ray-Coquard I (2005) Les cancers ovariens, Springer-Verlag France
4. Hackethal A, Brueggmann D, Bohlmann MK *et al.* (2008) Squamous-cell carcinoma in mature cystic teratoma of the ovary: systematic review and analysis of published data. Lancet Oncol 9(12): 1173-80. Erratum in: Lancet Oncol 2009 May;10(5): 446
5. McCluggage WG (2004) Ovarian neoplasms composed of small round cells: a review. Adv Anat Pathol 11: 288-96
6. **Ray-Coquard I, Pautier P, Pujade-Lauraine E *et al.* Rare ovarian tumours: therapeutic strategies in 2010, national website observatory for rare ovarian cancers and delineation of referent centers in France. Bull Cancer [Epub ahead of print])**
7. Reich O, Regauer S (2007) Hormonal therapy of endometrial stromal sarcoma. Curr Opin Oncol 19: 347-52
8. Segal R, DePetrillo AD, Thomas G (1995) Clinical review of adult granulosa cell tumors of the ovary. Gynecol Oncol 56: 338-44
9. **Stewart BW, Kleihues P eds (2005) WHO Worldwide cancer epidemiology. IARC Press**
10. **Tavassoli FA, Devilee P eds (2003) WHO Classification of Tumours. Pathology and genetics. Tumours of the Breast and Female Genital Organs. IARC Press Lyon**

Extraovarian primary peritoneal carcinoma

2

C. Nay Fellay, M. Fiche, J.-F. Delaloye and J. Bauer

Five Essential Points

1. *EOPPC should be considered in women presenting with peritoneal carcinomatosis of unknown primary site.*
2. *Risk factors for EOPPC are not known, excepting BRCA1 and 2 mutations.*
3. *An important prognostic factor is optimal cytoreductive surgery.*
4. *Treatment of EOPPC should be the same as for advanced epithelial ovarian cancer.*
5. *Keep in mind that EOPPC is a different entity than EOC and that, in this rare tumour, results in studies perhaps did not reach statistical difference because of the low number of patients.*

Introduction

In 1959, Swerdlow reported a case of a 27-year-old woman with a pelvic tumour that seemed to arise from the peritoneum, in the presence of normal ovaries, fallopian tubes and uterus, and that was histologically similar to papillary serous carcinoma of the ovary [52]. Since then several authors have described this disease using different names, such as extraovarian primary peritoneal carcinoma (EOPPC), peritoneal papillary serous carcinoma, peritoneal adenocarcinoma of Müllerian type, serous surface papillary carcinoma, normal sized ovary carcinoma syndrome, peritoneal mesothelioma, and primary peritoneal carcinoma. This illustrates the confusion about definition, histogenesis and clinicopathologic features of this entity. In 1993, in an attempt to sort out these confounding variables, the Gynecologic Oncology Group (GOG) developed criteria to define EOPPC:

1. Both ovaries must be either physiologically normal in size or enlarged by a benign process.
2. The involvement in extraovarian sites must be greater than the involvement on the surface of either ovary.
3. Microscopically, the ovarian component must be one of the following:
   a. non existent;
   b. confined to ovarian surface epithelium with no evidence of cortical invasion;
   c. involving ovarian surface epithelium and underlying cortical stroma but with tumour size less than 5x5mm within ovarian substance with or without surface disease.
4. The histological and cytological characteristics of the tumour must be predominantly of the serous type that is similar or identical to ovarian serous adenocarcinoma of any grade [8, 55].

In this chapter, we will try to clarify definition, differential diagnosis, and clinicopathologic features of EOPPC and discuss the principles of patient management.

2

Pathogenesis

The exact pathogenesis of EOPPC has still to be elucidated. However, it is suggested that its similarities to the papillary serous ovarian carcinoma may be due to their common embryologic heritage. The Müllerian ductal system is derived embryologically from coelemic epithelium and subcoelemic mesenchyma. Primary Müllerian epithelium is defined as the cell layer lining the fused and unfused portions of the müllerian ducts, which means tubal, endometrial and endocervical epithelium. The secondary müllerian system was first described by Lauchlan and is defined as the epithelium located external to the cavities of the original Müllerian ducts [31]. These cells are similar or identical to the primary Müllerian epithelium. It is postulated that the adult derivates of the secondary Müllerian system, i.e. the surface epithelium of the ovary or the peritoneal lining and its subjacent connective tissue, retain a potential for Müllerian differentiation. Therefore various tumours with histological types similar to epithelial ovarian cancer (EOC) can develop primarily in the peritoneum. Until now, no oncogenic stimulus that could explain the carcinogenesis in the mesoderm lining the abdominal cavity and ovaries, has been determined [25].

Tumorigenesis in the upper female genital tract is suggested to be multifocal [47]. Molecular analyses performed later confirmed that the origin of EOPPC is multifocal at least in some patients. Muto described 3 cases among 6 analysed, presenting different patterns of allelic loss at various anatomic sites in the same patient [37]. Schorge found 5 of 22 cases (23%) presenting patterns of selective loss of heterozygosity at the androgen receptor gene locus, consistent with multifocal, polyclonal disease origin [49]. In contrast, in EOC several molecular analyses suggest a unifocal origin [41,53]. Searching for similarities or differences between EOPPC and EOC, Chen found similar antigen expression patterns for HER-2/neu, p53, bcl-2 and nm23-H1 in EOC and in EOPPC, but Kowalski and Halperin identified different immunohistochemical (IHC) expression of ER, PR, Ki-67 and HER-2/neu between EOPPC and EOC suggesting distinct genetic events responsible for malignant transformation[11,27,30].

Differential diagnosis

Women presenting with a diffuse peritoneal tumour should be first considered to have a metastatic or advanced stage disease from another origin. The most frequent primary site is the ovary, but peritoneal metastases from other genital sites, gastro-intestinal tract, pancreas or breast are not rare. Less common are primary peritoneal carcinomas and mesotheliomas. The list of differential diagnosis (Table 1) is large and sometimes differences are slight and diagnosis difficult to make.

To differentiate EOPPC from metastatic disease, it is of prime importance to exclude a possible gastro-intestinal or breast cancer (see Diagnosis/Preoperative evaluation). If no primary tumour is detected, laparotomy and pathological examination of the ovaries, fallopian tubes and uterus should be performed to rule out the diagnosis of advanced stage female genital tract cancer rather than a primary peritoneal tumour.

Initially, EOPPC was classified as a mesothelioma due to the supposed common origin. However epidemiologic, clinical and pathologic differences are clear. Diffuse malignant mesotheliomas are more frequent in males and often associated with a history of asbestos exposure. Prognosis is poor, most patients dying within a year of

Table 1 – Differential diagnosis of extra-ovarian primary peritoneal carcinomas.

Metastatic tumours from another primary origin	
Primary ovarian carcinoma	No gross invasion of the ovaries as described in GOG criteria [8] Prognosis and management similar to EOPPC
Fallopian tube cancer	Prognosis and management similar to EOPPC
Gastro-intestinal cancer	Perform gastroscopy and colonoscopy Worse prognosis than EOPPC
Breast cancer	Perform mammography or breast MRI Worse prognosis than EOPPC
Pancreatic cancer	Perform MRI of the abdomen, if CT scan is inconclusive
Mesotheliomas	
Cystic mesothelioma	Benign or of low malignancy [24]
Well-differentiated papillary mesothelioma	Predominant in women, between 40-50 years Benign or of low malignancy [24]
Fibrous mesothelioma	Benign nature [24]
Diffuse malignant mesothelioma	Predominantly in males Exposure to asbestos Poor prognosis [24]
Other lesions of Müllerian type	
Endosalpingosis	Metaplastic lesion of benign nature Putative precursor of EOPPC Extremely common in women [24]
Primary peritoneal serous borderline tumour	Younger women (< 40 years) Good prognosis, but small risk for progression to serous carcinoma with fatal issue [54]
Primary peritoneal serous psammocarcinoma	Low-grade malignancy Favourable prognosis Progression in minority of patients [1]

initial diagnosis [24, 25]. Histologically, the proliferation of columnar neoplastic cells, the presence of psammoma bodies and the production of neutral mucin were thought to be specific for the diagnosis of EOPPC [56]. However, mesothelioma may closely resemble serous carcinoma, especially the well-differentiated papillary mesothelioma that predominates in women. The use of mucin staining and IHC analyses may help to differentiate malignant mesothelioma (MM) from EOPPC (Table 2).

Unlike EOPPC, MM virtually never stains for mucin. However, IHC stains for keratin and epithelial membrane antigen (EMA) are positive in both, but with a different pattern of staining [13]. To date, no single antibody with absolute speci-

Table 2 – Immunohistochemical markers in serous carcinomas (EOC and EOPPC) and malignant mesotheliomas (MM) [39,14].

Immunohistochemical marker	EOC and EOPPC	MM
BerEP4	+	-
ER	+	-
h-CD	-	+
Calretinin	-	+

Abbreviations : ER : estrogen receptor ; h-CD : h-caldesmon.

ficity and sensitivity for either MM or EOPPC has been identified. Ordonez found positive reactivity in immunostaining of estrogen receptor (ER) in 86% of women with EOPPC and 88% of women with EOC, whereas none of the examined mesotheliomas expressed ER, therefore making ER useful in distinguishing between serous carcinomas and MM [39]. Progesterone receptor (PR) expression has been found of less practical utility because of its low sensitivity (positivity in 60% of EOC and 56% of EOPPC). A recent study identified h-Caldesmon (h-CD) and calretinin to be the most sensitive and specific IHC positive markers for MM, and ER together with Ber-EP4 as positive markers for serous carcinomas (EOC and EOPPC). The combination of these four markers is currently considered as giving the best performance to differentiate MM from serous carcinoma [14].

Primary peritoneal lesions of Müllerian type constitute a spectrum of diseases with variable degrees of aggressivity. It is important to differentiate endosalpingosis, primary peritoneal serous borderline tumours and primary peritoneal psammocarcinomas from the much more aggressive EOPPC. The most common lesion within this spectrum is endosalpingosis, a benign lesion, probably metaplastic in nature. It usually occurs in females of reproductive age and is found in the omentum, but often not apparent on macroscopic examination. Endosalpingosis has however been proposed as a possible precursor of EOPPC [24].

Primary peritoneal serous borderline tumours have been reported to be similar to the non invasive implants of ovarian serous borderline tumours, with no tissue or lymphovascular invasion, and no cytonuclear atypia [54]. This very rare neoplasm occurs mostly in young women (mean age 40 years). Conservative surgery is the treatment of choice and adjuvant therapy is not indicated [24]. However, all tumour mass should be adequately debulked to avoid recurrence or bowel obstruction and to allow extensive sampling to rule out invasion. Prognosis is excellent, identical to ovarian serous borderline tumours. Although the risk of progression is small, careful clinical follow-up is warranted [54].

Psammocarcinoma is a variant of serous peritoneal carcinoma. It is of low malignant potential and should be considered in the diagnosis of primary peritoneal tumours. Mean age at presentation has been reported to be 48 years. Histological diagnostic criteria for peritoneal serous psammocarcinoma are presence of:

1. at least 75% of the epithelial proliferation associated with psammoma bodies;
2. no more than moderate cytologic atypia;
3. tissue or lymphovascular space invasion, or both;
4. no solid epithelial proliferation, except for occasional foci less than 15 cells [54].

Little is known about the prognosis of this rare tumour. It seems to be more favourable than EOPPC, but recurrences with progression and death have been reported [1]. No standard has been established in management of these patients, but authors recommend an optimal surgical debulking of the tumour, conservative surgery in fertile women and adjuvant chemotherapy [1,54].

Epidemiology

EOPPC occurs almost exclusively in women, with the exception of 2 cases reported in men [48,50]. The real incidence of EOPPC is not known. From 1992-1997, Roffers identified 139 women with EOPPC from the North American Association of Central Cancer Registries, corresponding to an incidence of 0.30 cases per million [46]. In the descriptions of small series, frequency of EOPPC is reported to be about 9-20% of all EOC [2,15,25,26,28] and up to 29% of advanced stage (III and IV) EOC [28]. This ratio increases with time, possibly due to the better knowledge of this disease and resulting in increased identification of EOPPC cases [26,28]. Most cases have been reported in Caucasians (94.2%) [46].

Mean age at presentation varies between 57.4 and 66 years as reported in the different series [2,4,6-9,12,17,22,23,25,26,28,38,42,44-46,51]. In several studies, women with EOPPC appear to be older at time of diagnosis than women with EOC with statistical difference reported by some authors [4,9,12,22]. When comparing age of menarche, oral contraceptive use, infertility, parity, menopausal status and hormonal replacement therapy, most authors did not observe any significant difference between these 2 groups. Only one report established a significant difference for later menarche (13.8 *vs* 12.8 years) and less use of perineal talc powder in women with EOPPC [22].

Several authors have also examined family and personal history of cancer [6,22,26,28,42]. They all report a trend for less cases of positive familial breast cancer history in women with EOPPC as compared to women with EOC. Barda found a significant difference in the frequency of personal history of breast cancer, being lower in women with EOPPC [6].

Reports of women developing EOPPC following prophylactic oophorectomy performed for a strong family history of ovarian carcinoma have led to speculation that EOPPC might be a part of the breast ovarian cancer syndrome [44]. Therefore Bandera analysed BRCA1 gene mutations in patients with EOPPC and compared them with those occurring in EOC patients [5]. Two of 17 patients with EOPPC showed germline BRCA1 mutation, a frequency comparable to EOC. Menczer confirmed these results in a larger study analysing 609 Jewish women with stage III-IV EOC and 68 with EOPPC [35]. The observed carrier rates of any BRCA1 or BRCA 2 mutation were 28% among the EOPPC group and 30% in advanced EOC. No differences were found between EOPPC and EOC, neither in the overall distribution of BRCA1/2 mutation carrier rates nor according to type of mutation, age, ethnic origin or histological subtype. In both groups however, carriers of a mutation were younger at diagnosis than non-carriers. For BRCA mutation carriers, the lifetime risk of developing EOPPC is estimated to be 1.3% [32]. These findings are important to consider when counselling patients with BRCA mutations for prophylactic oophorectomy.

Pathology

As already discussed in the introduction of this chapter, nomenclature and definition remained confusing until the Gynecologic Oncology Group (GOG) defined clear criteria for EOPPC [8]. These criteria especially help to distinguish EOPPC from EOC. Minimal involvement of the ovaries occurs in 80 to 95.8% patients with EOPPC, making the diagnosis of EOPPC in many cases possible only after surgery and complete pathological examination of the ovaries [25,42].

Serous well differentiated carcinoma is the predominant histology in EOPPC (>90%). Only isolated cases present as serous poorly differentiated [21], mucinous [15,21,51], endometroid [51] or clear cell carcinomas [2,21,38,51].

2

Staging

Until now no TNM or FIGO staging system has been developed for EOPPC. Consequently the FIGO staging system of ovarian cancer is used for EOPPC. Therefore, all EOPPC are at least stage III or IV at diagnosis (Table 3). Most patients present with stage III disease and stage IIIc is more frequent than stage IIIb [2,6-8,12,15,17,20,23,28,38,42]. In all reported series the proportion of stage III and stage IV disease was similar to that observed in EOC. Only one study that analysed 95 cases of EOPPC, reported a significant difference for less stage IV disease in patients with EOPPC compared to patients with EOC [6]. This result might indicate a slower evolution of EOPPC. The most frequent site of metastasis is the pleural cavity and the liver parenchyma, but other sites have been mentioned in isolated cases such as cervical, supraclavicular, axillar and inguinal lymph nodes, umbilic, or subcutaneous tissue and skin at other sites [16,25,45,51]. Lymphatic spread is frequent (63%-73%) and involves the pelvic and/or paraaortic lymph nodes, similar to EOC [18,20]. Distribution of tumour grade 2 or 3 is also similar in EOPPC and EOC [8,20,23].

Table 3 – FIGO Stages at diagnosis.

TNM categories (2006)	FIGO stages	Definitions	Frequencies
T3a, N0	IIIa	Microscopic peritoneal metastasis beyond pelvis (no macroscopic tumour)	71.4-96.8%
T3b, N0	IIIb	Macroscopic peritoneal metastasis beyond pelvis 2cm or less in greatest dimension	
T3c, N0	IIIc	Peritoneal metastasis beyond pelvis more than 2 cm in greatest dimension	
Any T, N1	IIIc	Regional lymph node metastases (pelvic and para-aortic)	
Any T, any N, M1	IV	Distant metastases: pleural effusion, liver parenchyma, lung, sub-clavicular and axillar lymph nodes, sub- and cutaneous metastases and brain metastases (excludes peritoneal metastases).	3.2-28.6%

Prognostic factors

Whereas several prognostic factors are well known in EOC, only few prognostic factors have been identified in EOPPC. In order to identify significant prognostic factors, Eltabbakh conducted a retrospective, clinicopathologic study of 75 women diagnosed with EOPPC [21]. Table 4 shows the identified prognostic factors and the clinical or pathological factors, which did not have any impact on overall survival. Optimal cytoreduction with residual disease ≤ 1 cm has been shown to be associated with a better survival as independent prognostic factor. These findings have been confirmed by other studies [4,38,44,51]. However, several authors could not identify optimal cytoreduction as a prognostic factor in EOPPC [6,7,23,25]. The small number of patients and confounding variables in treatment could explain these conflicting findings. Fromm also analysed prognostic factors and demonstrated in a group of 74 patients with EOPPC that patients receiving multi-agent chemotherapy expressed a significant longer survival than those treated with single-agent [25]. Among the pathological factors that these authors examined, only the absence of mitosis was significantly predictive of improved survival.

Table 4 – Prognostic factors [21].

Prognostic factors in multivariate analyses
Performance status ≤ 1 or > 1 Optimal primary cytoreduction (residual disease ≤ or >1 cm
Prognostic factors in univariate analyses
Age ≤ 70 or > 70 years Stage ≤ III or IV Performance status ≤ or > 1 Optimal primary cytoreduction (residual disease ≤ or > 1 cm
No prognostic value
Parity ≤ 1 or > 1 History of oophorectomy yes or no Abdominal distension yes or no Pain yes or no Dyspepsia yes or no Mass yes or no Ascites yes or no Architectural grade 1, 2 or 3 Nuclear grade 1, 2 or 3 Mitosis < or ≥ 20/10 HPF Histology serous or other Psamma bodies none, rare or occasional Estrogen receptors negative or positive Progesterone receptor negative or positive P53 over-expression negative or positive First-line chemotherapy Platin/Taxol or Platin/no Taxol

Of note, in the study of Eltabbakh, the median survival of EOPPC patients whose tumours were progesterone receptor positive, was almost twice as long as in negative patients (40.0 *versus* 21.2 months), but did not reach statistical difference. In the same way, tumours which demonstrated p53 overexpression translate to a shorter median survival than tumours which did not (11.0 *versus* 23.5 months, respectively) [21]. Nevertheless, one other study did not confirm this result [30].

Diagnosis

Symptoms and signs

Clinical presentation of EOPPC is similar to that of EOC and Table 5 lists the most common symptoms and signs of patients presenting with EOPPC. More than 50% of patients present with abdominal distension and pain. Gastrointestinal symptoms (dyspepsia, changing in bowel habits, nausea and vomiting), breathing difficulties or asymptomatic patients are less common. Clinical examination discloses abdominal or pelvic mass and ascites [6,7,12,22,23,25,26,28,38,42,45,51,56]. At laparotomy the presence of ascites is described in up to 81.5% of cases with EOPPC [38]. Barda and Halperin found that abdominal distension was more frequent in EOPPC than in EOC and palpation of a pelvic mass less common in EOPPC [6,26]. The second group of authors also found a significant higher proportion of clinical ascites none with negative cytology in EOPPC.

Table 5 – Clinical presentation of EOPPC.

Symptoms
Abdominal distension
Abdominal pain
Gastro-intestinal symptoms (dyspepsia, changing in bowel habits, nausea, vomiting)
No symptom
Weight loss
Cough, or breathing difficulties
Other
Signs
Abdominal mass
Pelvic mass
Ascites clinical
Ascites at laparotomy
Pleural effusion

Preoperative evaluation

Although EOPPC cannot reliably be distinguished from EOC by preoperative testing, radiological imaging revealing normal-sized ovaries with evidence of carcinomatosis should raise suspicion for EOPPC. Identifying a potential primary site is important in the preoperative assessment, because surgical management, postoperative treatment and prognosis differ radically in EOPCC as compared with carcinomatosis associated with other malignancies [13]. Gastroscopy and/or colonoscopy permits the exclusion of a primary tumour of the gastro-intestinal tract. Breast imaging (mammography or MRI) searching for primary tumour should be considered. A computed tomography (CT) scan provides an assessment of peritoneal disease, and putative retroperitoneal, hepatic and pulmonary lesions. Particular attention should be given to the pancreatic region and in inconclusive situations the examination should be completed with an MRI.

Paracentesis may provide short-term relief of symptoms caused by massive ascites. However, if the cytology is positive for malignancy, identification of the primary site is often not possible. Therefore, diagnostic paracentesis is not required in preoperative evaluation. Cytological evaluation of pleural effusion in women on the contrary is important for staging and consequently for prognosis [13].

Serum tumour markers

In most reported series, serum Ca-125 level was measured preoperatively and raised in almost all patients [2,6,12,26,28,38,42,56]. Several authors found a trend for Ca-125 levels being higher in EOPPC than in EOC [12,26], but only in one study did differences reach statistical significance [4]. Altaras mentioned a correlation between Ca-125 and disease stage [2]. Ca-125 is probably, as in EOC, a useful marker for the evaluation of tumour response to treatment and for the follow-up of patients.

Management of extraovarian primary peritoneal carcinoma

Multiple small series report similarities in the clinicopathologic features, response to treatment and prognosis between EOPPC and EOC. Even if there are some contradicting findings, all authors agree that EOPPC should be treated like EOC.

Surgical evaluation and debulking

Diagnosis and staging of EOPPC can only be performed by surgical assessment. Any woman with suspected EOPPC or EOC requires surgical exploration (Fig. 1). Diagnosis should be performed on the basis of frozen-section evaluation of the ovary and complete abdominal exploration. If the disease seems limited to the pelvis (macroscopic stage II), sampling of the omentum, abdominal peritoneal surfaces and retroperitoneal lymph nodes is important to rule out microscopic abdominal disease (stage III). If there is small volume disease (< 2 cm), abdominal and pelvic lymph node sampling is also recommended [13]. In EOC numerous phase III studies have demonstrated that primary optimal debulking with residual disease < 1 cm is an important prognostic factor [10]. As already discussed earlier, optimal cytoreduction in EOPPC appears also to be a prognostic factor. In advanced stage III and IV EOC the percentage of maximal cytoreductive surgery described in a meta-analysis was 41.9% with a range from 0% - 100% [10]. In EOPPC optimal debulking is reported in 28% - 67% of cases with most studies having described a rate of roughly 40% [2,6-8,12,21,23,25,26,28,38,42,45,51]. The optimal debulking rate in patients with EOPPC compared to EOC, was not significantly different [6,7,28,42], except in one study, where authors reported a trend that optimal cytoreduction is less often reached in EOPPC than in EOC [26]. In a similar manner, patients with EOPPC more often need neoadjuvant chemotherapy and optimal cytoreduction is completed only after two or three cycles of chemotherapy [17]. This is probably related to a more extensive peritoneal spread in the upper abdomen than in EOC. Complete cytoreductive surgery (initial or interval) is performed in 89% of patients with EOPPC comparable with EOC patients. In EOPPC, influence on survival with either initial or interval surgery is unknown. In EOC survival of patients without residual disease is similar whatever the timing of surgery (initial or interval surgery) [36].

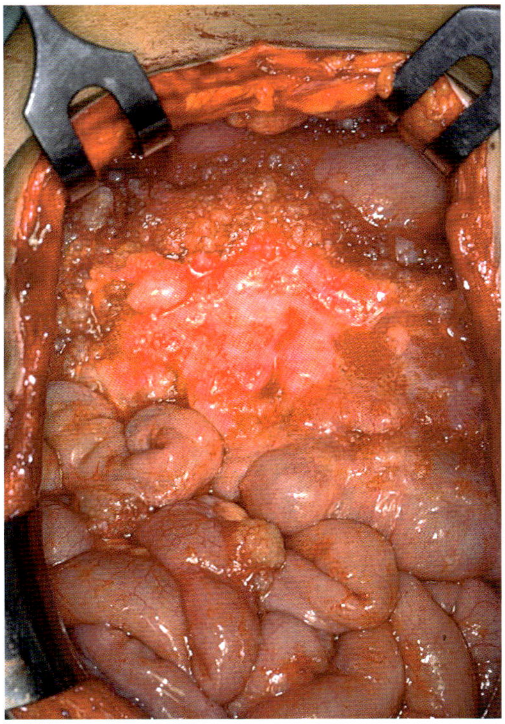

Fig. 1. Peritoneal carcinomatosis in EOPPC.

2

First-line chemotherapy

Similarities between EOPPC and EOC have led physicians to apply therapies for EOPPC which have proven effective in EOC. In the past twenty years, chemotherapy has consisted essentially of platinum-based regimens. During the nineties, paclitaxel added to either cisplatin or carboplatin showed superiority in response rate, progression free and overall survival [34]. Lower toxicity profile and comparable efficacy favoured carboplatin over cisplatin in combination with paclitaxel [40]. Currently, the standard treatment for EOC and EOPPC is carboplatin AUC 5-6 and paclitaxel 175mg/m2/3h administered every 21 days [19].

For patients with EOPPC, Fromm first reported that a chemotherapy with cisplatin versus no cisplatin prolonged survival (31.5 *vs* 19,5 months, $p < 0.02$) and that a multi-agent regimen was superior to a single-agent regimen (median survival 29.5 *vs* 16.5 months, $p < 0.01$) [25]. This was confirmed by Fowler in a study where EOPPC patients receiving a cisplatin regimen survived longer (23 to 92 months) than those treated with a non-cisplatin-regimen (≤ 25 months) [23]. In most series, patients receiving a cisplatin-based chemotherapy experienced response rates (complete responses and partial responses) ranging from 57% - 96.5% [4,6,8,9, 12,15,25,38,42,43] comparable to the response rate obtained in EOC [4,6,8,9,42]. A limited number of trials evaluated specific first-line chemotherapy in EOPPC. Piver first compared an induction with weekly cisplatin followed by the combination of cisplatin-doxorubicin-cyclophosphamide (PAC) or paclitaxel-cisplatin (TP). Both regimens were effective without significant difference in response, time to recurrence and survival. However, a trend for better response and prolonged time to progression was observed with TP [43]. Ayhan showed that paclitaxel combined with a platinum derivate had similar responses and overall survival in EOPPC and EOC patients [4]. The single prospective study is a phase II trial conducted by the Gynecologic Oncology Group (GOG) assessing clinical effectiveness of cisplatin and cyclophosphamide in EOPPC patients and comparing response to this treatment to a cohort of patients with EOC [9]. Cisplatin and cyclophosphamide combination demonstrated similar response rate (65% *vs* 59%) and overall survival (22 *vs* 27 months). Based on these findings and the fact that results of ovarian cancer trials are frequently extrapolated to patients with EOPPC, as from 2003 the GOG decided to include patients with EOPPC in advanced ovarian cancer trials.

Consequently, 48 patients presenting with EOPPC were included in a large GOG phase III trial that compared intravenous paclitaxel plus cisplatin with intravenous paclitaxel plus intraperitoneal cisplatin and paclitaxel in patients with optimally debulked stage III ovarian cancer [3]. The combination of intraperitoneal and intravenous chemotherapy was associated with an improved median progression-free survival (23.8 *vs* 18.3 months) and overall survival (65.6 *vs* 49.7 months). However, intraperitoneal therapy was associated with more additional side effects including catheter-related complications. The results of a recent meta-analysis of 8 randomized trials, comparing standard intravenous therapy with or without a component of intraperitoneal administration, support the survival benefit for intraperitoneal therapy [29]. Therefore, even if intraperitoneal therapy is still not a standard treatment, it should be considered in women with small residual tumour after maximal cytoreductive surgery and clear information about benefits and possible toxicities.

Second-line chemotherapy

Recurrent or persistent disease, that requires second line treatment, is common. Even after a complete response, up to 50% of patients will relapse and necessitate a second line treatment. In patients with EOPPC, the literature about second line treatment is limited. Bloss reported second-line treatments in 14 patients with EOPPC using agents such as adriamycin, methotrexate, paclitaxel, and 5-fluorouracil [8]. Unfortunately none of these patients achieved a complete and durable response. Eltabbakh described 43 patients with relapsing EOPPC [21]. Only 9 patients (20%) obtained a complete or partial response and 16 patients (37%) stable disease after second line chemotherapy. In this study paclitaxel was given in 50% of cases (either alone or combined with platinum) and 21 patients received various non-taxane treatments (cisplatin-based combination, intraperitoneal cisplatin/arabinoside C, topotecan and hexamethylmelamine). The median overall survival in these patients was 16 months. Piura analysed 10 patients with EOPPC and 23 patients with EOC, who received second-line chemotherapy with agents such as cisplatin, carboplatin, paclitaxel, etoposide, cyclophosphamide and hexylmethylmelamine [42]. Objective response was obtain in 2/10 (20%) EOPPC and in 8/23 (34.8%) EOC patients without significant difference. Response to second-line chemotherapy appears therefore similar in both diseases.

At relapse, it is important to consider treatment-free interval: patients who recur within 6 months of their last dose of platinum-based therapy are designated as "platinum resistant" and must be treated with a non-cross-resistant drug. Patients with disease-free interval greater than 6 months are "platinum sensitive". These patients can be retreated with their initial regimen, usually a platinum drug and a taxane. The duration of the disease-free interval directly correlates with the anticipated response rate and the duration of re-treatment with platinum [33]. For platinum resistant diseases several agents are available. These women generally have a poor prognosis and the goal of salvage therapy is palliation. An asymptomatic recurrence does not necessarily require immediate treatment. Benefits and side effects should be carefully evaluated and discussed with the patient. As all second-line chemotherapy regimens present similar response rates, the selection of drugs should be based on previous treatment, anticipated toxicities and way of administration. Generally single-agents are preferred. The different agents with activity include: paclitaxel, docetaxel, oral etoposide, liposomal doxorubicin, topotecan, gemcitabine, vinorelbine, ifosfamide and tamoxifen. Response rates with second-line treatment range from 15% - 30%. Most are of short duration, but responses can occasionally exceed 1 to 2 years, justifying the concept of second-line chemotherapy.

Prognosis

Median survival among women with EOPPC has been reported to vary from 17 to 41 months [2,4,6-9,15,21,23,25,26,28,38,42,45,51,56] and 3 and 5 years overall survival from 28% - 60% [4,17] and 18% - 52% respectively [7,21,38,42,56]. Virtually all studies suggest that EOPPC has similar survival rates to EOC. Only Halperin found a shorter median survival for EOPPC compared to EOC (17 *vs* 40 months) [26]. In contrast, Piura reported a trend for a better overall survival at 5 years for EOPPC patients (52% *vs* 20.5%) [42]. These results were not statistically significant, but patients alive with disease at 5 years were significantly more frequent in EOPPC (46.7% *vs* 11.5%). This illustrates that if relapse rate is identical in both diseases, evolution however could be slower in EOPPC than EOC. Dubernard reported similar findings without any difference at 3-year survival (60% *vs* 55%), but a significant difference in event-free survival (29% *vs* 16%), again in favour of EOPPC [17].

After complete response, disease-free survival ranges from 12.1 to 58.1 months and is comparable in EOPPC and EOC [7,8,12,21,44]. Long-term survivors are occasional [45,51].

Conclusion

EOPPC should be considered in women presenting with peritoneal carcinomatosis of unknown primary site. Clinicopathological features are similar in EOPPC and EOC, even if patients with EOPPC seem to be older than women presenting with EOC. EOPPC is also found in patients with BRCA1 or 2 gene mutations and patients undergoing prophylactic oophorectomy should be informed about the possibility of developing EOPPC. Risk factors like nulliparity or absence of oral contraception could not be identified for EOPPC in contrast to EOC. Only optimal cytoreductive surgery and performance status are reliable prognostic factors. Response to chemotherapy and survival are similar to EOC. Therefore the management of EOPPC should be the same as for advanced stage EOC.

For this relatively rare tumour, very few prospective studies exist; most of the present report is based on short case series. The largest one included 95 patients and was published 3 years ago [6]. It is possible that several results in the different studies did not reach statistical significance, due to of the low number of patients. Even if all authors agree that EOPPC should be treated like advanced stage EOC, it is important to keep in mind that it is a different entity.

References

1. Akbulut M, Kelten C, Bir F *et al.* (2007) Primary peritoneal serous psammocarcinoma with recurrent disease and metastasis: a case report and review of the literature. Gynecol Oncol 105: 248-51
2. Altaras MM, Aviram R, Cohen I *et al.* (1991) Primary peritoneal papillary serous adenocarcinoma: clinical and management aspects. Gynecol Oncol 40: 230-6
3. Armstrong DK, Bundy B, Wenzel L *et al.* (2006) Intraperitoneal cisplatin and paclitaxel in ovarian cancer. N Engl J Med 354: 34-43
4. Ayhan A, Taskiran C, Yigit-Celik N *et al.* (2006) Long-term survival after paclitaxel plus platinum-based combination chemotherapy for extraovarian peritoneal serous papillary carcinoma: is it different from that for ovarian serous papillary cancer? Int J Gynecol Cancer 16: 484-9
5. Bandera CA, Muto MG, Schorge JO *et al.* (1998) BRCA1 gene mutations in women with papillary serous carcinoma of the peritoneum. Obstet Gynecol 92: 596-600
6. Barda G, Menczer J, Chetrit A *et al.* (2004) Comparison between primary peritoneal and epithelial ovarian carcinoma: a population based study. Am J Obstet Gynecol 190: 1039-45
7. Ben-Baruch G, Sivan E, Moran O *et al.* (1996) Primary peritoneal serous papillary carcinoma: a study of 25 cases and comparison with stage III-IV ovarian papillary serous carcinoma. Gynecol Oncol 60: 393-6
8. Bloss JD, Liao SY, Buller RE *et al.* (1993) Extraovarian peritoneal serous papillary carcinoma: a case-control retrospective comparison to papillary adenocarcinoma of the ovary. Gynecol Oncol 50: 347-51
9. Bloss JD, Brady MF, Liao SY *et al.* (2003) Extraovarian peritoneal serous papillary carcinoma: a phase II trial of cisplatin and cyclophosphamide with comparison to a cohort with papillary serous ovarian carcinoma – a Gynecologic Oncology Group Study. Gynecol Oncol 89: 148-54

10. Bristow RE, Tomacruz RS, Amstrong DK (2002) Survival effect of maximal cytoreductive surgery for advanced ovarian carcinoma during the platinum era: a meta-analysis. J Clin Oncol 20: 1248-59
11. Chen LM, Yamada SD, Baldwin RL *et al.* (2003) Molecular similarities between primary peritoneal and primary ovarian carcinomas. Int J Gynecol Cancer 13: 749-55
12. Choi CH, Kim TJ, Kim WY *et al.* (2007) Papillary serous carcinoma in ovaries of normal size: a clinicopathologic study of 20 cases and comparison with extra-ovarian peritoneal papillary serous carcinoma. Gynecol Oncol 105: 762-8
13. Chu CS, Menzin AW, Leonard DG *et al.* (1999) Primary peritoneal carcinoma: a review of the literature. Obstet Gynecol Surv 54: 323-35
14. Comin CE, Saieva C, Messerini L (2007) h-Caldesmon, calretinin, estrogen receptor, and Ber-EP4: a useful combination of immunohistochemical markers for differentiating epitheloid peritoneal mesothelioma from serous papillary carcinoma of the ovary. Am J Surg Pathol 31: 1139-48
15. Cormio G, Di Vagno G, Di Gesù G *et al.* (2000) Primary peritoneal carcinoma: a report of twelve cases and a review of the literature. Gynecol Obstet Invest 50: 203-6
16. Cowan LJ, Roller JI, Connelly PJ *et al.* (1995) Extraovarian stage IV peritoneal serous papillary carcinoma presenting as an asymptomatic skin lesion: a case report and literature review. Gynecol Oncol 57: 433-5
17. Dubernard G, Morice P, Rey A *et al.* (2004) Prognosis of stage III and IV primary peritoneal serous papillary carcinoma. Eur J Surg Oncol 30: 976-81
18. Dubernard G, Morice P, Rey A *et al.* (2005) Lymph node spread in stage III or IV primary peritoneal serous papillary carcinoma. Gynecol Oncol 97: 136-41
19. Dubois A (2005) 2004 consensus statements on the management of ovarian cancer: final document of the 3rd International Gynaecologic Cancer Intergroup Ovarian Cancer Conference (GCIG OCCC 2004). Ann Oncol 16: viii7
20. Eltabbakh GH, Mount SL (2002) Lymphatic spread among women with primary peritoneal carcinoma. J Surg Oncol 81: 126-31
21. Eltabbakh GH, Werness BA, Piver S *et al.* (1998) Prognostic factors in extraovarian primary peritoneal carcinoma. Gynecol Oncol 71: 230-9
22. Eltabbakh GH, Piver MS, Natarajan N *et al.* (1998) Epidemiologic differences between women with extraovarian primary peritoneal carcinoma and women with epithelial ovarian cancer. Obstet Gynecol 91: 254-9
23. Fowler JM, Nieberg RK, Schooler TA *et al.* (1994) Peritoneal adenocarcinoma (serous) of müllerian type: a subgroup of women presenting with peritoneal carcinomatosis. Int J Gynecol Cancer 4: 43-51
24. Fox H (1993) Primary neoplasia of the female peritoneum. Histopathol 23: 103-10
25. Fromm GL, Gershenson DM, Silva EG (1990) Papillary serous carcinoma of the peritoneum. Obstet Gynecol 75: 89-95
26. Halperin R, Zehavi S, Langer R *et al.* (2001) Primary peritoneal serous papillary carcinoma: A new epidemiologic trend? A matched-case comparison with ovarian serous papillary cancer. Int J Gynecol Cancer 11: 403-8
27. Halperin R, Zehavi S, Hadas E *et al.* (2001) Immunohistochemical comparison of primary peritoneal and primary ovarian serous papillary carcinoma. Int J Gynecol Pathol 20: 341-5
28. Jaaback KS, Ludeman L, Clayton NL *et al.* (2006) Primary peritoneal carcinoma in a UK cancer center: comparison with advanced ovarian carcinoma over a 5-year period. Int J Gynecol Cancer 16 (Suppl 1): 123-8
29. Jaaback K (2006) Intraperitoneal chemotherapy for the initial management of primary epithelial ovarian cancer. Cochrane Database Syst Rev CD005340.
30. Kowalski LD, Kanbour AI, Price FV *et al.* (1997) A case-matched molecular comparison of extraovarian versus primary ovarian adenocarcinoma. Cancer 79: 1587-94
31. Lauchlan SC (1972) The secondary müllerian system. Obstet Gynecol Surv 27: 133-46
32. Levine DA, Argenta PA, Yee CJ *et al.* (2003) Fallopian tube and primary peritoneal carcinomas associated with BRCA mutations. J Clin Oncol 21: 4222-7
33. Markman M, Markman J, Webster K *et al.* (2004) Duration of response to second-line, platinum-based chemotherapy for ovarian cancer: implications for patient management and clinical trial design. J Clin Oncol 22: 3120-5

34. McGuire WP, Hoskins WJ, Brady MF *et al.* (1996) Cyclophosphamide and cisplatin compared with paclitaxel and cisplatin in patients with stage III and stage IV ovarian cancer. N Engl J Med 334: 1-6
35. Menczer J, Chetrit A, Barda G *et al.* (2003) Frequency of BRCA mutations in primary peritoneal carcinoma in Israeli Jewish women. Gynecol Oncol 88: 58-61
36. Morice P, Dubernard G, Rey A *et al.* (2003) Results of interval debulking surgery compared with primary debulking surgery in advanced stage ovarian cancer. J Am Coll Surg 197: 955-63
37. Muto MG, Welch WR, Chi-Ho Mok S *et al.* (1995) Evidence for a multifocal origin of papillary serous carcinoma of the peritoneum. Cancer Res 55: 490-2
38. Nam JH, Kim YM, Jung MH *et al.* (2006) Primary peritoneal carcinoma: experience with cytoreductive surgery and combination chemotherapy. Int J Gynecol Cancer 16: 23-8
39. Ordonez NG (2005) Value of estrogen and progesterone receptor immunostaining in distinguishing between peritoneal mesotheliomas and serous carcinomas. Hum Pathol 36: 1163-7
40. Ozols RF, Bundy BN, Greer BE *et al.* (2003) Phase III trial of carboplatin and paclitaxel compared with cisplatin and paclitaxel in patients with optimally resected stage III ovarian cancer: a Gynecologic Oncology Group study. J Clin Oncol 21: 3194-200
41. Park TW, Felix JC, Wright TC (1995) X chromosome inactivation and microsatellite instability in early and advanced bilateral ovarian carcinomas. Cancer Res 55: 4793-6
42. Piura B, Meirovitz M, Bartfeld M *et al.* (1998) Peritoneal papillary serous carcinoma: study of 15 cases and comparison with stage III-IV ovarian papillary serous carcinoma. J Surg Oncol 68: 173-8
43. Piver MS, Eltabbakh GH, Hempling RE *et al.* (1997) Two sequential studies for primary peritoneal carcinoma: induction with weekly cisplatin followed by either cisplatin-doxorubicin-cyclophosphamide or paclitaxel-cisplatin. Gynecol Oncol 67: 141-6
44. Piver MS, Jishi F, Tsukada Y *et al.* (1993) Primary peritoneal carcinoma after prophylactic oophorectomy in women with a family history of ovarian cancer. A report of the Gilda Radner familial ovarian cancer registry. Cancer 71: 2751-5
45. Ransom DT, Shreyaskumar R, Keeney GL *et al.* (1990) Papillary serous carcinoma of the peritoneum: a review of 33 cases treated with platin-based chemotherapy. Cancer 66: 1091-4
46. Roffers SD, Cheng Wu X, Hahn Johnson C *et al.* (2003) Incidence of extraovarian primary cancers in the United States, 1992-1997. Cancer 97: 2643-7
47. Russell P, Bannatyne PM, Solomon HJ *et al.* (1985) Multifocal tumorigenesis in the upper female genital tract – Implications for staging and management. Int J Gynecol Pathol 4: 192-210
48. Schmueli E, Leider-Trejo L, Schwartz I *et al.* (2001) Primary papillary serous carcinoma of the peritoneum in a man. Ann Oncol 12: 563-7
49. Schorge JO, Motu MG, Welch WR *et al.* (1998) Molecular evidence for multifocal papillary serous carcinoma of the peritoneum in patients with germline BRCA1 mutations. J Natl Cancer Inst 90: 841-5
50. Shah IA, Jayram L, Gani OS *et al.* (1998) Papillary serous carcinoma of the peritoneum in a man. a case report. Cancer 82: 860-6
51. Strnad CM, Grosh WW, Baxter J *et al.* (1989) Peritoneal carcinomatosis of unknown primary site in women. A distinctive subset of adenocarcinoma. Ann Intern Med 111: 213-7
52. Swerdlow M (1959) Mesothelioma of the pelvic peritoneum resembling papillary cystadenocarcinoma of the ovary: a case report. Am J Gynecol Obstet 77(1): 197-200
53. Tsao SW, Mok CH, Knapp RC *et al.* (1993) Molecular genetic evidence of a unifocal origin for human serous ovarian carcinomas. Gynecol Oncol 48: 5-10
54. Weir MM, Bell DA, Young RH (1998) Grade 1 peritoneal serous carcinomas: a report of 14 cases and comparison with 7 peritoneal serous psammocarcinomas and 19 peritoneal serous borderline tumors. Am J Surg Pathol 22: 849-62
55. World Health Organisation Clasification of Tumors. Tumors of the breast and female genital tract. Pathology and genetics. Lyon (France) 2003. Pages 113-197
56. Zhou J, Iwasa Y, Konishi I *et al.* (1995) Papillary serous carcinoma of the peritoneum in women: a clinicopathologic and immunohistochemical study. Cancer 76: 429-36

Uterine papillary serous carcinoma

3

V. Samouëlian, M.-C. Baranzelli and A. Lesoin[1]

Five Essential Points

1. *UPSC is a rare and unusually aggressive tumour with a poor prognosis due to early intra-abdominal and lymphatic spread, high recurrence rate and more frequent resistance to chemo- and radiotherapy.*
2. *Histological diagnosis, even on limited tissue samples such as biopsies, is essential.*
3. *Serum Ca125 in pre-operative evaluation and follow-up is useful.*
4. *Comprehensive surgical staging including total hysterectomy and bilateral salpingo-oophorectomy, peritoneal washings, multiple peritoneal biopsies, omentectomy, pelvic and para-aortic lymphadenectomies as well as aggressive cytoreduction in case of extra-uterine disease is recommended. If UPSC is diagnosed after hysterectomy, surgical restaging procedure, ideally by laparoscopy should be proposed.*
5. *UPSC requires surgery and adjuvant therapy in most cases. Several studies support the benefits of chemotherapy on overall survival and radiation on vaginal vault or pelvic recurrence. Prospective studies should help to clarify the modalities of adjuvant therapy.*

Introduction

Uterine papillary serous carcinoma (UPSC) was first identified as a distinct histological entity in 1981 by Lauchlan and Hendrickson [17, 22]. It represents up to 10% of all endometrial cancers [5, 11, 13, 28, 35] but accounts for 50% of the recurrences in patients diagnosed with disease thought to be confined to the uterus [15, 17]. It is an aggressive histological type of endometrial cancer with early intra-abdominal and lymphatic spread [11, 13, 28, 35], as observed in ovarian carcinomas. Therefore, a comprehensive surgical staging, optimal cytoreduction and adjuvant therapy are proposed to those women diagnosed with UPSC.

Clinical features (Table 1)

Endometrial cancer is the most prevalent of the gynecological malignancies. Based on etiological, clinical and biological features, they are classified into two types [2]. Type I uterine malignancy is represented by endometrioïd endometrial cancers. This pathological type accounts for about 80% of all endometrial carcinomas. It usually occurs among post-menopausal women with a history of hyperestrogenism, overweight, diabetes, hypertension and dyslipidemia. Atypical complex hyperplasia is generally associated. Often well or moderately differentiated, they typically have a good prognosis after appropriate therapy.

1. Acknowledgment: we thank Dr. Fabrice Norducci, Dr. Philippe Nickers and Dr. Éric Leblanc who contributed to this work.

3

Table 1 – Type I and type II endometrial carcinomas: clinical and pathological features.

Histological type	Endometrioid (Type I)	Papillary serous (Type II)
Incidence	Up to 80%	Up to 10%
Median age	59 years	70 years
Hyperestrogenism	Yes	No
Overweight	Yes	No
Stade I	80%	10%
Extrauterine disease	25-30%	70%
5 year survival	> 80%	50%
Adjacent endometrium	Hyperplasia	Atrophia
Precursor lesion	Atypical complex hyperplasia	EIC or ECIS*
ER / PR	Frequent	Possible
p53 mutation	Uncommon	Frequent
Microsatellite instability	Possible	Uncommon
k-RAS mutation	Possible	Uncommon
PTEN mutation	Possible	Uncommon

* EIC: endometrial intraepithelial carcinoma; ECIS: endometrial carcinoma *in situ*.
ER: estrogen receptor; PR: progesterone receptor.

Uterine papillary serous carcinoma (UPSC) and clear cell carcinomas belong to the type II endometrial carcinomas. UPSC represents up to 10% of all endometrial cancers [5, 11, 13, 28, 35]. It is still the second most common pathological type of endometrial cancer after the endometrioïd type.

Women with UPSC are non-obese and without hyperestrogenism. They are older and more likely black than patients with endometrial cancer [13]. A personal or familial history of breast cancer is reported in about 20% of UPSC cases [35]. Compared to endometrioïd tumours, UPSCs are more aggressive, have a higher propensity for extra-uterine spread and a poorer prognosis [13, 17, 22]. UPSC usually develops in an atrophic endometrium.

At the time of diagnosis, 50 to 70% of women with UPSC have extrauterine disease [10, 11, 13, 31, 38]. Depth of myometrial invasion is not predictive of disease outside the uterus. In a study by Goff *et al.*, lymph node metastases were found in 36% of women without myometrial invasion, in 50% with inner half myometrial invasion, and in 40% with outer half myometrial invasion. Intraperitoneal disease was found respectively in 43%, 37% and 35% [11]. In some UPSC patients, microscopic omental implants can be the only evidence of extrauterine disease [4, 39]. For this reason, "Stage I" UPSC can only be affirmed after comprehensive surgical staging. Olawaiye *et al.* showed that pre-operative serum Ca125 levels correlate with the stage of disease [29].

UPSC accounts for over 50% of all relapses and for most of the deaths caused by endometrial carcinomas [13, 17, 28, 35]. In the study of Kelly *et al.* (2005), 63% of surgical stage I women not receiving adjuvant therapy presented recurrence [19]. Five-year overall survival from type I endometrial cancers is higher than 80% [6, 13]. It is only about 50% when considering the type II cancers [5, 13, 35]. The main prognostic factors are age, surgical stage, lymph node status, presence of lymphatic/vascular space invasion (LVSI), and depth of myometrial invasion, [5, 12, 13, 35]. UPSC mixed with other histological types of endometrial carcinoma behave as pure UPSC [3, 8, 11, 19, 34].

Pathology (Table 1 & 2)

UPSC has specific pathological features. It resembles morphologically its ovarian counterpart. UPSC has a complex papillary architecture. The papillae fronds may be either short and densely fibrotic or thin and delicate. Usually the cells are detached and float in spaces between glands and papillae. Polyadenoïd structures may be found. Cells are rounded, often poorly differentiated with marked nuclear atypia. Hobnail cells are frequently observed. Clear cell, eosinophil polygonal cells and multinucleated cells are sometimes present. Mitoses, often abnormal, are numerous. Psammoma bodies are found in about 30% of cases. Nests of cells within the vascular spaces are frequent. The grading system is not applied to UPSCs which are, by definition, considered as high grade tumours. The adjacent endometrium is very often atrophic with endometrial intraepithelial carcinoma lesions [21].

As in other type II endometrial carcinomas, UPSCs usually do not express estrogen or progesterone receptors. In contrast to the usual situation in endometrioïd carcinoma, a strong immunoreactivity for p53 is observed in most cases of UPSC, as well as in the adjacent atrophic endometrium, reflecting a mutation on this tumour suppressor gene. Epidermal growth factor type II receptor (HER2) expression is frequent [32]. Microsatellite instability, mutations of k-RAS and PTEN are uncommon in UPSC [16, 18]. The different immunohistochemical profiles of endometrioïd and serous papillary endometrial carcinoma support the existence of different molecular pathways in their development [20]. The p53- driven model of carcinogenesis is responsible for the rapid development and progression of UPSC [26]. UPSC develops in an atrophic endometrium. A putative precursor lesion of UPSC is serous endometrial intraepithelial carcinoma (EIC) [1, 34], also called endometrial carcinoma in situ (ECIS) [36]. EIC or ECIS is characterized by a noninvasive replacement of benign endometrial surface and glandular epithelium (without myometrial or stromal invasion) by highly malignant cells that resemble those of the invasive UPSC [1, 34, 36].

Table 2 – Histological criteria.

Histological criteria of UPSC
1. Complex papillary architecture
2. Marked nuclear atypia
3. Hobnail cells
4. Numerous mitoses
5. Psammoma bodies in 30% of cases
6. Frequent p53 mutations
7. No expression of ER or PR
8. Unlike endometrioïd carcinoma, microsatellite instability, k-RAS and PTEN mutations are uncommon
9. High grade tumour by definition (no grading system applied)
10. Resembles microscopically papillary serous carcinoma of the ovary
11. Differential diagnoses: endometrial villoglandular carcinoma

Differential diagnosis with villoglandular carcinoma is important, because its prognosis is completely different: this carcinoma has a much better prognosis. In villoglandular carcinoma, cells look like endometrioïd carcinoma and lack high grade nuclear atypia. Moreover, the long papillary fronds do not harbour tufting and psammoma bodies are absent. These tumour cells usually express hormone receptors.

Management

Considering the rarity and the poor outcome of this pathological subtype of endometrial cancers, women diagnosed with UPSC should be referred to gynecologic oncologists for specific management. Mixed tumours with UPSC should be handled as pure UPSC.

Surgery: Staging, restaging, debulking surgery

Pre-operative assessment comprises abdominal and pelvic magnetic resonance imaging (MRI), serum Ca125 testing and anesthetic evaluation. Complete surgical staging, also referred to as comprehensive surgical staging, consists of total hysterectomy with bilateral salpingo-oophorectomy, pelvic and para-aortic lymph node dissection, omentectomy, peritoneal washings as well as multiple peritoneal biopsies [10, 19, 39]. UPSC staging should be similar to the procedure undertaken for patients with ovarian carcinoma. Pelvic and para-aortic lymph node dissection should be systematically performed as lymph node involvement is not correlated to myometrial invasion. Since microscopic omental implants sometimes represent the only evidence of extra-uterine disease, omentectomy should not be omitted [4, 19, 39]. If systematic comprehensive staging is not performed in UPSC patients, stage IV cases might be considered as stage I. About 65% of UPSC are diagnosed on pre-operative biopsy or after dilatation & curettage [8, 12]. When diagnosed after hysterectomy, patients should be surgically reassessed. Laparoscopic restaging can than be proposed. Laparoscopic retroperitoneal infrarenal para-aortic lymphadenectomy followed by transperitoneal pelvic lymph node dissection, omentectomy, peritoneal washings and multiple biopsies is a valuable option [23, 27, 30]. The laparoscopic approach has a lower morbidity than laparotomy [40, 41], allowing surgery in elderly patients. In case of preoperative MRI, suspected stage IA or IB, laparoscopic total hysterectomy, bilateral salpingo-oophorectomy, omentectomy, peritoneal and nodal staging is conceivable. In more advanced stages, UPSC patients should undergo debulking surgery by laparotomy with the aim of a complete surgery, as in ovarian carcinomas [10, 38].

Adjuvant chemotherapy and radiotherapy

Due to high risk of relapse, adjuvant therapy is often proposed in patients with UPSC. In the literature, many adjuvant therapies have been suggested, including abdominopelvic radiation, vaginal cuff radiation, chemotherapy and combinations of these. Due to the lack of randomized prospective trials, recommendations are still based on retrospective studies, some with a small number of patients and many with partially staged patients.

As in type I endometrial carcinomas, abdominopelvic radiation and vaginal cuff radiation are currently administrated. Although UPSC appears less radiosensitive than endometrioid endometrial carcinoma [25], radiation has been proven to reduce the risk of local recurrence [19]. It does not impact on overall survival. Thus, considering the high morbidity of vaginal vault or pelvic recurrence, the significant reduction of these recurrences with adjuvant radiation and the limited salvage options for patients with pelvic recurrence, adjuvant pelvic radiation should be considered in most cases of UPSC. High-dose rate vaginal cuff brachytherapy and pelvic radiation should be considered at all stages [12, 19]. Radiation extended to para-aortic nodes is indicated in patients with proven nodal involvement.

Several recent retrospective studies have reported improvement of survival with the addition of platinum-based chemotherapy after complete surgery [7, 14, 19, 37]. In a larger study, Kelly *et al.* described the experience of 74 patients with surgical stage I UPSC. Platinum-based chemotherapy improved the disease-free and overall survival and vaginal cuff radiation provided local control. The recurrence rate was reduced from 47% in patients without chemotherapy to 3% in those who received it. They concluded that most stage I UPSC, patients should be offered concomitant platinum-based chemotherapy and vaginal cuff radiation. Observation could be recommended in only stage IA UPSC patients with no residual uterine disease after hysterectomy [19]. Considering these studies, adjuvant platinum-based chemotherapy should be considered in most patients with UPSA, regardless of stage. The current regimen consisting of 6 cycles of paclitaxel (175 mg/m^2) and carboplatin (AUC 5) is usually well tolerated. In a phase II trial, Fields *et al.* reported the well-tolerated and efficacious regimen of radiation "sandwiched" between paclitaxel/platinum chemotherapy [9]. Nevertheless, hematologic toxicity may occur, especially when combining both chemotherapy and pelvic radiotherapy in elderly women.

Moreover, in the retrospective study of Golderg *et al.*, patients with gross residual disease or recurrence with no previous chemotherapy had a 37% response rate to platinum-based chemotherapy [12]. This is considerably lower than the response in ovarian carcinoma and representative of the moderate chemo-sensitivity of UPSC [24]. Other chemotherapies did not provide better results. New targeted therapies, against HER2 for example [33], may be available in the future. So far, optimal cytoreduction associated with chemotherapy should be undertaken as often as possible [38].

Conclusions

Considering these findings, all patients diagnosed with UPSC should undergo a complete surgical staging or restaging when pathological diagnosis is made on the hysterectomy sample. Adjuvant therapy including platinum based chemotherapy and radiation should then be offered. In order to improve our knowledge and understanding of this relatively rare disease, UPSC patients should be included in prospective studies. We expect much from the prospective PORTEC3 study, investigating adjuvant chemotherapy and radiotherapy in type II endometrial carcinomas.

References

1. Ambros RA, Sherman ME, Zahn CM *et al.* (1995) Endometrial intraepithelial carcinoma: a distinctive lesion specifically associated with tumors displaying serous differentiation. Hum Pathol 26(11): 1260-7

3

2. Bokhman JV (1983) Two pathogenetic types of endometrial carcinoma. Gynecol Oncol 15(1): 10-7
3. Carcangiu ML, Chambers JT (1992) Uterine papillary serous carcinoma: a study on 108 cases with emphasis on the prognostic significance of associated endometrioid carcinoma, absence of invasion, and concomitant ovarian carcinoma. Gynecol Oncol. 47(3): 298-305
4. Chan JK, Loizzi V, Youssef M *et al.* (2003) Significance of comprehensive surgical staging in noninvasive papillary serous carcinoma of the endometrium. Gynecol Oncol 90(1): 181-5
5. Cirisano FD, Jr., Robboy SJ, Dodge RK *et al.* (2000) The outcome of stage I-II clinically and surgically staged papillary serous and clear cell endometrial cancers when compared with endometrioid carcinoma. Gynecol Oncol 77(1): 55-65
6. Creasman WT, Odicino F, Maisonneuve P *et al.* (2001) Carcinoma of the corpus uteri. J Epidemiol Biostat 6(1): 47-86
7. Dietrich CS, 3rd, Modesitt SC, DePriest PD *et al.* (2005) The efficacy of adjuvant platinum-based chemotherapy in Stage I uterine papillary serous carcinoma (UPSC). Gynecol Oncol 99(3): 557-63
8. Faratian D, Stillie A, Busby-Earle RM *et al.* (2006) A review of the pathology and management of uterine papillary serous carcinoma and correlation with outcome. Int J Gynecol Cancer 16(3): 972-8
9. Fields AL, Einstein MH, Novetsky AP *et al.* (2008) Pilot phase II trial of radiation "sandwiched" between combination paclitaxel/platinum chemotherapy in patients with uterine papillary serous carcinoma (UPSC). Gynecol Oncol 108(1): 201-6
10. Geisler JP, Geisler HE, Melton ME, Wiemann MC (1999) What staging surgery should be performed on patients with uterine papillary serous carcinoma? Gynecol Oncol 74(3): 465-7
11. **Goff BA, Kato D, Schmidt RA, Ek M *et al.* (1994) Uterine papillary serous carcinoma: patterns of metastatic spread. Gynecol Oncol 54(3): 264-8**
12. Goldberg H, Miller RC, Abdah-Bortnyak R *et al.* (2008) Outcome after combined modality treatment for uterine papillary serous carcinoma: a study by the Rare Cancer Network (RCN). Gynecol Oncol 108(2): 298-305
13. **Hamilton CA, Cheung MK, Osann K *et al.* (2006) Uterine papillary serous and clear cell carcinomas predict for poorer survival compared to grade 3 endometrioid corpus cancers. Br J Cancer 94(5): 642-6**
14. Hamilton CA, Cheung MK, Osann K *et al.* (2006) The effect of adjuvant chemotherapy versus whole abdominopelvic radiation on the survival of patients with advanced stage uterine papillary serous carcinoma. Gynecol Oncol. 103(2): 679-83
15. Havrilesky LJ, Secord AA, Bae-Jump V *et al.* (2007) Outcomes in surgical stage I uterine papillary serous carcinoma. Gynecol Oncol 105(3): 677-82
16. Hecht JL, Mutter GL (2006) Molecular and pathologic aspects of endometrial carcinogenesis. J Clin Oncol 24(29): 4783-91
17. Hendrickson M, Ross J, Eifel P *et al.* (1982) Uterine papillary serous carcinoma: a highly malignant form of endometrial adenocarcinoma. Am J Surg Pathol 6(2): 93-108
18. Kanaya T, Kyo S, Maida Y *et al.* (2003) Frequent hypermethylation of MLH1 promoter in normal endometrium of patients with endometrial cancers. Oncogene 22(15): 2352-60
19. **Kelly MG, O'Malley D M, Hui P *et al.* (2005) Improved survival in surgical stage I patients with uterine papillary serous carcinoma (UPSC) treated with adjuvant platinum-based chemotherapy. Gynecol Oncol 98(3): 353-9**
20. Kounelis S, Kapranos N, Kouri E *et al.* (2000) Immunohistochemical profile of endometrial adenocarcinoma: a study of 61 cases and review of the literature. Mod Pathol 13(4): 379-88
21. Kurman RJ, Zaino RJ, Norris HJ (1994) Endometrial Carcinoma. In: Kurman RJ (4th ed) Blaustein's Pathology of the Female Genital Tract. Springer-Verlag, New York, p 439
22. Lauchlan SC. (1981) Tubal (serous) carcinoma of the endometrium. Arch Pathol Lab Med 105(11): 615-8
23. Leblanc E, Narducci F, Frumovitz M *et al.* (2007) Therapeutic value of pretherapeutic extraperitoneal laparoscopic staging of locally advanced cervical carcinoma. Gynecol Oncol 105(2): 304-11

24. Levenback C, Burke TW, Silva E *et al.* (1992) Uterine papillary serous carcinoma (UPSC) treated with cisplatin, doxorubicin, and cyclophosphamide (PAC). Gynecol Oncol 46(3): 317-21
25. Martin JD, Gilks B, Lim P (2005) Papillary serous carcinoma – a less radio-sensitive subtype of endometrial cancer. Gynecol Oncol 98(2): 299-303
26. Moll UM, Chalas E, Auguste M *et al.* (1996) Uterine papillary serous carcinoma evolves via a p53-driven pathway. Hum Pathol 27(12): 1295-300
27. Nicklin JL, Copeland LJ (1996) Endometrial papillary serous carcinoma: patterns of spread and treatment. Clin Obstet Gynecol 39(3): 686-95
28. Morice P, Leblanc E, Rey A *et al.* (2005) Conservative treatment in epithelial ovarian cancer: results of a multicentre study of the GCCLCC (Groupe des Chirurgiens de Centre de Lutte Contre le Cancer) and SFOG (Societe Francaise d'Oncologie Gynecologique). Hum Reprod 20(5): 1379-85
29. Olawaiye AB, Rauh-Hain JA, Withiam-Leitch M *et al.* (2008) Utility of pre-operative serum CA-125 in the management of uterine papillary serous carcinoma. Gynecol Oncol 110(3): 293-8
30. Querleu D, Leblanc E, Cartron G *et al.* (2006) Audit of preoperative and early complications of laparoscopic lymph node dissection in 1,000 gynecologic cancer patients. Am J Obstet Gynecol 195(5): 1287-92
31. Sagr ER, Denschlag D, Kerim-Dikeni A *et al.* (2007) Prognostic factors and treatment-related outcome in patients with uterine papillary serous carcinoma. Anticancer Res 27(2): 1213-7
32. Santin AD, Bellone S, Van Stedum S *et al.* 2005 Amplification of c-erbB2 oncogene: a major prognostic indicator in uterine serous papillary carcinoma. Cancer. 104(7): 1391-7
33. Santin AD, Zhan F, Cane S *et al.* (2005) Gene expression fingerprint of uterine serous papillary carcinoma: identification of novel molecular markers for uterine serous cancer diagnosis and therapy. Br J Cancer 92(8): 1561-73
34. Sherman ME, Bitterman P, Rosenshein NB *et al.* (1992) Uterine serous carcinoma. A morphologically diverse neoplasm with unifying clinicopathologic features. Am J Surg Pathol 16(6): 600-10
35. Slomovitz BM, Burke TW, Eifel PJ *et al.* (2003) Uterine papillary serous carcinoma (UPSC): a single institution review of 129 cases. Gynecol Oncol 91(3): 463-9
36. Spiegel GW (1995) Endometrial carcinoma in situ in postmenopausal women. Am J Surg Pathol 19(4): 417-32
37. Steed H, Manchul L, Rosen B *et al.* (2006) Uterine papillary serous carcinoma: evaluation of multimodality treatment with abdominopelvic radiotherapy and chemotherapy. Int J Gynecol Cancer 16 Suppl 1: 278-85
38. **Thomas MB, Mariani A, Cliby WA *et al.* (2007) Role of cytoreduction in stage III and IV uterine papillary serous carcinoma. Gynecol Oncol 107(2): 190-3**
39. **Thomas MB, Mariani A, Cliby WA *et al.* (2007) Role of systematic lymphadenectomy and adjuvant therapy in stage I uterine papillary serous carcinoma. Gynecol Oncol 107(2): 186-9**
40. Tozzi R, Malur S, Koehler C, Schneider A (2005) Laparoscopy versus laparotomy in endometrial cancer: first analysis of survival of a randomized prospective study. J Minim Invasive Gynecol 12(2): 130-6
41. Zullo F, Palomba S, Russo T *et al.* (????) A prospective randomized comparison between laparoscopic and laparotomic approaches in women with early stage endometrial cancer: a focus on the quality of life. Am J Obstet Gynecol. 193(4): 1344-52

Uterine sarcomas and rare endometrial carcinomas

4

H. Boussen, K. Rahal and N. Bouaouina

Five Essential Points

1. *US are rare tumours compared to the classical endometrial adenocarcinomas, representing less than 10% of uterine malignancies.*
2. *They occur at an age of 5 to 10 years younger than with endometrial adenocarcinomas.*
3. *US are associated like others sarcomas to a high metastatic (lungs and liver) and loco-regional risk of relapse.*
4. *US are more chemosensitive than endometrial carcinomas in regimes with anthracyclins and alkylating agents*
5. *US remain associated to a poor prognosis (less than 50% overall survival) compared to their carcinomatous counterpart.*

Introduction

More than 95% of cancers of the uterus are carcinomas and uterine sarcomas (US) represent less than 1% of gynecologic cancers and 3% to 8% of all uterine malignancies [17]. Three main types of US are recognized: malignant mixed Müllerian tumour (MMT), recently known as carcinosarcoma, endometrial stromal sarcoma (ESS), leiomyosarcoma (LMS) and a small cohort of unclassifiable high-grade tumours with sarcomatous elements [16]. LMS is observed in women of perimenopausal age, while carcinosarcoma (CS) and ESS occurs in postmenopausal women [4]. CS is associated with a high incidence of lymphatic spread, while LMS is linked with an early metastatic risk to lungs and liver [9,10]. Surgical management of US is based on a minimum of abdominal hysterectomy, bilateral salpingo-oophorectomy, careful inspection of the abdominal and pelvic contents, cytology of peritoneal washings and pelvic and/or para-aortic lymph node dissection [2]. Radiation therapy, chemotherapy, hormonal therapy and recently, biological or molecular targeted anticancer agents are used in the adjuvant or palliative setting (5, 15, 24, 30]). Adjuvant chemotherapy or radiation therapy remains however the subject of controversy, despite some prospective trials in resected stage I or II [15].

Epidemiology (Table 1)

Uterine sarcomas (US) are rare tumours that represent 3-8% of all invasive uterine cancers and have an annual incidence lower than 2 per 100,000 females and according to Olah [20], there is one US for every 11 adenocarcinoma cases [14, 16, 17]. Harlow *et al.* [11] reported an increased incidence of leiomyosarcoma (LMS) and

Table 1 – Epidemiology and histologic types of US.

Author	N	MA yrs	LMS	MMT	ESSI	Stage			
						I	II	III	IV
Livi [16]	52	55 (18-83)	47	30	19	50	11	21	18
Denschlag [8]	94	60 (20-93)	30	36	28	49	7	20	18
Benoit [3]	72	60.5 (33-91)	34	25	12	37	8	27	
Yoney [31]	105	50 (24-87)	43.8	27.6	28.6	55.2	13.3	19	

Abbreviations: MA: median age; LMS: leiomyosarcoma; MMT: malignant mixed Mullerian tumours; ESS: endometrial stromal sarcomas.

mixed mesodermal sarcoma (MMS) for in the African American population in comparison to caucasians. The Surveillance, Epidemiology, and End Results (SEER) studies aimed at determining the demographic characteristics, histological distribution, patterns of treatment, and survival in women with uterine sarcoma are of interest [4]. Their data concerned 2,677 women affected by US, 2,098 (78%) of whom were caucasian and 420 (16%) of whom were African American, from 1989-1999 and showed an overall age-adjusted incidence twice as high for African American. The overall age-adjusted incidence for African American women was twice that of caucasians and more than twice that of women of other races (7/105 *vs.* 3.6/105 *vs.* 2.7/105 with $p < 0.0001$). The etiology of US remains unknown, except in cases of prior pelvic radiation, administered for benign uterine bleeding 5 to 25 years earlier or long-term use of tamoxifen for breast cancer [7, 11]. The median age of US is around 50-65 years, while it is 50-55 years for LMS, 10 years younger than for patients with MMT [4]. Racial differences in the incidence of US existed for LMS ($1.51/10^5$ for African American *vs.* $0.91/10^5$ for caucasians *vs* 0.89 for women of other races ($p < 0.01$) and CS($4.3/10^5$) for African American *vs.* $1.7/10^5$ for caucasians, and 0.99 for women of other races with $p < 0.001$ [4].

Histology (Tables 1 and 2)

Increasingly, carcinosarcomas are recognised as no longer being true sarcomas, reflecting their probable epithelial origin and clinicopathological behaviour (Table 1). US derives from constitutional mesenchymatous elements of the uterine corpus such as the endometrial stroma and smooth muscle. The Gynecologic Oncology

Table 2 – Histologic classification of uterine sarcoma.

Old classification	New classification
Carcinosarcomas (MMMT)	Metaplastic carcinomas
Endometrial stromal sarcomas	Low grade High grade
Leiomyosarcomas	
Undifferentiated or unclassifiable	High grade

Abbreviation: MMT = malignant mixed Mullerian tumour.

Group (GOG) classifies these tumours into two categories: non-epithelial and mixed epithelial-non-epithelial. A second system was developed by the International Society of Gynecologic Pathologists and the World Health Organization, classifying US according to whether the tumour is purely nonepithelial or mixed epithelial-nonepithelial [18]. US can be separated into high-grade leiomyosarcomas (LMS), undifferentiated endometrial sarcomas, stromal sarcomas (ESS) and CS, covering all mixed Müllerian tumours (MMT) in the WHO classification [18]. The second group previously included low-grade endometrial stromal sarcomas and adenosarcomas. A new recent histological classification is currently used (Table 2). For a more accurate diagnosis, pathologic exam should include immunocytochemistry for differential diagnosis and LMS can be reviewed due its differential diagnosis with a gastrointestinal LMS stromal tumour requiring assessment for c-kit. Genetic differences observed indicate that myomas and leiomyosarcomas have distinct origins and leiomyosarcomas do not result from malignant degeneration of myomas [23]. LMS are frequently undifferentiated and associated to complex chromosomal rearrangements and aneuploid karyotypes [23]. Other types of US such as angiosarcomas, rhabdomyosarcomas and malignant fibrous histiocytomas are rarer and not specific to the uterine site.

Prognosis

Prognostic factors and survival of US (Table 3)

Due to the aggressive nature of US, prognosis remains poor with an overall survival of less than 50% at 2 years, even for early stage disease [4, 6, 4, 15, 17]. The main prognostic factors are histologic type, grade, stage and age [4, 14, 17]. In a review

Table 3 – Prognostic factors in US. Literature review.

	3 years	5 years	10 years	Prognostic factors
Livi [16]	39%	30%	20%	HG (p = 0.04), G (p = 0.003), Stage (p = 0.002), Age (p = 0.001) MMT < LMS < ESS DR at 3 years of 82%, 60% and 20% (HG, IG, LG) DR at 3 years of 44%, 55%, 67% and 95% (S I to IV)
Brooks [4]		53% (W) 42% (BA) 49% (O)		Adenosarcoma > Other types Combined S-RT < S alone (II to IV) Stage Race (B *vs* W)
Chauveinc [6]		45%	28%	For OS= HG (p = 0.001, Men (p < 0.003) RT → better local control (p < 0.005) CT → non significant MA → High HG, high FIGO stages, LMS, and Menop RT and ESS → better local control HG and LMS → more metastases
Denschlag [8]		47%		5 years OK, ESS (82%) *vs* MMT (40%) p < 0.0001 OS associated with age OS and ESS (p = 0.004) Adjuvant RT for MMT → p = 0.003 MA → Age and stage significant for OS in LMS or MMT

Abbreviations:
MA : Multivariate Analysis; HG : Histologic grade; S :Surgery; RT : Radiotherapy; CT : Chemotherapy; BA : Black African; W : White; MA : Multivariate analysis.

of about 1,396 cases of LMS, 5-year overall survival ranged from 29 to 67.4%, close to 65% for the recent cohort of patients [15]. Other important prognostic factors are age (menopausal status), mitotic index and p53 expression [4, 7]. Among the series of LMS reported by Kapp, prognosis is related to age, race, stage, grade and quality of primary surgery [15].

Treatment

Complete tumour resection is the optimal primary treatment for patients with US and can be curative when the tumour is confined to the uterus [5, 14, 15]. Surgery should include total abdominal hysterectomy, bilateral salpingo-oophorectomy, careful inspection of the abdomino-pelvic contents, cytology of peritoneal washings and pelvic and/or para-aortic lymph node dissection (PLND).

Radiotherapy is frequently used in the adjuvant setting, especially in stages I and II, early cases.

The EORTC study concerned 224 patients with LMS and CS, and showed no survival benefit for adjuvant radiotherapy, despite a trend for those with CS, without a survival advantage [24]. For CS, local control was 61% *vs.* 47% and for leiomyosarcoma 44% *vs.* 53%, while progression-free survival (PFS) was 6.2 years *vs.* 4.9 years and overall survival 8.5 years *vs.* 6.8 years [24].

Adjuvant chemotherapy with doxorubicin or ifosfamide has been also tested in the 1980's by the Gynecologic Oncology Group (GOG) and despite a reduction of the recurrence risk, no survival benefit was reported [27]. Another large study by the UK Medical Research Council concerned adjuvant chemotherapy in soft tissue sarcomas, including 264 US (17% of the total) and failed to show any evident benefit of adjuvant chemotherapy in sarcomas [29]. More recently a combined adjuvant radio- and chemotherapy regimen has been used with three cycles of cisplatin/doxorubicin/ifosfamide followed by external radiotherapy. This has shown a significant benefit compared to radiation alone with 76% *vs.* 43% PFS and 100% *vs.* 76% 5-year overall survival [21]. In recurrent disease, the most active agents are the anthracyclines, the platinum compounds, dacarbazine, taxanes and ifosfamide. In 1998, the GOG sudy demonstrated a better response rate (54%) for ifosfamide and cisplatin *vs.* 36% for ifosfamide alone [28]. A recent phase III trial of ifosfamide *vs.* ifosfamide and paclitaxel carried out by the GOG, reported a small advantage with the combination approach [13]. The combination of docetaxel and gemcitabine has been tested at the Memorial Sloan Kettering Cancer Centre in previously-treated patients, showing a 53% response rate in 34 patients including 29 with LMS [12]. Future treatment options are represented by Ecteinascidin/trabectedin (Yondelis or ET743) which is however not yet licensed for routine use [27]. New targeted agents are under further investigation in clinical trials [25].

Rare endometrial cancers

Excluding the most common endometrial cancer, the non-endometrioid histologies are papillary serous (10%), clear cell (2% to 4%), mucinous (0.6% to 5%) and squamous cell representing 0.1% to 0.5% of uterine cancers [19]. Primitive neuroectodermal tumours (PNET) arising from Kulchitsky cells are more rare [1]. Small cell carcinomas remain an exceptional situation with a poor prognosis due to the high risk of loco-regional and distant failures despite treatment by surgery and chemo-radiotherapy [22].

References

1. Akbayir O, Güngördük K, Rafio lu G *et al.* (2008) Primary primitive neuroectodermal tumor of the uterus: a case report. Arch Gynecol Obstet 277: 345-8
2. Amant F (2005) The rationale for comprehensive surgical staging in endometrial carcinosarcoma. Gynecol Oncol 99: 521-2
3. Benoit L, Arnould L, Cheynel N *et al.* (2005) The role of surgery and treatment trends in uterine sarcoma. Eur J Surg Oncol 31:434-42
4. **Brooks SE, Min Zhan B, Cote TC, Baquet C (2004) Surveillance, Epidemiology, and End Results analysis of 2677 cases of uterine sarcoma 1989-1999. Gynecol Oncol 93: 204-8**
5. **Chan JK, Wu H, Cheung MK *et al.* (2007) The outcomes of 27,063 women with unstaged endometrioid uterine cancer. Gynecol Oncol 106: 282-8**
6. Chauveinc L, Deniaud E, Plancher C *et al.* (1999) Uterine Sarcomas: The Curie Institut Experience. Prognosis Factors and Adjuvant Treatments. Gynecologic Oncol 72: 232-7
7. Curtis R, Freedman DM, Sherman ME, Fraumeni JF. (2004) Risk of malignant mixed mullerian tumors after tamoxifen therapy for breast cancer. J Natl Cancer Inst 96: 70-2
8. **Denschlag D, Masoud I, Stanimir G, Gilbert L (2007) Prognostic factors and outcome in women with uterine sarcoma. Eur J Surg Oncol 33: 91-5**
9. **Gadducci A, Cosio S, Romanini A, Genazzani AR (2008) The management of patients with uterine sarcoma: A debated clinical challenge. Critical Reviews in Oncology/Hematology 65: 129-42**
10. George M, Pejovic MH, Kramar A (1986) Gynecologic Cooperating Group of French Oncology Centers. Uterine sarcomas: prognostic factors and treatment modalities study on 209 patients. Gynecol Oncol 24: 58-67
11. Harlow B, Weiss N, Lofton S (1986) The epidemiology of sarcomas of the uterus. J Nat Cancer Inst 76: 399-402
12. Hensley ML, Maki R, Venkatraman E *et al.* (2002) Gemcitabine and docetaxel in patients with unresectable leiomyosarcoma: results of a phase II trial. J Clin Oncol 12: 2824-31
13. Homesley H, Filiaci G, Markman M *et al.* (2007) Phase III trial of ifosfamide with or without paclitaxel in advanced uterine carcinosarcoma: a Gynecologic Oncology Group study. J Clin Oncol 25: 526-31
14. Kapp DS, Shin JY, Chan JK (2008) Prognostic factors and survival in 1396 patients with uterine leiomyosarcomas. Emphasis on impact of lymphadenectomy and oophorectomy. Cancer 112: 820-30
15. Kong A, Johnson N, Cornes P *et al.* (2007) Adjuvant radiotherapy for stage I endometrial cancer. Available from: http://thecochranelibrary.com
16. Livi L, Andreopoulou E, Shah N *et al.* (2004) Treatment of uterine sarcoma at the Royal Marsden Hospital from 1974 to 1998. Clin Oncol (R Coll Radiol) 16: 261
17. Marchese MJ, Liskow AS, Crum CP *et al.* (1984) Uterine sarcomas: a clinicopathologic study, 1965 to 1981. Gynecol Oncol 18: 299.
18. Moinfar F, Azodi M, Tavassoli FA (2007) Uterine sarcomas. Pathology 39: 55-71
19. Mendivil A, Schuler KM, Gehrig PA (2009) Non-endometrioid adenocarcinoma of the uterine corpus: a review of selected histological subtypes. Cancer Control 16: 46-52
20. Olah KS, Dunn JA, Gee H (1992) Leiomyosarcomas have a poorer prognosis than mixed mesodermal tumours when adjusting for known prognostic factors: the result of a retrospective study of 423 cases of uterine sarcoma. Br J Obstet Gynaecol 99: 590
21. Pautier P, Rey A, Haie-Meder C *et al.* (2004) Adjuvant chemotherapy with cisplatin, ifosfamide, and doxorubicin followed by radiotherapy in localised uterine sarcomas: results of a casecontrolled study with radiotherapy alone. Int J Gynecol Cancer 14: 1112-7
22. Petru E, Pasterk C, Reich O *et al.* (2005) Small-cell carcinoma of the uterus and the vagina: experience with ten patients. Arch Gynecol Obstet 271: 316-9
23. Quade BJ, Wang TY, Sornberger K *et al.* (2004) Molecular pathogenesis of uterine smooth muscle tumors from transcriptional profiling. Genes Chromosomes Cancer 40: 97-108
24. Reed NS, Mangioni C, Malmstrom H *et al.* (2003) First results of a randomised trial comparing radiotherapy versus observation postoperatively in patients with uterine sarcomas, an EORTC GCG study. ESGO Congress. Int J Gynecol Cancer 13: 4

4

25. **Reed NS (2008) The Management of Uterine Sarcomas. Clinical Oncology 20: 470-8**
26. Schöffski P, Wolter P, Clement P *et al.* (2007) Trabectedin (ET-743): evaluation of its use in advanced soft-tissue sarcoma. Future Oncol 3: 381-92
27. Sutton GP, Blessing JA, Rosenshein N *et al.* (1989) Phase II trial of ifosfamide and mesna in mixed mesodermal tumors of the uterus (A Gynecologic Oncology Group study). Am J Obstet Gynecol 161: 309-15
28. Sutton G, Brunetto VL, Kilgore L *et al.* (2000) A phase III trial of ifosfamide with or without cisplatin in carcinosarcoma of the uterus: a Gynecologic Oncology Group study. Gynecol Oncol 79: 147-53
29. Tierney JF, Mosseri V, Stewart LA *et al.* (1995) Adjuvant chemotherapy for soft-tissue sarcoma: review and meta-analysis of the published results of randomised clinical trials. Br J Cancer 72: 469-75
30. Wolfson AH, Brady MF, Rocereto TF *et al.* (2007) A Gynecologic Oncology Group randomized trial of whole abdominal irradiation (WAI) *vs.* cisplatine-ifosfamide and mesna (CIM) as post surgical therapy in stage I-IV carcinosarcoma (CS) of the uterus. Gynecol Oncol 107: 177-85
31. Yoney A, Eren B, Eskici S *et al.* (2008) Retrospective analysis of 105 cases with uterine sarcomas. Bull Cancer 95: 1-8 (electronic)

Rare tumours of the uterine cervix

5

H. Lamallem, A. Toledano and P.G. Tsoutsou

Five Essential Points

1. Small cell cancer or neuroendocrine tumours of the cervix: *Conventional treatment is radical hysterectomy and bilateral pelvic and para-aortic lymphadenectomy, but a multimodality approach is also necessary. Distant metastasis is common, so the small cell lung cancer chemotherapy regimens, such as VAC/PE are beneficiary.*
2. Clear cell carcinoma: *Consists of 4% of adenocarcinomas. Most common in women exposed in utero to DES. Treatment is either radical hysterectomy with vaginectomy or radiotherapy. Prognosis of early tumours is no worse than squamous cell carcinoma but distant metastasis more common. Low risk patients can be spared radiotherapy.*
3. Sarcomas:
   Carcinosarcomas: *occur in post-menopausal women and tend to have early lymphatic spread.* Rhabdomyosarcomas: *occur in childhood mainly in the vagina. Suggested treatment is surgery and adjuvant chemotherapy.*
   Leiomyosarcomas: *occur in perimenopausal women and metastasize by haematogenous spread.*
4. Melanoma and Lymphomas: *A metastatic melanoma to the cervix has to be excluded. Bears very poor prognosis. Radical surgery (hysterectomy, salpingo-oophorectomy and retroperitoneal pelvic lymphadenectomy) followed by adjuvant radiotherapy is proposed.*
   Lymphoma and Leukaemia: *Very rare presence of extranodal lymphomas in the cervix, in women around 40 years old. Most stage IE with pelvic and paraaortic lymph node involvement: prognosis remains favourable, proposed treatment consists of CHOP and involved field radiotherapy.*
5. Adenoid cystic carcinoma: *consists of less than 1% of adenocarcinomas, most common in non-white patients. Bears a high risk of local recurrence and distant metastasis and should be treated as squamous cell carcinoma.*

Introduction

In 2008, only in the United States, there were 11,070 estimated new cases of invasive cancer of the uterine cervix. Over the last decades, there has been a decrease in the incidence and mortality in developed countries, whereas cervical cancer remains the second most frequent cause of cancer-related morbidity and mortality in developing countries; this discrepancy being largely due to the widespread implementation of cervical cancer prevention programs in the former.

Based on the SEER data, squamous cell carcinomas account for 70% of all cervical cancers, whereas adenocarcinomas (mucinous, endometrioid, clear cell, serous type) account for 25% and adenosquamous carcinomas for 3 to 5% of all cervical cancers, respectively. Neuroendocrine or small cell carcinomas originating in the cervix, primary lymphomas and sarcomas are rare tumours.

For each of these diseases, some general features and pathology characteristics will be examined first and then a therapeutic management will be proposed. Since in the literature only case reports and reviews with no data from clinical trials can be found, the standard of care has not been defined for these diseases.

Small cell carcinomas or neuroendocrine carcinomas

General features and pathology

Small cell carcinoma or neuroendocrine carcinoma is rare but aggressive. Small cell carcinoma represents 2 to 5 percent of all cervical carcinomas. In the US, between 1977 and 2003 the mean annual incidence was 0.06 per 100 000 women, compared with 6.6 and 1.2 for squamous cell carcinoma and adenocarcinoma [9]. The five-year survival rate (35.7%) was worse than squamous carcinoma (60.5%) and adenocarcinoma (69.7%). Neuroendocrine cervical cancer is considered to be an extrapulmonary variant of pulmonary small cell cancer. The cervix should always be considered as the site of origin in a woman with a neuroendocrine or small cell carcinoma of unknown primary site. Patients are the same age as, or younger than, women with ordinary forms of invasive cervical carcinoma. Noted for its aggressive behaviour [14,30,39,40] small cell carcinoma is occasionally associated with polypeptide hormone production. A few para-endocrine syndromes have been reported in association with small cell carcinomas of the cervix, including Cushing's syndrome [20] carcinoid syndrome, and Eaton-Lambert myasthenic syndrome [34]. Ectopic secretion of ADH, insulin, and calcitonin have also been described, but it has not been possible to determine whether the carcinomas responsible for that were small cell carcinomas, squamous cell carcinomas composed of small cells, or poorly-differentiated adenocarcinomas with carcinoid features. Although human papillomavirus type 18 has been found in most of the small cell carcinomas with endocrine granules, type 16 has also been reported [2].

Small cell carcinoma is composed of a uniform population of small cells with a high nucleus-cytoplasm ratio resembling small cell carcinoma (oat cell carcinoma) of the lung. It is highly cellular, composed of sheets of densely packed small cells with scant cytoplasm, and is identical to its counterpart in the vagina. In some examples, minor areas of glandular or squamous differentiation occur, but these, by definition, are less than 5 percent of the tumour. Nuclei are round-to-oval or slightly spindle-shaped and densely hyperchromatic to the degree that nucleoli are inconspicuous and the nuclei appear smudged, therefore obscuring nuclear detail. The cytoplasm is scant and finely stippled. Cell outlines, like the nuclei, are spindle to oval shaped. A few pleomorphic larger cells with more irregular nuclei and one or more nucleoli may be present. Mitotic activity is prominent, with three or more mitotic figures usually evident in each high-power field. Areas of necrosis are common. Capillary space invasion is observed in 60 to 90 percent of cases [39,40].

Nearly all neoplasms stain immunohistochemically for keratin. About one third to one half stain positively for one or more markers for endocrine granules such as chromogranin, serotonin, or somatostatin [37,40]. Neuron-specific enolase is too nonspecific to be a reliable marker for endocrine cells, since nearly all small cell carcinomas stain for it. In one study of 10 small cell carcinomas of the cervix that were positive with neuron-specific enolase, argyrophilia was evident in only 3 of 10, chromogranin immunostaining was positive in half, and serotonin positivity was evident in only 2 of 10. Immunostains for neurofilaments were negative [40]. Other investigators report an even higher degree of immunostaining for neuroendocrine granules [4].

Therapeutic management

The most usual treatment is radical hysterectomy and bilateral pelvic and para-aortic lymphadenectomy. As already mentioned, most published series contain only a few patients. Survival is poor with hysterectomy alone, but no optimal management has been described. A multimodality approach is probably necessary. Pelvic radiation is given to patients with nodal metastasis. Metastasis occurs relatively early and frequently in the course of the disease, compared with ordinary cervical carcinoma. Lymph node metastasis is present in more than half of the patients with small cell carcinomas less than 2 cm in diameter and in a higher proportion of those with larger lesions [39,40]. At least 40 percent of patients with stage I and II disease later present with a recurrence, compared to about 30 percent of patients with other forms of cervical carcinoma of the same stages [40]. Distant metastasis to lung, liver, brain, and bone is common. The small cell lung cancer chemotherapy regimens are mainly used in that situation.

In a series of 23 patients treated by radical hysterectomy, they received adjuvant chemotherapy with either PVB (cisplatin, vincristin, bleomycine) or VAC/PE (vincristine, doxorubicin, cyclophosphamide alternating with cisplatin and etoposide). At a median follow up of 41 months, 10/14 patients receiving VAC/PE were alive as compared to only 3/9 with PVB [8].

Another series reported the outcome and pattern of failure of 21 patients with neuroendocrine marker-positive small cell carcinoma of the uterine cervix treated locally with either surgery [34] or radiation therapy [10] and systemically with chemotherapy (cisplatin, doxorubicin and etoposide). The five-year overall survival rate was 29% with a mean time to first relapse of 8.4 months. None of the women with more extensive disease than stage IB1 survived for more than 30 months. Twelve of 14 relapses consisted of distant haematogenous metastases [41].

Glassy cell carcinoma

General features and pathology

Glassy cell carcinoma accounts for only 1 to 2 percent of all cervical carcinomas [22] but as much as 10 percent of adenocarcinomas [33]. First recognized by Cherry and Glucksmann [10] who classified it within the group of mixed (adenosquamous) carcinomas, it occurs in patients with a younger mean age (31-41 years) than patients with squamous cell or ordinary adenocarcinoma of the cervix, and has been associated with pregnancy in an unexpected number of cases in early reports, but not in more recent series.

This is a poorly differentiated carcinoma characterized by sheets of cells having a moderate amount of cytoplasm with a ground-glass or granular appearance, a distinct cytoplasmic membrane, and a large nucleus containing prominent single or multiple nucleoli. Low degrees of keratinisation, infrequent intercellular bridges, rare gland lumens, and intracellular mucin positivity may occur, but these are inconspicuous [22]. A striking inflammatory infiltrate is present in the stroma, usually containing numerous eosinophils and plasma cells.

Therapeutic management

Treatment is the same as for invasive squamous cell carcinoma and adenocarcinoma of the same stage (multimodality management), but the prognosis is not as good. In a study of 29 stage IB glassy cell carcinomas, the survival was only 55 percent, about 20 percent lower than that of squamous cell carcinoma [35]. The reputation of a poor prognosis, however, is based on only a few cases in each stage, so it can be questioned whether glassy cell carcinoma is worse than any other poorly differentiated carcinoma of the cervix [22]. The latest publications concern only case reports [29].

Clear cell carcinoma

General features and pathology

Clear cell carcinoma accounts for about 4 percent of adenocarcinomas of the cervix [28]. Almost two thirds of cases have occurred in women exposed *in utero* to diethylstilbestrol (DES) or a related substance. Those with a history of exposure have a median age of 19 years and a range of 7 to 31 years. Clear cell carcinoma of the cervix may also develop in the absence of *in utero* DES exposure, as demonstrated by its occurrence in women born before the use of DES during pregnancy [17]. Of the cervical tumours related to DES exposure, about 50 percent are associated with vaginal adenosis and about 20 percent with gross structural cervicovaginal mesenchymal abnormalities such as hypoplasia, strictures, bands, fibroepithelial polyps, and malformations of the cervicovaginal interface [31].

Papillary, microcystic, tubular, and solid patterns occur. The cells have clear or eosinophilic granular cytoplasm, and often have a hobnail shape. Hobnail cells have prominent nuclei but scant cytoplasm so that the nucleus appears to protrude into the lumen of neoplastic tubules and cysts. The tubules are typically lined by a single layer of relatively bland cells. The microscopic features are the same as in clear cell carcinoma of the vagina. As in the vagina, most clear cell carcinomas of the cervix are closely associated with vaginal adenosis or with tuboendometrial glands in the exocervix (cervical ectropion).

Therapeutic management

More than 85 percent of clear cell carcinomas are stage I or II when detected [31]. Treatment is either radical hysterectomy and vaginectomy or radiation. Metastasis occurs to pelvic nodes in about 18 percent of patients with stage I disease, but the frequency of metastasis reaches nearly 50 percent in stage II tumours [31].

Survival of patients with stage I disease is about 90 percent. Most recurrences occur within 3 years after primary therapy. Metastases are more often to distant sites than with squamous cell carcinoma; 36% of initial recurrences metastasize to the lung or supraclavicular nodes, in contrast to less than 10% in patients with squamous cell carcinoma. Features associated with a better prognosis include small tumour size, shallow depth of invasion, older age of the patient ($\geq$ 19 years), a tubulocystic microscopic pattern and lesser degrees of nuclear atypia. The last published series from the US (Mayo Clinic) between 1982 and 2004, describes 34 cases of cervical clear cell carcinoma, out of which 2 were previously exposed to DES. Even for early stages, nodes were often positive (25%), but the prognosis appears to be no worse than that of squamous carcinomas. Data suggests that the patients with low risk (negative pelvic nodes) may be managed with radical surgery alone. Radiation therapy should be reserved for patients with positive pelvic nodes [36].

Sarcomas of the cervix

General features and pathology

Sarcomas of the uterine cervix represent a diverse group of tumours. Sarcomas constitute less than 1% of all cervical malignancies. Carcinosarcomas (which have been called malignant mixed Müllerian tumours, and are most probably poorly differentiated epithelial carcinomas that tend to be highly aggressive and are generally associated with a poor prognosis [1]), rhabdomyosarcomas and leiomyosarcomas have been described in the uterine cervix. Clinical presentation often consists of vaginal bleeding, but other symptoms may occur depending on the age at presentation. Rhabdomyosarcomas (RMS) tend to occur in childhood in the vagina and in rare cases, RMS can originate in the uterine cervix, with a peak incidence in the second decade [13]. Leiomyosarcomas often occur in women of perimenopausal age, but carcinosarcomas tend to be associated with post-menopausal women [3,5]. There are important differences in the ways in which these tumours grow and metastasize, with carcinosarcomas tending to have a higher incidence of lymphatic spread and lymph node metastases, whereas leiomyosarcomas are more likely to have early haematogenous spread and the first metastases may well be in the lungs or the liver [12]. Therefore, this has important implications for the clinical work-up, staging and surgical management of these patients.

Therapeutic management

Clearly, there are no guidelines for the management of these tumours, and the majority of publications concerns uterine sarcomas. Only case reports and monocentric retrospective analyses exist on sarcomas of the cervix.

For rhabdomyosarcoma (RMS), the latest monocentric retrospective analysis was from Iran [13]. A hospital-based tumour registry found all patients with female genital tract RMS, who were treated between 1999 and 2004. The medical records of all patients were reviewed and a single pathologist reviewed all pathologic specimens. Among the 1,528 patients with genital tract malignancies, 6 RMS were found: 3 located in the vagina and 3 in the cervix with a mean age of 16 years. All patients were treated with surgery and adjuvant chemotherapy. One patient with cervical RMS was treated with adjuvant chemo-radiation. Primary therapy with wide local excision and chemotherapy can result in prolonged survival and cure in patients with early stage RMS. Vaginal lesions have a better prognosis than cervical lesions.

In the last monocentric retrospective analysis of all sarcomas of the cervix [42] published in 2005, carcinosarcomas are more frequent. Among 1,583 patients with cervical malignancies, 8 cervical sarcomas were identified. Five of the tumours were carcinosarcomas. Six patients were treated with curative intent and 5 received adjuvant therapy after surgery (chemotherapy, radiotherapy or chemoradiotherapy). Six patients remain alive after a mean follow-up of 2.5 years. Two died from disease progression. Two patients have recurred: one undergoing a thoracotomy for an isolated pulmonary metastasis, who is alive with no evidence of disease, while the second patient developed pulmonary metastases and is alive 8 months after recurrence.

To conclude, management of all of these rare entities should be considered within a multidisciplinary framework.

Adenoid cystic carcinoma

General features and pathology

Adenoid cystic carcinoma of the cervix is a rare tumour representing less than 1 percent of cervical adenocarcinomas [26]. Patients with adenoid cystic carcinoma tend to be elderly, with few of them being under 50 years of age. Reports from the United States contain a higher proportion of non- white patients than expected from the general population [26,38]. Ovarian epithelial tumours, particularly mucinous ones, are relatively common in women with adenoid cystic carcinoma.

Microscopically, the cells form clusters, cords, and trabeculae with a circular or spiral pattern formed with lumens containing hyaline eosinophilic material. The nuclei are small, dark, and relatively uniform and seldom show pleomorphism. Minor areas of squamous differentiation may be present. Mitotic figures and necrosis are common, and hyalinization of the stroma may be prominent. Overlapping patterns with ordinary adenocarcinoma and adenoid basal cells may be present. The mixture of patterns with ordinary forms of adenocarcinoma and the scarcity of myoepithelial differentiation indicates that most adenoid cystic carcinomas of the cervix are adenocarcinomas with adenoid cystic differentiation [11]. Lymphatic invasion is usually evident. Immunostaining for cytokeratins is usually strongly positive, whereas CEA and EMA staining is focal.

Therapeutic management

Adenoid cystic carcinoma of the cervix is an aggressive neoplasm for which there are no standardized treatment protocols. There is a high risk of local recurrence and distant metastasis. In some reports, the behaviour is similar to, or worse than, adenocarcinoma and squamous cell carcinoma of the cervix [11,38]. In the last case report it was proposed to follow the guidelines established for patients at similar stages with squamous cell carcinoma of the cervix [19]. In the elderly, if surgery is not possible, radiotherapy seems to be promising for local control [27].

Malignant melanoma

General features and pathology

At least 24 primary melanomas in the uterine cervix have been reported [32]. It is one fifth as common as primary melanoma of the vagina and vulva. Melanoma of the cervix occurs in women ranging in age from 26 to 74 years who present with vaginal bleeding or discharge, often of short duration [24]. About half of the melanomas of the cervix involve the vagina (stage II) when discovered [24]. Typically, melanomas appear as ulcerated greyish-blue or black protuberances or nodules. Microscopic examination reveals the tumour with a varied appearance similar to cutaneous melanomas and those arising in the vagina. Small cell and spindle cell variants are relatively common. Even in the usual epithelioid cell type, areas of relatively small undifferentiated cells may occur. Activity in the junction zone has been identified in less than half of the cases [32]. Melanin pigmentation may be evident in haematoxylin- and eosin-stained slides. Melanoma-specific HMB-45 and S-100 immunostains are helpful in distinguishing melanoma from carcinoma, although a few poorly differentiated carcinomas are S-100 positive. Immunoreactions for keratin are negative in melanoma. The differential diagnosis includes melanoma metastatic to the cervix, most of these being primary in the vagina or vulvar skin. Metastatic melanoma, in contrast to primary melanoma, lacks change in the junction zone.

Therapeutic management

Melanoma of the cervix has a poor prognosis. In summarizing melanomas of the cervix, Mordel *et al.* found a 5-year survival of 40% for patients with stage I disease, but only 14% for higher stages [24]. Most patients who die of the tumour do so within 1 year of diagnosis. The most common and earliest site of spread from melanoma of the cervix is by direct extension and metastasis to the vagina. A successful treatment has not yet been found.

The reviews published between 1999 and 2006 concerned reports including very few cases [6,25]. The main message from these reports is to recommend radical hysterectomy, bilateral salpingo-oophorectomy, and retroperitoneal pelvic lympadenectomy. Adjuvant radiotherapy is also proposed.

Lymphoma and leukaemia

General features and pathology

Both lymphoma and rarely leukaemia may manifest initially in the uterine cervix. More often, lymphoproliferative disorders involve the cervix secondarily in the course of systemic spread. More than 55 primary lymphomas of the cervix have been described [23]. Less than 1 in 175 extranodal lymphomas present, and possibly originate, in the uterus or vagina. In published reports, a distinction is seldom made between involvement of the cervix and involvement of the corpus. The cervix is more often affected as an initial manifestation of lymphoma than the uterine corpus or the vagina [16]. At post-mortem, 2-9% of women with lymphoma are found to have involvement of the uterus, about half of which is in the cervix.

Lymphomas of the cervix are staged by a modification of the Ann Arbor staging system for extranodal lymphomas [7] and by the International Federation of Gynecologists and Obstetricians (FIGO) system for staging of cervical carcinoma.

The median age of women with lymphoma or leukaemia is slightly over 40 years of age, with the age ranging from the third to the ninth decade of life [16]. More than 75% of patients present with a mass, 50% present with vaginal bleeding, and 33% have vaginal discharge. When the cervix is the initial site of the disease, some patients also have anaemia, splenomegaly, or other signs of lymphoma at the time of diagnosis. The duration of symptoms varies from 1 to 4 months. In about half of the patients, the disease is stage II or more by FIGO criteria, being beyond the cervix with extension to the pelvic wall or the lower third of the vagina. Most are stage IE by the modified Ann Arbor staging system for extranodal lymphomas; pelvic or para-aortic lymph node and ovarian involvement also occurs. Cervical cytology smears are usually negative [18,23].

Therapeutic management

There are no standard guidelines for treatment due to the rarity of the disease. The overall survival of patients with uterine lymphomas is often good. Patients with stage IE disease, have an overall survival at 5 years of around 75% [18].

5

The latest review in the literature that reported about 101 cases [15] of primary lymphoma of the uterine cervix included: 21 patients who received surgery plus radiotherapy, 19 who received chemotherapy plus radiotherapy, 12 surgery alone, 11 radiotherapy alone, 8 chemotherapy alone, 7 surgery plus chemotherapy, 2 surgery plus chemotherapy plus radiotherapy and 21 patients for whom the management was unknown. The recent studies used chemotherapy plus surgery, with or without radiotherapy. Another important issue concerns women of child-bearing age. There are a few cases reported of young women treated only with a chemotherapy combination such as CHOP, who are alive without disease at 3 and 5 years, one of whom having given birth to a normal baby [21]. The chemotherapy combination (CHOP) followed by involved field radiotherapy seems to be an effective treatment.

In summary

Table 1 shows the therapeutic options for each histology. More often surgery is radical hysterectomy, bilateral salpingo-oophorectomy, pelvic lymphadenomectomy. Retroperitoneal lymphadenomectomy has to be discussed for each case.

Table 1 – Therapeutic options for each histology.

Histology	Therapeutic propositions
Small cell carcinoma Neuroendocrine carcinoma	Surgery and chemotherapy Radiotherapy or radiochemotherapy?
Glassy cell carcinoma	Surgery and adjuvant treatment according to the stage (brachytherapy, radiotherapy or radiochemotherapy)
Clear cell carcinoma	Surgery Radiotherapy or radiochemotherapy
Sarcomas	Multimodality treatment with experts Surgery Adjuvant treatment?
Adenoid cystic carcinoma	Surgery Radiotherapy or radiochemotherapy
Melanomas	Surgery with retroperitoneal lymphadenectomy Adjuvant treatment has to be discussed
Lymphomas	Chemotherapy by CHOP + radiotherapy by involved field

References

1. Amant F, Cadron I, Fuso L *et al.* (2005) Endometrial carcinosarcomas have a different prognosis and pattern of spread compared to high risk epithelial endometrial cancer, Gynecol Oncol 98: 274-80
2. Ambros RA, Park J-S, Shah KV, Kurman RJ *et al.* (1991) Evaluation of histologic, morphometric, and immunohistochemical criteria in the differential diagnosis of small cell carcinomas of the cervix with particular reference to human papillomavirus types 16 and 18. Mod Pathol 586-93
3. Arrastia CD, Fruchter RG, Clark M *et al.* (1997) Uterine carcinosarcomas: incidence and trends in management and survival, Gynecol Oncol 65: 158-63

4. Barrett RJ II, Davos I, Leuchter RS, Lagasse LD (1987) Neuroendocrine features in poorly differentiated and undifferentiated carcinomas of the cervix. Cancer 60: 2325-30
5. **Brooks SE, Zhan M, Cote T *et al.* (2004) Surveillance, epidemiology, and end results analysis of 2677 cases of uterine sarcoma 1989-1999, Gynecol Oncol 93: 204-8**
6. Cantuaria G, Angioli R, Nahmias J *et al.* (1999) Primary malignant melanoma of the uterine cervix: case report and review of the literature. Gynecol Oncol 75(1): 170-4
7. Carbone PP, Kaplan HS, Musshoff K *et al.* (1971) Report of the Committee on Hodgkin's Disease Staging Classification. Cancer Res 31: 1860-1
8. Chan JK (2003) Prognostic factors in neuroendocrine small cell carcinoma: a multivariate analysis. Cancer 97: 568
9. **Chen J (2008) Incidence, Mortality, and prognostic factors of small cell carcinoma of the cervix. Obstet Gynecol 111: 1394**
10. Cherry CP, Glucksmann A (1956) Incidence, histology, and response to radiation of mixed carcinomas (adenoacanthomas) of the uterine cervix. Cancer 9: 971-9
11. Ferry JA, Scully RE (1988) "Adenoid cystic" carcinoma and adenoid basal carcinoma of the uterine cervix. A study of 28 cases. Am J Surg Pathol 12: 134-44
12. Gadducci A, Sartori E, Landoni F *et al.* (2002) The prognostic relevance of histological type in uterine sarcomas: a Cooperation Task Force (CTF) multivariate analysis of 249 cases, Eur J Gynecol Oncol 23: 295-9
13. Ghaemmaghami F, Karimi Zarchi M, Ghasemi M *et al.* (2008) Lower genital tract rhabdomyosarcoma: case series and literature review. Arch Gynecol Obstet 278(1): 65-9
14. Groben P, Reddick R, Askin F (1985) The pathologic spectrum of small cell carcinoma of the cervix. Int J Gynecol Pathol 4: 42-57
15. Hariprasad R, Kumar L, Bhatla DM *et al.* (2006) Primary uterine lymphoma: report of 2 cases and review of literature. Am J Obst and Gynecol 195: 308-13
16. Harris NL, Scully RE (1984) Malignant lymphoma and granulocytic sarcoma of the uterus and vagina. A clinicopathologic analysis of 27 cases. Cancer 53: 2530-45
17. Kaminski PF, Maier RC (1983) Clear cell adenocarcinoma of the cervix unrelated to diethylstilbestrol exposure. Obstet Gynecol 62: 720-7
18. Komaki R, Cox JD, Hansen RM *et al.* (1984) Malignant lymphoma of the uterine cervix. Cancer 54: 1699-704
19. **Koyfman SA, Abidi A, Ravichandran P *et al.* (2005) Adenoid cystic carcinoma of the cervix. Gynecol Oncol 99(2): 477-80**
20. Lojek MA, Fer MF, Kasselberg AG *et al.* (1980) Cushing's syndrome with small cell carcinoma of the uterine cervix. Am J Med 69: 140-4
21. Lorusso D, Ferrandina G, Pagano L *et al.* (2007) Successful pregnancy in stage IE primary non-Hodgkin's lymphoma of uterine cervix treated with neoadjuvant chemotherapy and conservative surgery. Oncology 72(3-4): 261-4
22. Maier RC, Norris HJ (1982) Glassy cell carcinoma of the cervix. Obstet Gynecol 60: 219-24
23. Mann R, Roberts WS, Gunasakeran S, Tralins A (1987) Primary lymphoma of the uterine cervix. Gynecol Oncol 26: 127-34
24. Mordel N, Mor-Yosef S, Ben-Baruch N *et al.* (1989) Malignant melanoma of the uterine cervix: case report and review of the literature. Gynecol Oncol 32: 375-80
25. Mousavi AS, Fakor F, Nazari Z *et al.* (2006) Primary malignant melanoma of the uterine cervix: case report and review of the literature. J Low Genit Tract Dis 10(4): 258-63
26. Musa AG, Hughes RR, Coleman SA (1985) Adenoid cystic carcinoma of the cervix: a report of 17 cases. Gynecol Oncol 22: 167-73
27. Nishida M, Nasu K, Takai N *et al.* (2005) Adenoid cystic carcinoma of the uterine cervix. Int J Clin Oncol 10(3): 198-200
28. Noller KL, Decker DG, Dockerty MB *et al.* (1974) Mesonephric (clear cell) carcinoma of the vagina and cervix. A retrospective analysis. Obstet Gynecol 43: 640-4
29. Nunez C, Abdul-Karim FWk, Sourak TM *et al.* (1985) Glassy-cell carcinoma of the uterine cervix. Cytopathologic and histopathologic study of five cases. Acta Cytol 29: 303-9
30. Pazdur R, Bonomi P, Slayton R *et al.* (1981) Neuroendocrine carcinoma of the cervix: implications for staging and therapy. Gynecol Oncol 12: 120-8

31. Robboy SJ, Young RH *et al.* (1982) Female genital tract changes related to prenatal diethylstilbestrol exposure. In: Blaustein A, ed. Pathology of the female genital tract. 2nd ed. New York: Springer-Verlag 99-118
32. Santoso JT, Kucera PR, Ray J *et al.* (1990) Primary malignant melanoma of the uterine cervix: two case reports and a century's review. Obstet Gynecol Surv 45: 733-40
33. Seltzer V, Sall S, Castandot MJ *et al.* (1979) Glassy cell cervical carcinoma. Gynecol Oncol 8: 141-51
34. Sutton GP, Siemers E, Stehman FB, Ehrlich CE (1988) Eaton-Lambert syndrome as a harbinger of recurrent small-cell carcinoma of the cervix with improvement after combination chemotherapy. Obstet Gynecol 72: 516-8
35. Tamimi HK, Ek M, Hesla J *et al.* (1988) Glassy cell carcinoma of the cervix redefined. Obstet Gynecol 71: 837-41
36. **Thomas MB, Wright JD, Leiser AL *et al.* (2008) Clear cell carcinoma of the cervix: a multi-institutional review in the post-DES era. Gynecol Oncol 109(3): 335-9**
37. Ulich TR, Liao SY, Layfield R *et al.* (1986) Endocrine and tumor differentiation markers in poorly differentiated small-cell carcinoids of the cervix and vagina. Arch Pathol Lab Med 110: 1054-7
38. Van Dinh T, Woodruff JD (1985) Adenoid cystic and adenoid basal carcinomas of the cervix. Obstet Gynecol 65: 705-9
39. Van Nagell JR Jr, Donaldson ES, Wood EG *et al.* (1977) Small cell cancer of the uterine cervix. Cancer 40: 2243-9
40. Van Nagell JR Jr, Powell DE, Gallion HH *et al.* (1988) Small cell carcinoma of the uterine cervix. Cancer 62: 1586-93
41. **Viswanathan AN (2004) Small cell neuroendocrine carcinoma of the cervix: outcome and patters of recurrence. Gyncecol Oncol 93: 27**

Tumours of the vagina and tumours of the vulva

6

C. Haie-Meder, R. Mazeron and P. Morice

Five Essential Points (vaginal tumours)

1. *Primary vaginal cancers occur mainly in post-menopausal women, except in cases of clear cell adenocarcinoma when diethylstilbestrol was given during maternal pregnancy.*
2. *Initial work-up is based on both clinical examination and MRI. PET-Scan has also been found relevant.*
3. *Treatment depends on stage (TNM/FIGO classification). Surgery is recommended for in situ tumours. In the other cases, treatment consists of a combination of external irradiation (usually 45 Gy) and brachytherapy up to 80 Gy total dose to the GTV. Concomitant chemoradiation is an option, similar to cervical cancers. Treatment time should not exceed 9 weeks. In patients with diethylstilbestrol exposure during maternal pregnancy, a more conservative strategy was proposed, consisting of ovarian transposition and pelvic lymph node dissection followed by BT with or without external beam irradiation according to the tumour size and nodal status, in order to maintain fertility.*
4. *Relative contribution of interstitial versus endocavitary brachytherapy remains controversial but it is generally considered that interstitial brachytherapy should be used when tumour thickness exceeds 15mm, but is contra-indicated in case of recto-vaginal septum infiltration.*
5. *Results highly depend on tumour stage, ranging from 50% to 100% in stage I, 50% to 85% in stage 2, 0% to 86% in stage III, and 0% to 67% in stage IV. FIGO stage, age, and overall treatment time are the main prognostic factors reported in the literature. Grade, length of vaginal involvement, and tumour location are more controversial prognostic factors.*

Primary cancers of the vagina are rare gynaecological tumours, accounting for approximately 1% to 2% of cancers of the female reproductive tract. Vulvar tumours are more frequent, accounting for 3% to 5% of the female reproductive tract cancers. As the treatment of vaginal and vulvar cancers differs dramatically, they will be approached in two different sections.

I. VAGINAL CANCERS

Introduction

To confirm the diagnosis of primary vaginal cancer, the cervix and the vulva must be clinically and pathologically free of cancer and with no history of cervix or vulvar cancer during the previous 5 years. Secondary vaginal cancers after treatment for a cervical or vulvar malignancy account for 80% to 90% of the tumours located in the vagina. Primary adult vaginal malignant tumours occur mainly in postmenopausal women (80%) and the mean age ranges from 60 to 65 years. One exception to this is clear cell adenocarcinoma, occurring in young patients whose mothers had received diethylstilbestrol (DES) during their pregnancies. Risk factors include HPV infection, DES exposure in utero, uterus prolapse treated with a pessary inducing chronic irritation [11]. Other possible risk factors are cigarette smoking and previous hysterectomy for a benign pathology.

Tumour location and spread; histological types

Primary vaginal cancers are usually located in the upper one third of the posterior part and the lower third of the anterior part of the vagina, and 40 to 50% of tumours are multifocal. The lymphatic extension of vaginal tumours correlates with the double embryologic origin of the vagina : the two upper thirds drain to iliac nodes while the lower third drains to hypogastric and inguinal nodes. The drainage of the posterior septum is located in the hemorroidal and sacral nodes. Histologically, most tumours are squamous cell carcinoma, including in situ and invasive tumours and account for 80% to 90% of vaginal cancers. Adenocarcinomas account for 8% to 15% of vaginal cancers, including post-DES clear cell adenocarcinomas and the remaining histological types include malignant melanomas, sarcomas and lymphomas (altogether 2%-3%); rhabdomyosarcomas are exceptional in adults.

Initial work-up and classification

Vaginal tumour extension requires a careful gynaecological examination, and general anaesthesia might be necessary. It is important to exclude a tumour from different origin involving the vagina (most often cervix cancer) or metastases into the vagina, *e.g.* from gynaecological tumours (endometrium, ovarian cancer) or other malignancies. The topographic situation of the tumour within the vagina, the macroscopic characteristics (exophytic and/or ulcerative growth), and the regional spread outside the vagina must be carefully documented. A systematic drawing is recommended at the time of diagnosis. A vaginal impression is also a good way to document the extent of the disease at the time of diagnosis with photographs. A second impression, taken at the time of brachytherapy (BT) allows an objective measurement of tumour regression after external irradiation. Transvaginal and/or transrectal sonography helps to check precisely the morphology, the location and the topography of the tumour within the vagina and moreover the tumour thickness which may have an impact on the technique used for BT. MRI identifies tumour dimensions, potential extension beyond the vagina (bladder, rectum) and displays enlarged pelvic and para-aortic nodes and metastases. Usually, most of these tumours give an iso-intense signal compared to muscle on T1-weighted images and hyper-intense compared to muscle on T2-weighted images 5 [39]. Taylor *et al.* concluded that MRI was able to identify over 95% of primary vaginal tumours in a series of 25 patients [39]. FDG-PET was found to be relevant to detect primary disease in all cases and nodal disease twice as often as CT and physical examination [22]. Further complementary examinations may be indicated, depending on the tumoral extension: rectoscopy and/or cystoscopy.

Tumours are staged according to the TNM/FIGO-classification: T0 for superficial non-invasive lesions; T1/stage I for lesions confined to the vaginal wall; T2/stage II for lesions extending into the paravaginal tissue; T3/stage III for lesions reaching the pelvic wall; T4/stage IVA for lesions involving bladder and/or rectum [20].

Treatment modalities

Surgery, external irradiation, brachytherapy (BT) and chemotherapy are the various treatment options, and the choice, often consisting of a combined approach, is highly stage- and histology-related.

Treatment of carcinoma

Given the rarity of primary carcinoma of the vagina, no randomized trial has been performed, particularly to assess the respective role of surgery and irradiation or to explore the value of concomitant chemoradiation as has been performed in cervical cancers.

Patients with *limited in situ tumours* are generally treated with surgery alone [41]. In a national cancer data base report, Creasman *et al.* reported an 84% rate of exclusive surgery in this type of tumours, with only 5% treated with irradiation and 4% with chemotherapy [6]. Surgery is of particular interest in young patients, preserving ovarian function. When irradiation is discussed, it generally consists of exclusive BT.

In *invasive tumours*, treatment combines external beam radiotherapy (EBR) and BT. In limited stage I tumours however, exclusive BT has been successfully used. Perez *et al.* reported no significant local control improvement in stage I when treatment combined EBR and BT compared to BT alone [32]. However, in a series reported by Frank *et al.*, a relapse rate of 18% was observed in stage I, all pelvic failures occurring in patients treated exclusively with BT [13]. In stages II-IV, all the authors recommend EBR and BT. Perez *et al.* found a 65% local control with EBR+BT *versus* 40% with only BT in stage II and III [32]. Similar findings were reported by MacNaught *et al.* [26].

Particular case of post DES clear cell adenocarcinoma of the vagina

Clear cell adenocarcinoma in the context of DES exposure during maternal pregnancy has occurred in young women, teenagers or even young children. The treatment first aimed at a local control of the disease and, in the first reported series, consisted of radical surgery. Later, a conservative procedure in order to maintain fertility was performed in some institutions. In order to achieve this goal, the therapeutic approach combined surgery and BT. Surgery consisted of pelvic lymphadenectomy and ovarian transposition. If pelvic nodes were negative, exclusive BT was performed, while in patients with positive pelvic nodes, treatment consisted of external irradiation and BT [15].

External beam radiotherapy

EBR delivers a standard dose of 45 Gy in 25 fractions to the pelvis. Some authors use midline shielding blocks, in order to increase the relative contribution of BT. Prophylactic inguinal irradiation is usually performed when the tumour extents to the lower third of the vagina. Concurrent cisplatin-based radio-chemotherapy is nowadays proposed to patients, based on the results of the different randomized trials in cervix cancer. This combined treatment has been published as being feasible in vaginal cancers and associated with excellent local control [8,12,13,35]. In case of inguinal nodes, a boost is performed on a more limited volume including the initial volume extension up to a total dose of 60 Gy.

Brachytherapy

BT plays an important role in the treatment of vaginal cancers.

Intracavitary BT

Different vaginal applicators have been described: metallic or plastic colpostats, cylinders of different diameters and sizes (with a central hollow metallic cylinder where the radioactive sources will be located), vaginal mould, the latter allowing an adaptation to the anatomy and the tumour extension [1]. Applicators specifically dedicated to vaginal cancers have been described. Perez *et al.* designed a vaginal applicator called MIRALVA (Mallinckrodt Institute of Radiology After Loading Vaginal Applicator) [31]. The Institut Gustave-Roussy technique consists of the use of customized intravaginal applicators, based on vaginal impression. This individualized applicator, designed for each patient, allows source position, space and length according to the tumour size, shape and extension. The vaginal mould by itself allows vaginal expansion, and increases the distance to organs at risk [1].

Interstitial BT

Different afterloading techniques can be used depending on the site and the size of the tumour. Tumoural thickness determination is a fundamental step when adding interstitial BT to endocavitary BT. The chosen technique is based on the experience of the different schools of BT. The most frequently used techniques are the plastic tube and the steel needles [36]. Templates have been designed to maintain parallel position and equidistance between the tubes and/or the needles. The templates used for interstitial BT in vaginal cancers are usually the same as for cervical cancers.

Relative place of endocavitary and interstitial BT

Tumoural thickness is determinant for interstitial BT. Depending upon the tumour site, interstitial BT is considered when tumour thickness exceeds 15 mm. The relative contra-indication to interstitial BT is infiltration of the recto-vaginal septum. Para-vaginal infiltration represents a good indication to combine intracavitary and interstitial techniques to increase the dose to the tumour while maintaining the dose to organs at risk at reasonable levels.

Dose, dosimetry

The aim is to deliver a total dose (integrating the dose of external irradiation) of at least 80 Gy to the GTV, assessed if possible by both clinical examination and MRI at the time of BT. A dose of 60 Gy is generally reached in the initial tumour volume. The dose to organs at risk must be taken into consideration with a maximal dose of 80-90Gy and 70-75Gy to the bladder and to the rectum, respectively, assessed by the 2cc dose. For interstitial implants, Paris system rules are applied for the implantation itself, and for dose calculations.

High dose-rate, low dose-rate or pulsed dose-rate BT is available nowadays, even if the majority of the series report experience with low dose-rate BT [9, 12, 13, 21, 23, 24, 26, 29, 32, 35, 38, 40, 42].

Results

According to stage, the five-year survival without pelvic recurrence ranges from 50% to 100% in stage I, 50% to 85% in stage 2, 0% to 86% in stage III, and 0% to 67% in stage IV. These discrepancies are explained by several factors. Indeed, published data may include different histological types (such as clear cell adenocarcinoma, small cell carcinoma), include invasive and *in situ* tumours, with a long period of time of observance (with more accurate staging using MRI and/or PET-CT and treatment modalities evolution).

Several prognostic factors have been reported in the literature: FIGO stage, age, and overall treatment time. In a series of 91 patients treated at the Institut Gustave-Roussy, de Crevoisier *et al.* reported a 5-year cause specific survival (CSS) of 83% in stage I, 76% in stage II, and 52% in stage III [9]. Frank *et al.* reported a 5-year disease-specific survival of 85% in stage I, 78% in stage II and 58% in stage III-IVA among 193 patients treated at MD Anderson [13]. Perez *et al.* found a correlation between stage and local control and disease-free survival [32]. Age usually has an impact on overall survival in this elderly population, but not on local control or CSS [9]. As in cervix cancer, Lee *et al.* and de Crevoisier *et al.* showed significant improvement in local control when treatment was completed in less than 9 weeks [9,23]. Tumour grade, length of vaginal involvement, and tumour location are more controversial prognostic factors. Chyle *et al.* found tumour site (upper versus middle or lower versus whole vagina; $p=0.047$), and circumferential location (posterior versus all other locations; $p=0.068$) to be significant prognostic factors [4].

The role of interstitial techniques in the treatment of vaginal cancers also remains controversial. Leung *et al.* reported a series of 103 patients treated between 1970 and 1989 [24]. After 1985, a better local control was achieved and the authors insist on the more systematic use of interstitial BT to explain this improvement. Stryker *et al.* also recommended the use of systematic interstitial techniques in vaginal cancers, based on their experience on 34 patients [38]. Tewari *et al.* in a series of 71 patients treated for vaginal primary cancers with interstitial BT using the Syed-Neblett applicator, also advocates the role of this technique [40].

In post DES clear cell adenocarcinoma, the age at diagnosis ranged from 7 to 34 years with the highest incidence from 14 to 22 years and a peak at 19 years. Fertility preservation was one of the major issues in this young population. The historically recommended treatment consisted of a non-conservative treatment such as radical hysterectomy and pelvic lymphadenectomy which caused infertility in all cases. A more conservative strategy with ovarian transposition and pelvic lymph node dissection followed by BT with or without external beam irradiation according to the tumour size and nodal status was secondarily proposed to maintain fertility. In a series of 61 patients treated for fertility preservation, the 5-year survival was 80% with 7 patients being pregnant but only 3 patients being able to deliver 4 normal children, the others having miscarriage [16].

6

Five Essential Points (tumours of the vulva)

1. *Vulvar vaginal cancers mainly occur in post-menopausal women with squamous cell carcinoma representing 90%-95% of vulvar carcinomas.*
2. *Standard treatment of the primary tumour is surgery, consisting of wide local incision if free microscopic margins can be achieved (at least 8 mm and preferably 20 mm). External irradiation, brachytherapy and chemotherapy are either adjuvant treatment options or exclusive treatment options in advanced disease.*
3. *Groin treatment is still a matter of debate. No randomized trial has compared surgery to irradiation in the absence of palpable inguinal nodes. When surgery is chosen, a unilateral inguino-femoral lymphadenectomy is generally performed if the tumour is lateralized while bilateral inguino-femoral lymphadenectomy remains the standard if the tumour is midline located. Sentinel node evaluation and mapping have been recently evaluated.*
4. *Results depend on tumour stage, ranging from 90% to 97% in stage I, 70% to 86% in stage II, 40% to 65% in stage III, and 10% to 27% in stage IV. Positive or close margins, presence of capillary space involvement, large invasion depth and large primary size are prognostic factors for local recurrence. Inguino-femoral lymph node status is the most important prognostic factor for survival.*
5. *High complication rates have been the rationale for more conservative therapeutic strategies.*

II. VULVAR CANCERS

Introduction

The diagnosis of primary malignant vulvar tumours is usually made in post-menopausal women between the ages 50 and 70 years [14] but an increase in young patients has also been reported [2,28]. Squamous cell carcinoma represents 90%-95% of vulvar carcinomas. Human papilloma virus is not reported as often as in cervical cancer and invasive cancer may arise from an area of lichen sclerosis [3]. The most common other histologies are represented by melanoma and basal cell carcinomas. These histologies will not be covered in this review.

Tumour location and spread

Delay in the diagnosis is a characteristic of the disease. The pattern of dissemination is mostly lymphogenic with inguino-femoral lymph node metastases. Lateralized tumours usually drain to the ipsilateral groin while median tumours (or less than 1cm from the midline) drain to either groin side. One particular case is represented by clitoris tumours with a possible direct drainage to pelvic nodes. Pelvic nodes are rarely involved if the inguinal area is free of nodes.

Initial work-up and classification

Vulvar tumours are easily accessible to clinical examination. Due to pain induced by the tumour, however, general anaesthesia might be necessary, especially to assess a potential extension into the vagina. Urethro-cystoscopy or anuscopy might be indicated depending on tumour extension. Lymph node status represents a fundamental prognostic factor and is integrated into the 1995 FIGO classification as well as the 2009 FIGO classification.

- Stage 0 : in situ tumour without nodal metastasis;
- Stage IA : tumour 2cm or less confined to the vulva or the perineum and with stromal invasion no greater than 1mm and without nodal metastasis;
- Stage IB : tumour 2cm or less confined to the vulva or the perineum and with stromal invasion greater than 1mm and without nodal metastasis;
- Stage II : tumour larger than 2cm confined to the vulva or the perineum without nodal metastasis;
- Stage III : tumour of any size with: (i) adjacent tumour spread of the lower urethra and/or vagina or anus and/or (ii) unilateral regional lymph node metastasis;
- Stage IV : tumour invades any of the following : upper urethra, bladder mucosa, rectal mucosa, pelvic bone and/or bilateral regional node metastasis:
- Stage IVB : any distant metastasis including pelvic lymph nodes.

Treatment modalities

Surgery is the standard treatment for squamous cell carcinoma of the vulva. External irradiation, BT and chemotherapy are either adjuvant treatment options or exclusive treatment options in advanced disease.

Surgery

Radical vulvectomy with "en bloc" bilateral inguino-femoral and pelvic lymphadenectomy used to be the standard treatment for many years. In order to reduce morbidity without compromising the result, the surgical procedure has become more conservative. Separate incisions do not appear to compromise survival. Wide local incision is nowadays recognized as an alternative to radical vulvectomy if free microscopic margins of at least 8 mm and preferably 20 mm can be achieved. In this situation, primary wound closure is generally possible. Metastases in pelvic lymph nodes are exceptional when the inguino-femoral nodes are free. No pelvic lymphadenectomy is routinely performed in patients with negative inguinal nodes. Given the rarity of contralateral inguino-femoral lymph nodes (3%-4%) in patients with lateralized tumours, a unilateral inguino-femoral lymphadenectomy is generally accepted. Bilateral inguino-femoral lymphadenectomy remains the standard if the tumour is located midline. The extent of groin dissection has been investigated as well. Superficial inguinal lymphadenectomy (in which the cribriform fascia is left intact) has been proposed as an alternative to inguino-femoral lymphadenectomy based on the anatomical supposition that no femoral node metastasis is possible if inguinal nodes are negative. In this situation however, groin recurrences have been reported. Some authors recommend that superficial and femoral lymph nodes medial from the femoral vein should be removed [10]. Sentinel node evaluation and mapping has been recently developed. One technique was initially validated with isosulfan blue injection [25]. Other approaches consist of a combination of either isosulfan blue dye or technetium-99 and lymphoscintigraphy [10]. Plante *et al.* reported a positive predictive value of 99% out of 12 series collecting 353 patients with vulvar cancer [33].

EBR

EBR to the primary tumour as *adjuvant therapy*

After wide local excision, EBR is indicated in case of positive margins or with margins < 3 mm if re-excision is not possible. In this situation, a total dose of 45-50 Gy in 25-28 fractions controls potential micro-metastases. The technique usually mixes electrons and photons. Interstitial BT can be combined with external irradiation depending on tumour location.

EBR to the *primary tumour as exclusive treatment*

In case of contra-indication to surgery or in advanced tumours, EBR has proven its efficacy. A total dose of 45 Gy is delivered to the pelvis, usually combined with interstitial BT to a total dose of 60-85 Gy. Concurrent chemoradiation consisting of cisplatinum or carboplatinum used alone or in combination with fluorouracil, has been shown to give a high response rate even in the absence of randomized trials.

EBR to the *groin as adjuvant treatment*

In case of involvement of two or more inguinal nodes, prophylactic external irradiation to the groin and to the pelvis compared to pelvic lymphadenectomy has been investigated in a randomized trial conducted by the GOG in 1986 [18]. The results showed a better prognosis in patients treated with external irradiation. A total dose of 45 Gy is generally recommended, using mixed electron and photon fields.

EBR to the *groin as exclusive treatment*

No randomized trial has been performed to compare groin dissection with groin irradiation. Radiation therapy has been shown to prevent regional recurrences in a retrospective series of 227 patients treated at M.D. Anderson with an overall 5-year inguinal recurrence rate of 15.4% [19]. Van der Velven *et al.* reported a literature review of three studies and their conclusion was that there was no evidence for a better control with external irradiation compared to dissection [43]. In case of contra-indication to surgery, external irradiation represents an alternative to treating inguinal nodes.

If external irradiation is to be performed prophylactically, a total dose of 45 Gy is recommended while this dose should reach 60-65 Gy in case of macroscopic nodes.

Results

According to stage, the five-year survival rates range from 90% to 97% in stage I, 70% to 86% in stage II, 40% to 65% in stage III, and 10% to 27% in stage IV.

Prognostic factors for local relapse are positive or close margins, presence of capillary space involvement, large invasion depth and large primary size [34]. Overall, the local recurrence incidence represents 50% of all the recurrences [27,37]. Maggino *et al.* individualized two patterns of recurrence: one far from the initial tumour site which is considered as a new primary and another located at the initial primary tumour site which correlates more with the margin status and the tumour characteristics than with the type of surgery [27]. Groin recurrences represent 6-30% of recurrences, depending upon groin nodal status at the time of diagnosis, and tend to occur sooner than local relapses [37].

The most important prognostic factor for survival is inguino-femoral lymph node status. Inguino-femoral metastases are present in 30% of the patients and among them 20% have pelvic metastases [7,17]. Nodal metastases correlate with primary tumour size, depth of invasion, capillary space involvement and clinical node status [18]. The number of involved nodes has a significant impact on survival: patients with one groin node metastasis have a better survival than patients with bilateral or with three or more groin metastases : 53% *versus* 23% [7,37].

Complications

Radical vulvectomy used to be associated with primary closure difficulty, wound breakdown and infection in up to 85% of the cases. Morbidity has significantly decreased with wide local incision. Groin complications include lymphocele, cellulitis and leg lymphoedema [10]. Leg oedema may significantly impair quality of life [30]. Risk factors for complications are frequently observed in the patient population with vulvar cancer: diabetes, obesity, age over 60, cardiovascular disease. The frequency of leg oedema can reach 65% after inguino-femoral lymphadenectomy and the incidence increases with combined treatment such as postoperative irradiation [5]. The high complication rate explains the attempt at a more conservative surgical strategy.

References

1. Albano M, Dumas I, Haie-Meder C (2008) Brachytherapy at the Institut Gustave-Roussy: Personalized vaginal mould applicator: technical modification and improvement. Cancer Radiother. Sept 08
2. Al Ghamdi A, Freedman D, Miller D *et al.* (2002) Vulvar squamous cell carcinoma in young women: a clinicopathologic study of 21 cases. Gynecol Oncol 84: 94-101
3. Carli P, De Magnis A, Mannone F *et al.* (2003) Vulvar carcinoma associated with lichen sclerosus. Experience at the Florence, Italy, Vulvar Clinic. J Reprod Med 48: 313-8
4. Chyle V, Zagars GK, Wheeler JA *et al.* (1996) Definitive radiotherapy for carcinoma of the vagina:outcome and prognostic factors. Int J Radiat Oncol Biol Phys 35: 891-905
5. Coit DG, Peters M, Brennan MF (1991) A prospective randomized trial of perioperative cefazolin treatment in axillary and groin dissection. Arch Surg 12: 1366-71
6. **Creasman WT, Phillips JL, Menck HR (1998) The national cancer data base report on cancer of the vagina. Cancer 83: 1033-40**
7. Curry SL, Wharton JT, Rutledge F (1980) Positive lymph node in vulvar squamous carcinoma. Gynecol Oncol 9: 63-7
8. Dalrymple JL, Russell AH, Lee SW *et al.* (2004) Chemoradiation for primary invasive squamous carcinoma of the vagina. Int J Gynecol Cancer 14: 110-7

6

9. **de Crevoisier R, Sanfilippo N, Gerbaulet A *et al.* (2007) Exclusive radiotherapy for primary squamous cell carcinoma of the vagina. Radiother Oncol 85: 362-70**
10. **De Hullu JA, van der Zee AGJ (2006) Surgery and radiotherapy in vulvar cancer. Crit Rev Oncol Hem 60: 36-58**
11. Duong TH, Flowers LC (2007) Vulvo-vaginal cancers:risks, evaluation, prevention and early detection. Obstet Gynecol Clin North Am 34: 783-802
12. Frank SJ, Deavers MT, Jhingran A *et al.* (2007) Primary adenocarcinoma of the vagina not associated with diethylstilbestrol (DES) exposure (2007) Gynecol Oncol 105: 470-4
13. **Frank SJ, Jhingran A, Levenback C *et al.* (2005) Definitive radiation therapy for squamous cell carcinoma of the vagina. Int J Radiat Oncol Biol Phys 62: 138-47**
14. Franklin EW, Rutledge FD (1972) Epidemiology of epidermoid carcinoma of the vulva. Obstet Gynecol 39: 165-72
15. Gerbaulet A, Charmeau L, Haie-Meder C *et al.* (1993) L'adénocarcinome à cellules claires du col et du vagin de la jeune fille: DES syndrome. Possibilité de traitement conservateur. Bull Cancer/Radiother 80: 291-305
16. Gerbaulet A, Escaillet B, Beral Y *et al.* (1995) Pregnancy after transposition and repositioning of the ovaries in a patient with clear cell adenocarcinoma. Rev Fr Gynecol Obstet 90(12): 534-8
17. Hacker NF, Nieberg RK, Berek JS *et al.* (1983) Superficially invasive vulvar cancer with nodal metastases. Gynecol Oncol 15: 65-77
18. Homesley HD, Bundy BN, Sedlis A *et al.* (1993) Prognostic factors for groin node metastasis in squamous cell carcinoma of the vulva (a Gynecologic Oncology Group study) Gynecol Oncol 49: 279-83
19. Katz A, Eifel P, Jhingran A *et al.* (2003) The role of radiation therapy in preventing regional recurrences of invasive squamous cell carcinoma of the vulva. Int J Radiat Oncol Biol Phys 57: 409-18
20. Kottmeier HL (1963) The classification and clinical staging of carcinoma of the uterus and vagina. J Int Fed Gynecol Obstet 1: 83-93
21. Kucera H, Mock U, Knocke TH *et al.* (2001) Radiotherapy alone for invasive vaginal cancer: outcome with intracavitary high dose rate brachytherapy versus conventional low dose rate brachytherapy. Acta Obstet Gynecol Scand 80: 355-60
22. Lamoreaux WT, Grigsby PW, Dehdashti F (2005) FDG-PET evaluation of squamous cell carcinoma of the vagina. Int J Radiat Oncol Biol Phys 62: 138-47
23. Lee WR, Marcus Jr RB, Sombeck MD *et al.* (1994) Radiotherapy alone for carcinoma of the vagina: the importance of overall treatment time. Int J Radiat Oncol Biol Phys 29: 983-8
24. Leung S, Sexton M (1993) Radical radiation therapy for carcinoma of the vagina-impact of treatment modalities on outcome: Peter Mac Callum Cancer Institute experience 1970-1990. Int J Radiat Oncol Biol Phys 25: 413-18
25. Levenback C, Burke TW, Gershenson DM *et al.* (1994) Intraoperative lymphatic mapping for vulvar cancer. Obstet Gynecol 84: 163-7
26. Mac Naught R, Symonds RP, Hole D *et al.* (1986) Improved control of primary vaginal tumours by combined external-beam and interstitial radiotherapy. Clin Radiol 37: 29-32
27. Maggino T, Landoni F, Sartori E *et al.* (2000) Patterns of recurrence in patients with squamous cell carcinoma. Cancer 89: 116-22
28. Messing MJ, Gallup DG (1995) Carcinoma of the vulva in young women. Obstet Gynecol 6: 51-4
29. Mock U, Kucera H, Fellner C *et al.* (2003) High-dose-rate (HDR) brachytherapy with or without external beam radiotherapy in the treatment of primary vaginal carcinoma: long-term results and side effects. Int J Radiat Oncol Biol Phys 56: 950-7
30. Pereira de Godoy JM, Braile DM, de Fatima Godoy M *et al.* (2002) Quality of life and peripheral lymphedema. Lymphology 3: 72-5
31. Perez C, Slessinger E, Grigsby PW (1990) Design of an afterloading vaginal applicator (MIRALVA). Int J Radiat Oncol Biol Phys 18: 1503-8
32. Perez C, Grigsby PW, Garipagaoglu M *et al.* (1999) Factors affecting long-term outcome of irradiation in carcinoma of the vagina. Int J Radiat Oncol Biol Phys 44: 37-45

33. Plante M, Renaud MC, Roy M (2004) Sentinel node evaluation in gynecologic cancer. Oncology 18: 75-87
34. Rouzier R, Haddad B, Plantier F *et al.* (2002) Local relapse in patients treated for squamous cell vulvar carcinoma: incidence and prognostic value. Obstet Gynecol 100: 1159-67
35. Samant R, Lau B, Choan E *et al.* (2007) Primary vaginal cancer treated with concurrent chemoradiation using cis-platinum. Int J Radiat Oncol Biol Phys 69: 746-50
36. Seeger AR, Windschall A, Lotter M *et al.* (2006) The role of interstitial brachytherapy in the treatment of vaginal and vulvar malignancies. Strahlenther Onkol 182: 142-8
37. Stehman FB, Look KY (2006) Carcinoma of the vulva. Obstet Gynecol 107: 719-33
38. Stryker JA (2000) Radiotherapy for vaginal carcinoma: a 23-year review. Br J Radiol 73: 1200-5
39. Taylor MB, Dugar N, Davidson SE *et al.* (2007) Magnetic resonance imaging of primary vaginal carcinoma. Clin Radiol 62: 549-55
40. Tewari KS, Cappuccini F, Puthawala AA *et al.* (2001) Primary invasive carcinoma of the vagina: treatment with interstitial brachytherapy. Cancer 91: 758-70
41. Tjalma WA, Monaghan JM, de Barros Lopes A *et al.* (2001) The role of surgery in invasive squamous carcinoma of the vagina. Gynecol Oncol 81: 360-5
42. Tran PT, Su Z, Lee P *et al.* (2007) Prognostic factors for outcomes and complications for primary squamous cell carcinoma of the vagina treated with radiation. Gynecol Oncol 105: 641-9
43. van der Velven J, Ansink A (2002) Primary groin irradiation versus primary groin surgery for early vulvar cancer (Cochrane Review). In: The Cochrane library, issue 1. Oxford:Update Sofware

Section 6
Breast

Invasive breast cancer and ductal carcinoma *in situ* in young women

1

G. Gruber and S. Aebi

Five Essential Points

1. *Young patients represent a small fraction of all cases of breast cancer; yet, at age 30 and beyond, breast cancer is the most frequent cancer in women.*
2. *The surgical therapy of invasive and ductal in situ breast cancer should be identical to that in older patients with special emphasis on achieving local control by adequate surgical margins.*
3. *Whole breast irradiation with an additional boost to the tumour bed has to be considered standard after breast conserving surgery.*
4. *Whereas the indication and the choice of chemotherapy do not depend on age, very young patients with ER-positive breast cancer should receive adjuvant endocrine therapy, preferentially in the framework of a clinical trial.*
5. *Recommendations for the local treatment (surgery and radiotherapy) of DCIS in young women are similar to those for invasive disease.*

Introduction

Despite continuous diagnostic and therapeutic improvements breast cancer remains a substantial clinical problem. In 2006, nearly 300,000 women were diagnosed in the United States and more than 40,000 patients died of their disease [46].

In many clinical situations age is an important parameter for treatment decision making. This is especially true for the elderly, but also at the other end of the age spectrum – in young or very young patients. The distinction between "young" and "very young" is arbitrary, but a cut-off of 35-40 years is chosen by most authors. Especially in the very young cohort, numerous additional problems arise: fertility, treatment-induced menopause and therapy-related side effects in the very long term have to be considered in very young patients. Furthermore, breast cancer in very young women is rare and often under-represented in clinical trials. Thus, it is hard to decide if general treatment recommendations are valid for the small subgroup of young patients.

According to the Surveillance, Epidemiology and End Results (SEER) Program between 1988 and 1997 only 5,869 out of 83,804 (7%) patients with T1/T2 breast cancer were diagnosed at the age 20-39 [49]. In recent years, the incidence of breast cancer in young patients has been slowly increasing [10]. A large European population-based series yielded similar results: only 3,197 out of 45,229 patients (7.1%) were 39 years old and under at diagnosis (< 35 years: 2.6%; 35-39 years: 4.4%) [45]. Nevertheless, there exist large geographical differences: in the 2002 annual report of the Saudi national cancer registry, 26.4% of all female breast cancers were diagnosed before age 40 [20].

This overview will focus on prognostic and therapeutic aspects of invasive breast cancer and ductal carcinoma *in situ* (DCIS) of the breast in young women.

1

Young age and prognosis

Traditionally, breast cancer in very young patients has been considered an aggressive disease with poor prognosis. In four randomised trials the International Breast Cancer Study Group (IBCSG) treated 3,700 pre- and peri-menopausal patients with adjuvant CMF chemotherapy; 314 patients (8.5%) were below 35 years of age. Relapse and death occurred earlier and more often in younger patients, and the 10-year disease-free (DFS) and overall survival (OS) was 35% and 49% *versus* 47% and 62% in older patients, respectively. Young age remained a significant predictor of poor outcome after adjusting for other risk factors [2]. The negative prognostic impact of young age has been documented in numerous population-based and single institutional studies. This was also true for a selected patient cohort with stage I breast cancer: after adjusting for tumour size, histological grade, estrogen receptor (ER) expression, and year of diagnosis, age was still a significant predictor with each year younger than 45 years increasing the relative risk of breast cancer death by 5% [1]. It is likely that age by itself is only a surrogate marker for adverse biological features which are finally responsible for the unfavourable outcome in young patients. Indeed, young women are more likely to have large, highly proliferating, lymph-node positive tumours with poor differentiation (G3) and ER and progesterone receptor (PgR) negativity [12]. This was confirmed in a prospectively collected database of 841 pre-menopausal node-negative patients $\leq$ 50 years operated between 1997 and 2001 at the European Institute of Oncology, of whom 101 patients (12%) were less than 35 years old [13]. In comparison to less young women, patients $<$ 35 had higher percentages of ER-negative (41.6% *vs* 17.4%) or PgR-negative (47.5% *vs* 23.2%) tumours, which were more often larger than 2 cm (35.6% *vs* 24.2%) and of high grade (48.5% *vs* 31.9%) with elevated Ki-67 labelling index (62.4% *vs* 50.7%). All differences were statistically highly significant [13]. A recent publication demonstrated that bone marrow micrometastases are also observed more frequently in young patients [9]. In some studies multivariate analyses could eliminate age as an independent prognostic factor [4,34,42], but in many others the known risk factors did not completely explain the higher likelihood of local [54] and distant recurrence in young patients [13].

In addition, the risk of contralateral breast cancer (CBC) seems to be affected by age: in a population-based study, the frequency of synchronous CBC was 1.4% and increased with age. However, the standardised incidence ratio (SIR) adjusted for age- and calendar-year yielded a more than 80-fold increased risk of synchronous CBC for Dutch patients $<$ 35 years old. This was much higher than the 9- to 17-fold increased risk for older patients [45]. The cumulative incidence of metachronous CBC was 2.1%, 4.2% and 5.9% at 5, 10 and 15 years, again with the highest risk for very young patients: the risk was increased more than 11-fold in patients $<$35, which is in contrast to the SIR of 1.5 in patients 60 years or older ($p<0.001$) [45]. These findings are in part explained by the fact that early onset is a well known feature of hereditary breast cancer and gene (e.g. BRCA1 and BRCA2) mutations are strongly linked with CBC [18].

Molecular gene signatures might help to improve the understanding of the underlying mechanisms for worse prognosis. A signature associated with poor prognosis was most frequently observed among the youngest women, and young age was not an independent factor in multivariate analysis including the gene signature [50]. The Recurrence Score (Oncotype Dx®) was validated in two trials of the NSABP; again, younger patients tended to have higher Recurrence Scores than older patients. Age was not a significant prognostic factor in a multivariate model incorporating the Recurrence Score [38].

Surgical aspects in young women with breast cancer

A positive family history and especially the finding of a BRCA1/2 gene mutation will influence the decision about the appropriate surgical management. Furthermore, the decision between breast conservation and mastectomy might be influenced by psychological factors, like disturbed femininity and diminished sexual attractiveness, but mainly by local failure rates and survival endpoints with each approach. The interpretation of older studies of breast conserving therapy is influenced by inadequate margin assessment as compared to contemporary standards [reviewed in 55]. Very young patients up to 35 years without extensive intraductal component experienced excellent local relapse rates of 3% at 10 years in case of negative margins compared to 34% in close or positive margins [22]. In the EORTC "boost trial" 5,318 patients who underwent microscopically complete excision for invasive carcinoma underwent breast conserving treatment [5,6]. However DCIS at the margin was no exclusion criterion. On central pathologic review 26% of patients ≤40 years old had microscopically positive resection margins for DCIS as compared to 15% in patients older than 40 ($p = 0.008$). Furthermore, young patients tended to have smaller excision specimens but had more frequent re-excisions [54]. There was a highly significant difference in local control between age groups, but unfortunately local relapse rates among age groups according to the margin status for DCIS were not analyzed [54].

Fewer data on the prognostic value of young age are available after mastectomy. Combined analyses of NSABP trials (B-15; B-16; B-18; B-22; B-25; n = 5758) as well as IBCSG trials (I to IX; n = 6660) in breast cancer patients treated with mastectomy but without radiotherapy revealed age < 40 years as significant and independent parameter for loco-regional failure in both node-negative [32] and node-positive disease [32,48].

Do young patients fare better with mastectomy rather than with breast conservation? Voogd *et al.* [53] demonstrated that young patients < 35 years had a more than nine-fold increased risk for local failure compared to patients aged 60 or older with BCT; in contrast, local failure risk was similar in younger and older patients after mastectomy.

In a recent report from British Columbia, patients between 20 and 49 years were either treated by BCT (n = 1597) or modified radical mastectomy (n = 801) [14]. While confirming the worse prognosis for the younger age group, results did not differ significantly according to treatment groups. Patients < 40 years with T1 node-negative breast cancer, negative margins and no reported DCIS had a slightly higher local failure rate with BCT compared to mastectomy ($p=0.3$), but distant relapse free survival and breast cancer specific survival were similar. Kroman *et al.* [36] reported on 9,285 pre-menopausal patients <50 years old treated within the protocols 82 + 89 of the Danish Breast Cancer Cooperative Group (DBCG), of whom 7,165 patients (77.2%) had radical mastectomy (RM) and 2,120 patients (22.8%) BCT. A total of 719 patients (RM: 500 patients; BCT: 219 patients) were < 35 years old. The median follow-up was 7.1 years. No increased risk of death was observed among women who received BCT compared with mastectomy, regardless of age at diagnosis, despite the increased risk of local recurrence among young women. Restricting the analysis to 5,195 women with small tumours (size ≤ 2 cm) brought similar results.

BRCA 1/2 carriers with breast cancer are at significantly higher risk for local failure after BCT. The 15-year actuarial rates of local failure was 21.5% in patients with breast conservation *vs* 7.1% in patients with mastectomy (HR 3.1; $p = 0.0043$).

However, there was no significant difference in distant failure (11.2% *vs* 12.7%; p = 0.29), CBC, breast cancer specific or overall survival [41].

Available data do not demonstrate a superior overall survival with mastectomy compared with BCT, but local failure rates tend to be higher in young patients with breast conservation compared to mastectomy. BCT with regular follow-up is an option, but young patients should be aware of a possible increased local failure rate.

Radiotherapeutic aspects in young women with breast cancer

The landmark trial of radiotherapy after breast conserving surgery is the EORTC "boost" trial. The impact of dose escalation ("boost") was most pronounced in patients aged <40 years and has to be considered standard treatment. The addition of a boost reduced the local recurrence rate at five years from 20% to 10% (p<0.002), and age and boost treatment were the only independent parameters in multivariate analysis [5,6,54].

Regardless of age, post mastectomy radiotherapy (PMRT) is well accepted in T3/T4 tumours or in patients with 4 or more positive axillary lymph nodes. Indications for PMRT in smaller tumours (T1/T2) with 1-3 positive lymph nodes are not clear, but some authors have advocated the routine use in patients < 45 years with T2 tumours [21]. Additionally, in a retrospective review of 107 patients < 35 years old treated with neoadjuvant chemotherapy and mastectomy for stage II/III breast cancer, young patients with additional PMRT had significantly better locoregional control (LRC) and overall survival than patients without PMRT (5-yrs-LRC: 88% *vs* 63%; p = 0.001; 5-yrs-OS: 67% *vs* 48%; p = 0.03) [23]. In patients with 1 to 3 positive lymph nodes, young age probably identifies a subgroup of patients who might benefit from additional radiotherapy after mastectomy [48].

Little is known about the different sites of loco-regional failure in young women. Age <40 years was a significant parameter for local, but not for axillary or supraclavicular failure in 933 premenopausal node-positive breast cancer patients treated within IBCSG trial VI [27]. Node-positive breast cancer patients at young age may be appropriate candidates for PMRT. Of concern are potential side effects, especially for the contralateral breast: young patients, especially those with a strong family history, had an increased risk of CBC with tangential field irradiation. The excess relative risk for medially located CBC was 37% per Gray radiation dose to the medial part of the contralateral breast [28].

Aspects of systemic treatments in young women with breast cancer

A recent analysis of SEER data demonstrated a reduction in breast cancer mortality from 1988 to 1997 for patients younger than 45 years with stage I breast cancer [1]. This is likely explained by an increased use of adjuvant systemic therapies in the same time period. It was argued that the impaired outcome of young patients is related to inadequate adjuvant therapy. Young patients < 35 and between 35-40 years old who did not receive adjuvant systemic treatment due to a presumed low-risk disease had a much higher probability of recurrence (hazard ratios 2.18 and 1.4) compared to the 45-49-year-old cohort with otherwise similar characteristics. This negative impact of young age was not observed in patients at higher risk who did receive adjuvant systemic therapy [35]. Information on differential treatment effects according to hormone receptor status was not given.

Some years ago it was common practice for many clinicians to prescribe young patients chemotherapy without endocrine treatment even in hormone-responsive disease. Findings from IBCSG [2] suggested an insufficient endocrine effect of chemotherapy alone in very young patients with endocrine-responsive disease. A possible interaction of age and ER-status in pre-menopausal patients treated with chemotherapy alone was tested and finally confirmed by a joint analysis in trial populations of the IBCSG (n = 2233), the National Surgical Adjuvant Breast and Bowel Project (NSABP; n = 5849), the Eastern Cooperative Oncology Group (ECOG; n = 1112) and the Southwest Oncology Group (SWOG; n = 670) [24]. In ER-positive disease, the 5-year DFS for patients < 35 years was much lower compared to older patients – 39% *vs* 60% (IBCSG), 49% *vs* 66% (NSABP), 53% *vs* 66% (ECOG) and 73% *vs* 89% (SWOG). These DFS differences according to age were not observed in patients with ER-negative tumours – 56% *vs* 59% (IBCSG), 59% *vs* 63% (NSABP), 55% *vs* 58% (ECOG) and 91% *vs* 88% (SWOG). These results contributed to a fundamental change in the St. Gallen Consensus Conference 2001: treatment selection was now based primarily on the responsiveness to endocrine therapy rather than on risk of recurrence [25].

Young patients with ER positive breast cancer should receive adjuvant endocrine therapy. Whereas on average oophorectomy and LHRH agonists are ineffective after chemotherapy, they might prevent recurrences in young women in whom chemotherapy does not induce amenorrhea [11,17]. Tamoxifen is effective in young patients after chemotherapy and in combination with ovarian function suppression [16]. The value of ovarian function suppression in addition to adjuvant tamoxifen is being investigated in an intergroup trial ("SOFT", IBCSG 24/02). For young patients, aromatase inhibitors should be used exclusively in the context of a clinical trial.

The impact of drug-induced amenorrhea on patients' outcome is still a matter of debate, but women with continuing menses had a significantly worse DFS both after CMF-based [30] and after anthracycline-containing chemotherapy [39]. It is therefore not possible to separately assess the effects of age and amenorrhea. However, the suppression of ovarian function for at least 2 years has been found to be at least as effective as CMF- and epirubicin-based chemotherapy without endocrine therapy in at least eight randomized controlled trials [3]; none of these trials reported differential effects of endocrine or chemotherapy by age, although some confirmed an inferior prognosis for very young patients [30]. Analyses from IBCSG VIII and from the ZEBRA trials demonstrated that the majority of young patients (< 40 years) treated with the LHRH analogue goserelin had a return of menses after treatment completion [11,33]. There is conflicting evidence of a possible protective effect of LHRH analogues against chemotherapy-induced permanent amenorrhea and loss of fertility [43], and results from several randomised trials are pending. One randomised clinical trial was stopped early, as the use of triptorelin did not appear to benefit patients to preserve their menstrual status [29].

While adjuvant chemotherapy (and trastuzumab) should not be chosen based on age, it became clear that adjuvant chemotherapy may act on at least two general pathways: while cytotoxicity is likely the main mechanism of action in hormone receptor-negative breast cancer, ovarian function suppression by chemotherapy may be the principal mode of action in ER and/or PgR-positive disease. However, adjuvant chemotherapy is less likely to produce permanent amenorrhea in very young patients. In an analysis of IBCSG trial VI evaluating adjuvant chemotherapy with 3-9 cycles of "classical" CMF, only 8% of patients < 35 experienced permanent

1

amenorrhea *vs* 59% in older pre-menopausal patients [24]. These figures vary substantially by the adjuvant treatment used [40], but the effect of age is no matter of controversy and was seen also in a very recent report using a more common chemotherapeutic regimen: 708 premenopausal patients treated with doxorubicin/cyclophosphamide followed by docetaxel within the NSABP-B30 trial were available for analysis. The estimated rate of resumption of menses at 2 years was 45% for women < 40 years, 11% for women 40-50, and 3% for women > 50 years. The rate of amenorrhea was also influenced by the use of tamoxifen [47], which reduces the risk of relapse and death from ER-positive breast cancer independent of age and its efficacy is not diminished by prior chemotherapy [19].

Young age and ductal carcinoma *in situ* (DCIS)

Similar to invasive breast cancer little is known about the optimal treatment in young patients with DCIS as they represent only a minority of the whole patient cohort. Only 6% (51 out of 863) were ≤ 40 years old in the EORTC study [7]. Of note, age ≤ 40 was one of the leading risk factors for local failure in the multivariable analysis (HR = 1.89, 95%CI: 1.18 – 2.90). Despite irradiation after breast conserving surgery, young patients had a 26% local recurrence rate at 10 years [8]. Only a few small studies specifically investigated the relationship between young patient age and outcome in patients with DCIS [15,52]. Similar to invasive breast cancer, young age is a risk factor for local relapse. The underlying reason is not clear, but young patients may have more local failures due to smaller excision volumes, a greater proportion of high nuclear grade, central necrosis [26] and HER-2 overexpression [44]. Overall, four large randomized trials demonstrated a highly significant risk reduction of about 50-60% for ipsilateral breast failure in patients with excision plus adjuvant radiotherapy in comparison to local excision alone for patients with DCIS [51].

In the randomised trials no boost irradiation was used. It is questionable if additional boost treatment improves local control [31]. A retrospective analysis from the Rare Cancer Network [37] included 373 women with DCIS age 45 years or younger. Fifty-seven patients (15%) had no radiotherapy after breast-conserving surgery, 166 (45%) had radiotherapy without boost (median dose 50 Gy), and 150 (40%) had radiotherapy with boost (median dose 60 Gy). Local relapse-free survival (LRFS) at 10 years was only 46% for patients without radiotherapy, 72% for those given radiotherapy without boost, and 86% for those given radiotherapy and boost. Age <40 years, margin status, and radiotherapy dose were significant predictors of LRFS. No difference was found between patients treated with excision followed by radiation therapy with a boost compared to patients with mastectomy in terms of LRFS (Rare Cancer Network, unpublished data).

In the absence of randomised trials, whole breast irradiation followed by a boost should be advised for breast conserving treatment in young patients with DCIS.

References

1. Aebi S, De Ridder M, Vlastos G *et al.* (2006) Young age is a poor prognostic factor in women with stage I breast cancer. Eur J Cancer (Suppl 4): 121
2. Aebi S, Gelber S, Castiglione-Gertsch M *et al.* (2000) Is chemotherapy alone adequate for young women with estrogen-receptor-positive breast cancer? Lancet 355: 1869-74

3. Aebi S (2005) Special issues related to the adjuvant therapy in very young women. Breast 14: 594-9
4. Albain KS, Allred DC, Clark GM (1994) Breast cancer outcome and predictors of outcome: are there age differentials? J Natl Cancer Inst Monogr 35-42
5. Bartelink H, Horiot JC, Poortmans P *et al.* (2001) European Organization for Research and Treatment of Cancer Radiotherapy and Breast Cancer Groups. Recurrence rates after treatment of breast cancer with standard radiotherapy with or without additional radiation. N Engl J Med 345: 1378-87
6. **Bartelink H, Horiot JC, Poortmans P *et al.* (2007) Impact of a higher radiation dose on local control and survival in breast-conserving therapy of early breast cancer: 10-year results of the randomized boost *versus* no boost EORTC 22881-10882 trial. J Clin Oncol 25: 3259-65**
7. Bijker N, Peterse JL, Duchateau L *et al.* (2001) Risk factors for recurrence and metastasis after breast conserving therapy for ductal carcinoma in situ: analysis of European Organization for Research and Treatment of Cancer Trial 10853. J Clin Oncol 19: 2263-71
8. Bijker N, Meijnen P, Bogaerts J, Peterse JL (2006) Breast-conserving treatment with or without radiotherapy for ductal carcinoma *in situ* (DCIS): ten-year results of European Organisation for Research and Treatment of Cancer (EORTC) randomized phase III trial 10853. Eur J Cancer 4 Suppl: 108
9. Braun S, Vogl FD, Naume B *et al.* (2005) A pooled analysis of bone marrow micrometastasis in breast cancer. N Engl J Med 353: 793-802
10. Brinton LA, Sherman ME, Carreon JD, Anderson WF (2008) Recent Trends in Breast Cancer Among Younger Women in the United States. J Natl Cancer Inst 100: 1643-8
11. Castiglione-Gertsch M, O'Neill A, Price KN *et al.* (2003) Adjuvant chemotherapy followed by goserelin *versus* either modality alone for premenopausal lymph node-negative breast cancer: a randomized trial. J Natl Cancer Inst 95: 1833-46
12. Colleoni M, Rotmensz N, Robertson C *et al.* (2002) Very young women (< 35 years) with operable breast cancer: features of disease at presentation. Ann Oncol 13: 273-9
13. Colleoni M, Rotmensz N, Peruzzotti G *et al.* (2006) Role of endocrine responsiveness and adjuvant therapy in very young women (below 35 years) with operable breast cancer and node negative disease. Ann Oncol 17: 1497-503
14. Coulombe G, Tyldesley S, Speers C *et al.* (2002) Is mastectomy superior to breast-conserving treatment for young women? Int J Radiat Oncol Biol Phys 67: 1282-90
15. Cutuli B, Cohen-Solal-le Nir C, de Lafontan B *et al.* (2002) Breast-conserving therapy for ductal carcinoma in situ of the breast: the French Cancer Centers' experience. Int J Radiat Oncol Biol Phys 53: 868-79
16. **Cuzick J, Ambroisine L, Davidson N *et al.* (2007) Use of luteinising-hormone-releasing hormone agonists as adjuvant treatment in premenopausal patients with hormone-receptor-positive breast cancer: a meta-analysis of individual patient data from randomised adjuvant trials. Lancet 369: 1711-23**
17. Davidson NE, O'Neill AM, Vukov AM *et al.* (2005) Chemoendocrine therapy for premenopausal women with axillary lymph node-positive, steroid hormone receptor-positive breast cancer: results from INT 0101 (E5188). J Clin Oncol 23: 5973-82
18. Dite GS, Jenkins MA, Southey MC *et al.* (2003) Familial risks, early-onset breast cancer, and BRCA1 and BRCA2 germline mutations. J Natl Cancer Inst 95: 448-57
19. Early Breast Cancer Trialists' Collaborative Group (2005) Effects of chemotherapy and hormonal therapy for early breast cancer on recurrence and 15-year survival: an overview of the randomised trials. Lancet 365: 1687-717
20. Elkum N, Dermime S, Ajarim D *et al.* (2007) Being 40 or younger is an independent risk factor for relapse in operable breast cancer patients: The Saudi Arabia experience. BMC Cancer 7: 222
21. Fodor J, Polgar C, Major T, Nemeth G (2003) Locoregional failure 15 years after mastectomy in women with one to three positive axillary nodes with or without irradiation: the significance of tumor size. Strahlenther Onkol 179: 197-202
22 Freedman GM, Hanlon AL, Fowble BL *et al.* (2002) Recursive partitioning identifies patients at high and low risk for ipsilateral tumor recurrence after breast-conserving surgery and radiation. J Clin Oncol 20: 4015-21
23. Garg AK, Oh JL, Oswald MJ *et al.* (2007) Effect of postmastectomy radiotherapy in patients < 35 years old with stage II-III breast cancer tretated with doxorubicin-

1

based neoadjuvant chemotherapy and mastectomy. Int J Radiat Oncol Biol Phys 69: 1478-83

24. **Goldhirsch A, Gelber RD, Yothers G *et al.* (2001) Adjuvant therapy for very young women with breast cancer: Need for tailored treatments. J Natl Cancer Inst Monogr 30: 44-51**
25. Goldhirsch A, Glick JH, Gelber RD *et al.* (2001) Meeting Highlights: International Consensus Panel on the Treatment of Primary Breast Cancer. J Clin Oncol 19: 3817-27
26. Goldstein NS, Vicini FA, Kestin LL, Thomas M (2000) Differences in the pathologic features of ductal carcinoma in situ of the breast based on patient age. Cancer 88: 2553-60
27. Gruber G, Cole BF, Castiglione-Gertsch M *et al.* (2008) Extracapsular tumor spread and the risk of local, axillary and supraclavicular recurrence in node-positive, premenopausal patients with breast cancer. Ann Oncol 19: 1393-401
28. Hooning MJ, Aleman BMP, Hauptmann M *et al.* (2008) Roles of radiotherapy and chemotherapy in the development of contralateral breast cancer. J Clin Oncol Oct 14th [epub ahead of print]
29. Ismail-Khan R, Minton S, Cox C *et al.* (2008) Preservation of ovarian function in young women treated with neoadjuvant chemotherapy for breast cancer: A randomized trial using the GnRH agonist (triptorelin) during chemotherapy. ASCO Proceedings I, Abstr. 524; p12s
30. Jakesz R, Hausmaninger H, Kubista E *et al.* (2002) Randomized adjuvant trial of tamoxifen and goserelin *versus* cyclophosphamide, methotrexate, and fluorouracil: evidence for the superiority of treatment with endocrine blockade in premenopausal patients with hormone-responsive breast cancer – Austrian Breast and Colorectal Cancer Study Group trial 5. J Clin Oncol 20: 4621-27
31. Julian TB, Land SR, Wang Y *et al.* (2008) Is boost therapy necessary in the treatment of DCIS? ASCO Proceedings I, Abstr. 537; p15s
32. Karlsson P, Cole BF, Price KN *et al.* (2007) The role of the number of uninvolved lymph nodes in predicting locoregional recurrence in breast cancer. J Clin Oncol 25: 2019-26
33. Kaufmann M, Jonat W, Blamey R *et al.* (2003) Survival analyses from the ZEBRA study. Goserelin (Zoladex®) *versus* CMF in premenopausal women with node-positive breast cancer. Eur J Cancer 39: 1711-7
34. Kollias J, Elston CW, Ellis IO *et al.* (1997) Early-onset breast cancer - histopathological and prognostic considerations. Br J Cancer 75: 1318-23
35. Kroman N, Jensen M-B, Wohlfahrt J *et al.* (2000) Factors influencing the effect of age on prognosis in breast cancer: population based study. BMJ 320: 474–9
36. Kroman N, Holtveg H, Wohlfahrt J *et al.* (2004) Effect of breast-conserving therapy *versus* radical mastectomy on prognosis for young women with breast carcinoma. Cancer 100: 688-93
37. **Omlin A, Amichetti M, Azria D *et al.* (2006) Boost radiotherapy in young women with ductal carcinoma in situ: a multicentre, retrospective study of the Rare Cancer Network. Lancet Oncol 7: 652-6**
38. Paik S, Tang G, Shak S *et al.* (2006) Gene expression and benefit of chemotherapy in women with node-negative, estrogen receptor-positive breast cancer. J Clin Oncol 24: 3726-34
39. Parulekar WR, Day AG, Ottaway JA *et al.* (2005) Incidence and prognostic impact of amenorrhea during adjuvant therapy in high-risk premenopausal breast cancer: analysis of a National Cancer Institute of Canada Clinical Trials Group Study – NCIC CTG MA.5. J Clin Oncol 23: 6002-8
40. Petrek JA, Naughton MJ, Case LD *et al.* (2006) Incidence, time course, and determinants of menstrual bleeding after breast cancer treatment: a prospective study. J Clin Oncol 24: 1045-51
41. Pierce LJ, Griffith KA, Buys S *et al.* (2008) Outcomes following breast conservation *versus* mastectomy in BRCA 1 / 2 carriers with early-stage breast cancer. ASCO Proceedings I, Abstr. 536; p15s
42. Rapiti E, Fioretta G, Verkooijen HM *et al.* (2005) Survival of young and older breast cancer patients in Geneva from 1990 to 2001. Eur J Cancer 41: 1446-52
43. Recchia F, Saggio G, Amiconi G *et al.* (2006) Gonadotropin-releasing hormone analogues added to adjuvant chemotherapy protect ovarian function and improve clinical outcomes in young women with early breast carcinoma. Cancer 106: 514-23

44. Rodrigues NA, Dillon D, Carter D *et al.* (2003) Differences in the pathologic and molecular features of intraductal breast carcinoma between younger and older women. Cancer 97: 1393-403
45. Schaapveld M, Visser O, Louwman WJ *et al.* (2008) The impact of adjuvant therapy on contralateral breast cancer risk and the prognostic significance of contralateral breast cancer: a population based study in the Netherlands. Breast Cancer Res Treat 110: 189-97
46. Smigal C, Jemal A, Ward E *et al.* (2006) Trends in breast cancer by race and ethnicity: update 2006. CA Cancer J Clin 56: 168-83
47. Swain SM, Land SR, Ritter MW *et al.* Amenorrhea in premenopausal women on the doxorubicin-and-cyclophosphamide-followed-by-docetaxel arm of NSABP B-30 trial. Breast Cancer Res Treat. 2008 Feb 27 [Epub ahead of print]
48. Taghian A, Jeong JH, Mamounas E *et al.* (2004) Patterns of locoregional failure in patients with operable breast cancer treated by mastectomy and adjuvant chemotherapy with or without tamoxifen and without radiotherapy: results from five National Surgical Adjuvant Breast and Bowel Project randomized clinical trials. J Clin Oncol 22: 4247-54
49. Tai P, Cserni G, Van de Steene J *et al.* (2005) Modelling the effect of age in T1-2 breast cancer using the SEER database. BMC Cancer 5: 130
50. Van de Vijver MJ, He YD, van't Veer LJ *et al.* (2002) A gene-expression signature as a predictor of survival in breast cancer. N Engl J Med 347: 1999-2009
51. Viani GA, Stefano EJ, Afonso SL *et al.* (2007) Breast-conserving surgery with or without radiotherapy in women with ductal carcinoma *in situ*: a meta-analysis of randomized trials. Radiation Oncology 2: 28
52. Vicini FA, Recht A (2002) Age at diagnosis and outcome for women with ductal carcinoma-in-situ of the breast: a critical review of the literature. J Clin Oncol 20: 2736-44
53. Voogd AC, Nielsen M, Peterse JL *et al.* (2001) Differences in risk factors for local and distant recurrence after breast-conserving therapy or mastectomy for stage I and II breast cancer: pooled results of two large European randomized trials. J Clin Oncol 19: 1688-97
54. Vrieling C, Collette L, Fourquet A *et al.* (2003) Can patient-, treatment- and pathology-related characteristics explain the high local recurrence rate following breast-conserving therapy in young patients? Eur J Cancer 39: 932-44
55. Zhou P, Recht A (2004) Young age and outcome for women with early-stage invasive breast carcinoma. Cancer 101: 1264-74

Tubular carcinoma of the breast

T. Sullivan and A.G. Taghian

2

Five Essential Points

1. *Tubular carcinoma is a rare breast malignancy associated with an excellent prognosis.*
2. *The histologic makeup of each tumour is an important prognostic factor, yet these criteria vary widely among published studies.*
3. *New histologic criteria may better predict patient outcomes.*
4. *The necessity of lymph node evaluation, adjuvant radiation therapy and systemic therapy for this disease have been questioned, but a less aggressive standard of care does not currently seem supported by the literature.*
5. *More evidence is needed to guide the future management of this disease.*

Introduction

Tubular carcinoma of the breast, first described by Cornil and Ranvier in 1869 [5], is a rare variant of invasive breast cancer, characterized by well-differentiated, orderly tubule formation and associated with excellent patient outcomes. The outstanding prognosis of this disease has led some to investigate if it could be safely managed less aggressively than standard invasive ductal carcinoma (IDC). In recent years, the necessity of lymph node evaluation [7, 16, 36], systemic therapy [7], and radiation therapy for these patients have all been questioned [18, 30]. Yet, while some have advocated a more restrained approach to the management of this cancer, others have expressed reluctance at deviating from a standard of care that has produced such exceptional outcomes [29].

Numerous cases of tubular carcinoma have been reported in the literature, however, deriving definitive treatment recommendations from this data is often not possible. Most cases have been reported in small retrospective series, and the histologic criteria for the diagnosis of this disease have varied widely among publications. As a result, cases can rarely be combined into more meaningful meta-analyses, and many of the important questions regarding the management of tubular carcinoma remain unresolved.

Although tubular carcinoma of the breast is a rare disease, making up less than 2% of all invasive breast cancers in the largest reports [7, 21, 26], recent findings indicate that its incidence may be rising by about 6% per year relative to other breast cancers [26]. As this disease becomes more common, and as the treatment of breast cancer continues to evolve, questions regarding the proper management of tubular carcinoma will likely persist. To address some of these uncertainties and to better inform the evidence-based management of this malignancy, this chapter presents an overview of the past research, recent developments and ongoing controversies in the treatment of tubular carcinoma of the breast.

Prognosis and histologic considerations

The excellent prognosis of tubular carcinoma has been demonstrated repeatedly in the literature. When compared to IDC, tubular carcinoma has often been linked to a higher rate of overall survival [4, 7], a lower rate of local recurrence [15], a lower incidence of lymph node involvement [15, 34], and a smaller primary tumour size

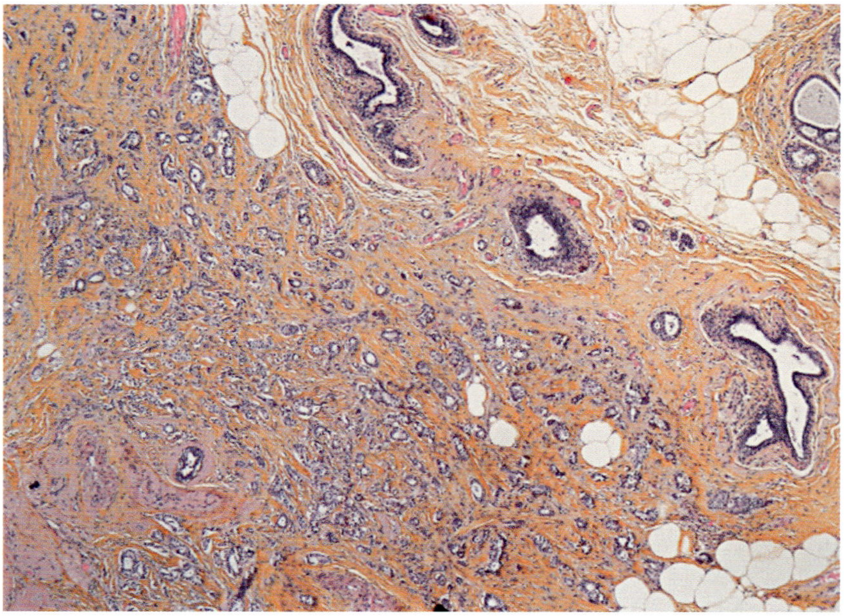

Fig. 1. 100% tubular carcinoma, × 50.

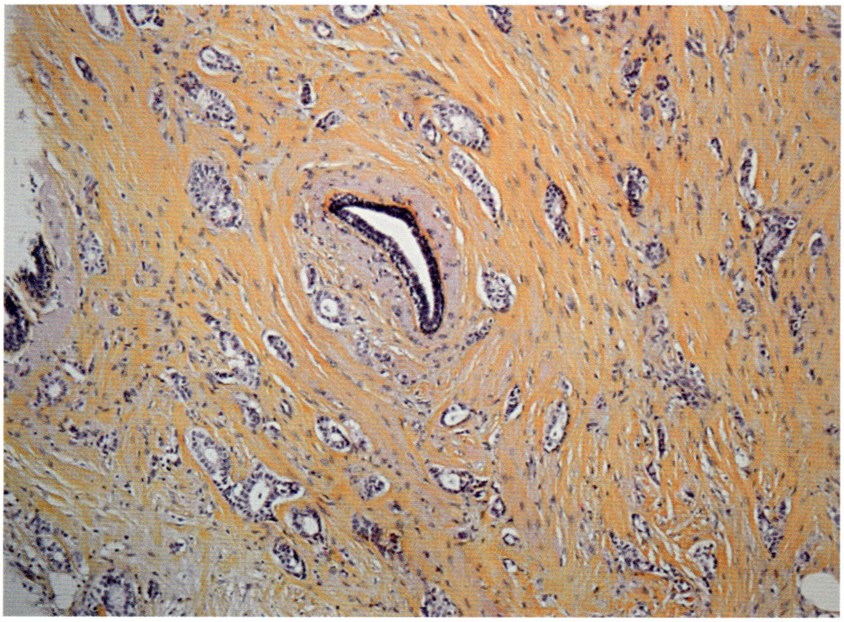

Fig. 2. 100% tubular carcinoma, × 100.

[7, 34]. One large review showed that the overall survival of tubular carcinoma patients was not significantly different from that of age-matched women from the general population, and that the majority of deaths among these patients were not due to their cancers [7].

Despite the established indolence of tubular carcinoma, it also has the potential to be a deadly disease, and multiple cases of metastasis and patient death have been reported [3, 15, 20]. Because poor outcomes are uncommon but possible among these patients, a number of studies have attempted to discern significant prognostic factors that may help identify high-risk patients.

One such prognostic factor is the histologic makeup of each patient's tumour. Histologically, tubular tumours are comprised of well-differentiated tubules containing a single layer of epithelial cells [Figs 1 and 2]. This well-differentiated tubular formation distinguishes tubular tumours from standard IDC, and may cause some tubular carcinomas to appear similar to benign lesions such as sclerosing adenosis or radial scars. However, tubular carcinomas can be distinguished from these lesions as tubular tumours lack myoepithelial cells [Figs 3 and 4].

Although tubular carcinoma and IDC are distinct entities, tubular carcinoma often occurs admixed with a component of standard IDC, and these mixed tumours have been associated with a poorer prognosis than pure tubular lesions. A greater percentage of IDC has been linked with a lower survival rate [3, 4, 25], higher rate of distant metastasis [25], and a higher rate of lymph node involvement [24].

Although the percent composition of IDC may be a significant predictor of patient outcomes, the published literature differs greatly in the proportion of IDC allowed before a tumour is not considered tubular. Some studies include only 100% tubular tumours [35], while others require a 90% [15], 75% [20, 30], or 50% minimum tubular component [6]. Some do not specify if this percent composition was even considered [16, 19]. This inconsistency among studies has precluded large meta-analyses of these cases, and may hinder the accurate prediction of patients' prognosis based on published reports.

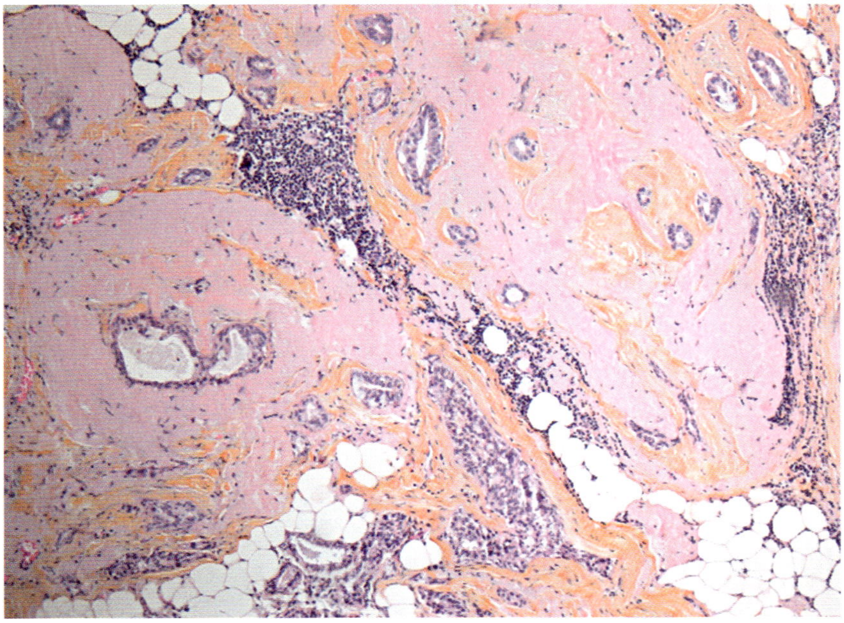

Fig. 3. Radial scar with calponin IHC stain demonstrating myoepithelial cells × 100.

2

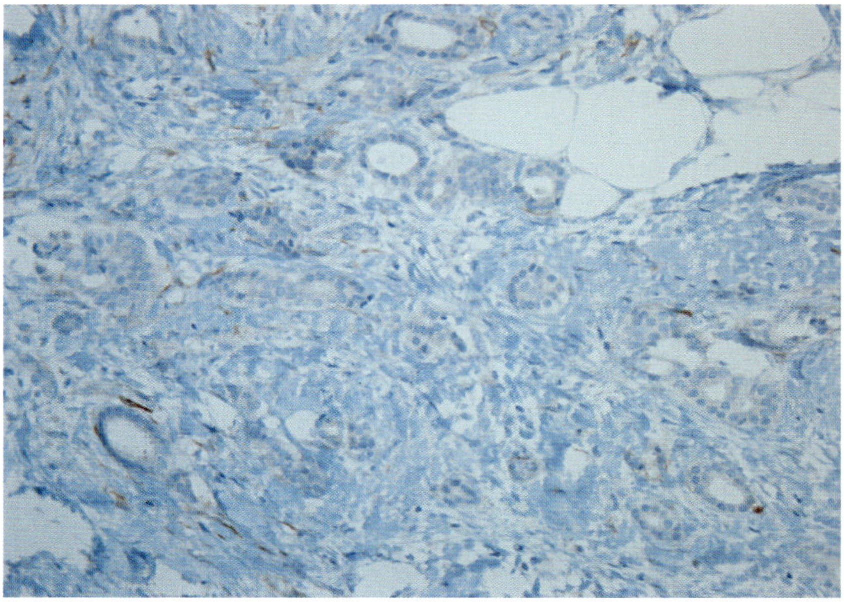

Fig. 4. Tubular carcinoma with calponin IHC stain demonstrating a lack of myoepithelial cells, × 200.

To better identify patients with favourable prognoses and to foster homogeneity among published series, some authors have advocated more stringently-defined morphologic criteria for the diagnosis of tubular carcinoma [11, 28]. By assessing not only the percent tubularity, but also the nuclear and mitotic grade of each tumour, these studies have been able to identify women at particularly low risk for lymph node involvement and death.

One of these groups has further argued that the survival advantage associated with tubular carcinoma may be diminishing, because, as the treatment of IDC has advanced, the good prognosis of tubular carcinoma patients has remained relatively constant [11]. Therefore, this group maintains that these new diagnostic criteria may be clinically useful for identifying patients with truly superior prognoses in this era of improved care.

Lymph node evaluation

Another prognostic factor that has received increased attention in recent years is regional lymph node involvement. Tubular carcinoma of the breast is not only associated with a low incidence of lymph node positivity, but, in some published series, spread to regional lymph nodes was not a significant predictor of patient outcomes [7, 16, 36]. One explanation for this diminished effect is that when positive lymph nodes are discovered in tubular carcinoma patients, more than three nodes are rarely involved [17, 36]. Because node-positivity may not predict outcomes, some have questioned whether lymph node evaluation may be unnecessary for these patients [7]. However, insufficient data currently exist to definitively disprove the value of node positivity for tubular carcinoma patients.

Others have proposed forgoing lymph node evaluation for tubular carcinoma not because of its lack of prognostic value, but because nodal involvement is so uncommon among these patients. Node-positivity is particularly rare among patients with pure tubular tumours, as one large review reported a 6.6% rate of lymph node positivity among patients with tumours that were > 90% tubular, *versus* a 25% rate in those with a 75-90% tubular component [24]. Patients with small primary tubular tumours, especially those with tumours of 1.0 cm or less, have also been shown to be at a low risk for lymph node-positivity [9, 24].

Although some have argued against the value of axillary evaluation for tubular carcinoma patients, it is important to recognize that most of these opinions were published before the widespread use of sentinel lymph node biopsy (SLNB). Recent studies have evaluated the efficacy of SLNB for tubular carcinoma and have concluded that it is a feasible, effective approach to the management of these patients [17, 37]. Until the prognostic implications of nodal involvement for tubular carcinoma are more firmly established, SLNB seems to be a reasonable means of axillary staging for these patients.

Surgery and radiation therapy

When compared to other types of breast cancer, tubular tumours treated with conservative surgery (CS) have been associated with a low rate of local failure, even without the use of adjuvant radiation therapy (RT) [19, 30]. This high rate of local control has prompted some to wonder if these patients could safely be treated by CS without RT [18].

A review of all published cases of tubular carcinoma treated by CS (Table 1) demonstrates that local failure may be uncommon among these patients, but adju-

Table 1 – Local failure among conservatively-treated tubular carcinomas[a].

	Minimum % Tubular Component	Local Failures		Follow-up
		CS no RT	CS + RT	
Deos *et al.* [6]	100%	3/8	–	144-month mean
Bradford *et al.* [35]	100%	0/17	0/21	48-month median[b]
Haffty *et al.* [12]	100%[c]	–	0/21	113-month median
Leonard *et al.* [18]	100%[c]	2/44	–	65-month mean
Winchester *et al.* [36]	80%	0/5	0/16	58-month median[b]
Peters *et al.* [25]	76%	0/1	0/2	84 month mean[b]
Sullivan *et al.* [30]	75%	0/13	3/49	93-month median
Oberman *et al.* [23]	75%	2/2	–	67-month mean
Cabral *et al.* [1]	75%	1/21	0/13	58-month mean
McDivitt *et al.* [20]	75%	1/12	0/3	36-month mean
Holland *et al.* [13]	75%	2/6	0/23	35-month median[b]
Carstens [2]	75%	2/5	–	24-month mean[b]
Thurman *et al.* [32]	N/S	–	2/28	120-month minimum
Kitchen *et al.* [16]	N/S	0/5	0/22	144-month median[b]
Livi *et al.* [19]	N/S	2/52	8/218	101-month median[b]
Weiss *et al.* [34]	N/S	–	2/18	61-month median[b]
Schnitt *et al.* [27]	N/S	0/7	–	56-month median[b]
Tobon *et al.* [33]	N/S	0/2	0/1	23-month mean[b]
Total		**15/200 7.5%**	**15/435 3.4%**	

[a] Tumors specified as less than 75% tubular carcinoma were not included.
[b] Given follow-up is from a larger study that included these tubular cases treated by CS.
[c] Cases reported as "pure" tubular carcinoma were considered 100% tubular.
Abbreviations: CS = conservative surgery; RT = radiation therapy; N/S = not specified.

vant RT may still increase local control. Among the cases reviewed, 7.5 % (15/200) of those treated by CS without RT recurred locally, *versus* 3.4 % (15/435) of those treated by CS + RT. Few conclusions can be drawn from this review, because these cases are compiled from heterogeneous retrospective reports with disparate inclusion criteria and varying follow-up times. Furthermore, some patients may have been selected for CS without RT due to other favourable prognostic factors. Nonetheless, when compared to the local failure rate of other breast cancers, these rates are markedly low. The Early Breast Cancer Trialists' Collaborative Group, for example, reported a 22% local recurrence rate for all breast cancers treated by CS without RT, and a 7.2% rate for those treated by CS + RT[8]. Therefore, although RT may reduce local failure following CS, even those treated without RT appear to have a low rate of local recurrence.

According to three recent retrospective reviews, the risk of local failure following CS may be even lower among elderly tubular patients [18, 19, 30]. It remains unclear if tubular carcinoma is especially indolent in older women, or if these patients are simply more likely to die of other causes before local failure can be detected.

Findings from two recent prospective trials that included all types of breast cancer may indicate that some elderly tubular patients may also not derive a survival benefit from RT. These studies found that although RT reduces local failure, it may not prolong survival in node-negative elderly women with small, estrogen-receptor (ER) positive tumours treated with CS and tamoxifen [10, 14]. Because tubular tumours are often small, ER positive [7, 34], and not associated with lymph node involvement, these findings may apply to many elderly tubular carcinoma patients. However, neither study specifically addressed this population, and the true effect of adjuvant RT on tubular carcinoma patient survival remains unknown.

Despite the low rate of local failure associated with tubular carcinoma, the evidence does not currently seem to support omitting RT following CS for all of these patients. More definitive data are needed to better determine the role of RT for this disease. However, the high rate of local control among these patients, particular elderly women with small, pure tubular tumours, may indicate that they are reasonable candidates for less aggressive approaches to RT, such as partial breast irradiation [31].

Systemic therapy

The necessity of systemic therapy for tubular carcinoma has also been questioned in the literature. However, the impact of systemic treatment on patient outcomes has been difficult to ascertain, because tubular carcinoma rarely metastasizes or causes death, and the effects of chemotherapy or hormonal therapy cannot be determined from small, retrospective reviews reporting few adverse outcomes. Furthermore, patients with lymph node involvement are often more likely to be treated systemically, obscuring the independent effects of systemic therapy [30].

Results from larger reviews addressing this topic have been conflicting. One review of 444 tubular carcinoma cases found that even patients with nodal involvement derived little benefit from systemic therapy [7], while another study concluded that systemic therapy may significantly improve patient outcomes [16]. More data are therefore needed to definitively determine the effects of systemic therapy, especially because many published cases have been treated with regimens that are no longer commonly in use.

Until the efficacy of systemic therapy for these patients can be further evaluated, many women with tubular carcinoma will likely be candidates for hormonal therapy, due to the high rate of ER-positivity associated with tubular tumours. These patients are, however, unlikely to benefit from trastuzumab therapy, as HER-2 gene amplification has been found to be exceedingly rare in tubular carcinomas [22].

Conclusions

As this chapter illustrates, the excellent prognosis of tubular carcinoma of the breast has led some to question the value of lymph node evaluation, RT following CS, and adjuvant systemic therapy for these patients. However, more evidence is needed to determine the necessity of these treatments and to guide the future management of this disease.

To foster more meaningful analyses of the literature and thereby answer some of these management questions, more stringent histologic criteria are needed in future publications. Such enhanced criteria may also enable the better identification of patients with superior prognoses, for whom less aggressive treatment may be appropriate.

Due to the lack of reliable data, the research evidence does not seem to currently justify a less thorough standard of care for tubular carcinoma. To insure the continued excellent prognosis of this disease, clinicians should avoid treating all tubular carcinoma patients less aggressively than similar women with other early breast cancers until such approaches are better supported by the literature.

Acknowledgment

We sincerely acknowledge Dr. Marie Christine Baranzelli for supplying us with the histological figures and Dr. Yazid Belkacémi for his helpful suggestions.

References

1. Cabral AH, Recine M, Paramo JC *et al.* (2003) Tubular carcinoma of the breast: an institutional experience and review of the literature. Breast J 9: 298-301
2. Carstens PH (1978) Tubular carcinoma of the breast. A study of frequency. Am J Clin Pathol 70: 204-10
3. Carstens PH, Greenberg RA, Francis D *et al.* (1985) Tubular carcinoma of the breast. A long term follow-up. Histopathology 9: 271-80
4. Cooper HS, Patchefsky AS, Krall RA (1978) Tubular carcinoma of the breast. Cancer 42: 2334-42
5. Cornil V, Ranvier L (1869). Manuel d'histologie pathologique. Germer Bailliere, Paris
6. Deos PH, Norris HJ (1982) Well-differentiated (tubular) carcinoma of the breast. A clinicopathologic study of 145 pure and mixed cases. Am J Clin Pathol 78: 1-7
7. **Diab SG, Clark GM, Osborne CK *et al.* (1999) Tumor characteristics and clinical outcome of tubular and mucinous breast carcinomas. J Clin Oncol 17: 1442-8**
8. Early Breast Cancer Trialists' Collaborative Group (2000) Favourable and unfavourable effects on long-term survival of radiotherapy for early breast cancer: an overview of the randomised trials. Lancet 355: 1757-70
9. Fein DA, Fowble BL, Hanlon AL *et al.* (1997) Identification of women with T1-T2 breast cancer at low risk of positive axillary nodes. J Surg Oncol 65: 34-9
10. Fyles AW, McCready DR, Manchul LA *et al.* (2004) Tamoxifen with or without Breast Irradiation in Women 50 Years of Age or Older with Early Breast Cancer. N Engl J Med 351: 963-70

11. Goldstein NS, Kestin LL, Vicini FA (2004) Refined morphologic criteria for tubular carcinoma to retain its favorable outcome status in contemporary breast carcinoma patients. Am J Clin Pathol 122: 728-39
12. Haffty BG, Perrotta PL, Ward B *et al.* (1997) Conservatively treated breast cancer: outcome by histologic subtype. Breast J 3: 7-14
13. Holland DW, Boucher LD, Mortimer JE (2001) Tubular breast cancer experience at Washington University: a review of the literature. Clin Breast Cancer 2: 210-4
14. Hughes K, Schnaper LA, Berry D *et al.* (2004) Lumpectomy plus tamoxifen with or without irradiation in women 70 Years of age or older with early breast cancer. N Engl J Med 351: 971-7
15. Kader HA, Jackson J, Mates D *et al.* (2001) Tubular carcinoma of the breast: a population-based study of nodal metastases at presentation and of patterns of relapse. Breast J 7: 8-13
16. Kitchen PR, Smith TH, Henderson MA *et al.* (2001) Tubular carcinoma of the breast: prognosis and response to adjuvant systemic therapy. ANZ J Surg 71: 27-31
17. Leikola J, Heikkilä P, Smitten KV *et al.* (2006) The prevalence of axillary lymph-node metastases in patients with pure tubular carcinoma of the breast and sentinel node biopsy. Eur J Surg Oncol 32: 488-91
18. Leonard CE, Howell K, Shapiro H *et al.* (2005) Excision only for tubular carcinoma of the breast. Breast J 11: 129-33
19. Livi L, Paiar F, Meldolesi E *et al.* (2005) Tubular carcinoma of the breast: outcome and loco-regional recurrence in 307 patients. Eur J Surg Oncol 31: 9-12
20. McDivitt RW, Boyce W, Gersell D (1982) Tubular carcinoma of the breast. Clinical and pathological observations concerning 135 cases. Am J Surg Pathol 6: 401-11
21. Northridge ME, Rhoads GG, Wartenberg D *et al.* (1997) The importance of histologic type on breast cancer survival. J Clin Epidemiol 50: 283-90
22. Oakley GJ, 3rd, Tubbs RR, Crowe J *et al.* (2006) HER-2 amplification in tubular carcinoma of the breast. Am J Clin Pathol 126: 55-8
23. Oberman HA, Fidler WJ Jr (1979) Tubular carcinoma of the breast. Am J Surg Pathol 3: 387-95
24. Papadatos G, Rangan AM, Psarianos T *et al.* (2001) Probability of axillary node involvement in patients with tubular carcinoma of the breast. Br J Surg 88: 860-4
25. Peters GN, Wolff M, Haagensen CD (1981) Tubular carcinoma of the breast. Clinical pathologic correlations based on 100 cases. Ann Surg 193: 138-49
26. Rescigno J, Schiff PB (1997) Tubular carcinoma: Analysis of 1,623 patients from the SEER database (Abstr. 142). Breast Cancer Res Treat 46: 40
27. Schnitt SJ, Hayman J, Gelman R *et al.* (1996) A prospective study of conservative surgery alone in the treatment of selected patients with stage I breast cancer. Cancer 77: 1094-100
28. Stalsberg H, Hartmann WH (2000) The delimitation of tubular carcinoma of the breast. Hum Pathol 31: 601-7
29. Sullivan T, Taghian AG (2006) Management of tubular carcinoma of the breast: general review. Curr Med Lit: Breast Cancer 18: 61-6
30. Sullivan T, Raad R, Goldberg S *et al.* (2005) Tubular Carcinoma of the Breast: a Retrospective Analysis and Review of the Literature. Breast Cancer Res Treat 93: 199-205
31. Taghian AG, Recht A (2006) Update on accelerated partial-breast irradiation. Curr Oncol Rep 8: 35-41
32. Thurman SA, Schnitt SJ, Connolly JL *et al.* (2004) Outcome after breast-conserving therapy for patients with stage I or II mucinous, medullary, or tubular breast carcinoma. Int J Radiat Oncol Biol Phys 59: 152-9
33. Tobon H, Salazar H (1977) Tubular carcinoma of the breast. Clinical, histological, and ultrastructural observations. Arch Pathol Lab Med 101: 310-6
34. Weiss MC, Fowble BL, Solin LJ *et al.* (1992) Outcome of conservative therapy for invasive breast cancer by histologic subtype. Int J Radiat Oncol Biol Phys 23: 941-7
35. Williamson Z, Bradford MD, Wayne N *et al.* (1998) Treatment of Pure Tubular Carcinoma of the Breast. Breast J 4: 437-40
36. Winchester DJ, Sahin AA, Tucker SL *et al.* (1996) Tubular carcinoma of the breast. Predicting axillary nodal metastases and recurrence. Ann Surg 223: 342-7
37. Wong SL, Chao C, Edwards MJ *et al.* (2002) Frequency of sentinel lymph node metastases in patients with favorable breast cancer histologic subtypes. Am J Surg 184: 492-8

Adenoid cystic carcinoma of the breast

K. Khanfir

3

Five Essential Points

1. *Mammary ACC is a rare slow-growing tumour accounting for 0.1% of all breast carcinomas.*
2. *Prognosis is good as axillary lymph nodes and distant metastasis are uncommon.*
3. *Treatment options include simple mastectomy, or lumpectomy followed by irradiation.*
4. *The value of adjuvant chemotherapy and or hormonotherapy is not established*
5. *Late recurrences can occur, thus long-term follow-up is mandatory*

Introduction

Mammary adenoid cystic carcinoma (ACC) is a rare breast cancer variant. It accounts for less than 0.1% of all cases of breast cancer. Fewer than 250 documented cases of ACC have been reported to date. These tumours have been described most frequently in salivary glands. However, the prognosis for ACC of the breast is generally better than ACC of the salivary glands and in comparison to other breast carcinomas [14, 16]. The histologic features of breast ACC are similar to that of ACC of other sites but this is not the case with regard to natural history. In this chapter, we describe epidemiology, clinical presentation, diagnosis, pathology, and management of breast ACC.

Clinical presentation

The age at diagnosis can range from 19 to 96 years but ACC is more common in the fifth and sixth decade. It usually affects female patients but rare cases have been described in males [8, 15].

The most common presenting symptom is a well-circumscribed palpable mass within the breast. Other presenting symptoms include breast tenderness and nipple retraction [11]. Nipple discharge and invasion of the pectoralis muscle are very rare. Most ACC are located in the subareolar region [8, 15]. Tumour size may range from 0.2 to 7 cm with an average of 2-3 cm [11]. Occasionally, ACC is multifocal [1,8]. Differential diagnosis of breast ACC includes cribriform ductal carcinoma *in situ*, invasive cribriform carcinoma, and collagenous spherulosis.

On mammography, the disease can appear as a low-density mass with well or poorly defined, borders [4, 11]. Areas of microcalcification are very rare.

Ultrasound features are those of an hypoechoic solid mass. Magnetic resonance mammography can reveal early enhancement suggesting malignant neoplasm. Preoperative fine-needle aspiration cytology can be useful for diagnosis [7].

Pathology

The cellular origin of this tumour in the breast remains unclear. On histological examination, ACC may show distinctive architectural growth patterns: trabecular-tubular, cribriform and solid. ACC is composed of two cell types, epithelial lining true glands and small basaloid myoepithelial surrounding pseudocystic spaces. Some authors grade these tumours according to a system for ACC of the salivary gland, based on the histological architectural pattern [8, 9, 16]. Ro *et al.* found that solid pattern was associated with a less favourable outcome in mammary ACC. He divided ACC into 3 grades based on the proportion of solid tumour (Grade I, no solid tumour; Grade II, less than 30% solid areas; Grade III, more than 30% solid areas). Recurrences and metastasis were seen only in Grade II or III tumours [16]. However, other studies did not confirm these results [8, 14]. Other authors suggest that the basaloid subtype of solid variant ACC is associated with a worse prognosis with more involvement of axillary lymph nodes [17]. Contrary to its salivary gland counterpart, perineural invasion is very rare in mammary ACC [3, 4].

Immunohistochemically, the epithelial cells are positive to cytokeratin and the myoepithelial cells are usually positive for vimentin, p63 and smooth muscle actin. In addition, ACC of the breast is positive for c-kit (CD117).

ACC is typically estrogen (ER) and progesterone receptor (PR) negative and does not show Her2 gene amplification [7, 11, 13, 19]. This status is related to a non-luminal differentiation in ACC and does not correlate with poor differentiation and high proliferation rate, unlike ductal and lobular breast cancers [19]. However, some tumours have been reported to be ER-positive (26 to 46%) [2, 8, 11].

More recently, molecular prognostic factors have been evaluated to determine their utility in predicting outcome. DNA ploidy, and S-phase fraction have been evaluated by flow cytometry in 28 patients [2]. Of these cases, 26 proved to be DNA diploid, whereas 2 were DNA aneuploid. In this study, ACC showed a very low proliferative activity [2]. None of these markers proved to have prognostic relevance.

Staging evaluation and prognosis

Many investigators have staged ACC according to the TNM system for adenocarcinoma of breast. Staging investigations included chest x-ray, abdominal ultrasound and an isotope bone scan. The prognosis of patients with ACC is much better than that for patients with other breast cancers. The 5-year survival rates ranged from 85-88% [2, 12]. In one of the largest reported series of breast ACC, Arpino and colleagues [2] noted 5-, and 10-year disease-free survival rates of 100% and 93% respectively.

Treatment options

Axillary nodal status is not a major determining factor in planning the treatment of this disease as axillary lymph nodes are infrequent with these tumours [11]. A review of 182 patients, who had axillary dissection identified only 4 cases (2%)

with axillary metastases [2]. Thus, axillary dissection is not indicated in most instances [18]. The sentinel node biopsy may therefore be appropriate for these patients [4, 11].

Distant metastases are uncommon, however the lung is the most frequent site. Metastases may also occur without primary involvement of axillary nodes. Other reported sites include liver, kidney, and bone. Metastases may be seen many years after the initial diagnosis. Even after the development of metastasis, patients have survived for many years in several series. Thus, long-term follow-up is required for these patients.

The best treatment of ACC remains the subject of controversy. Due to the rarity of this disease, results from randomized trials addressing treatment alternatives for breast ACC are not available.

Treatment strategies for the management of ACC of the breast have evolved over these few decades. There has been a trend away from radical mastectomy to simple mastectomy or lumpectomy with or without radiation therapy.

In the past, radical mastectomy then modified radical mastectomy were used for ACC of any size, because it was the standard treatment for breast cancers. In the late 80's, simple mastectomy became the preferred curative surgical option because of the low risk of axillary lymph node metastasis [3,14]. Some patients present with local recurrence following mastectomy [2].

During the same time period, local excision alone was used occasionally, even with large tumours [18]. Many of the reported cases have not included information on the status of margins. Recurrence after local excision alone has been reported by various authors [3, 8, 14-16]. The reported recurrence rate is variable. A review of the literature has identified 11 local recurrences in 182 (6%) patients. None of these patients received radiation therapy [2]. Local recurrence rates of 33% to 37% have been reported after local excision of these tumours in other studies [10, 12]. More than half of the ACC's had focal infiltration in the study of Kleer *et al.*, making free margins difficult to obtain [8]. Hence wide tumour resection with clear margins is recommended [8]. Local recurrence occurring 5 years or later after initial treatment is not a rare event [8, 12, 14]. As mentioned in the literature, the recurrence rate at 5 years was 6% compared to 31% at 10 years [12]. The large majority of recurrences are operable and the long-term outcome remains good [10, 12].

The need for radiotherapy after breast-conserving surgery in ACC is still questioned [8]. After initial local excision, some authors occasionally used radiation therapy in early studies [14, 18]. More recent published series have included patients with breast-conserving surgery and radiation therapy [2, 7, 12, 17]. The later cases (50% of patients) in the study of Millar *et al.* [12], underwent breast-conserving surgery plus radiotherapy rather than mastectomy. An improvement in relapse-free- survival was seen with a dose of 40 Gy in 16 fractions and a boost to the tumour bed of 12.5 Gy in 5 fractions. However, the number of patients in this report is too small to draw definitive conclusions. In early breast cancer, there is extensive evidence supporting the use of radiotherapy in preventing local recurrence after wide local excision or mastectomy [5, 6, 20]. Based on the results of randomized clinical trials, breast-conserving surgery followed by radiation therapy has largely replaced mastectomy for the majority of patients with stage I or II [6, 20]. Since ACC is not multicentic and has a better prognosis than other breast carcinomas, mastectomy is probably not needed for most small tumours. More advanced disease may require mastectomy.

The role of chemotherapy in treating patients with ACC has not been established. Reports of adjuvant systemic chemotherapy for these tumours are anecdotal [2, 12]. Very few patients received hormonal therapy based on the

3

hormone-receptor negativity status [2, 12, 17]. Consequently, few data for hormonal therapy is available.

Glivec therapy has been used in head and neck ACC expressing c-kit but has never been reported in breast ACC.

Due to the late onset of local relapse, as well as distant metastasis, a long-term follow-up for such patients is warranted.

References

1. Alis H, Yigitbas H, Kapan S *et al.* (2008) Multifocal adenoid cystic carcinoma of the breast: an unusual presentation. J Can Chir 51: 36-7
2. **Arpino G, Clarck G, Mohsin S *et al.* (2002) Adenoid cystic of the breast: molecular markers, treatment, and clinical outcome. Cancer 94: 2119-27**
3. Cavanzo FJ, Taylor HB (1969) Adenoid cystic carcinoma of the breast: an analysis of 21 cases. Cancer 24: 740-5
4. Delanote S, Vanden Broecke R, Schelfhout VR *et al.* (2003) Adenoid cystic carcinoma of the breast in a 19-year old girl. Breast 12: 75-7
5. Fisher B, Jeong JH, Anderson S, *et al.* (2002) Twenty-five-year follow-up of a randomized trial comparing radical mastectomy, total mastectomy, and total mastectomy followed by irradiation. N Engl J Med 347: 567-75
6. Fisher B, Anderson S, Bryant J *et al.* (2002) Twenty-year follow-up of a randomized trial comparing total mastectomy, lumpectomy and lumpectomy plus irradiation. N Engl J Med 347: 1233-41
7. Kasagawa T, Suzuki M, Doki T *et al.* (2006) Two cases of adenoid cystic carcinoma: preoperative cytological findings were useful in determining treatment strategy. Breast Cancer 13: 112-6
8. **Kleer CG, Oberman HA (1998) Adenoid cystic carcinoma of the breast value of histologic grading and proliferative activity. Am J Surg Pathol 22: 569-75**
9. Lamovec J, Us-Krasovec M, Zidar A *et al.* (1989) Adenoid cystic carcinoma of the breast. Semin Diagn Pathol 6: 153-64
10. Leeming R, Jenkins M, Mendelsohn G *et al.* (1992) Adenoid cystic carcinoma of the breast. Arch Surg 127: 233-5
11. McClenathan JH, de la Roza G (2002) Adenoid cystic breast cancer. Am J Surg 183: 646-9
12. **Millar BA, Kerba M, Youngston B *et al.* (2004) The potential role of breast conservation surgery and adjuvant breast radiation for adenoid cystic carcinoma of the breast. Breast Cancer Res Treat 87: 225-32**
13. Muslimani AA, Ahluwalia MS, Clark CT *et al.* (2006) Primary adenoid cystic carcinoma of the breast: case report and review of the literature. Int Semin Surg Oncol 3: 17
14. Peters GN, Wolff M (1983) Adenoid cystic of the breast: report of 11 new cases: review of the literature and discussion of biological behaviour. Cancer 52: 680-6
15. Quizilbach AH, Patterson MC, Oliveira KF (1977) Adenoid cystic carcinoma of the breast. Arch Pathol Lab Med 101: 302-6
16. **Ro JY, Silva EG, Gallager HS (1987) Adenoid cystic carcinoma of the breast. Hum Pathol 18: 1276-81**
17. **Shin SJ, Rosen PP (2002) Solid variant of mammary adenoid cystic carcinoma with basaloid features: a study of nine cases. Am J Surg Pathol 26: 413-20**
18. Sumpio BE, Jennings TA, Sullivan PD *et al.* (1987) Adenoid cystic carcinoma of the breast: data from the Connecticut tumor registry and a review of the literature. Ann Surg 205: 295-301
19. Trendell-Smith NJ, Peston D, Shousha S (1999) Adenoid cystic carcinoma of the breast: a tumor commonly devoid of oestrogen receptors and related proteins. Histopathology 35: 241-8
20. Veronesi U, Cascinelli N, Mariani L *et al.* (2002) Twenty-year follow-up of a randomized study comparing breast-conserving surgery with radical mastectomy for early breast cancer. N Engl J Med 347: 1227-32

Primary squamous cell carcinoma of the breast

4

L. Scandolaro

Five Essential Points

1. *BSCC, whose diagnosis follows strict criteria, is a very rare tumour constituting 0.04% to 0.075% of all breast cancers that affects particularly women in the fifth decade.*
2. *It is a form of metaplastic cancer whose risk factors and histogenesis are not well known.*
3. *It is usually found in the left breast and, at presentation, it can have size larger than 4 cm with negative hormone receptors.*
4. *Combination of surgery and radiation therapy is the gold standard therapy and chemotherapy, when needed also in neoadjuvant setting, is platinum based.*
5. *The clinical course is more aggressive and its prognosis is worse than typical breast cancers.*

Introduction

Breast cancer is the most frequent tumour and the second cause of death in women after lung cancer. Over the last 15 years, survival rates for this tumour, have risen to 80% with a 30% reduction in mortality. These important results have been reached with the application of new data emerging from clinical trials. The WHO Classification defines 23 types of malignant, invasive breast cancer but ductal carcinoma is the single largest entity taking in 75% of all breast cancers. Squamous-cell carcinoma of the breast (BSCC) is a very rare tumour. Very few series have been published in the literature and, for most of these, it is doubtful, due to the selection criteria used, that they concern true squamous-cell carcinoma (SCC). For some authors this tumour is a distinct entity, with separate histology from ductal carcinoma, while others feel that it is part of a squamous metaplasia spectrum that can occur with ductal cancers of the breast. Metaplastic tumours are considered a heterogeneous group with mixed features of adenocarcinoma and dominant areas of spindle cell, squamous and/or mesenchymal differentiation while sometimes the squamous component is present in a pure form. Inside this metaplastic group, broad subtypes are described: the pure squamous cell carcinoma (PSCC), referred to as homologous because it presents an epithelial character, and the pseudosarcomatous type, named heterologous because it presents similarity to tumours of mesenchymal origin [5]. This article aims at clarifying some of the pathological issues and verifying the diagnostic and therapeutic efforts in order to better understand the natural history and find the best way to treat this rare disease.

General considerations

Epidemiology

BSCC is a very rare tumour constituting 0.04% to 0.075% of all breast cancers. It can occur in women of all ages but its frequency is high in the fifth decade.

Risk factors

It is impossible to determine the risk factors for the rarity of this tumour. The disease was found in two women with previous breast silicone implants: one had a modified mastectomy for the presence of a 6 cm BSCC, contiguous with the implant's capsule, and the second had the implant surrounded by a thin layer of benign squamous epithelium. The origin of this benign epithelium is unclear but it is known that SCC can arise in tissues where chronic inflammation exists and the epithelialization of the breast implant capsule may be a possible precursor because the transection of ducts, and creation of cavity, can sustain a chronic inflammation that could be the pathogenetic factor responsible for squamous metaplasia and SCC. A similar case was described in another patient who had previous breast augmentation with silicone injected in the breasts.

Histogenesis

The tumour histogenesis is unexplained: the possible myoepithelial or glandular origin of this disease is not yet clear [3]. Keratinizing epithelium is not a normal constituent of breast glandular tissue so the presence of SCC in this organ must be regarded as a form of metaplasia. Squamous metaplasia has been observed in glandular epithelium associated with breast fibroadenoma, benign cystosarcoma phyllodes, papilloma and ginecomastia [5]. The tumour shows large sheets of well- to moderately-differentiated squamous cells that surround large cystic spaces containing nuclear debris and globoid atypical keratotic cells [7]. Pure SCC are often large tumours: more than 4 cm with cysts of variable size. The cysts, which are not always reported in pathology descriptions, seem to be the result of necrotic cavitation in the inner tumour core. One important feature has emerged recently: the squamous cells of pure BSCC express high molecular weight keratins while ductal cancer with epidermoid differentiation expresses low molecular weight keratin [6].

Clinical features

Table 1 summarizes some of general characteristics of patients abstracted from principal reports published in the literature. BSCC is usually found in the left breast and, macroscopically, there are no differences at presentation from other frequent histological types other than larger size: many reports describe tumour burden of 4 cm and more [4]. More than half of the patients are diagnosed in Stage II for the concomitant presence of axillary nodes, while only a small number has metastatic disease at diagnosis (9%).

Table 1 – Summary of primary BSCC principals reports.

Author	N° pts	Median age	T size cm	5 yr OS
Wargotz [7]	22	53	3.9 (1.5-12)	63
Jin [3]	14	62	4.7 (2-8)	54
Stevenson [6]	7	52	4.6 (3.5-6.5)	34
Hennessy [2]	33	52		37

Imaging

The tumour is indistinguishable from other breast cancers on mammography. There was a suggestion that SCC demonstrated more necrosis, with a particular cystic aspect on ultrasound, than ductal carcinomas but this is not a significant diagnostic feature. Application of scinti-mammography is anecdotal and the use of this radioisotope technique is incidental. Staging procedures are similar to those for common breast cancers.

Pathology

BSCC is a rare disease and its diagnosis follows these strict criteria [2, 3, 5, 7]:

1. Absence of extra-mammary primary SCC that may have metastasized and absence of possible deep invasion from skin cancer.
2. Presence of pure infiltrating epidermoid component or predominant infiltrating squamous component of between 50% and 90%.
3. Ductal or lobular component in the minority of the specimen.
4. Gross mass independent from the overlying skin.
5. Light microscopic findings of SCC with pale cytoplasm, keratin formation, intercellular bridges and absence of any invasive neoplastic glandular elements.
6. Ultrastructural demonstration of intracellular canaliculi suggesting that glandular features persist in these tumours.

When these criteria are met, the frequency of pure BSCC rises by 0.06%.

The negativity of hormonal receptors, in most of the patients, is consistent with what would be expected of a tumour with solely squamous cells [4].

Therapies

Treatment strategies are similar to those used for more common breast cancers and a combination of surgery and radiation therapy is the gold standard. As mentioned before, this cancer can have, at diagnosis, large dimension varying between a few centimetres to 10 or more centimetres. In these cases surgery, not only conservative, could be difficult to perform. The use of neoadjuvant chemotherapy is useful in obtaining downsizing and facilitates subsequent conservative surgery, otherwise surgery consists of radical mastectomy. Some series reported in literature have shown that this disease responds well to platinum based chemotherapy, such as the association of platinum and 5-Fluorouracil used in head and neck cancers, while it is less sensitive to a chemotherapy schedule used for common breast cancers. The recent wider use of taxanes and anti-EGFR therapies opens new frontiers, but their use must be validated in the clinical trial setting. In order to prevent locoregional recurrence, radiation therapy should be started earlier than is usual in the treatment of breast cancers. No difference in volume size or dose, compared to common breast tumours, is necessary.

Outcome

The prognosis of BSCC is worse than ductal or lobular breast carcinomas. Table 1 shows 5-year overall survival (OS) from series with large numbers of patients. In a group of 137 patients, collected in the SEER Data Base, the 5-year disease-free survival (DFS) and OS range between 8%-76% and 7%-71%, respectively, in function of disease stage [2]. Progression to distant sites is similar to common breast cancers and the more involved organs are lung and bone, followed by liver and brain. BSCC has two peculiar characteristics:

1. the development of distant metastases can bypass nodal localization [7];
2. relapses are rare 3-4 year after diagnosis.

Conclusions

BSCC is a rare tumour accounting for between 0.04 to 0.07% of all invasive breast cancers and it is frequent in women in their 5th decade. It must be considered a particular expression of metaplastic breast cancers and PSCC is the most frequent histology. This cancer, at presentation, has greater dimension than usual breast tumours and to date, there are no particular prognostic factors known. Surgery followed by radiotherapy, similar to other common breast cancers, is the best therapeutic sequence while chemotherapy, if requested, should be given with schedule similar to SCC of other sites with a platinum-based combination. Chemoradiotherapy is a safe option for those patients whose tumour at diagnosis is large: in these cases surgery should be delayed. This evidence, coupled with the fact that no event was seen in surviving patients 3 years after diagnosis and therapy, places BSCC outcome in the same category as that of common SCC of other sites and as in common SCC, its clinical course is more aggressive than typical breast cancers.

References

1. Dejager D, Redlich PN, Dayer AM *et al.* (1995) Primary squamous cell carcinoma of the breast: sensitivity to cisPlatinum based chemotherapy. J Surg Oncol 59: 199-203
2. Hennessy BT, Krishnamurthy S, Giordano S *et al.* (2005) Squamous cell carcinoma of the breast. J Clin Oncol 23: 7827-35
3. Jin Y, Campana F, Vilcoq JR *et al.* (1993) Carcinome épidermoide primitif du sein. Etude clinique, histopathologique et pronostique de 14 patientes. Bull Cancer 79: 675-9
4. **Menes T, Schachter J, Moregenstern S *et al.* (2003) Primary squamous cell carcinoma (SqCC) of the breast. Am J Clin Oncol 26: 571-3**
5. Rosen PP (1996) Invasive Mammary Carcinoma. Squamous carcinoma. In: Harris JR, Lippman ME, Morrow M, Hellman S (eds) Diseases of the breast. Lippincott-Raven Healthcare, Cedar Knoll, New Jersey, pp 416-417
6. **Stevenson JT, Graham DJ, Khiyami A, Mansour EG (1996) Squamous cell carcinoma of the breast: a clinical approach. Ann Surg Oncol 3: 367-74**
7. **Wargotz ES, Norris HJ (1990) Metaplastic carcinomas of the breast. IV Squamous cell carcinoma of ductal origin. Cancer 65: 272-6**

Primary breast lymphoma

W. Jeanneret Sozzi and R.-O. Mirimanoff

5

Five Essential Points

1. *PBL is a rare and distinct type of extranodal lymphoma; the majority is diffuse large B-cell lymphoma (DLBCL).*
2. *The most common presentation is a painless mass. Bilateral disease is not rare. A full lymphoma working is warranted.*
3. *Surgery should be limited to a biopsy; radiotherapy and anthracycline-based chemotherapy play a central role.*
4. *The best results are obtained with a combination of radiotherapy and chemotherapy, in low grade PBL, in which chemotherapy may be omitted.*
5. *Overall prognosis is relatively good, with 5-year survivals between 45% and 70%. Prognosis is related to stage, IPI score and combined treatment.*

Introduction

The term "primary breast lymphoma" (PBL) is used to define malignant lymphoma primarily occurring in the breast in the absence of other previously detected lymphoma localizations. The first definition was proposed by Wiseman and Liao in 1972 [49]. The clinical pathological criteria for the definition of PBL include: "the clinical site of presentation is the breast, the absence of disseminated lymphoma or preceding extra-mammary lymphoma at the time of diagnosis, adequate pathological specimen evaluation, histological evidence of a close association between the mammary tissue and the lymphomatous infiltrate, and presence of homolateral axillary lymph nodes that may be involved if they develop simultaneously with the primary breast tumour".

Thus, this definition of PBL comprises only tumours that are stage I (lymphoma limited to the breast) and stage II (lymphoma limited to the breast and axillary lymph nodes), excluding those tumours that may have originated at non-breast sites.

Incidence

PBL is a rare disease and represents only 0.38 to 0.7% of all non-Hodgkin's lymphoma (NHL) and between 1.7 and 2.2 % of all extranodal NHL [2, 11, 12, 23, 25, 27, 36, 39, 47, 49]. PBL accounts for only 0.04 to 0.5% of all breast malignancies [2, 10, 11, 12, 17, 23, 25, 27, 33, 39, 47, 49].

Secondary breast lymphoma is observed in association with extramammary non-Hodgkin lymphoma. It occurs more frequently than PBL but is less well studied in the literature. It represents the largest group of metastatic tumours in the breast [12, 19].

Anatomy and pathology

The breast is a mass of glandular, fatty and fibrous tissues positioned over the pectoral muscles of the chest wall. The parenchyma is divided into 15 to 20 segments that converge at the nipple. A lobe is made up of 20 to 40 lobules. The stroma and subcutaneous tissues of the breast contain fat, connective tissue, blood vessels, nerves and lymphatics.

The pathogenesis of PBL is still not clear. Dao *et al.* [15] and Zack *et al.* [53] suggest that PBL might originate in lymphatic tissue present within the breast adjacent to ducts and lobules or from intramammary lymph nodes. Some authors suggest that PBL may arise from mucosal-associated tissue (MALT) [20, 24, 31].

The size of PBL can vary from 1 cm to 20 cm with a median between 3-4 cm [12, 32, 35, 44, 50]. The majority of primary breast lymphomas are of B-cell origin [2, 4, 18, 29, 32, 35, 44, 50], and only few cases of T-cell lymphomas have been described [18, 32, 35, 50]. A large variety of different histologic subtypes have been reported in the literature.

According to Kuper-Hommel's review of the literature, the incidence of diffuse large B-cell lymphoma (DLBCL) is between 45% and 79% [32]. This type of lymphoma is generally unilateral and involves middle-aged women [2, 17, 23, 27, 33]. Burkitt's lymphoma is more aggressive with the capacity of disseminating rapidly and affecting young, pregnant or lactating women; its presentation is more often bilateral and diffuse [2]. These data are in agreement with those of Brogi *et al.* [11]. Kuper-Hommel found a highly variable frequency of MALT lymphoma, ranging from 0% to 75% [32].

Clinical presentation

In the literature, the median age at diagnosis is around 60 years (41-65 years) [1, 4, 12, 18, 22, 23, 29, 32, 35, 44]. There is of course a clear prevalence for female breast lymphoma, but some cases in men have been also reported [1, 25, 29, 44, 48, 50].

The most common symptom is a painless breast mass, whose incidence varies from 80% to 100% [12, 22, 25, 29, 37, 50]. The other symptoms are a painful mass and breast swelling [12]. Multifocal tumours or diffuse breast involvement have been reported by Baker *et al.* and by Lin *et al.* [6, 35]. Clinical signs of advanced breast malignancies are rare, such as inflammatory changes, nipple involvement, skin retraction or tumour fixation [27, 29]. Palpable ipsilateral lymphadenopathy has been noted in 30 to 70% of cases. The left breast is affected in 34% to 56% and the right breast in 32% to 61% [1, 12, 18, 21, 23, 25, 30, 32, 35, 44, 50]. This slight predominance of the right site has been reported without being statistically significant, which is in contrast to the left predominance for breast carcinoma and there is no clear explanation for this. Bilateral PBL are found from 0% to 30% [1, 2, 12, 18, 22, 23, 25, 30, 32, 44, 46, 50]. B symptoms are absent in the majority of the cases, namely from 82% to 96% [22, 23, 25, 32, 44].

Mammography is abnormal in only 9% to 24% of the cases [18, 22]. Thus PBL is generally detected first by the presence of a palpable mass in the breast rather than an abnormal mammography. Of all lymphomas which are diagnosed radiographically, the majority are low grade PBL [18]. The image revealed by mammography is generally a solitary mass without calcifications or spiculate margins [21, 34]. Lieberman *et al.* found in 69% of the mammograms a solitary and uncalcified mass, in 9% multiple masses and in 9% a diffuse increased opacity with skin thickening. Thirteen percent had no abnormal findings [34]. In Lyou *et al.*

study [38], a solitary mass was also the most common radiological pattern, with variable margins and without calcifications as observed in other series [34, 45].

According to Lyou *et al.* study, the echography shows generally a single lesion (75%), which is either circumscribed (50%), microlobulated (37.5%) or oval (50%) and the mass is hypoechogenic in 87.5% and hyperechogenic in 12.5% of the cases [38].

Staging procedure

As the majority of data are retrospective and many based on old series, various histological classifications are used such as the Kiel, the Working Formulation (WF), the Revised European-American Lymphoma (REAL) or the World Health Organization (WHO). With more recent data the WHO classification is now generally used.

The evaluation should include a history and physical examination, complete blood counts, serum chemistry, including lactic dehydrogenase level (LDH), β_2-microglobulin, an HIV test and a bone marrow aspiration and/or biopsy. Chest X-ray, bilateral mammography, CT scan of the thorax, abdomen and pelvis should be performed nowadays as a standard procedure. There are only few data on PET-CT, usually as case reports. Studies have shown that FDG PET scanning is a sensitive and cost-effective method for staging Hodgkin's and non-Hodgkin's lymphoma [16]. PET scan offers the advantage of screening the entire body, excluding the presence of metastases and confirming the origin of the breast lymphoma. Bakheet *et al.* describe a ring-shaped FDG uptake in the breast [7].

In the reported series, stage IE varied from 31% to 80% and stage IIE from 8% to 68% (Table 1).

Table 1 – Incidence of stage I or II according to Ann Arbor stage.

Authors	IE	IIE
Ryan *et al.*, 2008 [44]	67%	27%
Aviles *et al.*, 2005 [4]	31%	68%
Jeanneret Sozzi *et al.*, 2008 [29]	55%	39%
Kuper-Hommel *et al.*, 2003 [32]	58%	8%
Brustein *et al.*, 1987 [12]	54%	28%
Ganjoo *et al.*, 2007 [22]	35%	30%
Lin *et al.*, 2006 [35]	56%	44%
Giradini *et al.*, 1992 [23]	48%	52%
Wong *et al.*, 2002 [50]	80%	19%
Ha *et al.*, 1998 [25]	74%	22%

Treatment

As the majority of the data are derived from retrospective studies, patient management described in the literature shows considerable variations and includes surgery, chemotherapy, radiation therapy or a combination of these different modalities.

Surgery

Surgical procedure can vary from a simple biopsy to radical mastectomy. According to Jenning *et al.* review on 92 publications with data of 465 patients, mastectomy offers no benefit in the survival or on the recurrence risk in PBL [30]. Some authors have even found that surgery could be detrimental [21, 29, 44]. In any case, surgery should be limited to a biopsy large enough to ensure a reliable diagnosis regardless of the pathological classification used.

Chemotherapy and/or radiation therapy

Chemotherapy and/or radiation therapy are generally recognized as the treatment of choice in PBL even if no clear consensus exists regarding which modality, alone or in combination should be chosen, based on the type and stage of the breast lymphoma. Ryan *et al.* in their large retrospective study found that on multivariate analysis, anthracycline-containing chemotherapy and radiotherapy were significantly associated with longer overall survival, the combination of both offering the best outcomes ($P = 0.001$) [44]. In their unique prospective study, Aviles *et al.* found that the combined treatment (radiotherapy of 30 Gy and chemotherapy of 6 cycles with CHOP) was the best treatment, compared to either therapy alone, with an improvement in event-free survival and overall survival [4]. In this trial, 96 patients with PBL stage I and II were assigned to radiotherapy alone, chemotherapy alone or combined modality [4]. In the most recent reports, all patients with intermediate or high grade PBL received chemotherapy, alone or combined with radiotherapy [18, 29, 37, 44]. Radiotherapy alone has a positive and important impact on local control [29, 35, 44]. In low-grade lymphoma, the role of adjuvant chemotherapy is doubtful and patients with indolent lymphoma are generally treated with involved field radiation therapy alone [37].

Radiotherapy

No data on dose effect relationship have been clearly established in the literature. The reported median dose is about 40 Gy (35 Gy to 50.4 Gy) [4, 22, 29, 37, 44, 50]. Generally the radiation fields include breast and/or the chest wall and the regional lymph nodes, encompassing in the majority of cases the axilla and the supraclavicular fossa.

Chemotherapy

Chemotherapy regimens are numerous and have varied over the long period of time corresponding to the reported PBL series. In the latest years, anthracycline-containing chemotherapies like the CHOP regimen (CHOP = cyclophosphamide, adriamycin, vincristine, prednisolone) have emerged as the most effective systemic treatment in early-stage diffuse large B-cell lymphoma (DLBCL) [26, 41]. Ryan *et al.* found that anthracycline-containing chemotherapy had an impact on overall survival (OS) and progression free survival (PFS) [44]. The number of the cycles should be more than 3, depending of the stage of the disease, with or without RT. Chemotherapy appeared also to reduce the risk of controlateral breast involvement [44].

For patients with localized PBL, the current recommendations include the following:

1. For low grade lymphoma, local excision and/or radiation therapy, whereas the place of chemotherapy is controversial [32, 35, 50].

2. For intermediate and high grade PBL, 6-8 cycles of CHOP (or ideally inclusion in a prospective study for patients with high risk) combined to radiation therapy [32, 35, 37, 41, 43, 50].

Recently, anthracycline-containing chemotherapy with the addition of rituximab has provided an improved outcome for patients with DLBCL in a variety of sites [14, 40, 42]. Aviles *et al.* have studied rituximab with dose-dense chemotherapy in PBL on 32 patients. The treatment was well tolerated but the data did not suggest an improvement in event-free or overall survival [3].

Treatment results

The prognosis of PBL is difficult to assess due to the variety of lymphomas included in the same analyses, the variety of treatments and the small number of patients reported in the majority of the published articles. Table 2 summarizes treatment outcome in 17 series.

Ryan *et al.* have reported the results for 204 patients with primary diffuse large B-cell lymphoma, 80% of which have received chemotherapy (87% with anthracycline), and amongst these patients, 62% have also received radiation therapy [44]. Eighty-nine percent of the patients achieved a complete response and the 5- and 10-years overall survival rate was 63% and 47% respectively. The rate of progression and lymphoma-related death was highest in the first 3 years, and there was a continuing pattern of progression and death up to 14 years from the initial treatment [44].

Jennings *et al.* in their review, showed that radiation therapy had a positive impact on survival and recurrence rates for stage I ($P = 0.002$), while chemotherapy (CHOP regimen) had a positive effect on survival and recurrence rates for stage II ($P = 0.001$) [30].

The first sites of progression were the breast (16%), the regional nodes (3%), the central nervous system (CNS) (5%), and other extranodal or other nodal sites (11%) [44]. In our own series of the Rare Cancer Network with 84 patients, the 5-year overall survival was 53% and the 5-year disease-free survival 41% [29].

Aviles *et al.* have randomized 96 patients either to radiation therapy alone (30 patients), chemotherapy alone (32 patients) or a combined treatment (34 patients) [4]. A complete response was achieved in 71% overall of which 66% in the group of radiation therapy alone, 59% in the group of chemotherapy alone and 88% in the combined treatment. The 10-year event-free survival for the radiotherapy group was 50%, chemotherapy 56% and combined therapy 83% ($P < 0.01$). Overall survival at 10 years was 50%, 50% and 76% respectively ($P < 0.01$). Thus their results indicate that a combined treatment seems to be superior to either therapy alone [4].

Liu *et al.* have analyzed 7 studies with 93 patients, with a median follow-up of 34 months. The 3- and 5-year survival rates were 70% and 56% respectively. The combination of chemotherapy and radiation therapy offered a better survival and a lower relapse-free rate [36].

Several studies have reported a CNS relapse rate from 5% to 21% [4, 25, 27, 29, 36, 43, 44, 50, 52] whereas other have not found any CNS recurrences [17, 33, 49]. In the retrospective study by Kuper-Hommel *et al.* [32] on 38 patients, nodal relapses were observed in 17%, extranodal in 30% and nodal and extranodal in 39% of the patients. In 13% the relapse site was unknown. In Lin *et al.* study, the local-relapse-free survival [35] at 5 and 10-year was 80.6% and the distant-relapse-free survival was 58.6% and 47,1% respectively [35]. The distant-relapse-free survival was 67.8% for stage IE and 40.3% for stage IIE ($P = 0.002$). In the same study a group of patients treated with RT (20 cases) was compared to a group without RT (12 cases) [35].

Table 2 – Overall survival and disease-free survival in primary breast lymphoma.

Reference	Number of pts	5-y OS	10-y OS	DFS
Ryan *et al.*, 2008 [44]	204	63%	47%	Median PFS = 5.5 y
Aviles *et al.*, 2005 [4]	96**		 50% 50% 76%	10-y EFS 50% 56% 83%
Aviles *et al.*, 2007 [3]	32	Actuarial 3-y: 63%		EFS-3 y: 75%
Jeanneret *et al.*, 2008 [29]	84	53%		41% 5 y
Brustein *et al.*, 1987 [12]	53	74% 89% (I) 50% (II)	42% 42% (I) 50% (II)	RFS 5/10 y: 38%/33%
Kuper-Hommel *et al.*, 2003 [32]	38	45%, 5 y 63%, 2 y 72%, 2 y localized 46%, 2 y disseminated		
Ganjoo *et al.*, 2007 [22]	37	82% (estimated) Indolent: 92%	70%	PFS 61% (estimated)
Lin *et al.*, 2006 [35]	32	69.3% I: 78.6% II: 57.5%	55.4%	47.7%, 5 y 34.8%, 10 y I: 61.4% II: 22.3%
Giardini *et al.*, 1992 [23]	35	43% Stage I: 61% Stage II: 27%		Stage I: 50% Stage II: 26%
Ha *et al.*, 1998 [25]	23	74% DLCL*: 65%		73% DLCL: 70% (RFS)
Wong *et al.*, 2002 [50]		70% I: 83% I & H: 53% II: 20% L: 91%		RFS: 42% I & H: 29% L: 61%
Ribrag *et al.*, 2001 [43]	20	67% (follow-up 54 months)		50% (follow-up 54 months)
Brogi *et al.*, 1999 [11]		St.I : 60-70% St.II: 30-40%		
Jennings *et al.*, 2007 [30]	465	St.I : 78% St.II: 49%		44.5%
Fruchart *et al.*, 2005 [21]	19	38%		
Liu *et al.*, 2005 [36]	93/7studies	56%		
Vignot *et al.*, 2005 [48]	11/19	29%		Median EFS: 8.3 months

DLCL = diffuse large cell lymphoma.
Randomized trial: RT *versus* CT *versus* RT + CT.
PFS: progression-free survival; RFS: relapse-free survival; EFS: event-free survival; L: low grade; I: intermediate grade; H: high grade.

Prognostic factors

The International Prognostic Index (IPI) score was created to establish a reliable prognostic scoring system for aggressive NHL (The international non-Hodgkin's lymphoma prognostic factors project 1993). It includes five factors which predict treatment outcome: age ($\leqslant$ 60 *vs* > 60 years), performance status (0 or 1 *vs* $\geqslant$ 2), lactate dehydrogenase (< 1 *vs* $\geqslant$ 1 × normal), number of extranodal sites of disease ($\leqslant$ 1 *vs* $\geqslant$ 2) and tumour stage (stage I or II *vs* stage III or IV according to Ann Arbor staging). Thus, 4 risk groups are defined: low (0-1), low-intermediate (2), high

Table 3 – International Prognostic Index (IPI) in PBL.

<table>
<tr><th></th><th>IPI = 0</th><th>IPI = 1</th><th>IPI = 2</th><th>IPI = 3</th><th>IPI = 4</th><th>IPI = 5</th></tr>
<tr><td></td><td colspan="2">Low risk</td><td>Low intermediate risk</td><td>High-intermediate risk</td><td colspan="2">High risk</td></tr>
<tr><td>Ryan et al., 2008 [44]</td><td>26%</td><td>37%</td><td>15%</td><td>3%</td><td></td><td></td></tr>
<tr><td>Aviles et al., 2005 [4]</td><td colspan="2">36%</td><td>55%</td><td>8%</td><td></td><td></td></tr>
<tr><td>Kuper-Hommel et al., 2003 [32]</td><td colspan="2">53%</td><td>18%</td><td>11%</td><td colspan="2">11%</td></tr>
<tr><td>Ganjoo et al., 2007 [22]</td><td colspan="2">77%</td><td colspan="2">16%</td><td colspan="2">5%</td></tr>
<tr><td>Ha et al., 1998 [25]</td><td>48%</td><td>35%</td><td>13%</td><td>4%</td><td></td><td></td></tr>
<tr><td>Fruchart et al., 2005 [21]</td><td>90%</td><td>10%</td><td></td><td></td><td></td><td></td></tr>
</table>

intermediate (3) and high (4 or 5). Recent studies on PBL have shown that the majority of the patients presented a good IPI score of 0 or 1 as presented in Table 3.

Ryan *et al.* found that the prognostic factors which had the most statistical significance on overall survival were IPI ($P < 0.001$), anthracycline-containing chemotherapy ($P = 0.02$) and radiation therapy ($P = 0.03$) [44]. Regarding progression-free survival, IPI ($P = 0.01$), anthracycline-containing chemotherapy ($P = 0.001$) were significant. Thus IPI has been validated also in PBL in this large study. Conversely, radical mastectomy was associated with a statistically significantly poorer cause-specific survival ($P = 0.04$) [44]. Excluding stage, Lin *et al.* compared the groups IPI $\leqslant 1$ and IPI $\geqslant 2$. In these 2 prognostic classes the differences in 5-year overall survival (75.1% *vs* 43.4%, $P = 0.012$), relapse-free survival (58.8% *vs* 11.4%, $P = 0.004$) and distant-relapse-free survival (92.5% *vs* 50.3%, $P = 0.005$) were statistically significant. IPI had also an impact on local-relapse-free survival which was 87.9% and 77.6%, respectively ($P = 0.514$) [35]. Contrary to other investigators, Aviles *et al.* could not find a role of IPI on prognosis [4] whereas Ha *et al.* found an influence of IPI only on OS, but not on RFS [25].

The Ann Arbor staging was found to be a prognostic factor for overall survival ($P = 0.0021$) in Wong *et al.* study with 26 patients [50]. In Lin *et al.* study, Ann Arbor stage, KPS, IPI excluding stage, LDH and radiotherapy proved to be significant factors for OS. The same factors and radiotherapy had an impact on RFS and radiotherapy was significant for local control. Finally Ann Arbor stage, LDH and IPI excluding stage were related to distant control [35].

Some recent studies have found different cytogenetic patterns looking at the immunohistochemistry of primary breast DLCBCL, which may have prognostic implications and should be confirmed in future studies. Fruchart *et al.* have observed that breast lymphoma co-expressing Bcl6 and CD10 seemed to have a better prognosis as shown by others authors [5, 8, 9, 21]. Yoshida *et al.* have investigated 15 patients in using various markers, and have found that cases of DLCBCL with a negative expression of CD10 (0/15) and positive expression of MUM1 (15/15) correspond to a non-germinal centre B-cell phenotype, and have also a high MIB-1 index (mean 79%) which might be associated with a poor outcome [51].

Conclusions

Primary breast lymphoma is a rare entity. Clinically it appears as a well-defined mass, generally without calcification on mammography, and rarely discovered by screening. The symptoms are mostly non specific, with a painless palpable mass

5

which is usually unique. The most frequent histological type is the diffuse large B-cell lymphoma. The recommended treatment for primary breast lymphoma is a very limited surgery or biopsy, followed by anthracycline-containing chemotherapy and radiation therapy to the ipsilateral breast and/or chest wall, with or without treatment of the regional nodes. In low-grade PBL, radiotherapy alone may be sufficient.

The role of rituximab added to the standard chemotherapy in PBL has not yet been completely demonstrated, as is the case in other sites of DLCBL. It will be particularly important to evaluate its role in future prospective studies.

CNS recurrences are an issue in BL; however, experts do not agree on the possible benefit of CNS prophylaxis.

References

1. Abbondanzo SL, Seidman JD, Lefkowitz M *et al.* (1996) Primary diffuse large B-cell lymphoma of the breast. A clinicopathologic study of 31 cases. Pathol Res Pract 192(1): 37-43
2. Arber DA, Simpson JF, Weiss LM *et al.* (1994) Non-Hodgkin's lymphoma involving the breast. Am J Surg Pathol 18(3): 288-95
3. Avilés A, Castañeda C, Neri N *et al.* (2007) Rituximab and dose dense chemotherapy in primary breast lymphoma. Haematologica 92(08): 1147-8.
4. **Avilés A, Delgado S, Nambo MJ *et al.* (2005) Primary Breast Lymphoma: Results of a Controlled Clinical Trial. Oncology 69: 256-60**
5. Bai M, Agnantis NJ, Skyrlas A *et al.* (2003) Increased Expression of the bcl6 and CD10 Proteins Is Associated with Increased Apoptosis and Proliferation in Diffuse Large B-Cell Lymphomas. Mod Pathol 16: 471-80
6. Baker R, Slayden G, Jennings W *et al.* (2005) Multifocal primary breast lymphoma. South Med J 98: 1045-8
7. Bakheet SM, Bakheet R, Ezzat A *et al.* (2001) F-18 FDG Positron Emission Tomography in Primary Breast Non-Hodgkin's Lymphoma. Clin Nucl Med 26: 299-301
8. Barrans SL, Carter I, Owen RG *et al.* (2002) Germinal center phenotype and bcl-2 expression combined with the International Prognostic Index improves patient risk stratification in diffuse large B-cell lypmphoma. Blood 99: 1136-43
9. Barrans SL, O'Connor SJ, Evans PA *et al.* (2002) Rearrangement of the BCL6 locus at 3q27 is an independent poor prognostic factor in nodal diffuse B-cell lymphoma. Br J Haematol 117: 322-32
10. Bobrow LG, Richards MA, Happerfield LC *et al.* (1993) Breast lymphomas: a clinicopathologic review. Hum Pathol 24(3): 274-8
11. Brogi E, Harris NL (1999) Lymphomas of the breast: pathology and clinical behavior. Semin Oncol 26(3): 357-64
12. Brustein S, Kimmel M, Lieberman PH *et al.* (1987) Malignant Lymphoma of the Breast. A study of 53 patients. Ann. Surg vol 205(2): 144-50
13. Carbone PP, Kaplan HS, Musshoff K *et al.* (1971) Report of the Committee on Hodgkin's disease staging classification. Cancer Res 31: 1860-1
14. Coiffier B, Lepage E, Briere J *et al.* (2002) CHOP chemotherapy plus rituximab compared with CHOP alone in elderly patients with diffuse large-B-cell lymphoma. N Engl J Med 346: 235-42
15. Dao AH, Adkins RB Jr, Glick AD *et al.* (1992) Malignant lymphoma of the breast: a review of 13 cases. Am Surg 58(12): 792-6
16. Delbeke D (1999) Oncological applications of FDG PET imaging: brain tumors, colorectal cancer, lymphoma and melanoma. J Nucl Med 40: 591
17. Dixon JM, Lumsden AB, Krajewski A *et al.* (1987) Primary lymphoma of the breast. Br J Surg 74: 214-6
18. Domchek SM, Hecht JL, Fleming MD *et al.* (2002) Lymphomas of the breast. Primary and Secondary Involvement. Cancer 94: 6-13
19. **Duncan VE, Reddy VVB, Jhala NC *et al.* (2006) Non-Hodgkin's lymphoma of the breast: a review of 18 primary and secondary cases. Annals of Diagnostic Pathology 10: 144-8**

20. Farinha P, Saudade A, Cabecadas J *et al.* (2000) High frequency of MALT lymphoma in a series of 14 cases of primary breast lymphoma. Appl Immunol Mol Morpho 10: 115-26
21. Fruchart C, Denoux Y, Chasle J *et al.* (2005) High grade primary breast lymphoma: is it a different clinical entity? Breast Cancer Research and Treatment 93: 191-8
22. Ganjoo K, Advani R, Mariappan MR *et al.* (2007) Non-Hodgkin Lymphoma of the Breast. Cancer 110: 25-30
23. Giardini R, Piccolo C, Rilke F *et al.* (1992) Primary non-Hodgkin's lymphomas of the female breast. Cancer 69(3): 725-35
24. Gupta D, Shindham V, Zemba-Palko V, Keshgegian A (2000) Primary bilateral mucosa-associated lymphoid tissue lymphoma of the breast with atypical ductal hyperplasia and localized amyloidosis. A case report and review of the literature. Arch Pathol lab Med 124: 1233-6
25. Ha CS, Dubey P, Goyal LK *et al.* (1998) Localized Primary Non-Hodgkin Lymphoma of the Breast. Am J Clin Oncol 21(4): 376-80
26. Horning SJ, Weller E, Kim K *et al.* (2004) Chemotherapy with or without radiotherapy in limited-stage diffuse aggressive non-Hodgkin's lymphoma: Eastern Cooperative Oncology group Study 1484. J Clin Oncol 22: 3032-8
27. Hugh JC, Jackson FI, Hanson J *et al.* (1990) Primary breast lymphoma. An immunohistologic study of 20 new cases. Cancer 66: 2602-11
28. The International Non-Hodgkin's lymphoma Prognostic Factors Project (1993) A predictive Model for aggressive Non-Hodgkin's Lymphoma.N Engl J Med 329: 987-94
29. **Jeanneret Sozzi W, Taghian A, Epelbaum R *et al.* (2008) Primary breast lymphoma: Patient profile, outcome and prognostic factors. A multicentre Rare Cancer Network study. BMC Cancer 8: 86**
30. **Jennings WC, Baker RS, Murray SS *et al.* (2007) Primary Breast Lymphoma. The Role of Mastectomy and the Importance of Lymph Node Status. Ann Surg 245: 784-9**
31. Kambouchner M, Godmer P, Guillevin L *et al.* (2003) Low grade marginal zone B cell lymphoma of the breast associated with localized amyloidosis and corpora amylacea in a woman with long standing primary Sjogren's syndrome. J Clin Pathol 56: 74-7
32. Kuper-Hommel MJJ, Snijder S, Janssen-Heijnen MLG *et al.* (2003) Treatment and survival of 38 female breast lymphomas: a population-based study with clinical and pathological reviews. Ann Hematol 82: 397-404
33. Lavomec J, Jancar J (1987) Primary malignant lymphoma of the breast: lymphoma of the mucosa-associated lymphoid tissue. Cancer 60: 3033-41
34. Liberman L, Giess CS, Dershaw DD *et al.* (1994) Non-Hodgkin Lymphoma of the Breast: Imaging Characteristics and Correlation with Histopathologic Findings. Radiology 192: 157-60
35. Lin Y, Guo XM, Shen KW *et al.* (2006) Primary breast lymphoma: Long-term treatment outcome and prognosis. Leukemia & Lymphoma 47(10): 2102-9
36. Liu MT, Hsieh CY, Wang AY *et al.* (2005) Primary breast lymphoma: a pooled analysis of prognostic factors and survival in 93 cases. Ann Saudi Med 25(4): 288-93
37. Lyons JA, Myles J, Pohlman B *et al.* (2000) Treatment and Prognosis of Primary Breast Lymphoma: A Review of 13 Cases. Am J Clin Oncol 23(4): 334-6.
38. Lyou CY, Yang SK, Choe DH *et al.* (2007) Mammographic and sonographic findings of primary breast lymphoma. Clinical Imaging 31: 234-8
39. Mattia AR, Ferry JA, Harris NL *et al.* (1993) Breast lymphoma. A B-cell spectrum including the low grade B-cell lymphoma of mucosa associated lymphoid tissue. Am J Surg Pathol 17(6): 574-87
40. Miller T, Unger J, Spier C *et al.* (2004) Effect of adding rituximab to three cycles of CHOP plus involved field radiotherapy for limited stage aggressive diffuse large B-cell lymphoma (SWOG-0014) Blood 104: 48a-9a
41. Miller TP, LeBlanc M, Spier C *et al.* (2001) CHOP alone compared to CHOP plus radiotherapy for early stage aggressive non-Hogkin's lymphoma: update of the Southwest Oncology Group (SWOG) randomized trial. Blood 98: 72A
42. Pfreundschuh M. Trumper L, Osterborg A *et al.* (2006) CHOP-like chemotherapy plus rituximab *versus* CHOP-like chemotherapy alone in young patients with good-prognosis diffuse large B-cell lymphoma: a randomized controlled trial by the Mab Thera International Trial (MinT) Group. Lancet Oncol. 7: 379-91

5

43. Ribrag V, Bibeau F, El Weshi A *et al.* (2001) Primary breast lymphoma: a report of 20 cases. British Journal of Haematology 115: 253-6
44. Ryan G, Martinelli G, Kuper-Hommel M *et al.* (2008) Primary diffuse large B-cell lymphoma of the breast: prognostic factors and outcomes of a study by the International Extranodal Lymphoma Group. Annals of Oncology 19: 233-41
45. Sabaté JM, Gómez A, Torrubia S *et al.* (2002) Lymphoma of the Breast: Clinical and Radiologic Features With Pathologic Correlation in 28 Patients. The Breast Journal 8 (5): 294-304
46. Shouton JT, Weese JL, Carbone P *et al* (1981) Lymphoma of the breast. Ann Surg 194(69): 749-53
47. Topalovski M, Crisan D, Mattson JC *et al.* (1999) Lymphoma of the Breast. A Clinicopathologic Study of Primary and Secondary Cases. Arch Pathol Lab Med 123: 1208-18
48. Vignot S, Ledoussal V, Nodiot P et al (2005) Non-Hodgkin's Lymphoma of the Breast: a Report of 19 Cases and Review of the Literature. Clin Lymphoma 6(1): 37-42
49. Wiseman C, Liao KT (1972) Primary lymphoma of the breast. Cancer 29(6) 1705-12
50. Wong WW, Schild SE, Halyard MY *et al.* (2002) Primary Non-Hodgkin Lymphoma of the Breast: The Mayo Clinic Experience. Journal of Surgical Oncology 80: 19-25
51. Yoshida S, Nakamura N, Sasaki Y *et al.* (2005) Primary breast diffuse large B-cell lymphoma shows a non-germinal B-cell phenotype. Modern Pathology 18: 398-405
52. Young SD, Imrie K, Gospodarowicz M *et al.* (1999) Primary lymphoma of the breast: a 30 year retrospective analysis of the Toronto experience. Proc ASCO 18: 41a.
53. Zack RJ, Trevisan SG, Gupta M *et al.* (2001) Primary breast lymphoma originating in a benign intramammary lymph node. Am J Roentgenol 177: 177-8

Phyllodes tumours of the breast

6

G. Bousquet, J. Bonneterre and Y. Belkacémi

Five Essential Points

1. *The prognosis of phyllodes tumours of the breast is excellent, and only malignant forms have a metastatic potential. The major challenge in the management of these tumours is the local control.*
2. *Conservative surgery without axillary dissection is the standard of care for benign lesions, if the tumour size allows acceptable cosmesis. It may also be proposed for borderline tumours but with a persistent relapse risk rate of 20-30%.*
3. *Considering the high local relapse risk of conservative surgery, total mastectomy without axillary dissection should be proposed for malignant tumours, except if tumour size is less than 2 cm. The sentinel node biopsy has not been investigated in the phyllodes tumours.*
4. *For borderline and malignant tumours, conservative surgery with adjuvant radiation therapy may be an alternative to total mastectomy.*
5. *Adjuvant chemotherapy for malignant forms is not the standard of care.*

Introduction

Phyllodes tumours of the breast are rare tumours, accounting for 0.3-0.9% of breast tumours, and 2-3% of fibroepithelial tumours of the breast [3]. Phyllodes tumours have been described since 1982. The World Health Organization (WHO) proposed a classification with three distinct types: benign, borderline and malignant phyllodes tumours [11]. The pathological features classically used to distinguish these three categories are stromal cellularity, cell pleiomorphism, number of mitoses, margins, stromal pattern, and stromal differentiation. It is interesting to notice that malignant tumours have sarcomatous features with a metastatic potential, and although controversial, their prognosis is probably similar to that of non-phyllodes sarcomas of the breast [12]. The management of phyllodes tumours is mainly surgical, but controversies still remain concerning the type of surgery – conservative or not – especially for borderline and malignant forms. The role of adjuvant treatments (such as radiation therapy and chemotherapy) is also questioned. We propose to discuss these different pointsin this chapter.

Pathology

The WHO classification makes the distinction between three tumour types, using the pathological features described in Table 1 [11].

Table 1 – The three tumour types for phyllodes tumours according to WHO classification [11].

	Benign	Borderline	Malignant
Stromal hypercellularity	mild	mild	strong
Cell pleomorphism	weak	mild	strong
Mitosis	few	intermediate	> 10/10 hpf
Margin	"pushing"	intermediate	"invasive"
Stromal "pattern"	a uniform stromal distribution	heterogeneous stromal expansion	Strong "stromal overgrowth"
Stromal differentiation	rare	rare	frequent

Benign tumours are the most frequent phyllodes tumours and represent about 60% of all phyllodes tumours in recent published series, whereas malignant forms represent only 20% [2, 10]. While benign and borderline tumours have mostly a local relapse potential, malignant forms have a higher risk for metastatic dissemination in about 25% of the cases, mainly to the lung. On the other hand, benign and borderline forms may relapse in tumours with more aggressive histological features [1].

Prognosis

The prognosis of all phyllodes tumours is excellent with a 10-year survival rate of 96% in the large series of 443 patients published recently by the Rare Cancer Network (RCN) [2]. It is still excellent for malignant forms with a relative cumulative survival at 10 years close to 90% [4]. While controversial, histological type may be a prognostic factor for local relapse and survival [2]. Breast surgery without axillary dissection is the main treatment for phyllodes tumours, but type of surgery is still debated. In case of conservative surgery, tumour type, tumour size and margin status appear to be the most important prognostic factors for local relapse [1, 2, 8]. In fact, in a large review of several series, local relapse rate after wide tumorectomy with margins of 1-2 cm was 8%, 29% and 36% respectively in case of benign, borderline or malignant tumours, but also 21%, 46% and 69% respectively for the same groups if the margin status was uncertain [1]. In the RCN series in which 85% of the patients had a conservative surgery, the five-year local control of 74% for the combined group of borderline and malignant tumours [2]. In that series, the multivariate analysis revealed benign histology, negative margins (RR=2.13) and adjuvant radiation therapy (RR=2.32) as favourable prognostic factors for local control, whereas radiation therapy was the only prognostic factor for the sub-group of borderline and malignant tumours. The different pathological features such as stromal cellularity, cellular pleiomorphism, number of mitoses and necrosis are variably reported as independent prognostic factors for local control or survival, and may actually not be taken account for the management of phyllodes tumours. In fact, and despite the excellent prognosis of these tumours, other biological factors are required to better identify prognostic sub-groups, especially for malignant tumours [1, 2, 5, 8, 10].

Loco-regional therapy

It is widely accepted that conservative surgery without axillary dissection is a reasonable treatment for benign tumours, if breast volume and tumour size allow acceptable cosmesis. However, no consensus exists concerning management of cases where margins are positive after tumour excision. Considering the increased risk of local relapse, potentially with borderline or malignant histological features, it seems reasonable to systematically ensure adequate margins. In order to be able to avoid a perhaps unnecessary second surgery, it is recommended to have a histological diagnosis prior to surgery, in particular to make the distinction between benign phyllodes tumours and non-phyllodes fibroadenomas, which do not usually require wide surgical excision.

For borderline and malignant tumours, axillary dissection is also not recommended. In a series of 48 malignant tumours, axillary dissection was performed in 21 patients, with a mean number of 14 nodes, and none of them invaded [5]. According to this, the sentinel node biopsy has not been investigated in these indications. Contrary to benign tumours, the role of conservative surgery in borderline and malignant forms has not been clearly defined. In a series of 478 malignant tumours, 5-year local control rate was 79.4% and 91.2%, respectively in case of lumpectomy and total mastectomy. Local control was also correlated to tumour size, with a 5-year local control rate of 58% in tumours of 5-10 cm, with conservative surgery. It is interesting to note that the local relapse risk was 15% after mastectomy if the tumour size was more than 10 cm [8]. In their series of 159 borderline/malignant phyllodes tumours, Belkacémi *et al.* showed that total mastectomy was statistically correlated with a better local control and a trend for a better overall survival ($p = 0.06$) [2]. This observation was not confirmed in a large retrospective analysis of 821 malignant phyllodes tumours of the Surveillance Epidemiology and End Results (SEER) program [7]. Obviously, conservative surgery may be proposed for borderline tumours with a persistent local relapse rate of 20-30%, but care should be taken to have adequate margins in order to decrease the risk of recurrence [1]. For malignant phyllodes tumours, tumorectomy should also be discussed as an alternative to total mastectomy, if the tumour size allows conservative surgery with an acceptable cosmesis. Pezner *et al.* showed a 5-year local control of 91% after lumpectomy for tumours of less than 2 cm [8]. If total mastectomy is finally preferred to conservative surgery, the possibility of immediate breast reconstruction (IBR) may be discussed. Singh *et al.* recently published a series of 7 patients with phyllodes tumours and IBR after total mastectomy. Five of their patients had a maligant phyllodes tumour, and one of them developed a local recurrence one year after [9]. In fact, and considering a local relapse risk after total mastectomy of less than 10% for benign tumours, and of less than 15% for malignant forms of more than 10 cm insize, immediate reconstruction can reasonably be proposed to these patients [1, 8].

Despite the fact that local relapse being associated with a worse prognosis is still controversial, local control is the major challenge in phyllodes tumours, especially for borderline and malignant tumours. For this reason, adjuvant radiation therapy should be considered, particularly after conservative surgery. Nevertheless, there are very little data assessing the role of radiation therapy. The largest series published by Belkacémi *et al.* has described a sub-population of 39 patients among the 443 (9%) with phyllodes tumours who received adjuvant radiation therapy delivering a median total dose of 50 Gy; 37 patients had either a borderline or a malignant tumour. In this sub-group of patients with borderline/malignant tumours

6

who received radiation therapy, the 10-year local relapse rate was significantly improved compared to the sub-group of patients who did not, by 14% and 41% ($p = 0.02$), respectively. The local recurrence rate of 14% was comparable to that in the patients that have had only total mastectomy [2]. According to these results, which need to be confirmed, adjuvant radiation therapy may be proposed after conservative surgery for borderline and malignant tumours, particularly in large tumours. For malignant tumours, the role of adjuvant radiation therapy after total mastectomy is not known, and should be discussed for large tumours of more than 10 cm.

Systemic therapy

The last debate in the treatment of phyllodes tumours consists of systemic treatment in the adjuvant setting. As discussed, it seems that only malignant tumours have a metastatic potential, so that adjuvant chemotherapy should only be considered for this histological sub-type. In fact, malignant phyllodes tumours harbour sarcoma features, and should be properly characterized in terms of histological sub-type, but also in terms of grading using international systems of soft tissue sarcoma (STS). In their series of 83 women with primary breast sarcomas (PBS) including malignant phyllodes tumours, Zelek *et al.* showed that tumour size and histological grade according to the French classification were strong prognostic factors for survival. Their conclusion was that PBS and malignant phyllodes tumours have the same prognostic factors as STS of the extremities. Thus, similar treatment strategies should be used [12]. In fact, adjuvant chemotherapy for STS of the extremities is becoming less and less the standard of care. A recent pooled analysis of two large randomized trials including 819 patients with resected localized high grade STS failed to show a survival advantage of doxorubicin-based adjuvant chemotherapy compared to no treatment [6]. A better knowledge of molecular pathways implicated in the oncogenesis of phyllodes tumours as well as different histological subtypes of STS is required to better assess the question of the potential benefit of an adjuvant medical treatment for malignant phyllodes tumours. The role of new drugs and targeted therapies is still unknown in PBS.

References

1. **Barth RJ Jr (1999) Histologic features predict local recurrence after breast conserving therapy of phyllodes tumors. Breast Cancer Res Treat 57(3): 291-5**
2. **Belkacémi Y, Bousquet G, Marsiglia H *et al.* (2008) Phyllodes tumor of the breast. Int J Radiat Oncol Biol Phys 70(2): 492-500**
3. Geisler DP, Boyle MJ, Malnar KF *et al.* (2000) Phyllodes tumors of the breast: a review of 32 cases. Am Surg 66(4): 360-6
4. **Grabowski J, Salzstein SL, Sadler GR, Blair SL (2007) Malignant phyllodes tumors: a review of 752 cases. Am Surg 73(10): 967-9**
5. Kapiris I, Nasiri N, A'Hern R *et al.* (2001) Outcome and predictive factors of local recurrence and distant metastases following primary surgical treatment of high-grade malignant phyllodes tumours of the breast. Eur J Surg Oncol 27: 723-30
6. Le Cesne A, Van Glabbeke M, Woll PJ *et al.* (2008) The end of adjuvant chemotherapy (adCT) era with doxorubicin-based regimen in resected high-grade soft tissue sarcoma (STS): Pooled analysis of the two STBSG-EORTC phase III clinical trials. J Clin Oncol 26(suppl): abstr 10525
7. Macdonald OK, Lee CM, Tward JD *et al.* (2006) Malignant phyllodes tumor of the female breast: association of primary therapy with cause-specific survival from the

Surveillance, Epidemiology, and End Results (SEER) program. Cancer 107(9): 2127-33

8. **Pezner RD, Schultheiss TE, Paz IB (2008) Malignant phyllodes tumor of the breast: local control rates with surgery alone. Int J Radiat Oncol Biol Phys 71(3): 710-3**
9. Singh G, Sharma RK (2008) Immediate breast reconstruction for phyllodes tumors. Breast 17(3): 296-301
10. Tse GM, Lui PC, Lee CS *et al.* (2004) Stromal expression of vascular endothelial growth factor correlates with tumor grade and microvessel density in mammary phyllodes tumors: a multicenter study of 185 cases. Hum Pathol 35(9): 1053-7
11. **The world Health Organization Histological Typing of Breast Tumors – Second Edition. The World Organization. Am J Clin Pathol 1982 Dec;78(6): 806-16**
12. Zelek L, Llombart-Cussac A, Terrier P *et al.* (2003) Prognostic factors in primary breast sarcomas: a series of patients with long-term follow-up. J Clin Oncol 21(13): 2583-8

Primary breast sarcomas

7

L. Zelek, M. Spielmann, J. Grenier and A. Le Cesne

Five Essential Points

1. *Mastectomy remains the gold standard, only highly selected cases could be treated with conservative surgery.*
2. *Axillary dissection is not mandatory.*
3. *Adjuvant radiotherapy could improve local control.*
4. *Primary Breast Sarcomas usually behave as soft-tissue sarcomas of the extremities, pathological grade, tumor size and quality of margins being the most significant prognostic factors.*
5. *Angiosarcoma prognosis seems to be particularly poorer than for other breast sarcomas.*

Introduction

Primary breast sarcoma (PBS) is a rare entity, initially described in 1887 [14]. The annual incidence can be estimated at 45 new cases per 10 million women, and this incidence rate has remained constant during the past decades [19]. Due to the rarity of this tumour, the vast majority of publications are case reports or concern small series, and the data provided by these reports has not been sufficiently informative to enhance our understanding of the natural history of this malignancy.

A subject that has been debated is the confusion between cystosarcoma phyllodes and PBS. PBS arises from the mesenchymal tissue of the mammary gland and the pathologic definition of this entity is clear. Cystosarcoma phyllodes was initially defined according to its fleshy macroscopic appearance and encompasses a wide variety of tumours with mixed epithelial and benign or malignant mesenchymal proliferation [23]. Often the published series included PBS and cystosarcoma phyllodes, regardless of the histologic features of the mesenchymal component of the latter, making it impossible to obtain specific knowledge about these tumours [5,12,20]. However, there is now evidence that cystosarcoma phyllodes can be considered malignant when the stromal component exhibits a clear pattern of sarcoma (grade 3 phyllodes tumours) [30]. Several series have shown that the clinical course of PBS and phyllodes sarcomas as well as their survival rates are identical, leaving the practical value of this distinction open to doubt [8,30,34].

There is still no definitive consensus regarding the treatment of PBS. Even if simple mastectomy without axillary dissection is still widely regarded as the gold standard, there are major variations in the extent of local therapy, ranging from wide local excision [3,11] to radical mastectomy [2,3,5,8,11,12,18,20,26,30,34]. Recourse to chemotherapy and radiotherapy has also differed from one centre to another [3,15,26]. Finally, a significant proportion of PBS cases has been treated in the same manner as breast carcinomas by gynecologists or breast oncologists who are not necessarily experienced in the treatment of soft tissue sarcomas.

7

Prognostic factors

If angiosarcomas are excluded, there is evidence that the natural history of PBS does not differ significantly from that of soft tissue sarcomas arising at other sites. A major conclusion of recent studies [2,8,18,34] is that PBS has the same prognostic factors as common soft tissue sarcoma, including tumour size and histologic grade as it has previously been suggested [6,7,31,33]. Moreover, the survival curves obtained in each subgroup are comparable with those generally reported for sarcomas of the extremities and even the shape of the curve, which is characterized by a plateau after the fifth year, is comparable [6] (Figs 1 & 2). It is worth mentioning that the first recurrences were mainly local failures or lung metastases, which is consistent with what is already known about the clinical course of soft tissue sarcomas [6]. Finally, as we and others have reported [8,30,34], it is the malignant mesenchymal component that is decisive in the evolution of phyllodes sarcomas, and although the first steps of tumorigenesis may be different in phyllodes sarcomas and other breast sarcomas, this classic distinction is of marginal importance from a therapeutic point of view.

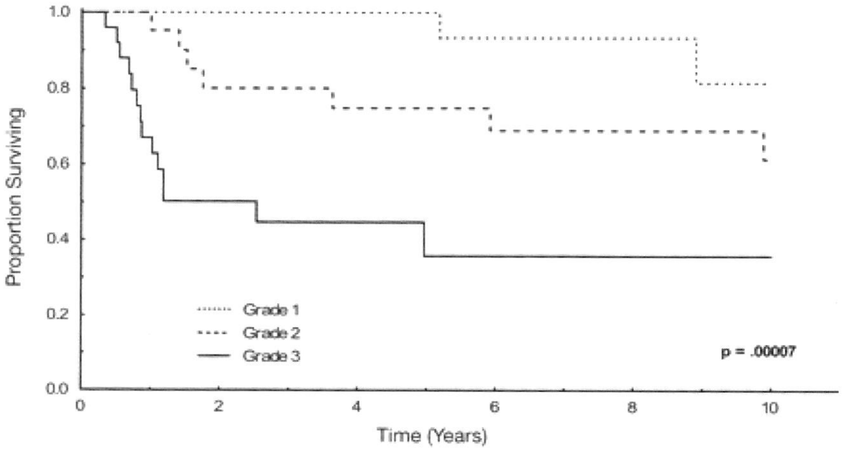

Fig. 1. Ten-year Overall Survival according to tumour FNCLCC grade [34, reprinted with permission. © 2008 American Society of Clinical Oncology. All rights reserved.]

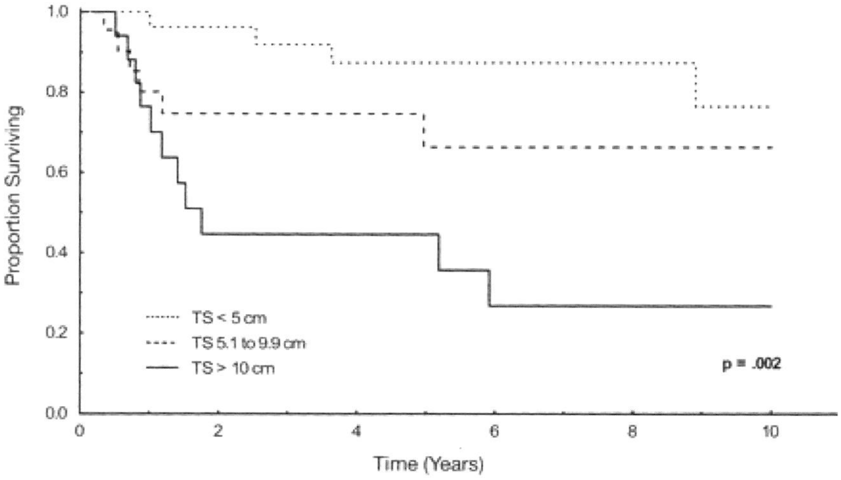

Fig. 2. Ten-year overall survival according to tumour size (TS) [34, reprinted with permission. © 2008 American Society of Clinical Oncology. All rights reserved.]

Distinguishing angiosarcomas from other histologic types is clinically more relevant because, in the majority of publications [2,4,8,9,13,18,21,34], the prognosis is dramatically poor, with lesions exhibiting diffuse and multicentric local extension rendering surgical resection difficult, and the majority of patients, if not all, develop early distant metastases.

Finally, the importance of the histologic grade must be underscored [17,34] because this grade is not an accurate prognostic factor in other specific sites where sarcomas arise, such as the uterus [22].

Local therapy

There is no doubt that wide surgery remains the cornerstone of soft tissue sarcoma treatment. Distant DFS rates exceeding 50% were obtained in series in which the majority of the patients underwent surgery alone [2,8,18,34]. In recent studies, the prognostic value of clear margins has been pointed out [2,8,29]. Mastectomy can still be considered the gold standard, but axillary dissection should not be recommended given the rareness of lymph node involvement reported by most authors [2,8,11,14,18,34]. A major concern regarding the extent of local treatment is whether conservative surgery can be proposed to a selected subgroup of patients. The rationale underlying this suggestion is that the majority of PBS (angiosarcomas excluded) is not multicentric. Because the histologic grade and the tumour size are the main prognostic factors, it seems reasonable to propose wide local excision to patients with grade 1 tumours smaller than 5 cm, provided that the margins of the operative specimen are free of disease. This approach has been demonstrated to be safe in selected patients and in our experience mastectomy has proven effective for most patients with local recurrence. Moreover, in our series a large proportion of the local recurrences occurred in patients with large tumours who refused mastectomy and who were thus not ideal candidates for breast preservation [34]. Although, like others, we were unable to demonstrate a detrimental effect of wide local excision on survival, the greater probability of distant metastases after local failure is a well-documented fact in soft tissue sarcomas [6] and wide local excision should not be recommended as the standard procedure. If carried out, margin status is of paramount importance.

Another debatable issue is the usefulness of postoperative radiotherapy. The main interest of this modality is that limb-sparing surgery can replace amputation for sarcomas of the extremities. Assuming that radical surgery is the gold standard for breast sarcomas, only a marginal benefit can be expected from adjuvant radiotherapy in PBS after mastectomy. However, like other authors [25], we are concerned by the significant rate of chest wall recurrences after mastectomy. Even if these local failures are surgically salvageable in most patients, they are certainly not trivial events and, in some cases, may have a deleterious impact on survival, an outcome already reported for extremity sarcomas [6]. If we consider three randomized studies in favour of local radiotherapy due to a significant decrease in local high-grade sarcoma recurrences [24,27,32], improved local control might be achieved by chest wall irradiation in high-grade PBS. The fact that Johnstone *et al.* [15] reported no local failures after adjuvant radiotherapy in high-grade PBS must be emphasized, but the small size of the population in that study precludes any definitive conclusion. The development of local recurrence in 20 of 59 patients after mastectomy in our series [34] underscores the need for improved local control. Furthermore, although most PBS are not multicentric and despite the lack of prospective studies, it seems reasonable to use this modality after conservative surgery, and after mastectomy, at least for larger or high-grade tumours [1,11].

Adjuvant chemotherapy

A further point that needs to be addressed is whether adjuvant chemotherapy is capable of increasing long-term survival in PBS, and in this respect, the poor 5-year survival rate of patients with grade 3 tumours must be stressed. A key article related to soft tissue sarcomas was the collaborative meta-analysis published in 1997, which showed that adjuvant chemotherapy with doxorubicin-based regimens yielded a statistically significant improvement in DFS but without a considerable impact on OS [28]. A randomized trial comparing intensive adjuvant epirubicin plus ifosfamide *versus* no treatment showed, despite its small size, a significant improvement in both DFS and OS [10]. Unfortunately, more recent data do not support the routine use of adjuvant chemotherapy in soft tissue sarcomas [16]. However, since there is evidence that, on the whole, PBS behaves like extremity sarcoma, there are clearly no grounds for excluding it from forthcoming adjuvant trials.

Neoadjuvant chemotherapy, finally, is not relevant in most patients because soft tissue sarcomas are poorly chemosensitive, with response rates ranging from 20% to 40% [6], and most PBS cases are amenable to surgery. Moreover, in our experience surgical resection is never possible after primary chemotherapy in patients presenting with locally advanced tumours [34]. Whether most recent schedules are capable of yielding enhanced response rates and improving breast preservation, remains an issue.

Breast angiosarcomas merit particular attention because the natural history of these tumours is fundamentally different. At the time of diagnosis, a great proportion of these tumours have already started to spread diffusely within the breast and even into the surrounding tissue, thus rendering surgical resection extremely difficult. Most authors have reported the grim prognosis of these tumours, with early distant relapses and a very poor short-term survival [2,4,8,9,13,18,21,34]. On an empirical basis, patients with angiosarcoma should be offered maximal therapy, including adjuvant radiotherapy and possibly chemotherapy.

In conclusion, the prognosis of PBS is dependent on margin status, tumour grade, size, and histologic type (angiosarcoma *v* others), and for most patients (excluding those with angiosarcoma), therapy can be similar to that administered for soft tissue sarcomas of other sites:

- whenever possible, patients should be referred to a reference centre for sarcoma,
- mastectomy without axillary dissection is the gold standard for the treatment of PBS, but wide local excision can be considered in highly selected patients,
- given the results of randomized trials, including trials of sarcomas of the extremities, adjuvant radiotherapy might improve local control at least for large or high-grade tumours or after conservative surgery,
- finally, adjuvant chemotherapy is not to be routinely recommended (except, perhaps, for breast angiosarcomas).

References

1. **Barrow BJ, Janjan NA, Gutman H *et al.* (1999) Role of radiotherapy in sarcoma of the breast: A retrospective review of the M.D. Anderson experience. Radiother Oncol 52: 173-8**
2. **Bousquet G, Confavreux C, Magné N *et al.* (2007) Outcome and prognostic factors in breast sarcoma: a multicenter study from the rare cancer network. Radiother Oncol 85: 355-61**

3. Chaney AW, Pollack A, McNeese MD *et al.* (2000) Primary treatment of cystosarcoma phyllodes of the breast. Cancer 89: 1502-11
4. Chen KT, Kirkegaard DD, Bocian JJ (1980) Angiosarcoma of the breast. Cancer 46: 368-71
5. Christiensen L, Schiodt T, Blichert-Toft M *et al.* (1993) Sarcomatoid tumors of the breast in Denmark from 1977 to 1987: A clinicopthological and immunohistochemical study of 100 cases. Eur J Cancer 29A: 1824-31
6. Clark MA, Fisher C, Judson I, Thomas JM (2005) Soft-tissue sarcomas in adults. N Engl J Med 353: 701-11
7. Coindre JM, Terrier P, Guillou L *et al.* (2001) Predictive value of grade for metastasis development in the main histologic types of adult soft tissue sarcomas: A study of 1,240 patients from the French Federation of Cancer Centers Sarcoma Group. Cancer 91: 1914-26
8. **Confavreux C, Lurkin A, Mitton N *et al.* (2006) Sarcomas and malignant phyllodes tumours of the breast – a retrospective study. Eur J Cancer 42: 2715-21**
9. Donnell RM, Rosen PP, Lieberman PH *et al.* (1981) Angiosarcoma and other vascular tumors of the breast. Am J Surg Pathol 5: 629-42
10. Frustaci S, Gherlinzoni F, De Paoli A *et al.* (2001) Adjuvant chemotherapy for adult soft tissue sarcomas of the extremities and girdles: Results of the Italian randomized cooperative trial. J Clin Oncol 19: 1238-47
11. Gutman H, Polock RE, Ross MI *et al.* (1994) Sarcoma of the breast: Implications for extent of therapy: The M.D. Anderson experience. Surgery 116: 505-9
12. Henry J, Norris MD, Herbert B *et al.* (1968) Sarcoma and related mesenchymal tumors of the breast. Cancer 22: 22-8
13. Hunter TB, Martin PC, Dietzen CD (1985) Angiosarcoma of the breast: Two case reports and a review of the literature. Cancer 56: 2099-106
14. Jardines L: Other cancers in the breast. In: Harris JR, Lippman S, Morrow M *et al.* (eds) (2000) Diseases of the Breast. Lippincott-Raven, Philadelphia, PA, pp. 76-882
15. **Johnstone PAS, Pierce LJ, Merino MJ *et al.* (1993) Primary soft tissue sarcomas of the breast: Local-regional control with post-operative radiotherapy. Int J Radiat Oncol Biol Phys 27: 671-5**
16. LeCesne A, VanGlabbeke M, Woll PJ *et al.* (2008) The end of adjuvant chemotherapy (adCT) era with doxorubicin-based regimen in resected high-grade soft tissue sarcoma (STS): Pooled analysis of the two STBSG-EORTC phase III clinical trials. J Clin Oncol 26(suppl) abstr 10525
17. MacGowan TS, Cummings BJ, O'Sullivan B *et al.* (2000) An analysis of 78 breast sarcoma patients without distant metastases at presentation. Int J Radiat Oncol Biol Phys 46: 383-90
18. Malard Y, DeLara CT, MacGrogan J *et al.* (2004) Primary breast sarcoma. A retrospective study of 42 patients treated at the Bergonié Institute during a 32-year period. J Gynecol Obstet Biol Reprod (Paris) 33: S89-99
19. May DS, Stroup NE (1991) The incidence of sarcomas of the breast among women in the United States, 1973-1986. Plast Reconstr Surg 87: 193-4 (letter)
20. McGregor GI, Knowling MA, Este FA (1994) Sarcoma and cystosarcoma phyllodes tumors of the breast: A retrospective review of 58 cases. Am J Surg 167: 477-80
21. Merino MJ, Carter D, Berman M (1983) Angiosarcoma of the breast. Am J Surg Pathol 7: 53-60
22. Pautier P, Genestie C, Rey A *et al.* (1998) Analysis of clinicopathological prognostic factors in 60 uterine leiomyosarcomas. Proc Am Soc Clin Oncol 17: 512a (abstr 1974)
23. Petrek JA: Phyllodes tumors. In: Harris JR, Lippman S, Morrow M *et al.* (eds) (2000) Diseases of the Breast. Lippincott-Raven, Philadelphia, PA, pp 863-869
24. Pisters PW, Harrison LB, Leung DH *et al.* (1996) Long-term results of a prospective randomised trial of adjuvant brachytherapy in soft tissue sarcoma. J Clin Oncol 14: 859-68
25. Pollard SG, Marks PV, Temple LN (1990) Breast sarcoma: A clinicopathologic review of 25 cases. Cancer 66: 941-4
26. Reinfuss M, Mitus J, Smolak K *et al.* (1993) Malignant phyllodes tumours of the breast: A clinical and pathological analysis of 55 cases. Eur J Cancer 29A: 1252-6
27. Rosenberg S, Tepper J, Galtstein E *et al.* (1982) The treatment of soft-tissue sarcoma of the extremities: Prospective randomized evaluation of (1) limb-sparing surgery plus radiation therapy compared with amputation and (2) the role of adjuvant chemotherapy. Ann Surg 196: 305-15

7

28. Sarcoma Meta-Analysis Collaboration (1997) Adjuvant chemotherapy for localised resectable soft-tissue sarcoma of adults: Meta-analysis of individual data. Lancet 350: 1647-54
29. Smola MG, Ratschek M, Amann W *et al.* (1993) The impact of resection margins in the treatment of primary sarcomas of the breast: A clinicopathological study of eight cases with review of the literature. Eur J Surg Oncol 19: 61-9
30. Terrier Ph, Terrier-Lacombe MJ, Mouriesse H *et al.* (1989) Primary breast sarcomas: A review of 33 cases with immunohistochemistry and prognostic factors. Breast Cancer Res Treat 13: 39-48
31. Trojani M, Contesso G, Coindre JM *et al.* (1984) Soft-tissue sarcomas of adults: Study of pathological prognostic variables and definition of a histopathological grading system. Int J Cancer 33: 37-42
32. Yang JC, Chang AE, Baker AR *et al.* (1998) Randomized prospective study of the benefit of adjuvant radiation therapy in the treatment of soft tissue sarcomas of the extremity. J Clin Oncol 16: 197-203
33. Zagars GK, Goswitz MS, Pollack A (1996) Liposarcoma: Outcome and prognostic factors following conservation surgery and radiation therapy. Int J Radiat Oncol Biol Phys 36: 311-9
34. **Zelek L, Llombart-Cussac A, Terrier P *et al.* (2003) Prognostic factors in primary breast sarcomas: a series of patients with long term follow-up. J Clin Oncol 21(13): 2583-8**

Angiosarcoma of the breast

Y.M. Kirova and A. Fourquet

8

Five Essential Points

1. *Sarcoma of the breast is a rare disease which can be divided into two main categories: primary breast sarcomas and treatment-associated breast sarcomas.*
2. *Primary soft tissue sarcoma of the breast represents less than 1% of breast malignancies and 10-25% of all breast sarcomas, their principal treatment is surgery.*
3. *Post irradiation sarcomas are rare but a recognized complication of radiation therapy for breast carcinoma, and are associated with poor prognosis.*
4. *They must fulfill Cahan's criteria: i) prior history of RT; ii) asymptomatic latent period of several years; iii) the occurrence of a sarcoma within a previously irradiated field; iv) histological confirmation of sarcomatous nature of the post-irradiation lesion.*
5. *Long and careful follow up is needed to detect these rare tumours and to propose radical surgical treatment.*

Introduction: breast sarcomas

Sarcoma of the breast is a rare disease. Different kinds of breast soft tissue sarcomas have been reported in the literature [1, 3-6, 10, 12, 13, 16, 18-26, 28-32, 34-42, 44-50] and can be divided into two main categories: primary breast sarcomas and treatment-associated breast sarcomas.

Primary soft tissue sarcoma of the breast represents less than 1% of breast malignancies [1, 24, 28, 49]. This group forms a heterogeneous array of histologic subtypes [1, 49]. Angiosarcomas are a relatively rare histological subtype of sarcomas and represent < 1% of all sarcomas [1]. Although rare, angiosarcomas display remarkable clinical heterogeneity. These tumours can occur anywhere in the body, but the breast is an important location.

Sarcomas are a recognized complication of radiation therapy for breast carcinoma, and are associated with poor prognosis [3-14, 16, 18-23, 26, 27, 29-32, 34-36, 38-48, 50]. Soft tissue sarcoma occurring in the treatment volume after breast cancer is a rare condition, described first by Warren and Sommer in 1936 [46]. In 1948, Cahan *et al.* [3] defined the criteria for the diagnosis of radiation-induced sarcoma (RIS): i) prior history of RT; ii) asymptomatic latent period of several years; iii) the occurrence of a sarcoma within a previously irradiated field; iv) histological confirmation of sarcomatous nature of the post-irradiation lesion.

Independent of RT, chronic lymphoedema is an important predisposing factor for angiosarcoma [2, 19, 15, 37]. Stewart and Treves in 1948 were the first to describe six cases of angiosarcoma occurring in lymphadoematous extremities after radical mastectomy [37].

Primary breast angiosarcoma

The incidence of primary breast angiosarcoma is about 10-25% of all breast sarcomas [1]. It is difficult to evaluate the incidence of primary breast angiosarcomas, due to their rarity and because heterogeneous retrospective series have been reported in the literature [1, 39, 49]. In a large number of published series, there is no clear border between primary breast angiosarcoma, radiation-induced angiosarcoma and/or Steward-Treves Syndrome [40]. A further problem is that most papers are case reports or small series. In the series of Zelek *et al.* [49], the authors reported 83 primary breast sarcomas with a follow-up of 7.8 years. Of these, 8 patients (10%) presented angiosarcomas. In this series angiosarcomas had a poorer prognosis (0.03) in comparison with other types of sarcoma. Distinguishing angiosarcomas from other histologic types is clinically more relevant because, in the majority of publications the prognosis is poor [1, 49]. In the Mayo Clinic series, angiosarcomas tended to be larger in size [1]. Another important problem, related to a small number of patients who experienced different treatment modalities (mastectomy, or breast conserving surgery, followed by radiotherapy, and/or chemotherapy) is that there is no consensus on standard treatment. It seems that in cases of primary breast angiosarcoma, mastectomy is the treatment of choice [1, 24]. In the published series no metastases were found when axillary lymph node dissection was performed [1, 49]. Other possible treatments have been reported by McGowan *et al.* who have studied 78 breast sarcomas (including 8 angiosarcomas) proposing breast conserving surgery followed by radiotherapy in case of negative surgical margins [28].

Treatment-associated breast angiosarcoma

Radiation-induced angiosarcoma (RIS)

The reported *incidence* of RIS ranges from 0.01% to 0.02% per year (Table 1). In the series of the Institut Curie the cumulative RIS incidence was 0.07% (± 0.02) at 5 years, 0.27% (±0.05) at 10 years and 0.48% (±0.11) at 15 years [21]. Different histological identities have been reported such as fibrosarcoma, malignant fibrous histiocytoma (MFH), liposarcoma, and angiosarcoma [10, 21, 23, 36, 39]. With the development of breast-conserving treatment, radiation-associated breast angiosarcoma became the most frequently reported type of breast sarcoma (Table 1). In the previously published series of the Institut Curie, 48% of radiation-induced sarcomas were angiosarcoma [21] (Fig. 1). In the series of Karlsson *et al.* who have studied the Swedish Cancer Register, the largest reported group of patients presented angiosarcoma [16].

The estimated incidence of treatment-associated breast angiosarcoma is 0.002% to 0.05% per year [5]. Yap *et al.* [48] reported that a cumulative incidence of angiosarcoma at 15 years post diagnosis was 0.9 per 1,000 for cases receiving radiation (SE = 0.2) and 0.1 per 1,000 for cases not receiving radiation (SE < 0.1). The authors found that the risk of subsequent angiosarcoma of the chest or breast was strongly and significantly increased among women with history of invasive breast cancer (OR 11.6, 95% CI = 1.7-5.8). The incidence of angiosarcomas in the largest published series is shown in Table 1.

Table 1 – Incidence of angiosarcomas (in red) in the largest published series of RIS after breast cancer treatment.

	Type of retrospective study	Total patients (N)	Total number of sarcomas (N)	RIS (N)	Incidence [95% conf. Intervals] after RT	Incidence without RT	Risk
Huang & Mackillop 2001 [13]	Cohort (SEER)	194,798	135	54 soft tissue sarcomas	SIR 26.2 [16.5-41.4] (angiosarcoma)	2.1	RR: 15.9
				20 angiosarcomas	2.5 [1.8-3.5] (other sarcomas)	1.3	RR: 2.2
Karlsson *et al.* 1998 [16]	Swedish Cancer Register (Case control study)	122,991	40 angiosarcomas 76 other sarcomas incl. STS		SIR: 1.9 [1.5-2.2]		AR: 1.3/10^4 person-yrs
Kirova *et al.* 2005 [21]	Single centre Institut Curie	16,705	36		Cumulative RIS incidence: 0.07% (± 0.02) at 5 years,	SIR 1.3 [0.3-3.6]	RR: 8 [4.98–12.7]
		13,472,RT	35	27 RIS (+ 2 STS)	0.27% (±0.05) at 10 years and 0.48% (±0.11)		
		3,233 without RT	1	13 angiosarcomas	at 15 years SIR 10.2 [9.03-11.59]		
Taghian *et al.* 1991 [40]	Single centre (Institut Gustave Roussy - IGR)	6 919	9 in field 2 STS	9 in field 3 angiosarcomas	Cumulative index: 0.2% at 10 yrs; 0.43% at 20 yrs; 0.78% at 30 yrs		
Zucali *et al.* 1994 [50]	Single center (Milan)	3,295		3 soft tissue sarcomas 2 angiosarcomas			

SIR: standardized incidence ratio; AR: absolute risk; RR: relative risk; SML: secondary malignancies; STS: Stewart-Treves syndrome.

1A

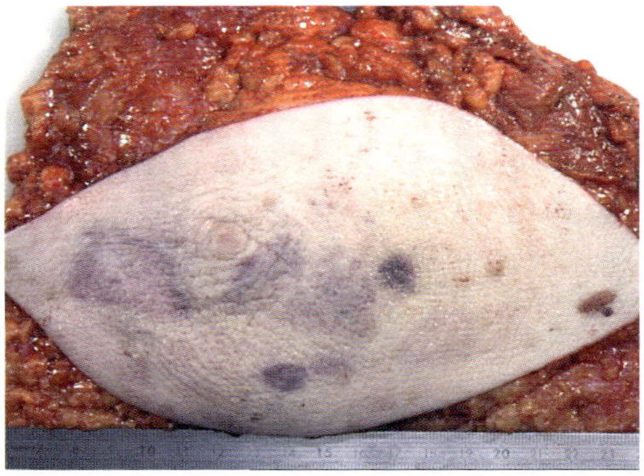

1B

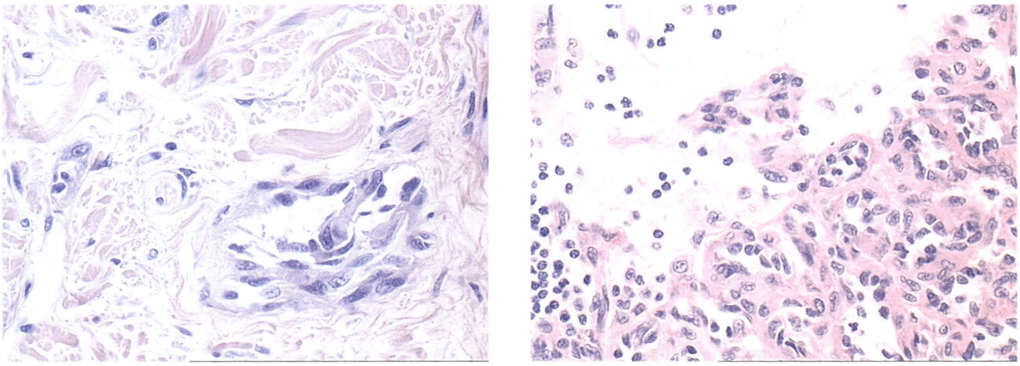

Fig. 1. Macroscopic and microscopic findings of radiation associated sarcoma, diagnosed 16 years after the initial treatment, treated by mastectomy.

1A: Mastectomy specimen with the typical clinical presentation;
1B: Microscopic presentation, pathological findings.

The prognosis of patients with RIS is poor with overall survival rates ranging from 10% to 30% [21, 22, 31, 40]. All 7 patients of the Kuten *et al.* series died within 6-36 months from the time of diagnosis of sarcoma [22]. Taghian *et al.* [44] reported a mean survival of 2.4 years (ranging from 4 months to 9 years).

Treatment and prognosis of RIS

The conventional treatment for RIS is surgery, and Robinson *et al.* [31] postulated, "...The radical surgical approach is the only chance of cure". RIS is associated with poor prognosis because most cases are diagnosed in advanced stage and frequently located in areas where radical surgery cannot be performed [31]. Some of the patients with RIS of the irradiated breast underwent radical surgery and they are long-term survivors [18-21]. Chemotherapy (CT) is often used in the treatment of RIS but the response rate has been reported to be poor [22]. In the literature there are reports of treatment of RIS with non-conventional methods, such as combination of RT and hyperthermia, but they are rare and no large series of published results is available.

Future development of treatment modalities will be possible with advances in the evaluation of genetic changes. Tarkkanen *et al.* [41] have analysed 27 RIS by comparative genomic hybridisation, which allows genome-wide screening of changes in the DNA sequence copy number. They have found that gains at 7q or 8q are associated with poor prognosis or large tumour size. Thus, the frequent gains at 7q and 8q might have been responsible in part for the poor prognosis of post-irradiation sarcomas [41].

Stewart-Treves syndrome (STS)

Post-mastectomy and radiotherapy-induced lymphoedema is an important predisposing factor for angiosarcoma. Numerous publications have reported cases with lymphoedema related exclusively to radical surgery [19, 37]. The incidence of Stewart-Treves syndrome decreases with the use of conserving surgery and radiotherapy [19, 33]. Schunemann *et al.* identified 107 cases (27%) of lymphoedema of the ipsilateral arm in a series 4101 patients undergoing radical surgery [33]. The authors reported 39.2% "oedema rate" after radical or modified mastectomy *versus* 9.5% in the patient group with breast-conserving surgery. Radiotherapy adds to the risk of lymphoedema. Some authors have evaluated the risk in relationship to treatment modalities, as follows: for radical mastectomy alone 22.7%; radical mastectomy and radiation therapy 44.7%; modified radical mastectomy alone 19.9%; modified radical mastectomy and radiation therapy 29.3%; breast conserving surgery alone 6.9%; breast conserving surgery followed by radiation therapy 10.4% [33]. At the same time, the oedema rate was decreased from 38% to 18% over the 20 year period with evaluation of surgical techniques [33]. The benefit of adjuvant radiotherapy to the chest wall has been controversial for many years. A recently updated meta-analysis showed that the radiotherapy regimens produced moderate but definite reductions not only in 15-year breast cancer mortality but also in 15-year overall mortality [8]. But as with the surgical techniques, there has been real progress in the development of new and less toxic techniques of radiotherapy to the chest wall [17]. Therefore, a real decrease in the incidence of Stewart-Treves syndrome has been observed over recent years. On the other hand, post-treatment oedema of the upper extremity is also related to other risk factors such as obesity, venous outflow obstruction, and hypertension. The prevention of Stewart-Treves syndrome is also the treatment for lymphangitis and lymphoedema of upper limb [19]. Different treatment modalities have been reported with various efficacies.

References

1. Adem C, Reynolds C (2004) Primary breast sarcoma: clinicopathologic series from the Mayo Clinic and review of the literature. Br J Cancer 91: 237-41
2. Balzarini A, Pirovano C *et al.* (1996) Ultrasound therapy of chronic lympoedema after surgical treatment of breast cancer. Lymphology 26: 128-34
3. **Cahan WG, Woodward HQ (1948) Sarcoma arising in irradiated bone: report of eleven cases. Cancer 1: 3-29**
4. Chauveinc L, Dutrillaux AM (1999) Cytogenetic study of eight new cases of radiation-induced solid tumors. Cancer Genet Cytogenet 114: 1-8
5. Cozen W, Bernstein L (1999) The risk of angiosarcoma following primary breast cancer. Br J Cancer 81: 532-6
6. Doherty MA, Rodger A (1986) Sarcoma of bone following therapeutic irradiation for breast carcinoma. Int J Radiat Oncol Biol Phys 12: 103-6
7. Dutrillaux B (1997) Ionizing radiation induced malignancies in man. Radioprotection 32: C1-431
8. Early Breast Cancer Trialists' Collaborative Group (EBCTCG) (2005) Effects of radiotherapy and of differences in the extent of surgery for early breast cancer on local recurrence and 15-year survival: an overview of the randomized trials. Lancet 366: 2087-106
9. Hall EJ: Principles of carcinogenesis. In: De Vita VT, Hellman S, Rosenberg SA (1993), eds. Cancer: Principles and Practice of Oncology, 4th edition Philadelphia, PA: Lippincott Co, p. 213-27
10. Hardy TJ, An T (1978) Postirradiation sarcoma (malignant fibrous histiocytoma) of axilla. Cancer 4: 118-24
11. Harris JR, Coleman CN (1989) Estimating the risk of second primary tumors following cancer treatment. J Clin Oncol 7: 5-6
12. Haselow RE, Nesbit M (1978) Second neoplasms following megavoltage radiation in a pediatric population. Cancer 42: 1185-91
13. Huang J, Mackillop WJ. (2001) Increased risk of soft tissue sarcoma after radiotherapy in women with breast carcinoma. Cancer 92: 172-80
14. Ishimaru M, Ishimaru T (1975) A review of 30 years study of Hiroshima and Nagasaki atomic bomb survivors. Biological effects. Leukemia and Related Disorders. J Radiat Res 16: S89-96
15. Kiricuta IC, Dammrich J (1992) Lymphangiosarcoma of arm after chronic lymphoedema: a rare long-term complication after radical mastectomy. Case report and overview. Strahlentherapie und Onkologie 169: 291-5
16. Karlsson P, Holmberg E (1998) Soft tissue sarcoma after treatment for breast cancer-a Swedish population – based study. Eur J Cancer 34: 2068-75
17. Kirova YM, Campana F *et al.* (2007) Postmastectomy Electron Beam Chest Wall Irradiation in Women with Breast Cancer: A Clinical Step Toward Conformal Electron Therapy Int J Radiat Oncol Biol Phys 69: 1137-44
18. Kirova YM, Feuilhade F (1998) Radiation-induced sarcomas following radiotherapy for breast cancer: six case reports and a review of the literature. The Breast 7: 277-82
19. Kirova Y, Feuilhade F (1999) Stewart-Treves syndrome after treatment for breast cancer. The Breast 8: 282-4
20. Kirova YM, Gambotti L (2007) Risk of second malignancies (SM) following adjuvant radiotherapy (RT) for breast cancer (BC): a large scale single institution review. Int J Radiat Oncol Biol Phys 68: 359-63
21. **Kirova Y, Vilcoq JR (2005) Radiation-induced sarcomas (RIS) following radiotherapy for breast cancer: a large-scale single institution review. Cancer 104: 856-63**
22. Kuten A, Sapir D (1985) Postirradiation soft tissu sarcoma occurring in breast cancer patients: report of seven cases and results of combination chemotherapy. J Surg Oncol 28: 168-71
23. Laskin WB, Silverman TA (1988) Postirradiation soft tissu sarcomas : an analysis of 53 cases. Cancer 62: 2330-40
24. Losanoff JE, Jaber S (2006) Primary angiosarcoma of the breast: do enlarged axillary nodes matter? The Breast Journal 12: 371-4
25. Maddox JC, Evans HL (1981) Angiosarcoma of skin and soft tissu. Cancer 48: 1907-24

8

26. **Mark PJ, Poen J (1994) Postirradiation sarcoma: a single institutional study and review of the literature. Cancer 73: 2653-62**
27. **Maruyama T, Kumamoto Y (1988) Reassessment of gamma doses from atomic bombs in Hiroshima and Nagasaki. Radiat Res 113: 1-14**
28. McGowan TS, Cummings BJ (2000): An analysis of 78 breast sarcoma patients without distant metastases at presentation. Int J Radiat Oncol Biol Phys 46: 383-90
29. Neglia JP, Friedman DL (2001) Second malignant neoplasms in five-year survivors of childhood cancer: childhood cancer survivor study. J Natl Cancer Inst 93: 618-29
30. Pierce SM, Recht A (1992) Long term radiation complications following conservative surgery and radiation therapy in patients with early stage breast cancer. Int J Radiat Oncol Biol Phys 23: 915-23
31. Robinson E, Neugut A (1988) Review: clinical aspects of postirradiation sarcomas. J Nat Cancer Inst 80: 233-24
32. Rosen PP, Kimmel M (1988) Mammary angiosarcoma-the prognostic significance of tumor differentiation. Cancer 62: 2145-51
33. Schunemann H, Willich N (1992) Secondary lymphoedema of the arm following primary therapy of breast carcinoma. Zentrablatt fur Chirurgie 117: 220-5
34. Schwarz RE, Hillebrand G (2002) Long-term survival after radical operations for cancer treatment-induced sarcomas. Am J Clin Oncol 25: 244-7
35. Sheppard DG, Libshitz HI (2001) Post-radiation sarcomas: a review of the clinical and imaging feature in 63 cases. Clinical Radiology 56: 22-9
36. Souba WW, McKenna R (1986) Radiation induced sarcomas of the chest wall. Cancer 57: 610-15
37. **Stewart FW, Treves N (1948) Lymphangiosarcoma in postmastectomy lymphedema: a report of six cases in elephanthiasis chirurgica. Cancer 1: 64-81**
38. Stokkel MPM, Peterse HL (1995) Angiosarcoma of the breast after lumpectomy and radiation therapy for adenocarcinoma. Cancer 6: 2965-8
39. Stout AP, Lattres R (1967) Tumors of the soft tissues. Atlas of tumor Pathology, 2nd series. Washington DC: Armed Forces institute of Pathology
40. Taghian A, de Vathaire F (1991) Long-term risk of sarcoma following radiation treatment for breast cancer. Int J Radiat Oncol Biol Phys 21: 361-7
41. Tarkkanen M, Wiklund TA (2001) Comparative Genomic hybridization of postirradiation sarcomas. Cancer 92: 1992-8
42. Travis EL, Kreuther A (1976) Unusual postirradiation sarcoma of chest wall. Cancer 38: 2269-73
43. Tubiana M (1983) Cancers par nuisance thérapeutiques : cancers et radiothérapie. Bull Cancer 70: 47-54
44. Valagussa P, Tancini G (1987) Second malignancies after CMF for resectable breast cancer. J Clin Oncol 5: 1138-42
45. Vries RA, de Brun M (1993) The biological effects of radiation. Int J Safety Med 4: 149-65
46. Warren S, Sommer GN (1936) Fibrosarcoma of the soft parts with special reference to recurrence and metastasis. Arch Surg 33: 425-50
47. Wiklund TA, Blomqvist CP (1991) Postirradiation sarcoma: analysis of a nation wide cancer registry material. Cancer 68: 524-31
48. **Yap J, Chuba PJ (2002) Sarcoma as a second malignancy after treatment for breast cancer. Int J Radiat Oncol Biol Phys 52: 1231-7**
49. Zelek L, Llombart-Cussac A *et al.* (2003) Prognostic factors in primary breast sarcomas: a series of patients with long-term follow-up. J Clin Oncol 21: 2583-8
50. Zukali R, Merson M (1994) Soft tissue sarcoma of the breast after conservative surgery and irradiation for early mammary cancer. Radiother Oncol 30: 271-3

Male breast cancer

B. Cuteli

9

Five Essential Points

1. *MRM (including axillary dissection) remains the optimal surgical treatment for MBC. Sentinel lymph node biopsy could be reserved for small lesions (T1) without clinical axillary lymph nodes.*
2. *Axillary nodal involvement (ANI) is very frequent (more than 50%) and is correlated to tumour size and SBR grading. It remains the most predictive factor both for local recurrence and metastases.*
3. *Locoregional radiotherapy (LR) is widely indicated, due to ANI frequency, central topography of the tumour (with high potential involvement of internal mammary chain), as well as high percentage of skin and/or muscle involvement. RT dramatically improves local control with a possible impact on survival.*
4. *Due to the very high level of estrogen and progestin receptors positivity, tamoxifen remains the best adjuvant treatment, but with some possible side-effects. Preliminary data on aromatase inhibitors seem equivalent in terms of effectiveness and side-effects. Chemotherapy (CT) seems to be used only in very high risk groups (e.g. pN > 3) and more particularly in young men (< 65 years old), due to a high rate of associated comorbidities in MBC patients.*
5. *Globally, when MBC and female BC are compared at the same stage, the overall and disease-specific survival rates are similar. However, due to late occurrence in men, the impact of comorbidities and second cancers can induce confusion in comparative results. For a better understanding of the disease, large multicentric prospective studies are strongly recommended.*

Introduction

In Western countries, male breast cancer (MBC) represents less than 1% of all breast cancers (BC) [10]. Only few series have included more than 200 cases [11, 15, 16, 20, 22, 27, 28, 41]. Median age at diagnosis was approximately 65 years, which is 8-10 years more than in women. More than one third of MBC occurred in elderly men (over 70 years), with an important rate of various comorbidities [10, 20].

Clinical and histopathological features

Retroareolar lump is the most frequent symptom, often associated with nipple retraction and sometimes serosanguineous discharge. Skin and/or muscle involvement is present in 20-25% of the cases (T_4 tumours).

Infiltrating ductal carcinoma (IDC) represents more than 90% of cases [12]. Infiltrating lobular carcinoma, medullar, tubular or neuroendocrine tumours are very rare, while ductal carcinoma in situ (DCIS) represents less than 10% of cases [4, 12, 29]. In a recent large multicentric French series including 489 MBC [14], the distribution according to Scarff Bloom Richardson grading was: SBR1 = 22%, SBR2 = 51% and SBR3 = 24%, quite similar to several other series both in men and in women. In the same series, estrogen receptors (ER) and progesterone receptors (PgR) were positive in 92% and 89% of the cases, with a 95.3% of positivity for at least one receptor. Other studies reported lower rates [32, 34]. Axillary nodal involvement (ANI) is frequent in MBC, accounting for 52% to 57% of the cases in the literature, with approximately 40% of "massive involvement" with more than three involved nodes (Table 1). ANI is significantly correlated to pathological tumour size [28] and SBR grading [10]. There are no specific data on internal mammary chain (IMC) involvement in MBC. However, due to high ANI rate, T_4 tumour frequency and central tumour location, this rate is probably very high. Indeed, a very large Chinese series precisely assesses IMC involvement according to size, age, tumour size and ANI [30].

Table 1 – Axillary nodal involvement (ANI) in the literature. (Series with more than 100 cases).

Author	Reference	N	pN^+
Cuturi	11	308	56%
Giordano	24	104	55%
Donegan	16	137	52%
Goss	27	161	57%
Salvadori	43	151	40%

Locoregional treatment

Surgery

Modified radical mastectomy (MRM) remains the surgical reference [10, 20]. In all series, 10 to 15% of patients underwent radical mastectomy (RM) for advanced tumours with large involvement of the pectoralis muscle. Very few teams use simple mastectomy [1] and some cases of lumpectomy generally followed by radiotherapy (RT) have been reported, especially in very old or frail patients.

For invasive MBC, axillary dissection (AD) is usually performed [20, 22, 28]. Indeed, AD (with at least 10 sampled nodes) allows optimal staging and ensures approximately 97% local control, even in case of ANI [14]. The impact of AD on survival is not clear, but several authors [44] confirmed that the number of histologically examined axillary lymph nodes had an impact on survival, especially in massive ANI ($pN_{>3}$). However, AD leads to 25-30% occurrence of side effects such as arm and/or shoulder pain or abduction limitation, sensitivity loss or arm edema. In order to avoid or minimize these symptoms, sentinel lymph node biopsy (SLNB) has been widely developed in women with clinically negative axilla. So far, very few papers have been published on SLNB in men [2, 21, 23, 37]. The most important is from Milan [23] reporting 23 tumours (90 pT_1). In all cases, SN was identified. Metastases were found in 6 cases (26%), resulting in AD. In four cases, SN was the only positive node. With a 30-month follow-up, no axillary recurrence was reported. Thus, SLNB seems indicated as a first approach in all T_1N_0 tumours.

Radiotherapy

Among women, locoregional irradiation (RT) provides a 60-70% reduction in locoregional recurrences and also clearly improves long-term survival [18, 33, 38, 46, 47]. The benefit is present in all pN^+ (both $pN_{1\text{-}3}$ and $pN_{>3}$) and in "advanced" tumours: T_3-T_4 and some T_2 (*i.e.* high grade tumours with vascular emboli, especially in young women) [46]. Thus, due to a high proportion of advanced tumours, retroareolar topography and ANI frequency, RT should be delivered in approximately 60-70% of MBC [10]. However, the literature reports are very heterogeneous (with regard to inclusion criteria and RT technique) and often with very few cases. In the above-mentioned French series including 489 cases, 85% of the patients underwent RT and the locoregional recurrence rate was only 2% [10, 14].

The most powerful predictive factor of locoregional recurrence (and survival) remains ANI. When extrapolating data from women, we can consider that the rates range between 15 to 18% for $pN_{1\text{-}3}$ and 30 to 40% for $pN_{>3}$ [18, 33, 46]. French and NCCN (National Comprehensive Cancer Network) guidelines recommend locoregional RT (at least chest wall and supraclavicular fossa) in all female patients with ANI. According to the European Institute of Oncology in Milan, such guidelines should also apply to men [10, 22]. To prevent long-term cardiovascular morbidity, modern RT techniques must be employed [25, 36], with computerized treatment planning including wide use of electron beams in order to spare the heart in case of IMC irradiation. In very elderly and/or frail patients, various hypofractionated schemes can be used (*i.e.* 45 Gy/15 fractions, 3 times a week).

Systemic treatment

Hormonetherapy

The median age for MBC occurrence is 65 years and hormone receptor (HR) positivity rates reach 90% [10, 14, 15, 20, 34, 41]. Thus, tamoxifen is generally considered a standard adjuvant therapy. Goss [27] and Ribeiro [40] showed an increase in DFS and OS with tamoxifen use. The results in other series were difficult to analyze due to concomitant use of CT. Despite this, tamoxifen use clearly increased from 39% in the period 1980 to 1989 to 63% in the period 1990 to 2001 [13]. In an English study including 161 men treated from 2002 to 2003, 126 (78%) received tamoxifen [31]. However, in several studies, tamoxifen treatment duration was often 1 or 2 years, and the 5-year optimal duration was not evaluated in men. On the other hand, several side-effects were observed during this treatment, especially hot flushes, depression, weight gain, impotence and thromboembolic accidents [5]. A recent report showed that in women, approximately 50% of the patients stopped tamoxifen for several reasons before completing the planned five years. Due to higher median age in men and frequency of comorbidities, prevention of thromboembolic accidents during tamoxifen treatment is mandatory, especially in all "risky situations", such as surgery and immobilization for various reasons.

The role of aromatase inhibitors (AI) in MBC is only documented in metastatic disease. In the French series, 43 patients received this treatment and the results seem similar to tamoxifen [13]. Further prospective studies are still needed on this specific setting.

9

Chemotherapy (CT)

Limited data suggest a CT benefit in some high risk subgroups and probably in younger patients [6, 20, 35, 48, 50]. However, it should be remembered that more than 30% of MBC occur in men who are older than 70 years, with high comorbidity rates; thus toxicity risk remains very high in these patients [26]. The use of CT has increased in recent years (Table 2). In the Texas series [24], among 71 patients treated after 1980, 27% received anthracyclines; in the French series [14] including patients treated between 1990 and 2005, 71% received anthracyclines. In both studies, CT was prescribed in 13% and 12% of pN_0 tumours and 45% and 54% of pN^+ tumours respectively. In older studies, the CMF protocol was more often used. On the other hand, the role of taxanes in MBC has not yet been evaluated. However, it is very difficult to evaluate the relative benefit of HT and CT. When extrapolating data from the latest overview of EBCTCG [17], CT should be proposed to men younger than 70 with ANI ($pN_{>3}$ and probably pN_{1-3}) and/or HR negative tumours. Her-2 neu overexpression in MBC varies from 9% to 29% in three series [39, 42, 49], but the role of trastuzumab in men is unknown.

Table 2 – Chemotherapy use in published series with more than 100 cases.

Author	Reference	n	Study period	PN^+	CT use (%)
Salvadori	43	170	1961-1990	40	14
Stierer	45	169	1970-1990	53	18
Donegan	16	215	1953-1995	52	24
Cutuli	14	489	1990-2005	53	34
Giordano	24	71	> 1980		44

Prognostic factors

As in women, tumour size, SBR grading, hormone receptor status and more particularly ANI are the main prognostic factors for local recurrence, disease specific survival (DSS) and overall survival (OS) in men. Due to MBC high median age, intercurrent deaths (especially from cardiovascular disease and second cancers) are frequent, and there are wide differences among DSS and OS rates.

In the French Cancer Center series [10, 13, 14], the 5-year OS and DSS rates were 81% and 89%, and the same 10-year rates were 59% and 72%, respectively. The 10-year OS according to tumour size were 70% for pT_1, 56% for pT_2 and 23% for pT_3T_4. The DSS rates were approximately 10% higher. The 10-year OS according to pN were 74% for pN_0, 54% for pN_{1-3} and 43% for $pN_{>3}$; the corresponding DSS rates were 78% (+ 4%), 71% (+ 17%) and 57% (+ 14%).

The major prognostic role of ANI was clearly confirmed by Guinee *et al.* [28]. Among 224 men undergoing AD, the 10-year DFS rates were 84%, 44% and 14% in pN_0, pN_{1-3} and $pN_{>3}$ groups, respectively. In the study by Donegan *et al.* [16], the 10-year survival rates were 51%, 44% and 33% for pN_0, pN_{1-3} and $pN_{>3}$ groups, respectively ($p = 0.006$).

In the Borgen study [8], the 10-year OS rates were 80% for pN_0 and 35% for pN^+. Similarly, in the Goss report [27] the 5-year OS rates were 68% for pN_0 and 47% for pN^+. According to Ribeiro *et al.* [41], grade is also a prognostic factor; among 125 cases (out of a total of 420), the 5-year survival rates were 76%, 66% and 43% for grades I, II, and III respectively ($p = 0.03$). Finally, hormone receptor status also influences survival rates. In the study by Donegan *et al.* [16], among 66 cases, the 5-year OS rates were 78% and 25% for ER^+ and ER^- patients ($p = 0.0001$).

Special situations

Metastatic disease

As a whole, 5-15% of men with BC present metastasis at diagnosis [9, 10, 15, 41, 45]. This rate is higher in African series [7, 19]. The sites of metastasis are similar to those in women, with bone and lung predominance. The first-line palliative therapy remains tamoxifen, with 25-58% response rates.

Aromatase inhibitors have been used in very few cases. CT was often used in men after failure of hormonal treatment, or in case of HR negativity, and/or visceral evolution. Response rates vary widely, but data are scarce [10, 20].

Ductal carcinoma in situ *(DCIS)*

DCIS average frequency in men is 7% [10, 12, 29]. The SEER (Surveillance, Epidemiology and End-Results) database (1973-2001) showed a 9.4% occurrence of DCIS in men *versus* 11.9% in women [4]. DCIS occurs in younger men (some less than 40). Retroareolar lump and blood nipple discharge are the most frequent symptoms, and more particularly papillary subtype. Simple mastectomy is the recommended treatment. In the French series, 3 out of 6 patients who underwent lumpectomy had local recurrence. AD is not useful, but SLNB could be proposed in case of suspicion of microinvasion.

Conclusions

Globally, when male and female BC are compared at the same stage, the overall and specific survival rates are similar [3]. However, MBC occurs approximately 8-10 years later than FBC [10, 15, 20]; consequently, the impact of comorbidities and second neoplasm is more important and can induce confusion in comparative results. Modified radical mastectomy with AD remains the standard treatment of MBC, but in selected cases ($T \leq 2$ cm without axillary palpable lymph nodes), SLNB could be proposed [2, 23]. Locoregional RT plays an important role to prevent local and regional recurrences, with a possible impact on survival [18, 33, 36, 38, 46, 47], although this fact cannot be clearly shown in men. Due to the high hormonal receptor positivity rate, tamoxifen remains the standard adjuvant treatment. The first results with AI (in adjuvant setting) in MBC seem very similar to those with tamoxifen [13], but more detailed studies are required in this field. Chemotherapy is useful in men under 70 with ANI, especially in case of negative hormone receptors [24, 26, 48]. In older men, the impact of comorbidities widely increases, and the benefit is probably limited to high-risk subgroups (*e.g.* $pN > 3$).

Finally, a comparison with two subsequent large cohorts of MBC in France confirmed that early diagnosis and use of adjuvant treatments (RT/CT/HT) dramatically increase survival rates in MBC reaching female rates (tables 3 and 4)

Table 3 – Comparison between two French cohorts (A: 1960-1986 and B: 1990-2005): histopathological features and treatment modalities (in %) [10, 11, 13].

	Cohort A	Cohort B	p
Number	397	489	
Median age	64	66	
Median delay to diagnosis	6 m	3 m	
Median tumour size (mm)	30	20	< 0.001
T_1	22	39	
T_2	41	41	< 0.0001
T_3T_4	26	7	
pN^+	56	53	NS
ER^+	79	92	
PgR^+	77	89	
RT	66	85	< 0.0001
CT	18	33	< 0.0001
HT	18	72	< 0.0001

RT: Radiotherapy.
CT: Chemotherapy.
HT: Hormonal treatment.

Table 4 – Comparison between two French cohorts (A: 1960-1986 and B: 1990-2005): Results (in %) [10, 11, 13].

	Cohort A	Cohort B	p
Number	397	489	
LR	8	2	< 0.0001
RR	3.7	5.6	0.21
M	42	23	< 0.0001
10-year OS	38	59	
10-year DDS	51	72	
10-year DDS:			
pN_0	77	81	
pN_{1-3}	50	62	
$pN_{<3}$	24	42	
Deatth rates:			
Breast cancer	60	63	
2nd cancer	10	11	NS
Complications	3	5	
Intercurrent	23	21	

[10, 11, 13]. The differences in 10-year DSS rates increase, especially in high-risk groups with a 12% gain (from 50 to 62%) and 18% (from 24 to 42%) in pN_{1-3} and $pN_{>3}$ groups, respectively (Table 4).

References

1. Agrawal A, Ayantunde AA, Rampaul R, Robertson (2007) Male breast cancer: a review of clinical management. Breast Cancer Res Treat 103: 11-21
2. Albo D, Ames FC, Hunt KK *et al.* (2003) Evaluation of lymph node status in male breast cancer patients. A role of sentinel lymph node biopsy. Breast Cancer Res Treat 77: 9-14

3. Anderson WF, Althuis MD, Brinton LA, Devesa PS (2004) Is male breast cancer similar or different than female breast cancer? Breast Cancer Res Treat 83: 77-86
4. Anderson WF, Devesa SS (2005) *In situ* male breast carcinoma in the Surveillance, Epidemiology and End results database of the National Cancer Institute. Cancer 104: 1733-41
5. Anelli TF, Anelli A, Tran KN *et al.* (1994) Tamoxifen administration in association with a high rate of treatment-limiting symptoms in male breast cancer patients. Cancer 74: 74-7
6. Bagley CS, Wesley MN, Young RC, Lippman ME (1987) Adjuvant chemotherapy in males with cancer of the breast. Am J Clin Oncol 10: 55-60
7. Ben Dhiab T, Bouzid T, Gamoudi A *et al.* (2005) Male breast cancer: about 123 cases collected at the Institute Salah-Azoiz of Tunis from 1979 to 1999. Bull Cancer 92: 281-5
8. Borgen PI, Wong GY, Vlamis V *et al.* (1992) Current management of Male Breast Cancer. A review of 104 cases. Ann Surg 215: 451-9
9. Ciatto S, Iossa A, Bonardi R, Pacini P (1990) Male breast carcinoma : review of a multicenter series of 150 cases. Tumori 76: 555-8
10. Cutuli B (2007) Strategies in treating male breast cancer. Expert Opin Pharmacother 8: 193-202
11. Cutuli B, Lacroze M, Dilhuydy JM *et al.* (1995) Male breast cancer. Results of the treatments and prognostic factors in 397 cases. Eur J Cancer 31A: 1960-4
12. Cutuli B, Dilhuydy JM, De Lafontan B *et al.* (1997) Ductal carcinoma in situ of the male breast: analysis of 31 cases. Eur J Cancer 33: 35-8
13. Cutuli B, Cohen-Solal-Le Nir C, Serin D *et al.* (2007) Male breast cancer: impact of early diagnosis and adjuvant treatments. Analysis of 983 cases. Breast Cancer Res Treat 2007, 106, Suppl 1, S222
14. Cutuli B, Cohen-Solal-Le Nir C, Serin D *et al.* (2008) Male breast cancer (MBC): analysis of 489 cases. Eur J Cancer 2008, 6, Supplement, 113 (Abs 219)
15. Donegan WL, Redlich PM (1996) Breast cancer in men. Surg Clin North Am 76: 343-63
16. Donegan WL, Redlich PN, Lang PJ Gall MT (1998) Carcinoma of the breast in males : a multi institutional survey. Cancer 83: 498-509
17. Early Breast Cancer Trialists' Collaborative Group (EBCTCG) (2005) Effects of chemotherapy and hormonal therapy for early breast cancer on recurrence and 15-year survival : an overview of the randomized trials. Lancet 365: 1687-717
18. Early Breast Cancer Trialists' Collaborative Group (EBCTCG) (2005) Effects of radiotherapy and of differences in the extent of surgery for early breast cancer on local recurrence and 15-year survival: an overview of the randomized trials. Lancet 365: 2087-106
19. El Omari-Alaoui H, Lahdiri I, Nejjar I *et al.* (2002) Male breast cancer. A report of 71 cases. Cancer Radiother 6: 349-51
20. Fentiman IS, Fourquet A, Hortobagyi G (2006) Male Breast Cancer. Lancet 367: 595-604
21. Gennari R, Renne G, Travaiani L *et al.* (2001) Sentinel node biopsy in male breast cancer: future standard treatment? Eur J Surg 167: 461-2
22. Gennari R, Curigliano G, Jereczec-Fossa B *et al.* (2004) Male breast cancer: a special therapeutic problem. Anything new? Int J Oncol 24(3): 663-70
23. Gentilini D, Chagas E, Zurrida S *et al.* (2007) Sentinel lymph node biopsy in male breast patients with early breast cancer. The Oncologist 12: 512-5
24. Giordano SH, Perkins GH, Broglio K *et al.* (2005) Adjuvant systemic therapy for male breast carcinoma. Cancer 104: 2359-64
25. Giordano SH, Kuo YF, Freeman JL *et al.* (2005) Risk of cardiac death after adjuvant radiotherapy for breast cancer. J Natl Cancer Inst 97: 419-24
26. Giordano SH, Duan Z, Kuo YF *et al.* (2006) Use and outcome of adjuvant chemotherapy in older women with breast cancer. J Clin Oncol 24: 2750-6
27. Goss PE, Reid C, Pintilie M *et al.* (1999) Male breast carcinoma. A review of 229 patients who presented to the Princess Margaret Hospital during 40 years: 1955-1996. Cancer 85: 629-63
28. Guinee VF, Olsson H, Moller T *et al.* (1993) The prognosis of breast cancer in males. A report of 335 cases. Cancer 71: 154-61
29. Hittmair AP, Lininger RA, Tavassoli FA (1998) Ductal carcinoma in situ (DCIS) in the male breast. A morphologic study of 84 cases of pure DCIS and 30 cases of DCIS associated with invasive carcinoma. A preliminary report. Cancer 83: 2139-49

9

30. Huang O, Wang L, Shen K *et al.* (2008) Breast cancer subpopulation with high risk of internal mammary lymph nodes metastasis: analysis of 2,269 Chinese breast cancer patients treated with extended radical mastectomy. Breast Cancer Res Treat 2008, 107: 379-87
31. Iredale R, Brain K, Williams B *et al.* (2006) The experiences of men with breast cancer in the United Kingdom. Eur J Cancer 42: 334-41
32. Nahleh ZA, Srikantiah R, Safa M *et al* (2007) Male breast cancer in the veterans affairs population: a comparative analysis. Cancer 109: 1471-7
33. Nielsen HM, Overgaard M, Grau C *et al.* (2006) Study of failure pattern amon high-risk breast cancer patients with or without post mastectomy radiotherapy in addition to systemic therapy: long term results from the Danish Breast Cancer Cooperative Group DBCG 82b and c randomized studies. J Clin Oncol 24: 2268-75
34. Olsson H (2000) Estrogen receptors content in malignant breast tumors in men. A review. J Mammary Gland Biol Neoplasia 5: 283-7
35. Patel HZ, Buzdar AV, Hortobagyi GN (1989) Role of adjuvant chemotherapy in male breast cancer. Cancer 64: 1583-5
36. Pierce LJ (2005) The use of radiotherapy after mastectomy : a review of the literature. J Clin Oncol 23: 1706-17
37. Port ER, Fey JV, Cody HS 3rd, Borgen PI (2001) Sentinel lymph node biopsy in patients with male breast carcinoma. Cancer 91: 319-23
38. Ragaz J, Olivotto IA, Spinelli JJ *et al.* (2005) Locoregional radiation therapy in patients with high-risk Breast Cancer Receiving adjuvant chemotherapy: 20-year results of the British Columbia randomized trial. J Natl Cancer Inst 97: 116-26
39. Rayson D, Erlichman C, Suman VJ *et al.* (1998) Molecular markers in male breast carcinoma. Cancer 83: 1947-55
40. Ribeiro GG (1985) Male breast carcinoma. A review of 301 cases from the Christie Hospital and Holt Radium Institute, Manchester. Br J Cancer 51: 115-9
41. Ribeiro GG, Swindell R, Harris M *et al.* (1996) A review of the management of the male breast carcinoma based on an analysis of 420 treated cases. The Breast 5: 141-6
42. Rudlowski C, Friedrichs N, Faridi A *et al.* (2004) Her-2/neu gene amplification and protein expression in primary male breast cancer. Breast Cancer Res Treat 84: 215-23
43. Salvadori B, Saccrozzi R, Mantzari A *et al.* (1994) Prognosis of breast cancer in males: an analysis of 170 cases. Eur. J. Cancer 30A: 930-5
44. Schaapveld M, De Vries EG, Van de Graaf WT *et al.* (2006) The prognostic effect of the number of histologically examined axillary lymph nodes in breast cancer: stage migration o rage association? Ann Surg Oncol 13: 465-74
45. Stierer M, Rosen H, Weitensfelder W *et al.* (1995) Male breast cancer: Austrian experience. World J Surg 19: 687-93
46. Truong PT, Woodward WA, Buchholz TA (2006) Optimizing locoregional control and survival for women with breast cancer: a review of current developments in post mastectomy radiotherapy. Expert Rev Anticancer Ther 6: 205-16
47. Wallgren A, Bonetti M, Gelber RD *et al.* (2003) Risk factors for locoregional recurrence among breast cancer patients ; results from International Breast Cancer Study Group Trials I through VII. J Clin Oncol 21: 1205-13
48. Walshe JM, Berman AW, Vatas U *et al.* (2007) A prospective study of adjuvant CMF in males with node positive breast cancer: 20-year follow-up. Breast Cancer Res Treat 103: 177-83
49. Wang-Rodriguez J, Cross K, Gallagher S *et al.* (2002) Male Breast carcinoma: correlation of ER, PR, KI-67, Her2-Neu and p53 with treatment and survival. A study of 65 cases. Med Pathol 15: 853-61
50. Yildirim E, Berberoglu U (1998) Male breast cancer: a 22-year experience. Eur J Surg Oncol 24: 548-52

Section 7

Lung and intrathoracic malignancies

Primary uncommon tumours of the lung: lymphomas, sarcomas and melanomas 1

K. Peignaux and P. Maingon

Five Essential Points

1. *Complete surgery remains the best curative treatment for primary pulmonary sarcoma and melanoma that have nevertheless a poor prognosis.*
2. *Lymphoma of the lung has a better prognosis. Surgery and chemotherapy are proposed for MALT lymphoma and anthracycline-based chemotherapy is the gold standard for diffuse large B-cell pulmonary lymphoma.*
3. *Melanomas, sarcomas and lymphomas of the lung are extremely rare. No radiological findings are specific for these diseases.*
4. *Surgery is the best treatment for primary pulmonary sarcomas and melanoma.*
5. *MALT lymphoma is an indolent pathology that can be treated by surgery and or chemotherapy. Diffuse large B-cell lymphoma requires chemotherapy.*

Introduction

Lymphoma, sarcoma and melanoma of the lung are extremely rare entites and account for about 1% of all primary pulmonary malignancies. Treatment of these uncommon tumours of the lung is mainly based on surgery.

Primary pulmonary lymphoma

Epidemiology, pathology and diagnosis

Primary pulmonary lymphoma (PPL) is rare, accounting for 3.6% of extranodal lymphoma and less than 1% of all primary lung neoplasms. PPL is defined as a clonal lymphoid proliferation, affecting one or both lungs in patients with no detectable extrapulmonary disease at diagnosis or during the subsequent three months. It is divided into Hodgkin's disease and non-Hodgkin's lymphoma. Primary Hodgkin's lymphoma is extremely rare, being reported in isolated cases. For non-Hodgkin's lymphoma of the lung, the WHO classification principally identifies 2 types of lymphoma: extranodal marginal zone lymphoma of Mucosa – Associated Lymphoid Tissue (MALT) and diffuse large B-Cell lymphoma. Seventy to ninety percent of PPL lymphoma cases are marginal zone lymphomas. The most common chromosomal translocation implicated in the development of MALT lymphoma is the translocation t(11;18)(q21;q21) found in more than one third of cases. Diffuse large B-cell lymphoma comprises about 5-20% of cases of lymphoma of the lung. The peak incidence of PPL is in the sixth decade. Presentation in young patients is rare without underlying immunosuppression.

Most of the patients are asymptomatic at diagnosis. When symptomatic, a patient suffers from cough, chest pain, dyspnoea and haemoptysis. The usual radiological aspect is a localised alveolar opacity in about half of the patients [2].

The diagnosis of pulmonary lymphoma requires an adequate biopsy specimen. Diagnosis can be made by bronchoscopic or transbronchial biopsy although surgical lung biopsy, either by laparoscopy or thoracotomy, is often required. The staging evaluations include CT of the chest, abdomen and pelvis, PET-scan, bone-marrow aspiration and laboratory tests.

Treatment

The treatment of PPL depends on the histological subtype, the extent of the disease and co-morbidities. For MALT lymphoma of the lung, different treatment strategies can be proposed: surgery, chemotherapy, radiotherapy and a policy of watchful waiting. However, the respective efficacy of these treatments cannot be confirmed due to the absence of comparative studies. Surgery can be useful at first to obtain diagnostic tissue. Some authors have also emphasized the therapeutic role of surgical resection. However, in most retrospective studies, surgery was often followed by chemotherapy. Ferraro *et al.* described a study group of 48 patients (73% MALT type and 27% non-MALT type) who underwent surgery, including 21 wedge excisions, 11 lobectomies, 2 pneumonectomies and 2 segmentectomies [6]. A complete resection was achieved in 19 patients (40%). It was followed by chemotherapy in 26 patients (54%) and by radiation therapy in 2 patients (4%). With a median follow up of 4.2 years, the survival rate at 5 and 10 years for patients with MALT lymphoma was 68% and 53% and for those with non-MALT type 65% and 64%. Cordier and colleagues reported a cohort of 42 patients with primary MALT pulmonary lymphoma who underwent a surgical resection [3]. Twenty one patients had no complementary treatment, 16 received chemotherapy, 3 had local radiation therapy and 2 received a combination of radio- and chemotherapy. Overall survival was 100% and 93.6% at two and five years respectively. With regard to adjuvant treatment, Nichols *et al.* recommend no adjuvant therapy after surgery for patients with localized MALT pulmonary lymphoma without bulky disease and chemotherapy for those with bulky disease [12]. Recommended chemotherapy includes chlorambucil, CHOP, or a fludarabine–containing regimen. Radiotherapy as exclusive treatment in MALT lymphoma is not be recommended. Tsang reported on 3 patients who underwent radiotherapy alone at a total dose of 30-35 Gy in 15 or 20 fractions [18]. Two of these patients had a partial response, defined as non-progressive radiographic abnormalities related to radiation fibrosis. The watch-and-wait policy is an option for MALT lymphoma of the lung which is an indolent disease with the potential for spontaneous regression. A retrospective study analysed 11 patients with MALT lymphoma of the lung who had no treatment after initial diagnosis [17]. The median time of observation without therapy was 28.1 months. Within this period, all patients had stable disease. Six of them had spontaneous regressions and wax–and-wane phenomena of the pulmonary lesions. Moreover, the Italian Society of Hematology suggests that pulmonary MALT lymphoma may not require treatment in the absence of symptoms [20].

Diffuse large B-cell pulmonary lymphomas have a worse prognosis and require anthracycline–based chemotherapy. Rituximab combined with chemotherapy has been evaluated in clinical trials. The Lymphome Non-Hodgkinien 98-5 study compared CHOP to rituximab plus CHOP in elderly patients with diffuse large

B-cell lymphoma [7]. The 5-year disease-free survival and overall survival was 66% and 58% respectively in rituximab-CHOP patients and 45% in CHOP patients. These results were statistically significant in favour of rituximab-CHOP.
The treatment of primary pulmonary Hodgkin's disease is no different from that of "classic" Hodgkin's lymphoma and is based on chemotherapy including doxorubicin, bleomycin, vinblastine and dacarbazine.

Primary pulmonary sarcoma

Epidemiology, pathology and diagnosis

Primary pulmonary sarcomas (PPS) account for less than 0.02% of all malignant pulmonary tumours. Pulmonary sarcomas, like soft tissue sarcomas, are categorized according to the normal tissue they mimic. They originate from the stromal elements of the bronchial or vascular wall or from the interstices of lung parenchyma. Considering that malignant mesenchymal tumours of the lung are often metastases, sarcoma of the lung should be considered as a primary tumour only if investigations have failed to discover a primary lesion elsewhere. For histological classification, the WHO classification of soft tissue tumours is applied [1]. In the literature, the most frequent histological types are leiomyosarcoma, fibrosarcoma and hemangiopericytoma.

Primary pulmonary sarcoma may affect any age group, although it is most commonly diagnosed in the elderly. Common presenting symptoms are dyspnoea, cough, chest pain, hemoptysis. The radiological findings are not specified. For diagnosis, lung biopsies are required and can be obtained by transcutaneous core biopsy or by surgical intervention.

Histological grade, tumour size and stage are identified as prognostic factors. For Jansen and colleagues, the grade of malignancy influenced the prognosis of the disease [8]. In this study, no patient with grade 1 sarcoma died because of malignancy, whereas median survival of patients with grade 2 tumours was 60 months and with grade 3 tumours 17 months (p=0.04). The influence of tumour size as a prognostic factor has been debated. For MacCormack, size did not influence survival [10]. Tumour size larger than 5 cm for Nascimento et al. and larger than 4 cm for Jansen et al., indicated poor prognosis [8,11]. Another prognostic factor identified by Regnard and Porte was the influence of the revised TNM international lung cancer staging system applied to primary pulmonary sarcoma [15,16]. The 5- and 10-year survival rate in stage IB was 83% whereas the 4-year survival in stage IIB was 30% (Table 1).

Table 1 – Resectability and survival in primary pulmonary sarcoma.

Authors	Periods	Number of patients	Operated patients (%)	Complete resection (%)	5-year overall survival (operated patients)	Prognostic factors
Jansen [8]	1959-1991	22	18 (82)	11 (50)	44	Size < 4 cm Grade
Regnard [16]	1973-1997	24	23 (96)	20 (83)	42	Stage
Porte [15]	1982-1998	18	18 (100)	19 (89)	43	Stage
Petrov [14]	1981-2000	48	43 (89)	43 (89)	49	Stage

Treatment

For PPS, a radical resection with pathological tumour-free margins is the best treatment. Consequently, surgery such as lobectomy or pneumonectomy with possible extension to the chest wall, pericardium or diaphragm (depending on tumour size) remains the gold standard. A systematic mediastinal lymphadenectomy is recommended because of potential node involvement. Petrov and colleagues found lymph node invasion in 23% of patients and Regnard *et al.* in 25% [14,16]. The survival of inoperable patients is very poor with death within 2 years. Regnard and colleagues reported 1-, 5-, and 10- year survival rates of 67%, 48% and 48% for patients who had complete resection, and a 1- and 2-year survival rate of 75% and 0% for non-operated patients.

Postoperative chemotherapy and radiotherapy are sometimes delivered. However, no evidence of benefit has been reported. According to Porte *et al.*, criteria that justify post operative treatment are incomplete resection, lymph node invasion, high grade or large tumours [15]. Neoadjuvant chemotherapy has been described in very few cases in order to facilitate surgery. No response was identified on imaging or at the time of surgery.

For unresectable disease, chemotherapy may have benefit. Chemotherapy regimens used are the same as those given to patients with traditional soft tissue sarcoma and usually include doxorubicin and ifosfamide. In a case report, chemotherapy including vincristine, dactinomycin, ifosfamide and doxorubicin was administrated to a child with a recurrent non-operable pulmonary leiomyosarcoma [5]. After 3 cycles of chemotherapy, a complete response was noted on surgical exploration. A total of 9 cycles was delivered followed by radiation therapy. No relapse was identified at 16 months.

Primary pulmonary melanoma

Epidemiology, pathology and diagnosis

Malignant melanoma commonly presents as a primary neoplasm of the skin but has been reported in non-cutaneous sites such as gastrointestinal tract, gall bladder, oral cavity, paranasal sinuses, oesophagus, vagina, vulva, and choroid. Primary melanoma of the lung is a very rare neoplasm, accounting for 0.01% for all lung tumours. In 2005, 53 cases were reported. Conversely, pulmonary metastases of melanoma are frequent and found at autopsy in 70% of patients dying from melanoma. It is often difficult to differentiate a primary melanoma of the lung from lung metastasis [4]. Supporting evidence of primary melanoma of the lung may be obtained from patterns of regional lymph node involvement which is consistent with the natural spread of common lung cancer. In order to identify cases of primary pulmonary melanoma with greater accuracy, criteria for the diagnosis have been proposed [9]. These include no history of previous melanoma, no demonstrable tumour elsewhere at the time of diagnosis, a solitary lung tumour, tumour morphology compatible with a primary tumour, no evidence at autopsy of a primary melanoma elsewhere.

Clinical manifestations of primary pulmonary melanoma are cough, hemoptysis, post-obstructive pneumonia, atelectasis or incidental finding on chest radiographs. Histological diagnosis can be obtained by bronchoscopy or by fine needle aspiration biopsy.

Treatment

The treatment of choice for primary melanoma of the lung is surgery, defined as lobectomy or pneumonectomy. Long-term survivors after radical surgery have been reported. Ost *et al.* reported on 20 patients with primary pulmonary melanoma [13]. In 15 of the 20 patients, surgical resection was performed consisting of 8 lobectomies, 5 pneumonectomies and 2 segmental resections. Six patients had lymph node involvement at the time of operation. Five patients did not undergo surgery, of whom 2 died at the time of diagnosis and 3 had unresectable tumours, dying within 4 months of diagnosis. Disease-free survival ranged from 18 months to 11 years. Recurrence was observed in 8 patients and 5 were alive without evidence of disease (2 with initial lymph node involvement and 3 without abnormal lymph nodes). Wilson analyzed a group of 8 patients treated with surgery (7 lobectomies and 1 wedge excision) [19]. One patient was alive without disease 108 months after radical surgery.

Long-term survivals after chemotherapy, immunotherapy or radiotherapy alone have not been documented.

References

1. Brambilla E, Travis WD, Shimosato Y *et al.* (2001) The new World Health Organisation classification of lung tumours. Eur Respir J 18: 1059-68
2. **Cadranel J, Wislez M, Antoine M *et al.* (2002) Primary pulmonary lymphoma. Eur Respir J 20: 750-62**
3. Cordier J.F., Chailleux E., Lauque D *et al.* (1993) Primary pulmonary lymphomas. A clinical study of 70 cases in nonimmunocompromised patients. Chest: 103: 201-8
4. De Wilt J, Farmer S, Thompson JF *et al.* (2005) Isolated melanoma in the lung where there is no known primary site: metastatic disease or primary lung tumour? Melanoma Research 15: 531-7
5. Ferrari A, Collini P, Mazza EA *et al.* (2002) Response to chemotherapy in a child with primary brochonpulmonary leiomyosarcoma. Med Pediatr Oncol 39: 55-7
6. **Ferraro P, Trastek VF, Pairolero P *et al.* (2000) Primary non-hodgkin's lymphoma of the lung. Ann Thorac Surg 69: 993-7**
7. Feugier P, Van Hoof A, Coiffier B *et al.* (2005) Long term results of the R-CHOP study in the treatment of elderly patients with diffuse large B-cell lymphoma: a study by the Groupe d'Etude des Lymphomes de l'Adulte. J Clin Oncol 23: 4117-26
8. Jansen JP, Mulder JJ, Van den Bosch JM *et al.* (1994) Primary sarcoma of the lung: a clinical study with long-term follow-up. Ann Thorac Surg 58: 1151-5
9. Jensen OA, Egedorf J (1967) Primary malignant melanoma of the lung. Scand J Respir Dis 48: 127-35
10. McCormack P.M., Martini N (1989) Primary sarcomas and lymphomas of the lung. In: Martini N., Vogt-Moykopf I (eds) Thoracic surgery: frontiers and uncommon neoplasms. St Louis, MO: Mosby, 261-83
11. Nascimento AG, Unni KK, Bernatz PE (1982) Sarcomas of the lung. Mayo Clin Proc 57: 355-9
12. Nichols FC, Stephen DC (2006) Primary lymphomas of the lung. Textbook of uncommon Cancer Third Edition
13. **Ost D, Joseph C, Menezes G *et al.* (1999) Primary pulmonary melanoma: case report and literature review. Mayo Clin Proc 74: 62-6**
14. Petrov DB, Vlassov VI, Danon SE *et al.* (2003) Primary pulmonary sarcoma and carcinosarcomas-postoperative results and comparative survival analysis. Eur J Cardiothorac Surg 23: 461-6
15. **Porte HL, Metois DG, Wurtz A *et al.* (2000) Surgical treatment of primary sarcoma of the lung. Eur J Cardiothorac Surg 18: 136-42**
16. Regnard JF, Icard P, Levasseur P *et al.* (1999) Prognostic factors and results after surgical treatment of primary sarcomas of the lung. Ann Thorac Surg 68: 227-31

1

17. Troch M, Streubel B, Raderer M *et al.* (2007) Does MALT lymphoma of the lung require immediate treatment? An analysis of 11 untreated cases with long-term follow-up. Anticancer Research 27: 3633-8
18. Tsang RW, Gospodarowicz MK, Crump M *et al.* (2001) Stage I and II Malt lymphoma: results of treatment with radiotherapy. Int J Radiation Oncology Biol Phys 50: 1258-64
19. Wilson RW, Moran CA (1997) Primary melanoma of the lung: a clinicopathologic and immunohistochemical study of eight patients. The Am Journal of Surgical Pathology 21: 1196-202
20. **Zinzani PL, Martelle M, Tura S *et al.* (2008) Practice guidelines for the management of extranodal non-hodgkin's lymphoma of adult non-immuno-deficient patients. Part I: primary lung and mediastinal lymphomas. A project of the Italian Society of haematology and the Italian Group for Bone Marrow Transplantation. Haematologica 93: 1363-71**

Thymoma and thymic carcinoma

2

N. Girard[1], F. Mornex, P. Van Houtte and J-F. Cordier

Five Essential Points

1. *Thymoma and thymic carcinoma are rare intrathoracic tumours. As a consequence of their rarity, knowledge regarding these diseases is mainly based upon case reports or small retrospective series, in which the respective role of each therapeutic modality is difficult to evaluate.*
2. *The most significant factor on survival is the invasiveness of the tumour. The most adopted staging systems are the Masaoka and the Groupe d'Etude des Tumeurs Thymiques (GETT) classifications, both based on per-operative and histo-pathological findings.*
3. *Surgery is the cornerstone of the management of thymic tumours, both being mandatory for histopathological diagnosis and staging, and in most cases indicating at the same time the first therapeutic step. Complete resection is, after tumour stage, the most constant and significant prognostic factor for progression-free and overall survival.*
4. *Adjuvant radiotherapy is recommended in incompletely resected thymomas. Completely resected stage II and III tumours may also benefit from adjuvant radiotherapy to reduce local recurrence rates, with no effect on survival.*
5. *In unresectable thymic tumours, multimodal strategies include neoadjuvant chemotherapy, extensive surgery, adjuvant radiotherapy, and, in some cases, adjuvant chemotherapy.*

Introduction

Thymoma and thymic carcinoma are rare intrathoracic tumours. Due to their rarity, knowledge regarding these tumours is mainly based on case reports or small retrospective series, most of which are outdated. Even if sometimes difficult to interpret, these studies nevertheless provide a good overview of the results of surgical resection, and many examples of the role of radiotherapy and chemotherapy. Publication bias regarding the recruitment of patients (medical, surgical or pathological studies) may hamper the estimation of the individual weight of each therapeutic option in the multimodal treatment of these tumours.

Thus, the objectives of this chapter are 1) to describe available therapeutic options for thymic tumours, 2) to review their indications in adults, and 3) to provide a comprehensive analysis of current treatment recommendations.

1. N. Girard is recipient travel grants from the Jean Walter-Zellidja foundation and the Lilly Institute.

Thymoma and thymic carcinoma: staging considerations in the clinic

Thymoma and thymic carcinoma are among the rarest malignant epithelial tumours, accounting for less than 0.5% of all cancers. Their main pathological characteristics include 1) a wide range of cytological patterns within thymic epithelial cells, from bland appearance in thymoma, to marked carcinomatous pattern in thymic carcinoma [49], and 2) the association with a non-tumoral lymphocytic component, whose relative proportion to neoplastic cells is the basis of the current *World Health Organisation* (WHO) histopathological classification (table 1) [49]. Thymic carcinoids, which require similar therapeutics to other neuroendocrine tumours are not discussed in the present review. Thymic carcinomas have been divided into low-grade tumours (basaloid, squamous, and mucoepidermoid subtypes) and high-grade tumours (adenocarcinoma, sarcomatoid, and lymphoepithelioma-like subtypes) [49].

Even if the WHO classification has been designed to assume some prognostic value (table 1) [10, 53], the most significant factor for survival is the invasiveness of the tumour [4, 7, 9, 34, 36-38, 41-43, 53]. Several staging systems have been described, but the most adopted are the Masaoka and the Groupe d'Étude des Tumeurs Thymiques (GETT) classifications, both based on per-operative and histopathological findings, the latter offering the advantage of being strikingly connected to therapeutic options (table 2) [7, 34]. Anyway, the correspondence between these two classification systems is higher than 85% [13].

Cooperation between surgeons and pathologists is mandatory to establish accurate staging of thymic tumours. Indeed, the pathological definition of invasive tumours may vary, referring either 1) to capsular invasion, as proposed in the original report from Masaoka *et al.* [34], which is, however, difficult to assess unless the capsule is completely breached, or 2) to invasion beyond the capsule in the mediastinal fat, then corresponding to microscopic invasion, which may also be hard to distinguish from persistent thymic remnants, especially in B1-B2 lymphocyte-rich subtypes. Moreover, per-operative clinical attributes of invasiveness, especially immovability and pleural adhesion, are not correlated with microscopic invasion [42].

Overall, invasive thymomas, referring to Masaoka stage II to IV tumours, account for 35-45% of cases. In most cases, invasion consists of direct local and regional spread within the lung, the pleura, and the pericardium, some patterns

Table 1 – The World Health Organisation histopathological classification of thymic epithelial tumours [49].

Type	Pathological features	Invasiveness	10-year disease-free survival
A	Spindle cell and medullary thymoma, lymphocyte-poor area	10-40%	100%
AB	Mixed pattern of type A (lymphocyte-poor) and type B (lymphocyte-rich) thymoma	30-40%	100%
B1	Thymoma ressembling the normal thymus	45-50%	85%
B2	Sub-types B1, B2, and B3 differenciated on the increasing epithelial/lymphocyte ratio and the emergence of atypia	65-70%	
B3		85-90%	35%
C	Thymic carcinoma: carcinoma cellular anaplasia - Low grade: basaloid, squamous carcinoma, mucoepidermoid - High grade: adenocarcinoma, sarcomatoid, lymphoepithelioma-like	90-95%	15%

Table 2 – Correspondence between the Masaoka and the Groupe d'Étude des Tumeurs Thymiques (GETT) staging classifications [7, 34, 49]. Overall survival and survival in completely resected tumours [7, 34, 42, 49].

Masaoka staging		GETT classification		Survival			
				Overall		Complete resection	
Stage	Description	Stage	Description	5-year	10-year	5-year	10-year
I	Macroscopically completely encapsulated	IA	Encapsulated tumour, totally resected	90-100%	85-95%	95-100%	90-100%
IIA	Macroscopic invasion into surrounding fatty tissue, mediastinal fat, or both	IB	Macroscopically encapsulated tumour, totally resected, per-operative suspicion of mediastinal adhesion or potential capsular invasion	75-90%	70-85%	85-100%	80-95%
IIB	Microscopic invasion into the capsule	II	Invasive tumour, totally resected				
III	Macroscopic invasion in neighbouring organs, such as pericardium, great vessels, or lung	IIIA	Invasive tumour, sub-totally resected	50-70%	25-60%	65-80%	45-70%
		IIIB	Invasive tumour, biopsy				
IVA	Pleural and pericardial dissemination	IVA	Supraclavicular metastasis or distant pleural droplets	30-40%	0-15%	30-60%	20-45%
IVB	Lymphogenous or hematogeneous metastasis	IVB	Distant metastasis				

rather considered as "droplet" local spread, thus classified as stage III, than true hematogenous or lymphogeneous dissemination. Rare droplet lesions may even occur within the peritoneum, by direct spread through the diaphragmatic orifices. Although designed for thymoma, these classifications have also been used for thymic carcinoma, although these tumours bear a higher potential for metastatic spread to the mediastinum and systemic organs, two locations of metastases which are not separated in the Masaoka classification [11, 49].

The WHO classification is highly correlated to stage, as 80-90% of A to B1 thymoma are stage I-II tumours, whereas 50-60% of B2, and 60-80% of B3 and C tumours are stage III-IV, a unique feature which may explain the prognostic value of the pathological classification (table 1) [42, 45].

Surgery for thymic tumours

Surgery as the prominent diagnostic tool for thymic tumours

The surgical management of thymoma and thymic carcinoma requires as a standard the wide opening of the mediastinum and the pleural cavities, which is in most cases achieved by median sternotomy [13]. Voluminous tumours for which parenchymal lung resection is anticipated, may be operated through an anterior bilateral thoracotomy and transverse sternotomy ("clamshell" incision). Regarding the need for a complete exploration of the thorax to achieve accurate staging, cervicotomy, described in ancient reports to spare patients with associated myasthenia gravis from high-risk anaesthesia, may no longer be indicated. Similarly, videothoracoscopy has been contra-indicated to avoid any per-operative tumour cell spread within the pleura.

The first step during surgery consists of a careful examination of the mediastinum and the pleural cavities, and of the macroscopic evaluation of the capsular invasion, the existence of peri-tumoral and pleural adhesions, and the involvement of surrounding tissues and of the mediastinum. The careful exploration of the mediastinal pleura, especially in the costo-diaphragmatic recesses, is needed to identify droplet metastases.

Current standards of surgery for thymic tumours

The second step is to evaluate the resectability of the thymic tumour. In stage I-II tumours, thymomectomy is in all cases associated with total thymectomy including total resection of the peri-thymic fat [53]. Capsular invasion may be subtle and not visible to the surgeon, so the tumour should not be shelled out but rather resected with all surrounding tissues. The surgical procedure for invasive stage III-IVA thymic tumours includes additional crucial issues: 1) *the extensive* en bloc *resection of the tumour*, the cervical and mediastinal fat, and all invaded local structures. Major vascular resections have also been reported feasible; 2) *the maximal preservation of phrenic nerves*, especially in patients with associated myasthenia gravis. The unilateral resection of the involved phrenic nerve is optional (5% of cases), and may be balanced with the positioning of surgical clips to plan subsequent adjuvant radiation boost; 3) *the possible need for lung parenchymal resection,* reported in almost 10% of cases, which consists in most cases of limited resection rather than traditional lobectomy or pneumonectomy [43], pleuro-pneumonectomy in selected patients with stage IVA lesions has also been reported; and 4) *the per-operative control of the clearance of resection margins* using fresh-frozen tissue sections, a meticulous ink-labelling of surgical specimens, and the placement of surgical clips to guide subsequent adjuvant radiotherapy. In recent series, overall reported morbidity and mortality rates range from 10% to 15% and 1% to 3%, respectively [4, 36, 43, 53].

Surgery as the most efficient therapeutic option for thymic tumours

Complete resection, which is obtained in 50-70% of cases, is, after tumour stage, the most constant and significant prognostic factor for progression-free and overall survival in thymic tumours (table 1) [4, 13, 26, 36-38, 41-43, 53]. The GETT classification, which takes into account the completeness of the initial surgery, may thus better reflect the aggressiveness of thymic tumours: for example, Masaoka-stage III tumours undergoing complete resection may achieve similar survival to stage I tumours, with 5-year progression-free survival of up to 95% [41]. These tumours are thus "up-classified" as stage II in the GETT system.

Conversely, the role for incomplete ("debulking") surgery in patients with stage III-IVA tumours has been debated for years, mainly following the report of small retrospective heterogeneous series, showing survival rates as low as 5-10%. However, an eventually incomplete resection significantly reduces local recurrence in comparison to a simple tumour biopsy: in the French series, Mornex *et al.* reported local control rates of 46% *vs* 16%, respectively [35, 38].

Radiotherapy for thymic tumours

Current standards for radiotherapy in thymic tumours

Current modalities of radiotherapy for thymoma and thymic carcinoma include 1) *the use of multi-field arrangement* conformal radiotherapy and three-dimensional treatment planning; 2) *a clinical target volume including the whole thymic space*, the tumour and its extensions, and the anterior, superior, and middle mediastinum (with field reduction after a total dose of 50-55 Gy). Prophylactic supraclavicular node irradiation is no more recommended, as isolated recurrences in this area are exceptional [41]. Some reports have indicated the feasibility and efficacy of delivering a 15 Gy prophylactic hemithoracic irradiation, with a reduction of pleural recurrence rates from 100% to 60%, without effect on overall survival [51]; 3) *a total dose ranging from 40 to 60 Gy*, including a boost to the tumour bed in incompletely or non-resected lesions – surgical clips may then be useful to plan the gross tumour volume –, with a standard fractionation scheme consisting of daily doses from 1.8 to 2 Gy over a 4 to 6 weeks period.

Although thymic tumours have been recognized as highly radiosensitive for years, the benefit of dose escalation on local control has not clearly been established. Arriagada *et al.* reported similar local control rates with total doses inferior to 48 Gy or superior to 60 Gy [2]. However, in the French series reported by Mornex *et al.*, the local recurrence rate in stage III-IV resected tumours was 80% after adjuvant radiotherapy delivered at median doses of 45 to 50 Gy. This led most investigators to increase radiation doses to 60-65 Gy [35].

Adjuvant radiotherapy to improve local control

The role of adjuvant radiotherapy in thymic tumours has been debated for years, and has to be discussed regarding both tumour stage and completeness of the surgical resection. Completely resected stage I thymoma carries a 0.9% overall recurrence risk and a 5-year survival of 100% after surgery only [25]. Adjuvant radiotherapy in these cases does not bring any additional survival benefit [44].

In completely resected Masaoka stage II and III (GETT stage II) thymomas, adjuvant radiotherapy reduced local recurrence rates from 28-36% to 0-5%, and from 53% to 28%, respectively [14, 35, 44]. In incompletely resected tumours, Curran *et al.* reported that adjuvant radiotherapy also increased mediastinal recurrence-free survival from 0% to 79%, a result which was better than the 47% recurrence-free survival of patients having received complete resection without adjuvant radiotherapy, suggesting that adjuvant radiotherapy might even salvage an incomplete resection [14]. However, adjuvant radiation has never been reported to increase overall local control and survival in these patients [13, 37, 44].

Overall, if adjuvant radiation to total doses above 50-55 Gy achieves relapse rates within the radiation field as low as 15-20% [37, 41], radiotherapy fails to control recurrent pleural dissemination, which may reflect the normal tumour dissemination pattern before or during surgery [37]. Some authors reported the use of hemithoracic prophylactic radiation, while others suggested that delivering radiation in a neoadjuvant setting may decrease the rate of pleural recurrences [23].

Neoadjuvant radiotherapy as an alternative approach

In reported series of thymic tumours, radiotherapy was delivered in a neoadjuvant setting in 10-20% of patients, mostly bearing stage IV primary unresectable tumours, in association with chemotherapy. The individualisation of the effect of neoadjuvant radiotherapy is then difficult to establish in these heavily treated patients. The feasibility and efficacy of pre-operative radiotherapy to a total dose of 18 Gy has also been reported in patients with invasion of the great vessels or mediastinal compression, to achieve subsequent complete resection [1].

2

Exclusive radiotherapy in the management of non-resectable tumours

The interpretation of reported data regarding exclusive radiotherapy for thymic tumours is difficult, as only small-accrual series have been published, most of which included patients with various tumour stages, heterogeneous performance status, and different total radiation doses and techniques. Overall, local control rates following exclusive radiotherapy in non-resectable tumours may not be over 45-50% [12].

Chemotherapy for thymic tumours

Exclusive chemotherapy in unresectable thymic tumours

The chemosensitivity of thymoma was established in several studies reporting the efficacy of single-agent chemotherapy regimens in non-resectable tumours (table 3). The highest response rates were observed in controlled studies with cisplatin [6] and ifosfamide [19]. Non cisplatin-containing regimens have been abandoned for many years. Current standard regimens include the following multiple agent protocols, which have actually never been compared to these single-agent regimens in a randomized setting: cisplatin and etoposide (PE) [16]; cisplatin, adriamycin, cyclophosphamide (PAC) [30]; adriamycin, cisplatin, vincristine, cyclophosphamide (ADOC) [15]; etoposide, ifosfamide, cisplatin (VIP) [29] (table 3). Response rates range between 32% and 92%, including 10% to 43% of complete responses (table 3). In the 10-year observational study reported by Giacone *et al.*, the PAC and the VIP regimens were the most used in an exclusive setting, and the overall response rate was 32% [17]. The VIP regimen, even if showing slightly lower responses rates, is significantly less toxic than the PAC regimen.

Targeted therapies have been disappointing, despite the overexpression of Epidermal Growth Factor and c-Kit especially by thymic carcinoma. Reported

Table 3 – Prospectively evaluated chemotherapy regimens in thymic tumours.

Regimen	Drugs	Doses	Response rate		Reference
			Overall	Complete	
Single agent					
Cisplatin		50 mg/m²/3 weeks	10-62%	10%	[6]
Ifosfamide		1.5 g/m² × 5 days/3 weeks	46-54%	38%	[19]
Multiple agents					
PE	Cisplatin	60 mg/m²/3 weeks	56-60%	31%	[16]
	Etoposide	120 mg/m² × 3/3 weeks			
PAC	Cisplatin	50 mg/m²/3 weeks			
	Adriamycin	50 mg/m²/3 weeks	51%	10%	[30]
	Cyclophosphamide	500 mg/m²/3 weeks			
ADOC	Adriamycin	40 mg/m²/3 weeks			
	Cisplatin	50 mg/m²/3 weeks	85-92%	40-43%	[15]
	Vincristine	700 mg/m²/3 weeks			
	Cyclophosphamide	0.6 mg/m²/3 weeks			
VIP	Etoposide	75 mg/m² × 4 days/3 weeks			
	Ifosfamide	1.2 g/m² × 4 days/3 weeks	32%	0%	[29]
	Cisplatin	20 mg/m² × 4 days/3 weeks			

response rates for gefitinib, bevacuzimab, and imatinib are as low as 1-4%, what may be explained by the exceptional presence of activating mutations of the corresponding genes in these tumours [46, 54].

Finally, in all these studies, the evaluation of response to chemotherapy rarely takes into account (1) the short-term effect of associated corticoids on the lymphocytic cells, which may be important in AB and B lymphocyte-rich subtypes, without efficacy on the epithelial tumoral component, and (2) the possible rebound thymic hyperplasia after chemotherapy.

Adjuvant chemotherapy in selected patients

Adjuvant chemotherapy has been reported to favourably influence survival in patients with Masaoka stage III-IV thymic tumours [13, 35]. Main regimens were cisplatin-based protocols [35], including CEE [52] and PAC. In incompletely resected tumours, response rates were higher when chemotherapy was administered before radiotherapy, than after radiotherapy (60-62% *vs* 40-55%, respectively). In sequential association with chemotherapy, radiotherapy has been delivered to total doses ranging from 30 to 70 Gy.

Neoadjuvant chemotherapy in potentially resectable thymic tumours

The main objective of neoadjuvant chemotherapy, delivered in stage III and IV thymic tumours, is to reduce the tumour volume either to allow subsequent surgical resection with higher chances of achieving negative margins, or to spare more normal tissues during radiotherapy. The main protocol used in a neoadjuvant setting is the VIP regimen [30]. Response rates of 50% are higher than in an exclusive setting [17]. Other regimens used in a neoadjuvant setting are the association of cisplatin, epirubicin, etoposide (CEE) [31], or of PAC and methylprednisolone [55], with response rates of up to 92%.

Combined multimodal treatments: one future direction in the treatment of thymic tumours

Exclusive chemoradiation

Chemotherapy and radiotherapy in stage III-IV unresectable tumours has always been administered in a sequential setting to avoid the combination of treatment toxicities, especially the high risk of radiosensitization with anthracyclines. Exclusive chemoradiation combining PAC chemotherapy with standard radiation to total dose of 54 Gy allowed an overall response rate of 70%, and a 5-year survival of 53%, favourably comparing with the results of incomplete resection [28].

Neoadjuvant chemotherapy, surgery, adjuvant radiotherapy

In primary unresectable stage IIIB-IV thymic tumours, several recent series (including no more than 7 to 22 patients), reported the feasibility of extensive resection after response to neoadjuvant chemotherapy with CEE, ADOC, or PAC regimens and followed by adjuvant radiotherapy to total doses from 30 to 60 Gy [3, 52, 55], and by adjuvant chemotherapy in some cases [22]. The high response rates to neoadjuvant chemotherapy, ranging from 77% to 100%, associated with survival rates ranging from 77% to 95%, may lead us, as in locally-advanced non-small cell lung cancer, to question the need for surgical resection in such multimodal approaches. However, local control was achieved in more than 80% of cases in these series.

Current therapeutic recommendations in thymic tumours

Masaoka-stage I tumours

The treatment of Masaoka stage I thymoma consists of upfront surgery. In the absence of capsular invasion at pathological examination (stage IA tumours in the GETT classification), no adjuvant treatment is recommended [25]. In all cases, mandatory follow-up may be longer than 10 years, as late recurrences may occur up to 15 years after initial resection.

In non-operable patients, exclusive radiotherapy may hamper tumour growth for a prolonged time, although overall survival may not be influenced.

Masaoka-stage II-III resectable tumours

The treatment of Masaoka stage II-III resectable thymic tumours also consists of upfront surgery. When complete resection is obtained (GETT stage IB-II tumours), delivering adjuvant radiotherapy to a total dose of 50-55 Gy is controversial [14, 35, 44]. In case of incomplete resection (GETT stage IIIA tumours), adjuvant radiotherapy is systematically recommended to a total dose of 60 to 65 Gy including a boost to areas of macroscopic invasion (marked with surgical clips).

Masaoka-stage III marginally and non-resectable tumours

These tumours correspond to GETT stage IIIB tumours. Surgical biopsy is performed to obtain the pathological diagnosis of the mediastinal tumour. Induction chemotherapy based on the CAP-VIP combination allows the subsequent feasibility either of surgical resection followed by adjuvant radiotherapy (total doses between 50 and 65 Gy depending on the completeness of surgery), or of sequential radiotherapy to a total dose of 65 Gy [52].

Masaoka-stage IVA tumours

In case of resectable pleural droplet metastases, surgical resection, although controversial, may also be discussed, possibly after induction chemotherapy [3, 28]. Adjuvant radiotherapy to a total dose of 50 to 65 Gy to selected volumes is recommended. In non-resectable tumours, the recommendation is exclusive sequential chemoradiation to a total dose of 65 Gy.

Masaoka-stage IVB tumours

Exclusive chemotherapy is the treatment for stage IVB tumours; the PAC and ADOC chemotherapy regimens may be the most efficient to achieve significant response rates [17]. Subsequent surgery of residual masses and radiotherapy may be feasible in case of major response to first-line treatment [3, 28].

Treatment of associated auto-immune manifestations

Associated parathymic manifestations occur in association with thymoma in 50-70% of cases, but are exceptional in case of thymic carcinoma, which is a less differentiated and more immunologically inert lesion. The most frequent parathymic disease is myasthenia gravis, found in 30-50% of cases. Treatment of thymoma, mainly thymectomy, but also chemoradiation, has been reported to lessen myasthenia gravis symptoms in 50-60% of cases, with achievement of complete remission in 8-30% of cases [26]. Specific treatments for myasthenia are effective in other cases. Recurrence of myasthenia rarely heralds recurrence of the tumour, but may rather be associated with any other transient medical stress.

Although more than 25 additional parathymic manifestations have been described, few data exist regarding their evolution after thymectomy: only hypogammaglobulinemia (10% of thymomas), pure red cell aplasia (5-10% of thymomas), and stiff-person syndrome have been reported to improve with the treatment of the thymic tumour [21, 24]. Especially, pure red cell aplasia, rather than hypogammaglobulinemia, may hamper the completion of the therapeutic strategy, especially chemotherapy, due to increased haematological toxicity.

Local and locoregional recurrences of thymoma

Late recurrences occurring more than 5 or 10 years after resection are not uncommon in thymoma. If local control mostly depends on the completeness of initial surgery, pleural "droplet" recurrences are rather related to local spread than to hematogeneous metastazing spread. Surgery, when feasible, remains then the major therapeutic option in case of recurrent thymoma. Complete re-resection, obtained in as many as 68% of local recurrences [43], even allows patients to recover a similar outcome than those not experiencing tumour recurrence after first resection, with 5-year survival ranging from 65% to 80% [43, 45]. Adjuvant radiation is feasible [45].

In non-resectable recurrences, exclusive radiotherapy has been reported as an efficient treatment, especially on pleural recurrences, even if irradiation had previously been delivered, with response rates as high as 80% 5-year survival rates in small retrospective series.

Specific issues regarding thymic carcinoma

Due to the paucity of cases, specific treatment options for thymic carcinoma remain undefined. In most reported studies, these aggressive tumours have been treated with multimodal approaches, including neoadjuvant chemotherapy, surgery when feasible (30% of cases [11]), and adjuvant chemoradiation (table 4) [20]. Complete resection has been achieved in 25-70% of cases in surgical series (table 4). In the prospective trial reported by Loehrer *et al.*, response rate and overall survival after induction chemotherapy with VIP were 25%, and 50%, respectively [23, 29]. In case of systemic metastases, treatment is exclusive chemotherapy, consisting of VIP, CAP, or ADOC combinations in case of high-grade subtypes, and of cisplatin-based regimens in low-grade tumours [23, 29].

Future directions

The management of thymic tumours is a paradigm of cooperation between clinicians, surgeons, and pathologists from establishing the diagnosis to organizing the therapeutic strategy and evaluating the prognosis. As a consequence of their rarity,

Table 4 – Selected surgical series of thymic carcinoma.

Author	n	Complete resection (%)	Adjuvant treatment: Chemotherapy (%)	Adjuvant treatment: Radiotherapy (%)	Adjuvant treatment: Chemoradiation (%)	Local control rate (%)	Overall survival: Median (mois)	Overall survival: 5-year (%)	Prognosis factors
Suster *et al.*, 1991 [47]	60	80	10	35	33	44	17	33	Complete resection, grade
Chang et al., 1992 [10]	16	29				77	30	31	Squamous subtype
Blumberg *et al.*, 1998 [5]	43	67	9	33	47	52	73	65	Vascular invasion
Lucchi *et al.*, 2001 [32]	13	46	54 (neoadjuvant)	69	23	77	38	61	
Liu *et al.*, 2002 [27]	38	21	9	49	29		24	27	Stage, grade, resection
Hsu *et al.*, 2002 [20]	26	65	0	65	0	91		77	Stage
Ogawa *et al.*, 2002 [40]	40	40	10 (neoadjuvant)	43	10	100		38	Complete resection, radiotherapy
Kondo *et al.*, 2003 [25]	186	51	6	18	13	49	71	51	Complete resection
Tseng *et al.*, 2003 [50]	38	71	0	71	18	52	81	68	Vascular invasion
Nonaka *et al.*, 2004 [39]	14	71	40	100	0	43	36	25 (3-year)	
Takeda *et al.*, 2004 [48]	15	60	11	44	0	89	25	39	
Chalabreysse *et al.*, 2004 [8]	19	52	58	84	0		16	15	
Hernandez-Ilizaliturri *et al.*,2004 [18]	22	23	56	72	39	11		41	
Magois *et al.*, 2007 [33]	9	33	44 (neoadjuvant)	11	22	75	20		

collaborative studies are warranted in order to evaluate and improve current therapeutic standards, taking into account recent improvements in techniques, such as radiotherapy, and supportive treatments. Furthermore, among the large variety of questions relative to the therapeutic strategy, thymic tumours represent a model of therapeutic implementation and achievement in oncology, showing how the advent of new results leads to new questions, as well as diversifying clinical research directions.

References

1. Akaogi E, Ohara K, Mitsui K *et al.* (1996) Preoperative radiotherapy and surgery for advanced thymoma with invasion to the great vessels. J Surg Oncol 63: 17-22
2. Arriagada R, Bretel JJ, Caillaud JM *et al.* (1984) Invasive carcinoma of the thymus. A multicenter retrospective review of 56 cases. Eur J Cancer Clin Oncol: 20: 69-74
3. Berruti A, Borasio P, Gerbino A *et al.* (1999) Primary chemotherapy with adriamycin, cisplatin, vincristine and cyclophosphamide in locally advanced thymomas: a single institution experience. Br J Cancer 81: 841-5
4. Blumberg D, Port JL, Weksler B *et al.* (1995) Thymoma: a multivariate analysis of factors predicting survival. Ann Thorac Surg 60: 908-13
5. Blumberg D, Burt ME, Bains MS *et al.* (1998) Thymic carcinoma: current staging does not predict prognosis. J Thorac Cardiovasc Surg 115: 303-8
6. Bonomi PD, Finkelstein D, Aisner S, Ettinger D. (1993) EST 2582 phase II trial of cisplatin in metastatic or recurrent thymoma. Am J Clin Oncol 16: 342-5
7. Bretel JJ. Sarrazin, Vrousos, Vincent, eds. (1989) Staging and preliminary results of the Thymic Tumour Study Group – in: 7th cancer research workshop. Basel (Swiss): Kargel
8. Chalabreysse L, Etienne-Mastroianni B, Adeleine P *et al.* (2004) Thymic carcinoma: a clinicopathological and immunohistological study of 19 cases. Histopathology 44: 367-74
9. **Chalabreysse L, Roy P, Cordier JF *et al.* (2002) Correlation of the WHO schema for the classification of thymic epithelial neoplasms with prognosis: a retrospective study of 90 tumors. Am J Surg Pathol 26: 1605-11**
10. Chang HK, Wang CH, Liaw CC *et al.* (1992) Prognosis of thymic carcinoma: analysis of 16 cases. J Formos Med Assoc 91: 764-9
11. Chung DA. (2000) Thymic carcinoma-analysis of nineteen clinicopathological studies. Thorac Cardiovasc Surg 48: 114-9
12. Ciernik IF, Meier U, Lütolf UM. (1994) Prognostic factors and outcome of incompletely resected invasive thymoma following radiation therapy. J Clin Oncol 12: 1484-90
13. **Cowen D, Richaud P, Mornex F *et al.* (1995) Thymoma: results of a multicentric retrospective series of 149 non-metastatic irradiated patients and review of the literature. FNCLCC trialists. Fédération Nationale des Centres de Lutte Contre le Cancer. Radiother Oncol 34: 9-16**
14. Curran WJ Jr, Kornstein MJ, Brooks JJ, Turrisi AT 3rd (1988) Invasive thymoma: the role of mediastinal irradiation following complete or incomplete surgical resection. J Clin Oncol 6: 1722-7
15. Fornasiero A, Daniele O, Ghiotto C *et al.* (1990) Chemotherapy of invasive thymoma. J Clin Oncol 8: 1419-23
16. Giaccone G, Ardizzoni A, Kirkpatrick A *et al.* (1996) Cisplatin and etoposide combination chemotherapy for locally advanced or metastatic thymoma. A phase II study of the European Organization for Research and Treatment of Cancer Lung Cancer Cooperative Group. J Clin Oncol 14: 814-20
17. Giaccone G, Wilmink H, Paul MA, van der Valk P. (2006) Systemic treatment of malignant thymoma: a decade experience at a single institution. Am J Clin Oncol 29: 336-44
18. Hernandez-Ilizaliturri FJ, Tan D, Cipolla D *et al.* (2004) Multimodality therapy for thymic carcinoma (TCA): results of a 30-year single-institution experience. Am J Clin Oncol 27: 68-72
19. Highley MS, Underhill CR, Parnis FX *et al.* (1999) Treatment of invasive thymoma with single-agent ifosfamide. J Clin Oncol 17: 2737-44

2

20. Hsu HC, Huang EY, Wang CJ *et al.* (2002) Postoperative radiotherapy in thymic carcinoma: treatment results and prognostic factors. Int J Radiat Oncol Biol Phys 52: 801-5
21. Iwata T, Inoue K, Mizuguchi S *et al.* (2006) Thymectomy for paraneoplastic stiff-person syndrome associated with invasive thymoma. J Thorac Cardiovasc Surg 132: 196-7
22. Kim ES, Putnam JB, Komaki R *et al.* (2004) Phase II study of a multidisciplinary approach with induction chemotherapy, followed by surgical resection, radiation therapy, and consolidation chemotherapy for unresectable malignant thymomas: final report. Lung Cancer 44: 369-79
23. Kitami A, Suzuki T, Kamio Y, Suzuki S (2001) Chemotherapy of thymic carcinoma: analysis of seven cases and review of the literature. Jpn J Clin Oncol 31: 601-4
24. Thompson CA, Steensma DP (2006) Pure red cell aplasia associated with thymoma: clinical insights from a 50-year single-institution experience. Br J Haematol 135: 405-7
25. **Kondo K, Monden Y (2003) Therapy for thymic epithelial tumors: a clinical study of 1,320 patients from Japan. Ann Thorac Surg 76: 878-84**
26. Kudva GC, Maliekel K, Kim HJ *et al.* (2002) Thymoma and myotonic dystrophy: successful treatment with chemotherapy and radiation: case report and review of the literature. Chest 121: 2061-3
27. Liu HC, Hsu WH, Chen YJ *et al.* (2002) Primary thymic carcinoma. Ann Thorac Surg 73: 1076-81
28. Loehrer PJ Sr, Chen M, Kim K *et al.* (1997) Cisplatin, doxorubicin, and cyclophosphamide plus thoracic radiation therapy for limited-stage unresectable thymoma: an intergroup trial. J Clin Oncol 15: 3093-9
29. Loehrer PJ Sr, Jiroutek M, Aisner S *et al.* (2001) Combined etoposide, ifosfamide, and cisplatin in the treatment of patients with advanced thymoma and thymic carcinoma: an intergroup trial. Cancer 91: 2010-5
30. Loehrer PJ Sr, Kim K, Aisner SC *et al.* (1994) Cisplatin plus doxorubicin plus cyclophosphamide in metastatic or recurrent thymoma: final results of an intergroup trial. The Eastern Cooperative Oncology Group, Southwest Oncology Group, and Southeastern Cancer Study Group. J Clin Oncol 12: 1164-8
31. Lucchi M, Melfi F, Dini P *et al.* (2006) Neoadjuvant chemotherapy for stage III and IVA thymomas: a single-institution experience with a long follow-up. J Thorac Oncol 1: 308-13
32. Lucchi M, Mussi A, Basolo F *et al.* (2001) The multimodality treatment of thymic carcinoma. Eur J Cardiothorac Surg 19: 566-9
33. Magois E, Guigay J, Blancard PS *et al.* (2007) Multimodal treatment of thymic carcinoma: Report of nine cases. Lung Cancer (in press)
34. **Masaoka A, Monden Y, Nakahara K, Tanioka T. (1981) Follow-up study of thymomas with special reference to their clinical stages. Cancer 48: 2485-92**
35. **Mornex F, Resbeut M, Richaud P *et al.* (1995) Radiotherapy and chemotherapy for invasive thymomas: a multicentric retrospective review of 90 cases. The FNCLCC trialists. Fédération Nationale des Centres de Lutte Contre le Cancer. Int J Radiat Oncol Biol Phys 32: 651-9**
36. Murakawa T, Nakajima J, Kohno T *et al.* (2000) Results from surgical treatment for thymoma. 43 years of experience. Jpn J Thorac Cardiovasc Surg 48: 89-95
37. Myojin M, Choi NC, Wright CD *et al.* (2000) Stage III thymoma: pattern of failure after surgery and postoperative radiotherapy and its implication for future study. Int J Radiat Oncol Biol Phys 46: 927-33
38. Nakagawa K, Asamura H, Matsuno Y *et al.* (2003) Thymoma: a clinicopathologic study based on the new World Health Organization classification. J Thorac Cardiovasc Surg 126: 1134-40
39. Nonaka T, Tamaki Y, Higuchi K *et al.* (2004) The role of radiotherapy for thymic carcinoma. Jpn J Clin Oncol 34: 722-6
40. Ogawa K, Toita T, Uno T *et al.* (2002) Treatment and prognosis of thymic carcinoma: a retrospective analysis of 40 cases. Cancer 94: 3115-9
41. Ogawa K, Uno T, Toita T *et al.* (2002) Postoperative radiotherapy for patients with completely resected thymoma: a multi-institutional, retrospective review of 103 patients. Cancer 94: 1405-13
42. Okumura M, Miyoshi S, Fujii Y *et al.* (2001) Clinical and functional significance of WHO classification on human thymic epithelial neoplasms: a study of 146 consecutive tumors. Am J Surg Pathol 25: 103-10

43. Regnard JF, Zinzindohoue F, Magdeleinat P *et al.* (1997) Results of re-resection for recurrent thymomas. Ann Thorac Surg 64: 1593-8
44. Singhal S, Shrager JB, Rosenthal DI *et al.* (2003) Comparison of stages I-II thymoma treated by complete resection with or without adjuvant radiation. Ann Thorac Surg 76: 1635-41
45. Ströbel P, Bauer A, Puppe B *et al.* (2004) Tumor recurrence and survival in patients treated for thymomas and thymic squamous cell carcinomas: a retrospective analysis. J Clin Oncol 22: 1501-9
46. Ströbel P, Hartmann M, Jakob A *et al.* (2004) Thymic carcinoma with overexpression of mutated KIT and the response to imatinib. N Engl J Med 350: 2625-6
47. Suster S, Rosai J. (1991) Thymic carcinoma. A clinicopathologic study of 60 cases. Cancer 67: 1025-32
48. Takeda S, Sawabata N, Inoue M *et al.* (2004) Thymic carcinoma. Clinical institutional experience with 15 patients. Eur J Cardiothorac Surg 26: 401-6
49. Travis WB, Brambilla A, Muller-Hermelinck HK, Harris CC (2004) World Health Organization Classification of Tumours. Pathology and Genetics of Tumours of the Lung, Pleura, Thymus and Heart. Lyon, IARC Press
50. Tseng YL, Wang ST, Wu MH *et al.* (2003) Thymic carcinoma: involvement of great vessels indicates poor prognosis. Ann Thorac Surg 76: 1041-5
51. Uematsu M, Yoshida H, Kondo M *et al.* (1996) Entire hemithorax irradiation following complete resection in patients with stage II-III invasive thymoma. Int J Radiat Oncol Biol Phys 35: 357-60
52. Venuta F, Rendina EA, Longo F *et al.* (2003) Long-term outcome after multimodality treatment for stage III thymic tumors. Ann Thorac Surg 76: 1866-72
53. Wilkins KB, Sheikh E, Green R *et al.* (1999) Clinical and pathologic predictors of survival in patients with thymoma. Ann Surg 230: 562-72
54. Yamaguchi H, Soda H, Kitazaki T *et al.* (2006) Thymic carcinoma with epidermal growth factor receptor gene mutations. Lung Cancer 52: 261-2
55. Yokoi K, Matsuguma H, Nakahara R *et al.* (2007) Multidisciplinary treatment for advanced invasive thymoma with cisplatin, doxorubicin, and methylprednisolone. J Thorac Oncol 2: 73-8

Large cell neuroendocrine carcinoma of the lung

3

J.-Y. Perentes and H.-B. Ris

Five Essential Points

1. *Large cell neuroendocrine lung tumours (LCNETs) are rare and its diagnosis is difficult.*
2. *While the clinical presentation of LCNETs is comparable to NSCLCs, their biological behaviour is similar to small c ell cancers.*
3. *Only sparse data is available concerning the management of LCNETs.*
4. *Surgery combined with adjuvant chemotherapy is generally applied in early stage LCNETs.*
5. *Definitive radiotherapy is generally applied in late stage LCNETs.*

Introduction

Neuroendocrine cancers of the lung are a broad category of tumours that have distinct biological features and behaviours. An initial classification from the early 1970s based on histology, included three types of neuroendocrine tumours: typical carcinoid tumours, atypical carcinoid tumours and small cell carcinomas (SCC) [2]. In 1991, large cell neuroendocrine tumours (LCNETs) were first described as a distinct type of neuroendocrine cancer [24]. Histological characteristics of LCNET included a high mitotic rate, cellular palisading with rosette like areas, an organoid growth pattern and a cell size at least three times bigger than that of SCCs [24,25]. Because of the similar prognosis and behaviour, LCNETs were initially classified with SCCs [7]. However, in 1999, the World Health Organization (WHO) and International Association of Staging of Lung Cancer (IASLC) classified LCNETs as one of the four subtypes of "large cell carcinomas (LCCs)" [26]. This classification, based on morphology and often used as a diagnosis of exclusion, has brought much confusion in the characterization and treatment management of LCNETs. Indeed, while LCNETs share comparable morphological features with NSCLCs, their biology seems more comparable to SCCs. This is further supported by genetic expression studies which have shown comparable profiles between LCNETs and SCCs [11,19,20]. A considerable debate has since emerged as to whether LCNETs should be classified and treated as NSCLCs or as SCCs.

Incidence and epidemiology

Because the histopathological diagnosis of LCNETs is difficult and the fact that different entities can be classified as LCCs, there is little accurate epidemiological data for LCNETs in the literature. In various reports, the incidence of LCNET was shown to be low and range from 2.1 to 3.5% of all surgically resected lung cancers [3,13,17]. Because the accurate differentiation of LCNETs from other lung cancers

3

requires generous and well-preserved histopathological material for careful examination, LCNETs are rarely diagnosed on tumour through-cut biopsies (such as obtained by bronchoscopy or transthoracic puncture). Thus the incidence of LCNET in non-surgically treated lung cancers is unknown.

As with other variants of lung cancer, smoking appears to be the primary cause of disease and is found in 85% to 98% of patients [3,13,17]. The mean age of patients at diagnosis ranges from 62 to 68 years with a median of 65.8 years [3,13,17]. Patients with LCNET are in majority men [3,13,17]. Current ongoing studies focus on environmental and genetic predisposition factors for LCNETs.

Pathological characterization and molecular biology

The diagnosis of large cell neuroendocrine tumours is made when obvious neuroendocrine light microscopy features are found and that typical and atypical carcinoid or SCC characteristics are excluded. Tumour cells have an organoid growth pattern with palisading or rosette-like areas and patches of geographic necrosis (Fig. 1) [25]. A high mitotic rate comparable to SCC is often found. In some situations, foci of squamous and adenomatous differentiation may be observed [25]. Ultrastructure

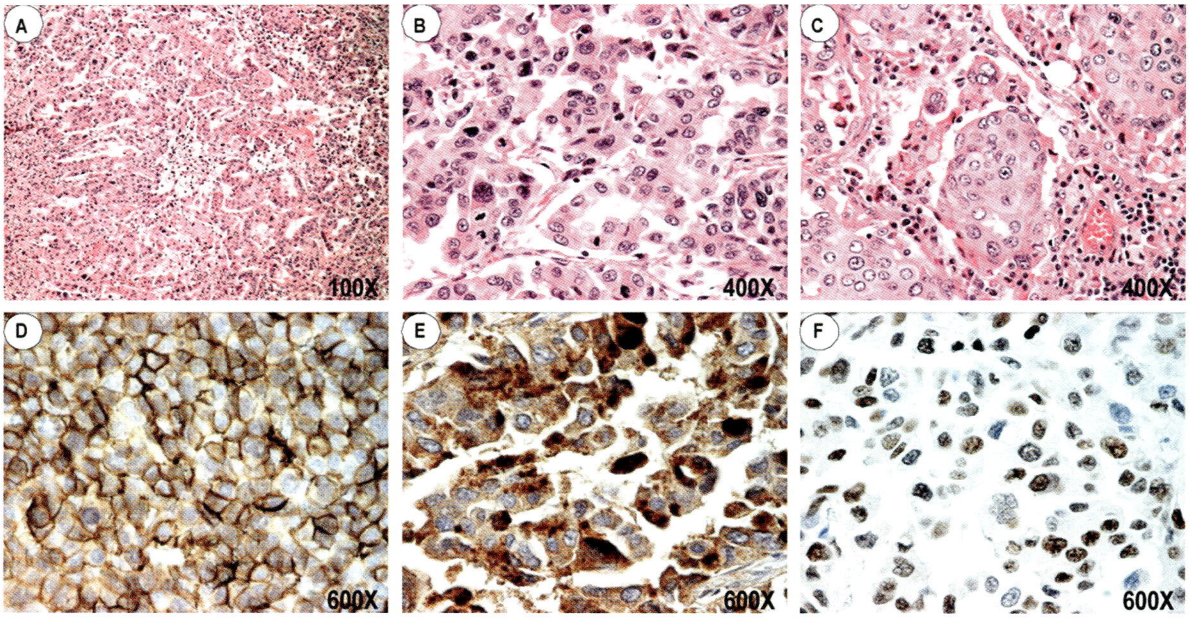

Fig. 1. Large cell neuroendocrine carcinomas do not have the cytologic and architectural features of small cell carcinoma and do not present features of glandular or squamous differentiation (A). In some cases these tumours can show basaloid differentiation with a palissading architecture, an organoid growth pattern with rosette like areas (B). These large cell tumours may also show neurodocrine features, such as nuclear molding, vesicular chromatine and large nuclei (at least 3 times the diameter of a small resting lymphocytes, C). These tumours also express neuroendocrine markers such as synaptophysine, chromogranine and CD56. Immunostaining for Neural Cell Adhesion Molecule (CD56) shows a typical membranous pattern (D). Also, immunostaining for Synaptophysin shows a granular cytoplasmic pattern (E). Around 50% of LCNEC express Thyroid Transcription Factor 1 (TTF-1) which can confirm a pulmonary origin of the tumour (F).

Images provided by Dr S. Rotman, Institute of Pathology, University Hospital of Lausanne (CHUV), Lausanne, Switzerland.

analysis reveals the presence of neurosecretory granules with intercellular junctions and granular differentiation suggestive of squamous differentiation [24]. Tumours express neuron-specific enolase, carcinoembryonic antigen and keratin which can be detected by immunohistochemistry. Less common markers include chromagranin, Leu-7, synaptophysin and adenocorticotropin hormone and can in some cases help with the diagnosis of LCNET [22,27].

Recent studies have compared genetic/epigenetic profiles between LCNETs and SCCs. High levels of Ki67 (an oncogene), abnormal p53 (a tumour suppressor gene) and the absence of Rb (a tumour suppressor gene) have been described in LCNET and SCC but not in other neuroendocrine or LCC subtypes [20]. This could explain the high rate of proliferation in these tumours. Interestingly, low stage LCNETs were also shown to express more p21 (an oncogene), higher Ki67 levels and high Bcl2 (an apoptosis inhibitor) levels compared to low stage LCCs [1,12]. Finally, studies on the loss of heterozygosity, the methylation patterns of p16 and the expression of p53, K-Ras-2 (a proncogene) and C-raf-1 (a proncogene) have suggested a close relationship between LCNETs and SCCs but not with NCSLCs [11]. This could explain why surgically-resected LCNETs are associated with high recurrence rates.

Clinical presentation

Large cell neuroendocrine tumours often present as spiculated peripheral asymptomatic lung lesions [17]. This differs from the typical perihilar masses observed in SCCs. Patients usually have no complaints but can, in some cases, present cough, hemoptysis and/or postobstructive pneumonia [28]. Other rare symptoms can include chest pain (depending on location), dyspnea, night sweats and paraneoplastic syndrome [28]. Large cell neuroendocrine tumours are thus often incidentally identified in patients with high lung cancer risk profiles.

Diagnosis

Large cell neuroendocrine tumours are misdiagnosed in most cases because their differentiation from other subtypes of NSCLCs and SCCs requires large amounts of tumour material and a careful microscopy examination. The first step consists in confirming the presence of neuroendocrine differentiation by light microscopy which is distinct from typical carcinoma, atypical carcinoma and SCC [24]. To further confirm the diagnosis of LCNETs, immunohistological staining of tumours for neuroendocrine markers such as chromagranin, synaptophysin, neuron-specific enolase and CD56 can be useful [22,27]. In rare cases, the use of electron microscopy may be necessary. For example, the presence of secretary nodules and of intercellular junctions in cells is compatible with the neuroendocrine origin of a tumour [25].

Clinically, because neuroendocrine tumours often express somatostatin receptors, octreoscans can be useful for screening, preoperative staging and postoperative surveillance (recurrence risk and/or systemic treatment response) of LCNETs [8]. Finally, some studies have shown that PET-scans can be useful for the detection, staging and follow-up of LCNETs [6,21].

Staging

Because specific staging systems for LCNETs are unavailable, these tumours are evaluated based on the SCC or NSCLC classification systems. For example, the Veterans Affairs Lung Study Group (VALSG) is widely utilized in the staging of SCCs. Tumours can fall into two distinct categories: limited disease defined as a tumour confined to the ipsilateral hemithorax and extensive disease defined as evident metastatic disease outside the ipsilateral hemithorax (Table 1).

Other systems include the TNM/IASLC staging system. This system describes the extent and burden of disease more accurately than the VALSG. Its value in LCNETs has not been determined. In SCCs, the TNM is of limited value as a large overlap in prognosis exists between the different staging subgroups (Table 1).

Clinical staging should include by a physical examination, chest, abdominal computed tomography, brain MRI and PET scan to help identify mediastinal and extrapulmonary sites.

Table 1 – TNM/IASLC staging system which describes the extent and burden of disease and the VALSG localized and extensive disease classification system.

<table>
<tr><th>T</th><th>N</th><th>M</th><th colspan="3">Stage</th></tr>
<tr><td>T1
< 3cm diam without lobar invasion</td><td>N0
No regional lymph node involvement</td><td rowspan="3">M0
No distant metastasis</td><td rowspan="6">Localized disease</td><td>IA</td><td>T1N0M0</td></tr>
<tr><td rowspan="2">T2
> 3cm or invades visceral pleura or atelectasis lobe</td><td rowspan="2">N1
Ipsilateral hilar or ipsilateral peribronchial node</td><td>IB</td><td>T2N0M0</td></tr>
<tr><td>IIA</td><td>T1N1M0</td></tr>
<tr><td rowspan="2">T3
Chest wall, diaphragm, mediastinal pleura, atelectasis lung</td><td rowspan="2">N2
Ipsilateral mediastinal or subcarinal nodes</td><td rowspan="4">M1
Distant metastasis</td><td>IIB</td><td>T2N1M0 or T3N0M0</td></tr>
<tr><td>IIIA</td><td>T3N1M0
or T1-3N2M0</td></tr>
<tr><td rowspan="2">T4
Mediastinum, great vessels, trachea, vertebra, carina or effusion</td><td rowspan="2">N3
Controlateral nodes or scalene or subclavicular nodes</td><td>IIIB</td><td>TxN3M0
or T4NxM0</td></tr>
<tr><td>Extensive</td><td>IV</td><td>TxNxM1</td></tr>
</table>

Management and prognosis

Because the diagnosis of LCNET is so difficult, many of these tumours are initially managed as NSCLCs or SCCs. Some studies have shown that the survival of patients with LCNETs is worst compared to equally staged cases of NSCLCs [3,4]. Large cell neuroendocrine tumours are relatively infrequent and the exact roles of surgery, neoadjuvant and adjuvant radio-chemotherapy are still debated.

The general practice for early stage LCNETs consists of combined surgery and adjuvant chemotherapy as these tumours have a significant risk of local failure and distant metastasis [7,9,10,23]. A recent study has shown a survival advantage of early stage surgically-treated LCNETs following adjuvant chemotherapy with cisplatin, carboplatin or cyclophosphamide [13]. Interestingly, it is also known that neuroendocrine lung cancers may express high levels of a multidrug resistance receptor which could limit the response to chemotherapy in some cases [15].

Little data is available for advanced stage LCNETs. The role of neoadjuvant chemoradiotherapy is uncertain [5]. For unresectable LCNETs, some studies have shown that definitive radiation could induce tumour response [18]. Also, in most neuroendocrine tumours, palliative radiation has demonstrated efficacy for symptomatic lesions. Interestingly, a somatostatin analog (octreotide) was shown to control metastatic growth and to be well tolerated in other neuroendocrine tumours but never tested in LCNETs [8,16]. Therefore, more investigation is required to determine its role in the treatment of LCNETs. This can most likely be achieved by multicentre group trials to increase the number of LCNET cases.

At presentation, some reports have shown that 35% of patients with LCNETs have extensive stage disease and 65% have limited stage disease [4,5]. The 5-year overall survival of resectable LCNETs was reported to range from 13 to 57% in various series (Table 2) [7,14,25,28]. This survival is worse than that observed in LCCs with no neuroendocrine differentiation. Also, it was shown that LCNETs have worse overall survival compared to LCCs and NSCLCs at early stages of disease progression when treated surgically [3].

Table 2 – Five-year overall survival rate after resection for LCNETs of the different series reported in the literature between 1997 and 2006 (see references therein).

Author	Five-year overall survival rate	Year of study
Dresler *et al.* [7]	13%	1997
Travis *et al.* [23]	27%	1998
Iyoda *et al.* [13]	35.3%	2001
Takei *et al.* [22]	57%	2002
Paci *et al.* [17]	21%	2004
Zacharias *et al.* [28]	4%	2003
Battafarano *et al.* [3]	30.3%	2005

Conclusion

Large cell neuroendocrine lung cancer is a rare but aggressive neoplasm with poor prognosis. Its accurate identification is in some cases challenging and further investigation is required to test novel approaches of combined therapy to improve prognosis. The aggressiveness of LCNET is comparable to SCCs although it shares many morphological and clinical features with LCC and NSCLC. Future investigation is required for accurate diagnosis and staging and systematization of therapy and its evaluation.

3

References

1. Ab' Saber AM, Massoni Neto LM, Bianchi CP *et al.* (2004) Neuroendocrine and biologic features of primary tumors and tissue in pulmonary large cell carcinomas. Ann Thorac Surg 77: 1883-1890.
2. Arrigoni MG, Woolner LB, Bernatz PE (1972) Atypical carcinoid tumors of the lung. J Thorac Cardiovasc Surg 64: 413-21
3. Battafarano RJ, Fernandez FG, Ritter J *et al.* (2005) Large cell neuroendocrine carcinoma: an aggressive form of non-small cell lung cancer. J Thorac Cardiovasc Surg 130: 166-72
4. Battafarano RJ, Piccirillo JF, Meyers BF *et al.* (2002) Impact of comorbidity on survival after surgical resection in patients with stage I non-small cell lung cancer. J Thorac Cardiovasc Surg 123: 280-7
5. Cagirici U, Cakan A, Samancilar O, Veral A, Ozhan M (2006) [Surgical results of large cell neuroendocrine carcinoma of the lung.] Tuberk Toraks 54: 30-3
6. **Chong S, Lee KS, Kim BT *et al.* (2007) Integrated PET/CT of pulmonary neuroendocrine tumors: diagnostic and prognostic implications. AJR Am J Roentgenol 188: 1223-31**
7. Dresler CM, Ritter JH, Patterson GA *et al.* (1997) Clinical-pathologic analysis of 40 patients with large cell neuroendocrine carcinoma of the lung. Ann Thorac Surg 63: 180-5
8. Filosso PL, Ruffini E, Oliaro A *et al.* (2002) Long-term survival of atypical bronchial carcinoids with liver metastases, treated with octreotide. Eur J Cardiothorac Surg 21: 913-7
9. Garcia-Yuste M, Matilla JM, Alvarez-Gago T *et al.* (2000) Prognostic factors in neuroendocrine lung tumors: a Spanish Multicenter Study. Spanish Multicenter Study of Neuroendocrine Tumors of the Lung of the Spanish Society of Pneumonology and Thoracic Surgery (EMETNE-SEPAR). Ann Thorac Surg 70: 258-63
10. Hage R, Seldenrijk K, de Bruin P *et al.* (2003) Pulmonary large-cell neuroendocrine carcinoma (LCNEC). Eur J Cardiothorac Surg 23: 457-60
11. **Hiroshima K, Iyoda A, Shibuya K *et al.* (2004) Genetic alterations in early-stage pulmonary large cell neuroendocrine carcinoma. Cancer 100: 1190-8**
12. Iyoda A, Hiroshima K, Shiba M *et al.* (2004) Clinicopathological analysis of pulmonary sclerosing hemangioma. Ann Thorac Surg 78: 1928-31
13. Iyoda A, Hiroshima K, Toyozaki T *et al.* (2001) Clinical characterization of pulmonary large cell neuroendocrine carcinoma and large cell carcinoma with neuroendocrine morphology. Cancer 91: 1992-2000
14. Jiang SX, Kameya T, Shoji M *et al.* (1998) Large cell neuroendocrine carcinoma of the lung: a histologic and immunohistochemical study of 22 cases. Am J Surg Pathol 22: 526-37
15. Lai SL, Goldstein LJ, Gottesman MM, Pastan I, Tsai CM, *et al.* (1989) MDR1 gene expression in lung cancer. J Natl Cancer Inst 81: 1144-50
16. O'Byrne KJ, Schally AV, Thomas A, Carney DN, Steward WP (2001) Somatostatin, its receptors and analogs, in lung cancer. Chemotherapy 47 Suppl 2: 78-108
17. Paci M, Cavazza A, Annessi V *et al.* (2004) Large cell neuroendocrine carcinoma of the lung: a 10-year clinicopathologic retrospective study. Ann Thorac Surg 77: 1163-7
18. Petrovic M, Tomic I, Ilic S (2007) [Neuroendocrine differentiation as a survival prognostic factor in advanced non-small cell lung cancer]. Vojnosanit Pregl 64: 525-9
19. Przygodzki RM, Finkelstein SD, Langer JC *et al.* (1996) Analysis of p53, K-ras-2, and C-raf-1 in pulmonary neuroendocrine tumors. Correlation with histological subtype and clinical outcome. Am J Pathol 148: 1531-41
20. Rusch VW, Klimstra DS, Venkatraman ES (1996) Molecular markers help characterize neuroendocrine lung tumors. Ann Thorac Surg 62: 798-809; discussion 809-710
21. Song YS, Lee WW, Chung JH *et al.* (2008) Correlation between FDG uptake and glucose transporter type 1 expression in neuroendocrine tumors of the lung. Lung Cancer 61: 54-60

22. Takei H, Asamura H, Maeshima A, Suzuki K, Kondo H *et al.* (2002) Large cell neuroendocrine carcinoma of the lung: a clinicopathologic study of eighty-seven cases. J Thorac Cardiovasc Surg 124: 285-92

23. Travis WD, Gal AA, Colby TV *et al.* (1998) Reproducibility of neuroendocrine lung tumor classification. Hum Pathol 29: 272-9

24. Travis WD, Linnoila RI, Tsokos MG *et al.* (1991) Neuroendocrine tumors of the lung with proposed criteria for large-cell neuroendocrine carcinoma. An ultrastructural, immunohistochemical, and flow cytometric study of 35 cases. Am J Surg Pathol 15: 529-53

25. Travis WD, Rush W, Flieder DB *et al.* (1998) Survival analysis of 200 pulmonary neuroendocrine tumors with clarification of criteria for atypical carcinoid and its separation from typical carcinoid. Am J Surg Pathol 22: 934-44

26. WHO (2007) International statistical classification of disease, 10th revision

27. Wick MR, Berg LC, Hertz MI (1992) Large cell carcinoma of the lung with neuroendocrine differentiation. A comparison with large cell "undifferentiated" pulmonary tumors. Am J Clin Pathol 97: 796-805

28. Zacharias J, Nicholson AG, Ladas GP, Goldstraw P (2003) Large cell neuroendocrine carcinoma and large cell carcinomas with neuroendocrine morphology of the lung: prognosis after complete resection and systematic nodal dissection. Ann Thorac Surg 75: 348-52

Neuroendocrine tumours of the lung

4

A. Bonnichon, H. Le Floch, F. Rivière, J. Margery and F. Vaylet

Five Essential Points

1. *Neuroendocrine tumours are represented by a broad spectrum of tumours of increasing aggressiveness, from typical carcinoid tumours to small cell cancers: included are carcinoid tumours, usually of good prognosis and poorly radiochemosensitive, small and large cells tumours, chemosensitive but of poor prognosis, including the strong link with smoking that may explain the different oncogeneses.*
2. *Surgery remains the treatment of choice for carcinoid tumours even if an adjuvant treatment, the modalities of which remain to be defined, might be considered for atypical forms with node invasion, particularly N2.*
3. *Somatostatin analogues are useful for the scintigraphic control of carcinoid symptoms in case of hyperfixation; they might in the future be associated with targeted treatments (i.e. everolimus, bevacizumab, sorafenib, SUFITNIB) or temzolomide that is giving encouraging results.*
4. *Large cell neuroendocrine tumours justify a systemic combination therapy of the platin-etoposide type, even after an early stage surgical treatment because of frequent and rapid metastatic relapse.*
5. *To improve local control, large cell neuroendocrine tumours might benefit from a supplementary radiotherapy the modalities of which are yet to be defined through prospective studies.*

Introduction

Neuroendocrine tumours of the lung (NETL) are rare, representing some 20 % of lung tumours. This term groups different entities, covering a wide histological spectrum: typical (TC) and atypical (AC) carcinoid tumours, large cell neuroendocrine carcinomas (LCNEC) as well as small cell carcinomas (SCLC), the frequency of which is high (15% of lung tumours and nearly 80% of neuroendocrine tumours of the lung), the latter not described in this chapter. The clinical presentation and progressive profile of NETL are different and reflect a growing aggressiveness. The knowledge of the oncogenesis and natural history of these tumours has greatly evolved in recent years and the histological criteria that allow their individualisation have been refined; however, their rarity has as yet prevented the definition of an optimal treatment. Nonetheless, encouraging therapeutic prospects are creating renewed interest in clinical research on these little-known tumours.

General Features

Pulmonary endocrine cells originating from the endodermic sheet are scattered over the respiratory tract or in the form of small clusters. They possess common chemical properties such as secretion of peptides.

Classification

After almost 30 years evolution of NETL classification, Travis has defined the widely accepted classification [43]. TC tumours present an architecture that is mostly organoid or trabecular, more rarely with clear, spindle or melanocytic cells. The cytology is monomorphic with nuclei containing fine granular chromatin, invisible nucleoli and an eosinophilic cytoplasm of moderate size. Mitoses are rare ($< 2/mm^2$) and necrosis is absent. AC tumours are distinguished by the existence of foci of necrosis and more frequent mitoses but less than $10/mm^2$. Cellular peculiarities are more marked and the architecture more disorganised. The LCNEC are high-grade tumours presenting a neuroendocrine architecture (trabecular, palissading, in islets or pseudorosettes) and having cellular characteristics similar to those of non-small cell cancer except in size. Associated with this is the number of mitoses at $> 10/mm^2$ and foci of necrosis, extensive and confluent, sometimes in large plaques. The cells have high nucleocytoplasmic content, a vesicular or coarse chromatin and voluminous nucleoli. Concerning the immunophenotype, neuroendocrine tumours express pancytokeratins and neuroendocrine markers (e.g. Neural Cell Adhesion Molecular, synaptophysin, chromogranin A). Twenty percent of LCNEC are combined with adenocarcinoma and squamous cell carcinoma and 10% to 20% of non-small cell lung cancers (NSCLC) show neuroendocrine differentiation (especially adenocarcinomas) the significance of which is still unclear, although it appears that there exists a different impact on survival and chemosensitivity. Composite carcinoid tumours are, however, quite rare, never associated with high-grade tumours, probably because of different oncogenesis [1].

Histological diagnosis is difficult, based on small fragments such as bronchial biopsies or puncture-biopsies, even for experienced histologists. Poor fixation, extent of necrosis, too thick sections and poor quality of immunofixation are confounding factors [3, 43]. The frequent overlap of nuclear and cellular sizes sometimes makes the differential diagnosis of small or large cell neuroendocrine tumours difficult [42].

This new classification into four types and three grades of malignancy (Table 1) allows for better individualisation of neuroendocrine tumours, good reproducibility and thus better prediction of the prognosis [38].

Table 1 – Classification of neuroendocrine tumours of the lung (WHO 1999).

Variable	TC	AC	LCNEC	SCLC
Microscopy	Carcinoid features	Carcinoid features	Neuroendocrine features[1] immunostaining[2], cytologic caracteristics of LCC[3]	Small size (< 3 lymphocytes), scant cytoplasm nucleoli: finely granular nuclear chromatin, absent or faint nucleoli
Mitosis/2 mm^3 (10HPF)	< 2	≥ 2 and < 10	≥ 10	≥ 10
Necrosis	No	Focal	Often large zones	Large zones
Grade	Low	Intermediate	High	High

TC: typical carcinoid; AC: atypical carcinoid; LCNEC: large cell neuroendocrine carcinoma; SCLC: small cell lung cancer; LCC: large cell carcinoma; HPF: high power field × 40.

[1]: palissading, rosette, trabecular, islet.

[2]: one or more positive staining for neuroendocrine markers, except Neuron Specific Enolase.

[3]:large cell size, low nucleolocytoplasmic count, fine or vesicular chromatine and/or frequent nucleoli.

Epidemiology

Carcinoid tumours are rare tumours that represent less than 2% of pulmonary tumours [14,17]. They are mainly of typical histology (80–85% of cases) and affect women in particular [14,15,49]. Most often centrally located, they are endobronchial in 75% of the cases and then appear as well-delineated tumours, raspberry or beige-pink-coloured, richly vascularised with a possible iceberg-type of extension [17]. TC tumours can also occur on a DIPNECH (Diffuse Idiopathic Pulmonary Neuroendocrine Cell Hyperplasia) ground, especially in women with peripheral tumours. The annual incidence has increased steadily over the past thirty years, to about 6% per year [39], multiplied by two for women (between 8.9 to 13 per million) and by three for men (2 to 5.2 per million) in the United States [49]. The peak incidence occurs in the fifth decade for typical carcinoids, in the sixth for atypical ones [15,23], but a few non-rare cases occur before the age of 40. Familial forms also exist which, although rare, are classically associated with a Multiple Endocrine Neoplasia type 1 (MEN) [31].

LCNEC are rare with a reported incidence of 0.9% to 5.1%, most frequently around 3% of operated tumours [4,7,13,15,32,35]. The link with smoking is strong (75% to 100%) [12,13], unlike carcinoid tumours, explaining a predominance of male patients (85% to 98%) as well as the classical age of onset in the seventh decade with an average age of 65 years [3, 7, 32].

Prognosis

Overall 5-yr survival is 87% to 100% for TC tumours and 44% to 78% for AC tumours; overall 10-yr survival is from 82% to 92% and 35% to 67% respectively [14, 15, 17, 37, 39]. Identified prognostic factors include the histological type and completeness of resection whereas lymphatic invasion also seems relevant, at least for atypical forms.

Thus the cellular aggressiveness reflected by histological grade has the most important prognostic weight as evidenced by the overall survival rate at 5 and 10 years for both types of carcinoid tumours. Moreover, the recurrence rate at 5 years is significantly higher for early stages having undergone surgery in cases of atypical histology: 3.26% locally and 16.3% at distance against 0.88% and 1.58%, respectively for TC tumours. Finally, mortality is higher in case of recurrence in AC tumours compared to TC tumours: 80% *versus* 45% [15].

The value of the TNM classification for carcinoid tumours is positive with a different survival rate depending on the stage. Thus, the overall survival rate at 5 years is only 22% for metastatic AC tumours at diagnosis [16]. The nodal status also seems to be correlated to the prognosis in different surgical series, at least in AC tumours [6, 23, 26, 27], which is confirmed by the Spanish cohort study in which the lymphatic extension at diagnosis is also more frequent [15]: overall survival at 10 years is 92% for TC tumours, dropping to 66% in case of lymph node involvement, while overall survival is 60% at 10 years for AC N+ tumours against 70% in the absence of lymph node invasion. This data remains controversial, particularly for TC tumours[13].

High-grade aggressive tumours with a 10-yr survival rate of 9% [23, 43], LCNEC have poorer prognosis than carcinoid tumours and other large cell lung tumours, including those of early stages [19]. In the North American endocrine tumours study, including all primary tumours, median overall survival for poorly

4

differentiated neuroendocrine tumours is 10 months [9-11], with variations depending on localized stages (34 months [27-41]), with lymphatic (14 [13-15]) or metastatic (5 [4,5-5,5]) invasion, with a probability of survival at 5 years of 38%, 21% and 4%, respectively [49]. The overall survival at 5 years reported in the literature is almost always less than 45%, all stages included (Table 2). In the majority of these series, the observed difference in overall survival is inversely proportional to the proportion of early stages. There is no significant difference in survival with SCLCs of the same stage [23, 32, 42]. Progression-free survival is of short duration and relapse occurs in 50% to 75% of cases within the first six months and in only 9% of cases after a year [42]. Relapse is most often metastatic (50% to 75%) [3, 4, 13], the most frequent site being the brain (23% to 43%) [35, 42, 45].

Falling under the group of high-grade neuroendocrine tumours represents a very important prognostic factor, including for stage I, with a relative risk > 17 [3]. Other markers are proposed as prognostic factors, including mitotic index with an overall survival rate inversely proportional for advanced stages [11]. Neuroendocrine marking is a controversial prognostic factor: the more a tumour appears differentiated on the neuroendocrine plane, the better the prognosis. In contrast, neuroendocrine differentiation within the framework of combined non-small cell tumours is a decreasing prognostic factor for overall survival and progression-free survival [11].

Table 2 – Overall survival for LCNEC.

Authors	Reference	Number of patients	5-years OS (%)	5-years OS stage I only (n/%)
Travis	(43)	37	27%	NE
Garcia-Yuste [a, c]	(15)	22	21%	33% (13/59%)
Hage [a]	(17)	7	0%	0% (5/71%)
Takei [a, c]	(42)	87	57%	67% (41/47%)
Paci	(32)	48	21%	27% (29/60%)
Daddi	(7)	18	37.5%	NE
Battafarano [a]	(4)	45	30%	43% (30/66%)
Filosso [a, c]	(13)	18	35%	NE (5/28%)
Iyoda [c, d]	(19)	15	88.9% (1 year)	NE
Veronesi [b]	(45)	144	43%	52% (74/51%)
Rossi [a, c]	(35)	83	27%	33% (54/65%)
Asamura [b]	(3)	141	41%	58% (63/45%)

LCNEC: large cell neuroendocrine carcinoma; OS: overall survival; a: monocentric study; b: retrospective multicentric study; c: neo – or adjuvant treatment; d: prospective study; NE: non evaluated.

Clinical presentation and initial evaluation

Clinical features

Half of the patients presenting carcinoid tumours are asymptomatic at diagnosis [14]. The majority of clinical signs are related to the endobronchial location of the tumour: cough, haemoptysis, repeated infections in the same area, sometimes unilateral wheezing [37]. Lymphatic invasion is more common for AC (20% to 57%) than for TC (0% to 14%) tumours and is also greater in the case of atypical histology. There is an increased rate of N2 (ranging from 27% to 58% for AC against 2% to 3.5% for TC tumours) and a ratio of N2/N1 always greater than 1 for the atypical forms [14, 15, 23, 39]. The same applies for the metastatic character at diagnosis, representing about 1% of TC, but 16% to 30% of AC tumours. The most frequently affected sites are bone, liver, lung, adrenals, brain and soft tissues [17, 39, 46]. The TNM classification, thus, indicates more advanced stages at diagnosis in atypical forms: 25% stages III-IV as *versus* 5% for TC tumours and only 57% of stage I *versus* 87% [15].

Paraneoplastic syndrome is independent of the existence of metastasis or of the tumour mass. It is of haematological, hormonal, dermatological or neurological origin. Carcinoid syndrome is classical but rare and is present in about 1 to 5% of the cases, whereas there is some ectopic hormonal secretion, such as Cushing's syndrome by the secretion of ACTH (25% of paraneoplastic Cushings relate to slow progressing carcinoid tumours) or acromegaly detected by the determination of GHRH. Some authors have reported hormonal hypersecretion in nearly 15% of patients through systematic preoperative determination in patients who are carriers of neuroendocrine tumours. In case of hormonal hypersecretion, one may consider an association of a type 1 NEM, autosomal dominant disorder that increases mortality, including pancreatic, parathyroid and pituitary impairment.

Carcinoid syndrome is produced by low or intermediary grade endocrine tumours [3, 7, 11, 13, 32, 35, 42].

The presentation of LCNEC appears to be less frequently symptomatic compared to carcinoid tumours, which may seem surprising given the aggressive nature of these tumours. The most likely explanation is the high number of early stages listed, discovered on poorly symptomatic peripheral lesions. Thus, while the presentation is central in 75% of cases of carcinoid tumours, most series of LCNEC report only exceptional cases of central presentation [7, 32]. On the other hand, when the proportion of stage IV cases or nodal invasion is more significant (N2-3), the rate of central presentation is higher (23% to 33%), approaching that of small cell carcinomas [15,35] and suggesting that the central presentation is certainly more frequent.

Extension evaluation

Radiologically, carcinoid tumours present most often a central location, more or less associated with an atelectasis. Peripheral locations are more frequent in the case of atypical forms [34]. Conventional imaging does not show particular characteristics except for the existence of calcification or a fatty component in 10% of the cases [17].

Positive diagnosis is most often achieved by lung fibroscopy, performed in the presence of recurring pulmonary infections or atypical asthma. Bronchial biopsies of these richly vascularised tumours present a potential risk for bleeding, usually without complications. Serum chromogranin A appears to be a good neuroendocrine marker, more efficient than the determination of neuron-specific enolase or the alpha sub-unit of glycoprotein hormones, by setting the threshold at 300 μg/l. It is indeed correlated to the tumour mass and may prove useful in monitoring but, due to this fact, it underestimates low secreting small tumours [30]. Hormone determinations are not systematically recommended in the absence of carcinoid syndrome, where serotonine and 5'HIAA rates are determined [37].

The rest of the extended evaluation does not carry any specificity compared with that of another broncho-pulmonary tumour. Imaging with somatostatin analogues (such as octreoscan) is classical. Different tracers exist (e.g. octreotide, lanreotide, pentreotide) and their efficacies are broadly similar. Scintigraphy with meta-iodo-benzyl guanidine or MIBG is less efficient. These techniques are useful to explore possible extrathoracic locations but fixation is not strictly correlated with the prediction of response to treatment with somatostatin analogues. Their implementation is thus especially useful for monitoring in case of initial fixation, sometimes allowing the detection of relapse well before the recurrence of symptoms. The negative predictive value of these examinations, however, is poor.

PET-CT is classically known for its poor contribution in carcinoid tumours. This statement is, in fact, partially incorrect since if fixing to 18-FDG is usually low in TC tumours [25, 40], it is more often positive for AC tumours [8]. Positivity of this tracer is indeed correlated to the level of Glut-1, a receptor more frequently present in AC tumours. Recently, preliminary results obtained with ^{68}Ga DOTATATE seem promising, but the low availability of this tracer remains an obstacle to its large scale development.

The radiological presentation of LCNEC does not carry any specificity compared to non-small cell cancers of the lung [35]. Data relative to the PET by 18-FDG are patchy but seem to show a strong affinity for this tracer, consistent with that of SCLC. In cases of localised presentation and in the absence of suggestive radiological signs, it has every significance for the assessment of potential metastatic sites. Indeed, scintigraphy with somatostatin analogues shows conflicting results in LCNEC [11, 13].

Treatment

Localized disease

Surgery remains the treatment of choice, with modalities varying according to histological type. For AC tumours, the more frequent existence of nodal invasion and the pejorative prognosis favour the recommendation of a technique similar to that for any lung cancer surgery: systematic resection to healthy margins of the lobectomy- or pneumonectomy-type according to localisation, and complete mediastinal clearance. Thus Garcia-Yuste finds a better prognosis among patients who are carriers of an AC tumour, having undergone a complete surgical clearance in his prospective series, as compared to retrospective results, in agreement with other authors [13, 15].

For TC tumours, a systematic complete surgical clearance does not guarantee any certainty. Thus, some authors recommend a functional conserving surgery with segmentectomy in peripheral forms and anastomosis resection in the central locations in young adults. For the same reasons, in the central locations and under certain conditions, an exclusive endobronchial treatment may be proposed: typical histology, central endoluminal tumours without any evidence of invasion of the bronchial wall by endoscopy and absence of lymph node invasion. This technique is still controversial and carries a risk of relapse in case of incomplete resection (in the absence of lymph node clearance) and must be performed exclusively by teams well trained in interventional endoscopy [5, 24].

Metastatic disease and recurrence

Metastases occur in 5% to 70% of cases depending on the series and the histology. They can occur long after surgery and justify a prolonged surveillance. In the absence of randomised prospective studies, no clear strategy has yet been defined and the modalities of the treatment depend on the tumour histology, disease progression, evolutive kinetics and importance of the symptoms, particularly the existence of carcinoid syndrome.

Most data reported in the literature relate to neuroendocrine tumours of the digestive system and are extrapolated to lung tumours even if the latter have a poorer response to conventional radiochemotherapies. Furthermore, carcinoid tumours depict the particularity of a low response to imaging data and the evaluation of the effectiveness of the treatment presently relies on the reduction of symptoms, endocrine markers and fixation in metabolic imaging. Finally, the naturally long doubling time of these tumours does not enable an easy assessment whether stabilisation is rather related to treatment or to the natural course of the disease.

Historically, the first chemotherapy trials were performed with doxorubicin, 5-fluorouracil (5 FU) and streptozocin (STZ) followed by interferon and somatostatin analogues with disappointing response rates, ranging from 15% to 20% [29]. More recently, a Swedish study reported 20% to 25% of responders to chemotherapy with platinum-etoposide in some carriers of TC and AC tumours without any correlation with the expression of Ki67 [16]. In the same publication, the paclitaxel–doxorubicin combination conferred a stability of several months in four patients who received this treatment. The efficacy of paclitaxel has been reported in other publications [46]. The rate of overall response for first line treatment is about 15-20%, whether the 5FU is associated with doxorubicin or streptozocin, but the median survival was better in the scheme associating 5FU-STZ rather than 5FU-doxorubicin: 24.3 *versus* 15.7 months [41]. If effectiveness is moderate as evaluated by the usual criteria, the treatment may still lead to a significant improvement in the survival of advanced carcinoids from 39% to 70% at 5 years and 48% at 10 years. These results are obtained by combining temozolomide, a promising molecule currently being studied in multiple associations, to conventional chemotherapy of 5FU-STZ or 5FU-doxorubicin type, in the third or fifth line treatment with response rates of around 14% and 53% of stabilisation [10,20].

New treatments also open some hope in the treatment of carcinoid tumours. These tumours are richly vascularised and tumour size and progression-free survival are correlated with the level of VEGF in typical carcinoids [33]. Thus, several antiangiogenics have been efficient in phase II: sufitinib [21], bevacizumab [22,44], vatalanib [2], sorafenib being less efficient [18]. Bevacizumab gave superior results compared to pegylated interferon alpha 2b in 44 patients presenting carcinoid tumours of the digestive system with a decrease in intratumoural blood flow, an improved response rate and progression-free survival [48]. Recently, everolimus has also given interesting results in association with octreotide LAR in a phase II study in pre-treated carriers of pancreatic carcinoids, obtaining 22% of partial response and 70% stabilisation, resulting in an overall survival at 1, 2 and 3 years of 83%, 81% and 78%, a median progression-free survival at 60 weeks, and a biological response with a decrease in the level of CgA in 70% of patients and Ki67 in 7% of patients having undergone histological control at 2 weeks pre- and post-treatment [50]. These results obtained for tumours of the digestive system must be confirmed in pulmonary carcinoids and in more numerous series.

In the absence of radiological response, the treatment may help control symptoms, particularly carcinoid syndrome. It may bring in somatostatin analogues with

4

similar effectiveness according to the form of octreotide and or type of administration. This efficiency has been reported in other studies with 73% of symptom control associated with a 77% biochemical response, but the results are very disappointing on tumour regression: 3% response only [9]. In the case of secondary locations, particularly hepatic, hepatic embolisation or ablation by radiofrequency can sometimes bring clinical benefits, to be repeated if necessary. Finally, these tumours are known to be poorly radiosensitive even if complete and lasting responses have been reported in secondary cerebral and bone localisations [36].

Adjuvant therapy

In tumours with a high risk of relapse, the principle of adjuvant chemotherapy is to obtain a better progression-free-overall survival with an acceptable toxicity profile. Therefore, it should not be given in TC tumours with excellent prognosis and with a minimal risk of relapse.

The clinical translation of the histological prognostic factor is the greater proportion of lymph node invasion, the worst overall survival and more frequent relapses in AC tumours, including those after surgery [23]. These data question the need for adjuvant treatment for AC tumours with mediastinal invasion. However, studies are contradictory as some authors propose it for N1, others for N2 or else for N3 [15]. So far, there is no indication for an adjuvant treatment, but this remains to be defined in prospective studies for AC N + tumours, with perhaps new modalities using targeted treatments.

Large cell neuroendocrine carcinoma

The worst LCNEC prognosis indicates the need for an adjuvant treatment, including those cases in early stages, unlike the results observed in histologies of the NSCLC type. The importance of the latter has been demonstrated by Iyoda in retrospective series, and then confirmed by a small prospective series, showing an overall survival of 89% at 2 years, thanks to a cisplatin-etoposide chemotherapy regime, always for stages IA [19]. The choice of this first line treatment is based on knowledge of the chemosensitivity of SCLCs and is confirmed by a 1999 study on LCNEC [28].

The reported objective response rate to chemotherapy based on cisplatin and etoposide is from 30% to 80%. This response is better in chemonaïve subjects (64% *vs* 17% statistically significant) [35, 45, 47]. Rossi reports an increase in median survival, but the survival curve of patients having received chemotherapy of NSCLC type can be matched with that of patients not having received adjuvant chemotherapy [3, 35, 42].

The radiosensitivity of these tumours has not been the subject of any randomised study. However, individual data from various series tend to suggest that radiotherapy may increase local control of the disease, whether mediastinal or metastatic and should possibly be proposed in addition to chemotherapy, according to modalities which remain to be specified.

Conclusion

Neuroendocrine tumours of the lung are rare, making up a wide histological spectrum of growing aggressiveness. Carcinoid tumours are poorly metastatic with a good prognosis and the elective treatment is surgery. However, AC are tumours that metastase more frequently, both at lymphatic and systemic levels, therefore justifying systematic lymph node dissection. They might benefit from an adjuvant treatment, the modalities of which remain to be specified. Systemic treatment of carcinoid tumours in case of metastatic invasion is based on chemotherapy, the effectiveness of which remains modest, such as that of interferon. First results obtained with temozolomide and targeted treatments are encouraging. Somatostatin analogues are efficient in controlling symptoms. LCNEC are more aggressive tumours, with a prognosis close to that of SCLC, with which they share many similarities. Treatment is surgery with clearance if feasible, followed by adjuvant chemotherapy irrespective of the stage. The chemotherapy of reference is the platinum-etoposide combination. Radiotherapy might be beneficial for local control.

The rarity of these tumours complicates clinical research and knowledge of optimal treatments. More than ever, it is necessary to register patients who suffer from them so as to optimise their management through prospective trials at a time when certain new treatments show encouraging effects.

References

1. Anbazhagan R, Tihan T, Bornmann DM *et al.* (1999) Classification of small cell lung cancer and pulmonary carcinoid by gene expression profile. Cancer Res 59: 5119-22
2. Anthony L, Chester M, Michael S *et al.* (2006) Phase II open-label clinical trial of vatalanib (PTK/2K) in patients with progressive neuroendocrine cancer. ASCO Meeting Abstracts 24: 4044
3. Asamura H, Kameya T, Matsuno Y *et al.* (2006) Neuroendocrine neoplasms of the lung: a prognostic spectrum. J Clin Oncol 24(1): 70-5
4. Battafarano RJ, Fernandez, FG, Ritter J (2005) Large cell neuroendocrine carcinoma: an aggressive form of non-small cell lung cancer. J Thorac Cardiovasc Surg 130(1): 166-71
5. Bertoletti L, Elleuch R, Kaczmarek D *et al.* (2006) Bronchoscopic cryotherapy treatment of isolated endoluminal typical carcinoid tumour. Chest 130: 1405-11
6. Cardillo G, Sera F, Di Martino M *et al.* (2004). Bronchial carcinoid tumours: nodal status and long-term survival after resection. Ann Thorac Surg 77: 1781-5
7. Daddi N, Ferolla P, Urbani M *et al.* (2004) Surgical treatment of neuroendocrine tumours of the lung. Eur J Cardiothorac Surg 26: 813-7
8. Daniels CE, Lowe VJ, Aubry MC *et al.* (2007) The utility of fluorodeoxyglucose positron emission tomography in the evaluation of carcinoid tumours presenting as pulmonary nodules. Chest 131: 255-60
9. Di Bartolomeo M, Bajetta E, Buzzoni R *et al.* (1996) Clinical efficacy of octreotide in the treatment of metastatic neuroendocrine tumours. A study by the Italian Trials in Medical Oncology Group. Cancer 77: 402-8
10. Ekeblad S, Sundin A, Janson ET *et al.* (2007) Temozolomide as monotherapy is effective in treatment of advanced malignant neuroendocrine tumours. Clin Cancer Res 13: 2986-91
11. Faggiano A, Sabourin JC, Ducreux M *et al.* (2007) Pulmonary and extrapulmonary poorly differentiated large cell neuroendocrine carcinomas. Diagnostic and prognostic features. Cancer 110(2): 265-74
12. Fernandez FG, Battafarano RJ (2006) Large cell neuroendocrine carcinoma of the lung. Cancer Control 13: 270-5
13. Filosso PL, Rena O, Donati G *et al.* (2002) Bronchial carcinoid tumours: surgical management and long-term outcome. J Thorac Cardiovasc Surg 123: 303-9
14. Fink G, Krelbaum T, Yellin A *et al.* (2001) Pulmonary carcinoid: presentation, diagnosis and outcome in 142 cases in Israel and review of 640 cases from the literature. Chest 119: 1647-51
15. **Garcia-Yuste M, Matilla JM, Cueto A *et al.* (2007) Typical and atypical carcinoid tumours: analysis of the experience of the Spanish Multi-centric Study of Neuroendocrine Tumours of the Lung. Eur J CardioThorac Surg 31: 192-7**

16. Granberg D, Eriksson B, Wilander E (2001) Experience in treatment of metastatic pulmonary carcinoid tumours. Ann Oncol 12: 1383-91
17. **Hage R, Brutel de la Rivière A, Seldenrijk CA, van den Bosch JMM (2003) Update in pulmonary carcinoid tumours: a review article. Ann Surg Oncol 10: 697-704**
18. Hobday TJ, Rubin J, Holen K *et al.* (2007) MCO44h, a phase II trial of sorafenib in patients with metastatic neuroendocrine tumours (NET): a Phase II Consortium (P2C) study. ASCO Meeting Abstracts 25: 4504
19. Iyoda A, Hiroshima K, Moriya Y *et al.* (2006) Prognostic impact of large cell neuroendocrine histology in patients with pathologic stage Ia pulmonary non small cell carcinoma. J Thorac Cardiovasc Surg 132(2): 312-5
20. Kulke MH, Stuart K, Earle CC *et al.* (2006) A phase II study of temzolomide and bavacizumab in patients with advanced neuroendocrine tumours. ASCO Meeting Abstracts 24: 4044
21. Kulke MH, Lenz HJ, Meropol NJ *et al.* (2008) Activity of sufitinib in patients with advanced neuroendocrine tumours. J Clin Oncol 26: 3403-10
22. Kunz PL, Kuo T, Kaiser HL *et al.* (2008) A phase II study of capecitabine, oxaliplatine and bevacizumab for metastatic or unresectable neuroendocrine tumours: Preliminary results. ASCO Meeting Abstracts 26: 15502
23. Lim E, Yap YK, De Stavola BL *et al.* (2005). The impact of stage and cell type on the prognosis of pulmonary neuroendocrine tumours. J Thorac Cardiovasc Surg 130(4): 969-72
24. Luckraz H, Amer K, Thomas L *et al.* (2006). Long-term outcome of bronchoscopically resected endobronchial typical carcinoid tumours. J Thorac Cardiovasc Surg 132: 13-5
25. Marom EM, Sarvis S, Herndon JE (2002) Lung cancers: sensitivity of diagnosis with fluorodeoxyglucose PET. Radiology 223: 453-9
26. Martini N, Zaman M, Bains M *et al.* (1994) Treatment and prognosis in bronchial carcinoid involving regional lymph nodes. J Thorac Cardiovasc Surg 107: 1-7
27. Mezzetti M, Raveglia F, Panigalli T *et al.* (2003) Assessment of outcomes in typical and atypical carcinoids according to latest WHO classification. Ann Thorac Surg 76: 1838-42
28. Mitry E, Baudin E, Ducreux M *et al.* (1999) Treatment of poorly differentiated neuroendocrine tumours with etoposide and cisplatin. Br J Cancer 81: 1351-5
29. Moertel CG, Hanley JA (1979) Combination chemotherapy trials in metastatic carcinoid tumour and the malignant carcinoid syndrome. Cancer Clin Trials 2: 327-34
30. Nobels FR, Kwekkeboom DJ, Coopmans W *et al.* (1997) Chromogranin A as serum marker for neuroendocrine neoplasia: comparison with neuron-specific enolase and the alpha-subunit of glycoprotein hormones. J Clin Endoc Metabol 82: 2622-8
31. Oliveira AM, Tozelaar HD, Wentzlaff KA (2001) Familiar pulmonary carcinoid tumours. Cancer 91: 2104-9
32. Paci M, Cavazza A, Annessi V *et al.* (2004). Large cell neuroendocrine carcinoma of the lung: A 10-year clinicopathologic retrospective study. Ann Thorac Surg 77: 1163-7
33. Phan AT, Wang L, Xie K *et al.* (2008). Association of VEGF expression with poor prognosis among patients with low-grade neuroendocrine carcinoma. ASCO Meeting Abstracts 24: 4091
34. Rosado de Christenson M, Abbott G, Kirejezyk W (1999) Thoracic carcinoids: radiologic-pathologic correlation. Radiographics 19: 707-36
35. **Rossi G, Cavazza A, Marchioni A *et al.* (2006). Role of chemotherapy and receptor tyrosyne kinases KIT, PDGFR alpha, PDGFR beta, and MET in large cell neuroendocrine carcinoma of the lung. J Clin Oncol 23(34): 8774-85**
36. Schupak KD, Wallner KE (1991) The role of radiation therapy in the treatment of locally unresectable or metastatic carcinoid tumours. Int J Radiat Oncol Biol Phys 20: 489-95
37. Scott WJ (2003) Surgical treatment of other bronchial tumours. Chest Surg Clin North Am 13: 111-28
38. Skov BG, Krasnik M, Lantuejoul S *et al.* (2008). Reclassification of neuroendocrine tumours improves the separation of carcinoids and the prediction of survival. J Thorac Oncol 12: 1410-5

39. Skuladottir H, Hirsch FR, Hansen HH, Olsen JH (2002) Pulmonary neuroendocrine tumours: incidence and prognosis of histological subtypes. A population-based study in Denmark. Lung Cancer 37: 127-35
40. Squerzanti A, Basteri V, Antinolfi G (2002) Bronchial carcinoid tumours: clinical and radiological correlation. Radiol Med 104: 273-84
41. Sun W, Lipsitz S, Catalano P *et al.*, Eastern Cooperative Oncology Group (2005) Phase II/III study of doxorubicin with fluorouracil compared with streptozocin with fluorouracil or dacarbazine in the treatment of advanced carcinoid tumours: Eastern Cooperative Oncology Group study E1281. J Clin Oncol 23: 4897-904
42. Takei H, Asamura H, Maeshima A *et al.* (2002) Large cell neuroendocrine carcinoma of the lung: a clinicopathologic study of eighty-seven cases. J Thorac Cardiovasc Surg 124(2): 285-92
43. Travis WD, Rush W, Flieder DB *et al.* (1998). Survival analysis of 200 pulmonary neuroendocrine tumours with clarification of criteria for atypical carcinoid and its separation from typical carcinoid. Am J Pathol 22(8): 934-44
44. Venook AP, Ko AH, Tempero MA *et al.* (2008). Phase II trial of FOLFOX plus bevacizumab in advanced, progressive neuroendocrine tumours. ASCO Meeting Abstracts 26: 15545
45. Veronesi G, Morandi U, Alloisio M *et al.* (2006) Large cell carcinoma of the lung: A retrospective analysis of 144 surgical cases. Lung Cancer 53: 111-5
46. Wirth LJ, Carter MR, Jänne PA, Johnson BE (2004) Outcome of patients with pulmonary carcinoid tumours receiving chemotherapy or chemoradiotherapy. Lung Cancer 44: 213-20
47. Yamazaki S, Sekine I, Matsuno Y *et al.* (2005) Clinical responses of large cell neuroendocrine carcinoma of the lung to cisplatin-based chemotherapy. Lung Cancer 49(2): 217-23
48. Yao JC, Phan A, Hoff PM *et al.* (2008) Targeting vascular endothelial growth factor in advanced carcinoid tumour: a random assignment phase II study of depot octreotide with bevacizumab and pegylated interferon alpha-2b. J Clin Oncol 26: 1316-23
49. Yao JC, Hassan M, Phan A *et al.* (2008) One hundred years after "carcinoid": Epidemiology and prognostic factors for neuroendocine tumours in 35,852 cases in the United States. J Clin Oncol 26: 3063-72
50. Yao JC, Phan AT, Chang DZ *et al.* (2008) Efficacy of RAD001 (everolimus) and octreotide LAR in advanced low-to intermediate-grade neuroendocrine tumours: results of a phase II study. J Clin Oncol 26: 4311-7

Pleural mesothelioma

E. Dansin, S. Dewas, C. Ferté and H. Porte

5

Five Essential Points

1. *Correlation has been clearly established between development of pleural mesothelioma and exposure to asbestos*
2. *Diagnosis of pleural mesothelioma should be based on large biopsies and confirmed by immunohistochemical studies*
3. *Surgical resection should be performed only on selected patients (cardio-respiratory function, comorbidities, PS 0-1, epithelioid histology, N0...) by experienced surgeons*
4. *Multimodality treatment of pleural mesothelioma should be evaluated in prospective clinical trials*
5. *First-line chemotherapy for pleural mesothelioma should be based on cisplatin and pemetrexed or raltitrexed regimen*

Introduction

Mesothelioma is a malignant tumour of the serous membranes that principally affects the pleura. Pleural localisation of mesothelioma is five times more frequent than other localisations (peritoneal, pericardial). It has clearly been established that the risks of pleural mesothelioma (PM) and lung cancer are associated with exposure (professional, environmental, domestic) to asbestos. Nowadays, the demolition, renovation and even maintenance of buildings containing asbestos can represent a risk of exposure. PM may manifest itself up to 30 or 40 years after exposure to asbestos. Certain forecasts suggest a strong increase in incidence of PM in the years 2020 to 2040 [24]. Research on mesothelial carcinogenesis has recently been completed, showing mutation of the NF2 gene, inactivation of *p16* and of RASSF1A, dysregulation of *Wnt1*and *Wnt2*.

Diagnostic – pretherapeutic assessment

Clinical signs of PM are non-specific (chest pain, dyspnea, impairment of the general state of health, hemi-thoracic retraction, parietal mass, pleural effusion). Diagnostic assessment should include a thoraco-abdominal tomodensitometry to search for a tumoral pleura (nodularity, pleural thickening...) and/or a parietal, mediastinal, pericardial, diaphragmatic even subphrenic extension. Magnetic Resonance Imaging (MRI) does not provide supplementary diagnostic information. Lymph node and tumour lesions are generally under-evaluated by CT scan and

MRI. Positron Emission Tomography (PET) more often uncovers pleural and/or mediastinal hyperfixations. The prognostic value of PET still remains to be demonstrated. A positive diagnosis of PM is based on the anatomopathological examination of large pleural biopsies obtained through video-assisted thoracoscopic surgery (VATS) or minithoracotomy. There are three main histological types: epithelioid (60%), sarcomatoid (10%) and biphasic (30%). Diagnosis may be difficult with pleural metastases of adenocarcinomas and immuno-histochemical analyses are useful (anti-EMA, anti-claretinin, anti-WT1, anti-CK5/6, anti-mesothelin, Ber-EP4, TTF1, CEA, anti-Ro/Rp...). [11]. When surgery is considered, it is imperative to take into account the comorbidities, cardiorespiratory capacity (PFT, ventilation/perfusion lung scan, cardiopulmonary exercise testing), mediastinal staging (PET, mediastinoscopy, EBUS) and eventual transdiaphragmatic extension (MRI, scannographic reconstruction, even laparoscopy). Evaluation is ongoing to specify accuracy of PET/CT scan for mediastinal lymph node (N) and extra-thoracic metastases (M) staging.

Thoracoscopy also enables talc pleurodesis to avoid recurrent effusions. The classification to be used in pleural mesothelioma is that of the International Mesothelioma Interest Group (IMIG) [25] (Table 1).

Osteopontin and soluble mesothelin-related peptides (SMRP) are the new serous and/or pleural markers being evaluated for the diagnosis of PM and for the follow up of patients at risk [19, 26]. Mesothelin inhibition by monoclonal antibodies or immunotherapy is opening new therapeutic perspectives [12].

Table 1 – IMIG classification for pleural mesothelioma [22]

Stage	Description
Stage I	
Ia	T1aN0M0
Ib	T1bN0M0
Stage II	T2N0M0
Stage III	Any T3M0 Any N1M0 Any N2M0
Stage IV	Any T4 Any N3 Any M1

Treatments

The prognosis of PM is poor (median survival time of 4 to 12 months, 5-year survival in the order of 5%) and therapeutic management is still the subject of much debate, namely for the potentially resectable forms (Fig. 5).

Treatments for resectable forms

Numerous controversies have revolved around the type of surgery to be chosen for resectable forms of PM from opposing pleurectomy to extrapleural pneumonectomy (EPP) [8]. Stewart's non-randomised retrospective series indicate the benefits in terms of median survival time after treatment with EPP over pleurectomy (364 days *versus* 233 days) [30]. EPP is an extensive and complex intervention (block resection of the lung, pleura, pericardium and diaphragm) requiring sophisticated reconstruction techniques where surgical experience is an essential element (Fig. 1). EPP is marked by a mortality rate of 5 to 15% and with morbidity in the order of 60%. The main post-operative complications include atrial fibrillation, venous thrombosis, cardiac tamponade, empyema, pulmonary embolism, bronchopleural fistula [32] (Fig. 2). EPP should only be undertaken in experienced centres that are involved in the evaluation of innovative multimodality strategies.

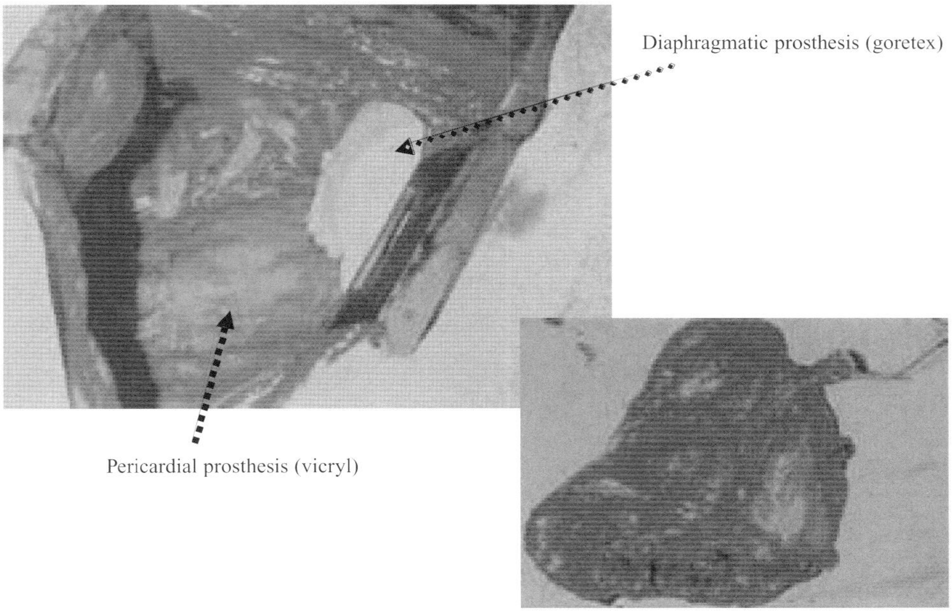

Fig. 1. Extrapleural pneumonectomy (patchs for reconstruction of the pericardium and diaphragm, specimen) (photo by Pr Porte, CHRU, Lille, France).

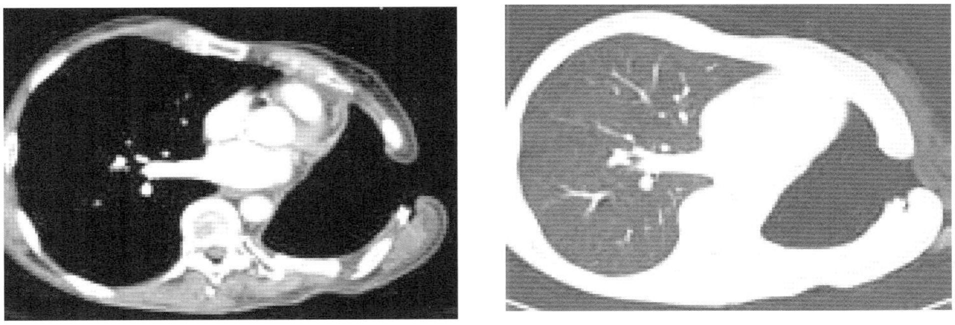

Fig. 2. Complication of extrapleural pneumonectomy: empyema imposing a pleurotomy (photo by the Centre Oscar-Lambret, France).

Multimodality strategies

In 1999, Sugarbaker reported his experience of a multimodal treatment with EPP followed by chemotherapy and adjuvant radiotherapy. Out of 183 patients, this author reported a median survival time of 19 months, a 5-year survival rate of 15% and identified a sub-group of good prognosis for 17% of the patients (epithelioid subtype, absence of lymph node involvement (pN0) and complete resection (R0)). Within this sub-group, the median survival time was 51 months with a 5-year survival rate of 46% [31]. Selection of candidates for multimodality treatment is based on these results and aims at identifying these favourable prognostic factors before surgery. Compliance to chemotherapy after an EPP being limited, some teams have developed a multimodality approach, integrating chemotherapy before an EPP with adjuvant radiotherapy. Within this framework, patient selection remains essential since morbidity of EPP is high after preoperative chemotherapy [17] (Figs 3 and 4). This multimodality approach remains experimental with published series having between 19 to 72 patients. In 2004, Weder reported results obtained from 19 patients with no surgical mortality and a median survival time of 23 months for the whole group [37]. Weder, Rea, Flores, de Perrot and Krug respectively report median survival times of 23, 27.5, 33.5, 59 and 29.1 months for some patient subgroups [7, 16, 20, 22, 38]. These multimodality treatments are still subject to feasibility with international clinical studies. On this subject, the EORTC phase II feasibility study reported by Van Schil and the British randomised trial aiming at the inclusion of 700 patients, following 3 chemotherapy cycles, randomising between surveillance and EPP followed by adjuvant radiotherapy should be mentioned [33, 35]. Modalities for adjuvant radiotherapy are also evolving fast with conformational techniques and stereotactic intensity-modulated radiation therapy (IMRT).

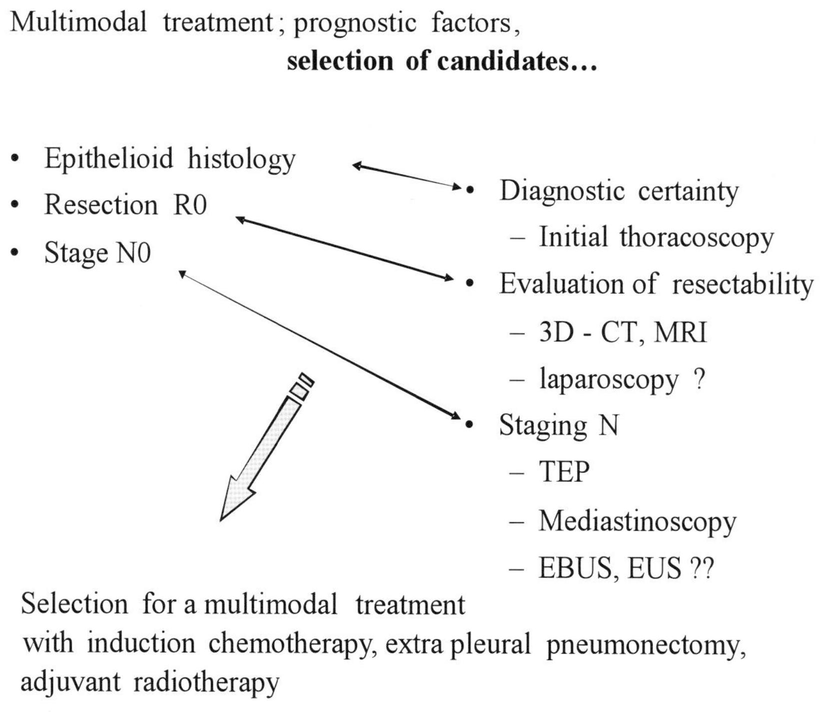

Fig. 3. Selection criteria for a multimodality treatment in experienced centres (clinical trial is recommended).

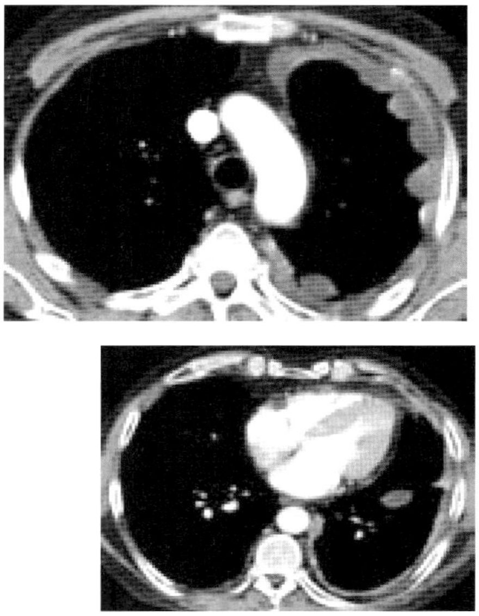

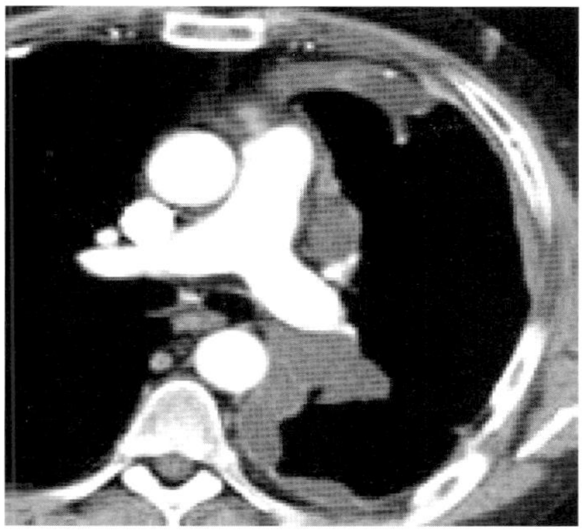

Fig. 4. Left pleural mesothelioma (epithelioid histology, cN0 (PET) M0). Selected patient for multimodality treatment with induction chemotherapy/surgery/adjuvant radiotherapy in a clinical trial.

Adjuvant radiotherapy concerns the entire hemithorax with the lower insertion areas of the diaphragm, the pericardium, the mediastinum and the areas difficult to resect as indicated by the surgeon with the help of clips. This adjuvant radiotherapy under these conditions of an extended resection is always a difficult technical achievement [2]. IMRT is still under supplementary investigation in terms of efficacy and of tolerance, given the appreciable toxicity risks [1, 23].

Treatment of inoperable forms

Numerous heterogeneous phase II trials have used different drugs either in monotherapy or in combination and the response rate has varied between 5% and 30%. The meta-analysis of Berghmans identified the cisplatin/doxorubicin combination as the optimal scheme with a response rate of 28% [3]. Until the year 2000, this combination was considered to be the treatment of reference. Vogelzang in 2003 and Van Meerbeeck in 2005 have published results of phase III trials randomising patients with non resectable PM, between monotherapy with cisplatin and bitherapy respectively with cisplatin/pemetrexed or cisplatin/raltitrexed with vitamin supplementation using folic acid and B12 [34, 36]. The cisplatin and multi-target antifolate (MTA)-based combinations gave better response rates and significantly superior median survival times compared to the cisplatin alone arm (12.1 months *vs* 9.3 and 11.4 *vs* 8.8). The rates of 1-year survival were superior in the double chemotherapy arms (50% *vs* 38% and 46% *vs* 40% (Table 2 and fig. 5).

The combination of cisplatin and MTA such as pemetrexed or raltitrexed is now recommended as first-line treatment with a high level of evidence [27, 29]. For patients who cannot receive a platinum-based chemotherapy, the pemetrexed/gemcitabine combination represents an active but particularly hematotoxic alternative [28]. There is no recommendation for second-line chemotherapy after failure of a cisplatin/pemetrexed-based first-line treatment. When these agents have not been used in first-line treatment, pemetrexed in second-line treatment proves to be superior to palliative care in terms of time to progression according to Jassem's

5

Table 2 – Chemotherapy in mesothelioma, review of phase III randomised trials [30, 31].

	VOGELZANG		VAN MEERBEECK	
	Cisplatin + Pemetrexed	**Cisplatin**	**Cisplatin**	**Cisplatin + Raltitrexed**
N	226	222	124	126
OR (%)	41% p<.001	17%	14%	24% p<.056
MS (months)	12.1 p<.02	9.3	8.8	11.4 p<.04
Survival 1 year (%)	50% p<.012	38%	40%	46%
QoL	>		=	=

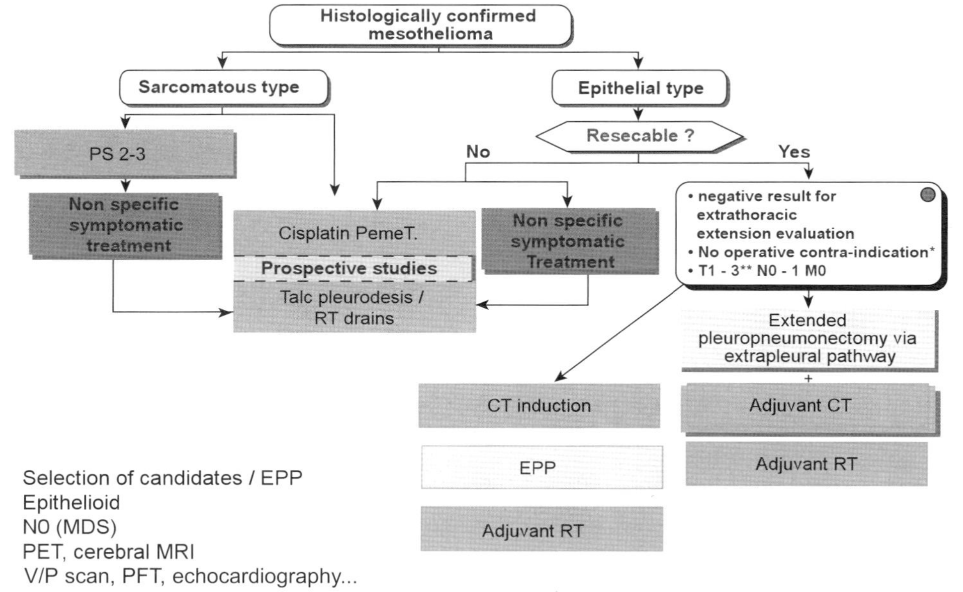

Fig. 5. Proposal for a therapeutic algorithm in mesothelima. Favour therapeutic trials namely in multimodal strategies and experienced centers. EPP: Extra pleural pneumonectomy; MDS: Mediastinoscopy; PFT: Pulmonary function tests.

randomised trial [14]. Several targeted agents are under evaluation in this situation of second-line treatment (erlotinib, vorinostat, ranpirnase, bortezomib, belinostat...) but none has demonstrated any significant activity [13, 21]. A North-American trial did not reveal any benefit from the addition of bevacizumab to a cisplatin/gemcitabine chemotherapy [15]. Combination of this anti-VEGF agent to a cisplatin/pemetrexed chemotherapy is currently under evaluation in North-American and French phase II trials (trial IFCT0701).

Prophylactic radiotherapy for pleural procedures sites: surgical or biopsy

Boutin's historic study carried out on 40 patients showed a significant decrease in permeation metastases in the irradiated arm [4]. In some countries, to prevent permeation nodules on the sites of pleural procedures it is recommended to carry out an irradiation of 3 fractions of 7 Gy during 3 consecutive days within the four weeks by using electron irradiation adapted to the depth [27]. However, two recent randomised trials did not confirm the efficacy of prophylactic irradiation to prevent surgical or biopsy site metastasis [5, 18]. A strategy of surveillance and treatment only if needed has also been proposed [6].

The therapeutic strategy in PM is still under discussion and evaluation (EPP within a multimodality approach, adjuvant radiotherapy by IMRT, second-line chemotherapy, targeted therapies...). This absence of therapeutic reference justifies the setting up of clinical studies. In spite of the progress made, the poor prognosis of PM underlines the importance of nutritional, antalgic and psychological palliative care. Medico-social support taking into account the occupational pathology and its compensation is an equally essential component in the management of PM patients and their families.

References

1. Allen AM, Czerminska M, Jänne PA *et al.* (2006) Fatal pneumonitis associated with intensity-modulated radiation therapy for mesothelioma. Int J Radiat Oncol Biol Phys 65(3): 640-5
2. Allen AM, Den R, Wong JS *et al.* (2007) Influence of radiotherapy technique and dose on patterns of failure for mesothelioma patients after extrapleural pneumonectomy. Int J Radiat Oncol Biol Phys 68(5): 1366-74
3. Berghmans T, Paesmans M, Lalami Y *et al.* (2002) Activity of chemotherapy and immunotherapy on malignant mesothelioma: a systematic review of the literature with meta-analysis. Lung Cancer 38(2): 111-21
4. Boutin C, Rey F, Viallat J (1995) Prevention of malignant seeding after invasive diagnostic procedures in patients with pleural mesothelioma. A randomized trial of local radiotherapy. Chest 108: 754-8
5. Bydder S, Phillips M, Joseph DJ *et al.* (2004) A randomised trial of single-dose radiotherapy to prevent procedure tract metastasis by malignant mesothelioma. Br J Cancer 91(1): 9-10
6. Davies HE, Musk AW, Lee YC (2008) Prophylactic radiotherapy for pleural puncture sites in mesothelioma: the controversy continues. Curr Opin Pulm Med 14(4): 326-30
7. Flores RM, Krug LM, Rosenzweig KE *et al.* (2006) Induction chemotherapy, extrapleural pneumonectomy, and postoperative high-dose radiotherapy for locally advanced malignant pleural mesothelioma: a phase II trial. J Thorac Oncol 1(4): 289-95
8. Flores RM, Pass HI, Seshan VE *et al.* (2008) Extrapleural pneumonectomy versus pleurectomy/decortication in the surgical management of malignant pleural mesothelioma: results in 663 patients. J Thorac Cardiovasc Surg 135(3): 620-6
9. Flores RM, Routledge T, Seshan VE *et al.* (2008) The impact of lymph node station on survival in 348 patients with surgically resected malignant pleural mesothelioma: implications for revision of the American Joint Committee on Cancer staging system. J Thorac Cardiovasc Surg 136(3): 605-10
10. **Flores RM, Zakowski M, Venkatraman E *et al.* (2007) Prognostic factors in the treatment of malignant pleural mesothelioma at a large tertiary referral center. J Thorac Oncol 2(10): 957-65**
11. Galateau-Sallé F, Brambilla E, Cagle P *et al.* (2005) Pathology of malignant mesothelioma; an update of the international mesothelioma panel. In: Galateau-Sallé (ed) Springer-Verlag New York, 1st edition

5

12. Hassan R, Ho M (2008) Mesothelin targeted cancer immunotherapy. Eur J Cancer 44(1): 46-53
13. Jackman DM, Kindler HL, Yeap BY *et al.* (2008) Erlotinib plus bevacizumab in previously treated patients with malignant pleural mesothelioma. Cancer 113(4): 808-14
14. Jassem J, Ramlau R, Santoro A *et al.* (2008) Phase III trial of pemetrexed plus best supportive care compared with best supportive care in previously treated patients with advanced malignant pleural mesothelioma. J Clin Oncol 26(10): 1698-704
15. Karrison T, Kindler H, Gandara D *et al.* (2007) Final analysis of a multi-center double-blind, placebo-controlled, randomized phase II trial of gemcitabine/cisplatin plus bevacizumab or placebo in patients with malignant mesothelioma. J Clin Oncol 25(18s): abstract 7526
16. Krug LM, Pass HI, Rusch VW *et al.* (2009) Multicenter phase II trial of neoadjuvant pemetrexed plus cisplatin followed by extrapleural pneumonectomy and radiation for malignant pleural mesothelioma. J Clin Oncol 27(18): 3007-13
17. Opitz I, Kestenholz P, Lardinois D *et al.* (2006) Incidence and management of complications after neoadjuvant chemotherapy followed by extrapleural pneumonectomy for malignant pleural mesothelioma. Eur J Cardiothorac Surg 29(4): 579-84
18. O'Rourke N, Garcia JC, Paul J *et al.* (2007) A randomised controlled trial of intervention site radiotherapy in malignant pleural mesothelioma. Radiother Oncol 84(1): 18-22
19. Pass HI, Wali A, Tang N *et al.* (2008) Soluble mesothelin-related peptide level elevation in mesothelioma serum and pleural effusions. Ann Thorac Surg 85(1): 265-72
20. de Perrot M, Feld R, Cho BC *et al.* (2009) Trimodality therapy with induction chemotherapy followed by extrapleural pneumonectomy and adjuvant high-dose hemithoracic radiation for malignant pleural mesothelioma. J Clin Oncol 20;27(9): 1413-8
21. Ramalingam SS, Belani CP, Ruel C *et al.* (2009) Phase II study of belinostat (PXD101), a histone deacetylase inhibitor, for second line therapy of advanced malignant pleural mesothelioma. J Thorac Oncol 4(1): 97-101
22. Rea F, Marulli G, Bortolotti L *et al.* (2007) Induction chemotherapy, extrapleural pneumonectomy (EPP) and adjuvant hemi-thoracic radiation in malignant pleural mesothelioma (MPM): Feasibility and results. Lung Cancer 57(1): 89-95
23. Rice DC, Smythe WR, Liao Z *et al.* (2007) Dose-dependent pulmonary toxicity after postoperative intensity-modulated radiotherapy for malignant pleural mesothelioma. Int J Radiat Oncol Biol Phys 69(2): 350-7
24. Robinson BW, Lake RA (2005) Advances in malignant mesothelioma. N Engl J Med 353(15): 1591-603
25. Rusch VW (1995) A proposed new international TNM staging system for malignant mesothelioma. From the International Mesothelioma Interest Group. Chest 108: 1122-8
26. Scherpereel A, Grigoriu B, Conti M *et al.* (2006) Soluble mesothelin-related peptides in the diagnosis of malignant pleural mesothelioma. Am J Respir Crit Care Med 173(10): 1155-60
27. Scherpereel A, Astoul P, Baas P *et al.* (2009) Guidelines of the European Respiratory Society and the European Society of Thoracic Surgeons for management of Malignant Pleural Mesothelioma. Eur Respir J
28. Simon GR, Verschraegen CF, Jänne PA *et al.* (2008) Pemetrexed plus gemcitabine as first-line chemotherapy for patients with peritoneal mesothelioma: final report of a phase II trial. J Clin Oncol 26(21): 3567-72
29. **Stahel RA, Weder W, Felip E (2008) ESMO Guidelines Working Group. Malignant pleural mesothelioma: ESMO clinical recommendations for diagnosis, treatment and follow-up. Ann Oncol 19 Suppl 2: ii43-4**
30. Stewart DJ, Martin-Ucar A, Pilling JE *et al.* (2004) The effect of extent of local resection on patterns of disease progression in malignant pleural mesothelioma. Ann Thorac Surg 78(1): 245-52
31. **Sugarbaker DJ, Flores RM, Jaklitsch MT *et al.* (1999) Resection margins, extrapleural nodal status, and cell type determine postoperative long-term survival in trimodality therapy of malignant pleural mesothelioma: results in 183 patients. J Thorac Cardiovasc Surg 117(1): 54-63**

32. Sugarbaker DJ, Jaklitsch MT, Bueno R *et al*. (2004) Prevention, early detection, and management of complications after 328 consecutive extrapleural pneumonectomies. J Thorac Cardiovasc Surg 128(1): 138-46
33. Treasure T, Waller D, Tan C *et al*. (2009) The Mesothelioma and Radical Surgery Randomized Controlled Trial: The MARS Feasibility Study. J Thorac Oncol
34. Van Meerbeeck JP, Gaafar R, Manegold C *et al* (2005) European Organisation for Research and Treatment of Cancer Lung Cancer Group; National Cancer Institute of Canada. Randomized phase III study of cisplatin with or without raltitrexed in patients with malignant pleural mesothelioma: an intergroup study of the European Organisation for Research and Treatment of Cancer Lung Cancer Group and the National Cancer Institute of Canada. J Clin Oncol 23(28): 6881-9
35. Van Schil P, Baas R, Gaafar AP *et al*. (2009) EORTC Lung Cancer Group. Phase II feasibility trial of induction chemotherapy (ICT) followed by extrapleural pneumonectomy (EPP) and postoperative radiotherapy (PORT) for cT3N1M0 or less malignant pleural mesothelioma (MPM) (EORTC 08031). American Society of Clinical Oncology. Process. Abstract #7509
36. Vogelzang NJ, Rusthoven JJ, Symanowski J *et al*. (2003) Phase III study of pemetrexed in combination with cisplatin *versus* cisplatin alone in patients with malignant pleural mesothelioma. J Clin Oncol 121(14): 2636-44
37. Weder W, Kestenholz P, Taverna C *et al*. (2004) Neoadjuvant chemotherapy followed by extrapleural pneumonectomy in malignant pleural mesothelioma. J Clin Oncol 22(17): 3451-7
38. Weder W, Stahel RA, Bernhard J *et al*. (2007) Swiss Group for Clinical Cancer Research. Multicenter trial of neo-adjuvant chemotherapy followed by extrapleural pneumonectomy in malignant pleural mesothelioma. Ann Oncol 18(7): 1196-202

Bronchioloalveolar carcinoma and adenocarcinoma with bronchioloalveolar carcinoma features: a clinico-pathological spectrum

6

J. Cadranel, M. Antoine and M. Wislez

Five Essential Points

1. *The definition of BAC in the WHO pathological classification is highly restrictive and corresponds to the single nodular form, of small size, surgically resected. Pneumonic, multifocal and diffuse forms correspond, for the most part, to ADC-BAC.*
2. *BAC and ADC-BAC can be distinguished from other NSCLC by an increased frequency of onset in women, non-smokers and persons of Asian descent.*
3. *Evolution of BAC and ADC-BAC is slower and prognosis is better than for other NSCLC.*
4. *In localized forms of BAC, the treatment of choice is surgery.*
5. *In extended forms, some patients show a strong response to EGFR-TKI (non-mucinous) while others seems to react better to taxane-based chemotherapy (mucinous/mixed).*

Introduction

Over the last five years, bronchioloalveolar carcinoma (BAC) has been arousing growing interest for several reasons – first of all because its definition was modified in 1999 when the World Health Organization (WHO) updated the pathological classification of bronchial cancers (BC) [18], but also because of its epidemiological, biological, clinical, prognostic and treatment particularities which distinguish it from other non-small-cell lung carcinomas (NSCLC) [2, 10, 20]. The aim of the present chapter is to elucidate these different aspects by enlarging the concept of BAC to that of adenocarcinoma (ADC) with BAC features (ADC-BAC) and by focusing on recent developments in therapeutic management.

Definition of BAC and cytological types

In the WHO 1999 pathological classification, revised in 2004, BAC was strictly defined [18, 19]. It was considered a primitive pulmonary ADC which developed from the epithelial cells of the terminal respiratory unit, and which respected pulmonary architecture in its tumoral progression, thereby defining so-called "lepidic" progression. Thus, this diagnosis could only be confirmed on a surgical specimen which revealed its clear-cut histological BAC subtype (*i.e.* possessing no other subtype component, such as papillary or acinar) and the absence of histological signs of stromal, pleural or vascular invasion throughout the entire sample [2, 10, 18, 19, 20]. This strict definition was justified by the demonstration that pure BAC, smaller than 2 cm, could be cured by surgery alone [11].

According to the WHO 2004 classification, tumours for which the absence of histological invasion cannot be demonstrated must be referred to as ADC, and their histological subtype must be described (BAC, papillary, acinar, etc.) [19]. When several histological subtypes are associated, which is the most frequent situation, the tumours must then be referred to as mixed ADC and the various histological components must be detailed, starting with the predominant component (papillary-BAC, BAC-papillary) [19]. Although stage IIIB-IV tumours are excluded from BAC according to the strict WHO definition, the first international workshop devoted to this tumour, held in 2004, emphasized the pathological and clinical continuum existing between BAC, as defined by the WHO classification, and ADC-BAC [2, 10, 20].

At the cytological level, we distinguish three types of BAC: non-mucinous (the most common), mucinous and mixed (non-mucinous and mucinous) [19] (Fig. 1). It has become increasingly important to take this distinction into consideration, since the carcinogenic role of tobacco, tumour biology, radiological appearance, risk of relapse, sensitivity to molecules targeting the membrane receptor of the epidermal growth factor (EGFR) and also sensitivity to taxanes, may differ between non-mucinous and mucinous or mixed BAC [2].

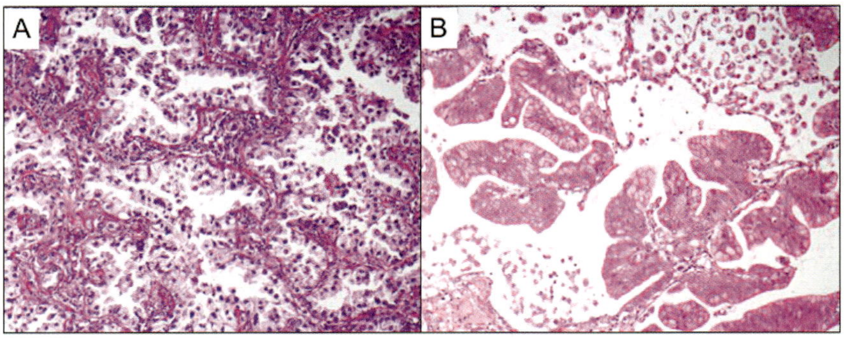

Fig. 1. Two main cytologic types of bronchioloalveolar carcinoma. Non mucinous (A) and mucinous (B) types.

Mucinous BAC, most frequently observed in non-smokers, would appear to arise from the mucinous metaplasia of bronchiolar cells [2, 10, 19, 20]. They show strong intra- and extracellular mucosecretion and generally do not express TTF1. Non-mucinous BAC include two, often intricately combined cell types, the most frequently found deriving from Clara cells, while the other is derived from type II pneumocytes [2, 19]. They do not show intracellular mucosecretion and most often express TTF1. They sometimes present strong mitotic activity and thickening of alveolar compartments due to fibrosis and T lymphocyte, plasmocyte and dendritic cell infiltration [2, 10, 19, 20]. Nevertheless, the presence of desmoplastic fibrosis (tumour-induced) is an exclusion factor according to the current WHO definition of BAC, and these tumours should henceforth be classified as ADC-BAC (*cf.* above).

Tumour biology

Specific aspects of BAC and ADC-BAC biology warrant close attention, since some of them are the cause of early evaluation of molecules targeting EGFR for first-line treatment of these tumours [2, 10].

Tumour progression is essentially lepidic, but also aerogenous, thereby explaining radiological images which may be diffuse, pneumonic or multifocal, as well as the fact that death is more frequently linked to bilateral pulmonary diffusion than to the occurrence of extrathoracic metastases. The presence of a neutrophilic alveolar inflammatory reaction in certain tumours may favour lepidic and aerogenous progression by facilitating desquamation of tumour cell motility [26, 27].

Such tumours are distinct from other types of ADC because of their higher EGFR protein overexpression and by the presence of EGFR gene amplification and or mutation [3, 4, 6]. The latter include deletions, insertions and substitutions located at exons 18-21 of the EGFR gene that confer upon it a functional advantage [7, 12]. Amplification and mutations in the EGFR gene are essentially described in non-mucinous BAC and are more frequent in ADC-BAC than in pure BAC [4]. Another member of the EGFR family, ErbB2, is also overexpressed in non-mucinous forms [4]. Finally, these tumours may also present a K-*ras* proto-oncogene mutation, more frequent in the mucinous cytologic types than in the non-mucinous types [2]. The type of mutation would seem to differ according to the geographic origin and tobacco exposure of the patients [2]. Nevertheless, we must emphasize that EGFR and K-*ras* mutations seem to be only very rarely associated [3, 6]. Thus, they would appear to indicate differing oncogeneses, as suggested, for example, by the rather specific association of each of these mutations to one of the two cytological types [2].

Epidemiology

BAC is a rare tumour, and represented only around 5% of the 11,969 consecutive NSCLC in a very recent American epidemiological series, if we judge them according to the WHO 1999 classification [30]. The apparent increase in its incidence, which has been suggested in recent years, remains subject to debate [2]. Nevertheless, around 30 to 50% of peripheral pulmonary ADC include a BAC component of a non-mucinous type, and the proportion of BAC is much higher in Asian epidemiological series and those of lung cancer screening by computed tomography scan (CT-scan) [7].

BAC and ADC-BAC are associated with specific epidemiological characteristics which distinguish them from other ADC subtypes, but which remain controversial [2], including an earlier age at onset and a higher prevalence of women. In contrast, the higher prevalence of non-smokers (30 to 50%) and of light smokers among patients with BAC was confirmed by case-control studies [2]. Such epidemiological characteristics are also more clear-cut for southeast Asian populations.

Clinical and radiological presentation

Single nodular form

This is the most frequent form and has been particularly well described in a surgical series of peripheral ADC [2]. In most cases, it is discovered by accident during routine x-ray. Physical examination is normal. Radiologically [17, 20, 21], it presents as a single peripheral round opacity which can measure up to 10 cm in diameter, in

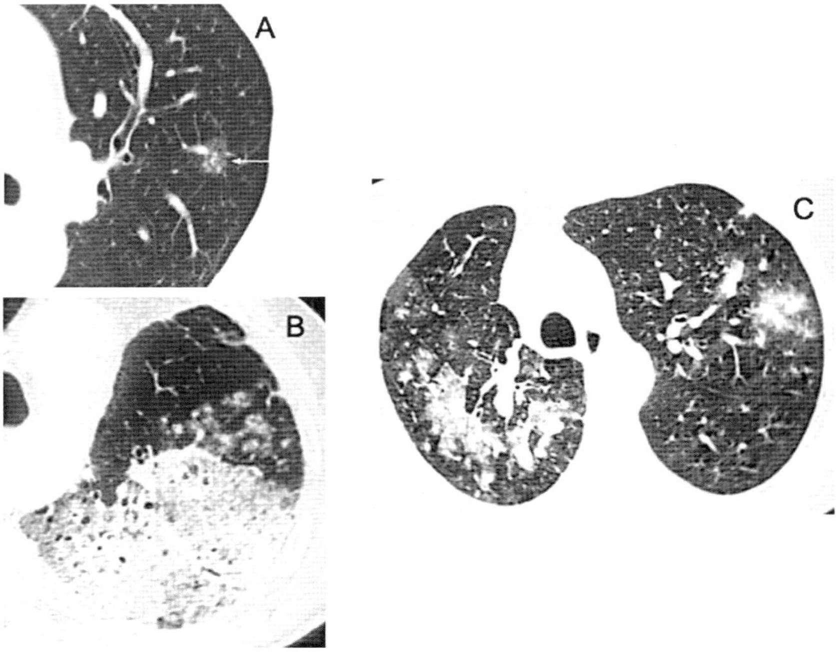

Fig. 2. Three main CT scan patterns of bronchioloalveolar carcinoma. Pure ground glass nodule (A), chronic alveolar condensation also called "pneumonic type BAC" (B) and multiple nodular and diffuse form (C).

general clearly delimited but with possibly spicular contours. The ground-glass or subsolid nodule in CT-scan is highly specific of a diagnosis of BAC. Such forms are often non-mucinous (Fig. 2).

Pneumonic, multiple nodular and diffuse forms

By definition, most of these tumours are not pure BAC, but rather ADC-BAC. They are usually symptomatic [2]. Symptoms are non-specific. However, we should point out the evocative nature, fairly rare, of bronchorrhea [2]. This is a mucous expectoration which may be very abundant (up to 500 ml/day) and is sometimes responsible for progressive respiratory insufficiency. Physical examination may reveal crepitant rales and on rare occasions clubbings (< 10%) [2]. Surprisingly, the performance status of such patients is usually good [2].

Radiological examination may reveal multiple nodules or chronic alveolar condensation (pneumonic BAC), frequently with an air bronchogram [2, 17, 21] (Fig. 2). Condensation may be either single or multiple, associated with one or several ground glass nodules. In these forms, which are generally mucinous, the air bronchogram may have a cystic appearance related to copious intra-alveolar production of mucin, and may be associated with an angiogram sign indicating that vascularization has been preserved.

Diagnostic approach

In isolated nodules, only complete analysis of the surgical specimen can confirm the diagnosis of BAC or ADC-BAC according to WHO criteria [2, 20]. Diagnosis of inoperable ADC-BAC is based on a compatible clinical and radiological appearance (peripheral lung radiological ground glass or subsolid lesion), the absence of endobronchial lesions, and type ADC-BAC histology on a lung biopsy sample obtained by surgery and videothoracoscopy or CT-scan-guided transthoracic or per-endoscopic transbronchial pulmonary biopsy [2, 20]. Cytological diagnosis (examination of sputum, fibroaspiration, bronchioloalveolar lavage, cytological puncture guided by TDM) can be considered adequate in case of relapse of an earlier operated tumour or if the radiological presentation shows diffuse opacities or a single or multiple alveolar condensation(s) (pneumonic ADC) [2, 20]. Indeed, centralized re-reading of surgical samples of patients presenting with a pneumonic ADC, included in the French multicentric prospective IFCT-0401 trial, confirmed that they were BAC according to the WHO classification or ADC-BAC in 73% of cases; in the other cases, they were ADC, most often having a papillary component with aerogenous tumour progression [28]; similar results had previously been reported by our group on a retrospective series of 52 pneumonic ADC [25].

Pre-therapeutic staging approach

Tumour progression is essentially of an intrapulmonary nature, uni- and then bilateral [2, 20]. We must also emphasize the low frequency of pleural loco-regional and mediastinal lymph node extension, the predominance of bone metastatic localizations rather than cerebral, and the rarity of hepatic and adrenal gland metastases [2].

Thus, the pre-therapeutic staging approach recommended for BAC and ADC-BAC should not differ from that for other NSCLC [2]. Nevertheless, we underline the importance of carrying out a high-resolution lung CT-scan to detect the presence of ground glass densities distant from the primary lesion which could modify initial staging, thus affecting the prognosis and treatment [2].

The sensitivity and possible prognostic value of fluorodeoxygluose positron emission tomography (PET) are currently being evaluated [2]. In any case, it should be kept in mind that BAC are frequently responsible for false-negatives on PET scan [2].

Survival and prognostic factors

In the epidemiological series of Zell *et al.*, which included 11,969 consecutive NSCLC, the presence of BAC was an independent criterion for better survival (HR = 1.71) [30]. Moreover, average survival for all categories of BAC and ADC-BAC taken together was over 53 months compared to 10 months for other NSCLC. Finally, it remained significantly higher for the different TNM stages (I-IIIA: 98 *vs* 4 months; IIIB: 47 *vs* 16 months; and IV: 10 *vs* 5 months, $p < 0.0001$).

Independent of the TNM stage, certain characteristics of BAC and ADC-BAC which are easy to collate for some of them at the time of diagnosis, constitute prognostic factors for survival. Female sex and the absence of smoking seem to play a favourable role [2, 30]. Tumours with a multiple nodular-type presentation have a better prognosis than those with a single or multifocal diffuse pneumonic presentation (Tx) [2, 20]. The presence of bronchorrhea or crepitant rales is a sign of an unfavorable prognosis [2, 25]. Within the IIIB stages, we should distinguish tumours classed as T4 due to multiple lesions within the same lobe, which have a better prognosis than tumours having pleural or N3 lymph node involvement. Likewise, tumours classified as M1 because of pulmonary involvement affecting more than one lobe, have a better prognosis than those classified as M1 because of an extrathoracic metastasis [30]. Elsewhere, patients having involvement of several lobes within the same lung (unilateral involvement) have a better prognosis than patients with both lungs affected (bilateral involvement) [30].

Certain cytological and pathological characteristics would also appear to have prognostic value, but their systematic collectior at the time of diagnosis is more difficult to obtain and their analysis necessitates confirmation by centralized re-reading of histological specimens. The presence of tumour cells in samples of respiratory secretions, as well as evaluation, in biopsy samples, of the intensity of aerogenous progression and an inflammatory reaction associated with the tumour, appear to constitute a poor prognosis [8,25,29]. The non-mucinous cytological type, associated with strong expression of TTF1 by tumour cells, has a better prognosis than mucinous and mixed cytological types [2, 14, 17].

Finally, the prognostic value of some biological tumour markers was studied in short retrospective series [2]. Their validity warrants confirmation in prospective series that include a sufficient number of cases, and confrontation with classical prognostic factors. Finally, their feasibility must also be evaluated before such markers can be introduced as prognostic factors in the framework of prospective therapeutic trials [2].

Therapeutic management

When possible, the treatment of choice for BAC and ADC-BAC is surgery [2, 20, 10]. Indeed, only lobectomy would seem to be carcinogenically effective, but intrapulmonary relapses are possible, though often delayed [2]. Atypical resections carry the risk of early relapse within the same lobe, and pneumonectomy may lead to a contralateral relapse [2].

Therapeutic management of extended BAC and ADC-BAC basically consists of chemotherapy and therapies targeting the EGFR [2, 10, 23]. Radiotherapy is used only rarely in treatment of ADC-BAC. Indeed, ADC-BAC at stage III are rarely associated with lymph node involvement (< 25% of cases) [2], and stage IV ADC-BAC for pulmonary lesions are generally impossible to irradiate because of the bilaterality of the lesions (around 75% of cases) [2, 30]. In contrast, the role of surgery has been re-evaluated, especially in nodular, multilobar and bilateral forms, because of its favourable impact upon prognosis [2, 30].

The frequent observation of EGFR protein overexpression and amplification and/or mutation of its gene, as well as the observation of several cases of a major response to EGFR tyrosine kinase inhibitors (EGFR-TKI), have led to several therapeutic clinical trials using these molecules (gefitinib and erlotinib) [1, 4, 5, 9, 13, 15, 24]; likewise, chemotherapy, after having been abandoned, has also been the object of two phase II therapeutic trials using paclitaxel [16, 22]. Results obtained with EGFR-TKI in treatment of ADC-BAC were not nearly as satisfactory as expected, and paclitaxel in monotherapy seems to give similar results in terms of the objective response rate (10-25% *vs* 9-14%), stabilized disease rate (17-31% *vs* 40-50%), time to progression (2.9-4 months *vs* 2.2-5 months) and 1-year survival (50-71% *vs* 35-50%). Nevertheless, there clearly appears to exist heterogeneity in the tumoral response to EGFR-TKI and to paclitaxel in patients with ADC-BAC. Thus, certain patients show a strong response to EGFR-TKI or else are stable over a long period, while others seems to react better to chemotherapy. Unfortunately, the role of epidemiological (tobacco, gender), pathological (cytological type, expression of TTF1) and biological factors (K-*ras* mutation, overexpression, amplification or mutation of EGFR [3, 4, 6, 28] which might enable predicting therapeutic responses, remains to be elucidated. Thus, at present, neither EGFR-TKI nor paclitaxel can be considered as the reference treatment for ADC-BAC, and there is no simple criterion for choosing the better of these two treatments in a given patient.

Conclusion

The definition of BAC in the WHO pathological classification is highly restrictive and corresponds to the single nodular form, of small size, surgically resected. Pneumonic, multifocal and diffuse forms correspond, for the most part, to ADC-BAC. BAC and ADC-BAC can be distinguished from other NSCLC by an increased frequency of onset in women, non-smokers and persons of Asian descent. The basically lepidic and aerogenous tumour progression explains the often pneumonic, multifocal or diffuse presentation and the fact that death is most often associated with bilateral pulmonary diffusion rather than the onset of extra-thoracic metastases. Evolution is slower and prognosis is better than for other ADC. In localized forms, the treatment of choice is surgery. Treatment of extended forms raises specific problems: the possibility of having recourse to surgery under certain conditions; the chemosensitivity of certain tumours; and also, in certain cases, the sometimes very high sensitivity to EGFR-TKI. These novel therapeutic strategies based on our improved knowledge of the natural history of BAC should lead to the elaboration of specific therapeutic trials.

References

1. Cadranel J, Quoix E, Baudrin L *et al.* (2009) IFCT-0401 Trial Group. IFCT-0401 Trial: a phase II study of gefitinib administered as first-line treatment in advanced adenocarcinoma with bronchioloalveolar carcinoma subtype. J Thorac Oncol 4(9): 1126-35. PubMed PMID: 19574932
2. Garfield D, Cadranel J, Wislez M *et al.* (2006) The bronchioloalveolar carcinoma and peripheral adenocarcinoma spectrum of diseases. J Thoracic Oncol 1: 340-59
3. Gumerlock PH, Holland WS, Chen H *et al.* (2005) Mutational analysis of K-RAS and EGFR implicates K-ras as a resistance marker in the Southwest Oncology Group (SWOG) trial S1026 of bronchioloalveolar carcinoma (BAC) patients (pts) treated with gefitinib. J Clin Oncol 23: 7008S – abstr
4. Hirsch FR, Varella-Garcia M, McCoy J *et al.* for Southwest Oncology Group (2005) Increased epidermal growth factor gene copy number detected by FISH associates with increased sensitivity to gefitinib in patients with bronchioloalveolar carcinoma subtypes. J Clin Oncol 23: 6838-45
5. Kris MG, Sandler A, Miller V *et al.* (2004) Cigarette smoking predicts sensitivity to erlotinib: Results of a phase II trial in patients with bronchioloalveolar carcinoma (BAC). J Clin Oncol 22: 631S – abst
6. Kris MG, Sandler A, Miller V *et al.* (2005) EGFR and KRAS mutations in patients with bronchioloalveolar carcinoma treated with erlotinib in a phase II multicenter trial. J Clin Oncol 23: 7029S – abstr
7. Lynch TJ, Bell DW, Sordella R *et al.* (2004) Activating mutations in the epidermal growth factor receptor underlying responsiveness of non-small-cell lung cancers to gefitinib. N Eng J Med 350: 2129-39
8. Makimoto Y, Nabeshima K, Iwasaki H *et al.* (2005) Micropapillary pattern: a distinct pathological marker to subclassify tumours with a significantly poor prognosis within small peripheral lung adenocarcinoma (</= 20 mm) with mixed bronchioloalveolar and invasive subtypes (Noguchi's type C tumours). Histopathology 46: 677-84

9. **Miller VA, Kris MG, Shah N *et al.* (2004) Bronchioloalveolar pathologic subtype and smoking history predict sensitivity to gefitinib in advanced non-small-cell lung cancer. J Clin Oncol 22: 1103-9**
10. Miller VA, Hirsch FR, Johnson DH (2005) Systemic therapy of advanced bronchioloalveolar carcinoma: challenges and opportunities. J Clin Oncol 23:3288-93
11. Noguchi M, Morikawa A, Kawasaki M *et al.* (1995) Small adenocarcinoma of the lung: histologic characteristics and prognosis. Cancer 75: 2844-52
12. Pao W, Miller V, Zakowski M *et al.* (2004) EGF receptor gene mutations are common in lung cancers from "never smokers", and are associated with sensitivity of tumors to gefitinib and erlotinib. Proc Natl Acad Sci 101: 13306-11
13. Patel J, Miller VA, Kris MG *et al.* (2003) Encouraging activity and durable responses demonstrated by the EGFR-tyrosine kinase inhibitors, Erlotinib (Tarceva®), in patients with advanced bronchioloalveolar cell (BAC) carcinoma. Lung Cancer 41: S46 – abstr
14. Saad RS, Liu YL, Han H *et al.* (2004) Prognostic significance of thyroid transcription factor-1 expression in both early-stage conventional adenocarcinoma and bronchioloalveolar carcinoma of the lung. Hum Pathol 35: 3-7
15. Sandler A, Kris M, Miller V *et al.* (2005) Phase II trial of erlotinib in patients with bronchioloalveolar carcinoma. Lung Cancer 49: S38 – abstr
16. Scagliotti GV, Smit E, Bosquee L *et al.* European Organisation for Research and Treatment of Cancer (EORTC) Lung Cancer Group (LCG): A phase II study of paclitaxel in advanced bronchioloalveolar carcinoma (EORTC trial 08956). Lung Cancer 50: 91-6
17. Shah RM, Balsara G, Webster M *et al.* (2000) Bronchioloalveolar cell carcinoma. J Thorac Imaging 15: 180-6
18. Travis WD, Colby TV, Corrin B *et al.* (1999) Histological typing of lung and pleural tumors. 3rd ed. Berlin, Springer
19. **Travis WD, Brambilla E, Muller-Hermelink HK *et al.* (2004) Pathology and Genetics of Tumors of the Lung, Pleura, Thymus, and Heart. World Health Organization Classification of Tumours. Lyon IARC Press.**
20. Travis WD, Garg K, Franklin WA *et al.* (2005) Evolving concepts in the pathology and computed tomography imaging of lung adenocarcinoma and bronchioloalveolar carcinoma. J Clin Oncol 23: 3279-87
21. Trigaux JP, Gevenois PA, Goncette L *et al.* (1996) Bronchioloalveolar carcinoma computed tomography findings. Eur Respir J 9: 11-6
22. **West HL, Crowley JJ, Vance RB *et al.* Southwest Oncology Group (2005) Advanced bronchioloalveolar carcinoma: A phase II trial of paclitaxel by 96-hour infusion (SWOG 9714): A Southwest Oncology Group Study. Ann Oncol 16: 1076-80**
23. West H (2006) Emerging approaches to advanced bronchioloalveolar carcinoma. Curr Treat Options Pharmacol 7: 769-76
24. **West H, Franklin WA, McCoy J *et al.* (2006) Gefitinib therapy for advanced bronchioloalveolar carcinoma: Southwest Oncology Group Study S0126. J Clin Oncol 24: 1807-13**
25. Wislez M, Massiani MA, Milleron B *et al.* (2003) Clinical characteristics of pneumonic-type adenocarcinoma of the lung. Chest 123: 1868-77
26. Wislez M, Rabbe N, Marchal J *et al.* (2003) Hepatocyte growth factor production by neutrophils infiltrating bronchioloalveolar subtype pulmonary adenocarcinoma: role in tumor progression and death. Cancer Res 63: 1405-12
27. Wislez M, Antoine M, Rabbe N *et al.* (2007) Neutrophils promote aerogeneous spread of lung adenocarcinoma with bronchioloalveolar features Clin Cancer Res 13: 3518-27
28. Wislez M, Antoine M, Baudrin L *et al.* (2009) Non-mucinous and mucinous subtypes of adenocarcinoma with bronchioloalveolar carcinoma features differ by biomarker expression and in the response to gefitinib. Lung Cancer. 2009 Jul 4. [Epub ahead of print] PubMed PMID: 19581016
29. Yokose T, Suzuki K, Nagai K *et al.* (2000) Favorable and unfavorable morphological prognostic factors in peripheral adenocarcinoma of the lung 3 cm or less in diameter. Lung Cancer 29: 179-88
30. **Zell JA, Ou S-H I, Ziogas A *et al.* (2005) Epidemiology of bronchioloalveolar carcinoma: improvement in survival after release of the 1999 WHO classification of lung tumors. J Clin Oncol 23: 8396-405**

Primary adenoid cystic carcinoma of the trachea and bronchus

7

M. Roelandts and P. Van Houtte

Five Essential Points

1. *ACC is a slow growing tumour with a long delay before diagnosis.*
2. *Airway control is often an emergency, requiring endobronchial treatment.*
3. *Surgery remains the cornerstone of the curative treatment for well-selected patients operated by very skilful and specialized teams.*
4. *Radio-chemotherapy with high radiation dose is a good alternative for inoperable patients.*
5. *A long follow-up is necessary due to late relapse (after 5 years).*

Introduction

Adenoid cystic carcinoma (ACC) was known in the past as cylindroma and is a variant of adenocarcinoma with specific histopathologic and clinical features. The most common localisation is within the salivary glands but ACC has been reported in many other sites including skin, cervix and trachea.

Incidence

Tracheal cancers are rare: they represent less than 0.2% of all respiratory tract cancers and 0.02 to 0.04% of all cancers in the United States. Adenoid cystic carcinoma (ACC) represents only a few percent of all tracheal cancers: this entity is very uncommon (Table 1) [14, 18, 21, 24, 27, 31, 38].

Table 1 – Percentage of ACC amongst tracheal tumours.

Author	Year	Duration	Number of cases	ACC (%)s
Licht [24]	2001	17	109	7
Yang [38]	1997	15	67	8
Manninen [27]	1993	18	95	6
Gelder [14]	1993	20	321	11
Kurien [21]	1981	27	97	3
Mornex [31]	1998	30	106	2
Honings [18]	2006	13	308	8
Bhattacharyya [3]	2004	12	99	20.7

Median age at diagnosis is in the fifties with a range from 20 to 90 years. There is no sex prevalence but in some series a few more women. ACC are not associated with cigarette smoking and have a propensity to spread along both submucosal and perineural planes.

Anatomy and pathology

The adult trachea is around 12 cm in length and 1.5 to 2 cm wide. It connects the larynx to the carina: the distal two-thirds is located within the thorax. It is composed of c-shaped cartilage rings with a posterior membrane and fibrous tissue. ACC tumours arise from the small salivary glands located within the submucosa of the tracheal wall and rarely in the bronchus. They progress usually slowly through the submucosa and along the nerve sheets. They tend to stay localized for a long time.

The pathological presentation is as cylindrical structures lined by small cuboidal cells with deeply eosinophilic cores of basement-membrane-like material. Mucinous material may be seen as a cribriform pattern. Cytological features of malignancy are not often seen but the malignant behaviour is manifest by its insidious growth pattern [13].

Clinical presentation

The most common symptom is wheezing or stridor. Haemoptysis is seen in less than 25% of patients explaining the long delay before a definitive diagnosis. This delay may reach 24 months as observed by Gaissert [13]. Extra-thoracic metastases are rare and often diagnosed late in the course of the disease. The most common site is the lung but they may occur in the liver, brain, bone, and kidneys.

Staging procedure

ACC is usually diagnosed by a fiberbronchoscopy allowing the possibility of pathological confirmation. Differential diagnosis may include a muco-epidermoid cancer or a carcinoid especially in case of a small biopsy. The workup should include a chest CT scan or more rarely a NMR. Nowadays, an endobronchial echography is helpful to determine the extension through the bronchial wall. Due to the presentation with a marked obstruction of the lumen, a laser photoresection via rigid bronchoscope is often required before completing the workup to search for distant metastases. A PET scan may be useful in selected cases but in our own experience, there was no FDG uptake by the tumour in our two last cases [4].

TNM classification

There is no specific UICC classification for tracheal tumours. According to the lung classification, a tumour invading the trachea should be a T4. Different authors have proposed their own staging system. They are based for the T on the length of the tumour, its localisation within the trachea and its extension within the wall. Macchiarini *et al.* proposed the following classification: a T1 tumour is limited to the mucosa and is either a T1a if less than 3 cm and a T1b if more than 3 cm; a T2 tumour extends through the tracheal wall, a T3 tumour invades the larynx, a T4 tumour invades the carina, main bronchus or neighbouring structures [25]. The Licht classification is slightly different: a T1 tumour is less than 3 cm not growing through the tracheal wall; a T2 tumour is less than 3 cm growing through the tracheal wall; a T3 tumour is more than 3 cm, including larynx or growing onto the mediastinum but not fixed to nearby organs; a T4 tumour is more than 3 cm involving the carina and/or main bronchus or fixed to nearby organs [24]. For Bhattacharyya, the cut-off is 2 cm [3].

Treatment

Airway management

An important issue is certainly the ability to control the airway; ACC may present as a true emergency due to an obstructive lesion of the trachea. Intubation may not even be possible. The initial evaluation should be done with a rigid bronchoscope. Endobronchial removal of a tumour may be done mechanically or by laser and may require the insertion of a prosthesis (Figure 1). This is only a temporary measure for an emergency situation [33]. In the series of Albers, a marked obstruction of the tracheal lumen was seen in 7 out of 14 patients, ranging from 60 to 98%; 12 of the 14 patients had a laser photoresection and 4 had subsequently a stent to maintain airway patency [1].

Surgery

Surgery remains the cornerstone of the curative treatment of ACC. It requires experienced surgeons and very specialized teams. The possibility to perform a complete resection is determined by tumour extent especially the length of the ACC but also by patient-related factors: old age, short neck, and thoracic kyphosis. ACC would seem to be more often operable than other histological types: in the nationwide study of the Netherlands, 50% of patients with ACC were operated compared to only 8% of those with other histological types [18]. In the MGH experience, the resection rate reached 75% for ACC [12].

During surgery, there are two important principles in the achievement of a successful resection: no tension on the two anastomoses and the preservation of blood supply. The latter is particularly important to avoid necrosis. This may lead to some compromise between leaving paratracheal tissues, perhaps containing some positive lymph node, and avoiding a devascularization. Furthermore, the classic concept of complete resection is difficult due to the immediate vicinity of very vital structures located in the mediastinum (oesophagus, great vessels, superior vena cava) and the limited length of the airway. In case of transmural growth, there will be a problem of radial margins due to the vicinity of the oesophagus and great vessels. In the longitudinal axis of the airway, there may be also a problem of free margin: if the resected segment of trachea is too long, there is a problem of tension on the anastomosis and a risk of dehiscence.

The choice of surgical approach depends on tumour location, anatomical variations in neck and chest and on previous surgery. The most common operation is a sleeve resection of the trachea with end-to-end anastomosis; carinal resection is a more complicated procedure due to the two anastomoses and is used for lower tracheal tumours. Grillo and Mathisen have described the different techniques [15, 28]. Usually upper tracheal tumours are explored through a cervical collar incision.

For mid-tracheal tumours, the incision may extend through a full median sternotomy. Lower tracheal tumours are more often approached through a right thoracotomy. Frozen sections are important to obtain clear margin as ACC may extend far away from the bulk of the disease. Systematic lymph node dissection is not routinely performed in order to preserve blood supply. In ACC, lymph node metastases are rare: in the Regnard series, 6 out of 65 patients and in the Gaissert series, 13 patients out of 101 had positive lymph nodes; in 45 resected patients no lymph nodes were found in the surgical specimen [12, 32]. In contrast, Molina *et al.* reported a rate of positive lymph nodes reaching 31% [30]. In the large series of Gaissert *et al.* including 101 patients with an ACC, 9 patients had a laryngotracheal resection, 51 a tracheal resection and 41 carinal resection including a pulmonary resection in 18 patients; the mean tumour length in was 3.2 cm ranging from 2.9 to 3.5 cm [12]. In the Regnard experience, the length of resection was 3.8 cm [32]. Operative mortality is between 5 and 10% in various series and decreases with surgical experience. It is lower for resection with end-to-end anastomosis and is higher (10% or more) in case of carinal reconstruction.

One of the main problems with ACC is its infiltrative growth. In the MGH experience, 59% of the patients had positive surgical margins [12]. In the Toronto experience, 16 out of 32 resected patients had residual tumour [29]. The question for the surgeon is to extend the resection with the risk of anastomotic tension or to leave an incomplete resection, most often containing microscopic disease. Several authors have showed that an R1 resection had no adverse effect on long term survival nor on wound healing [12, 15, 29, 32].

Postoperative radiotherapy is advocated either systematically [9, 15] or in case of positive margins [30, 32, 36]. ACC is considered to be a radiosensitive and slow growing tumour. RT should be given 2 months after surgery and after a repeated fiberbronchoscopy to assess the anastomosis. The doses vary between 45 and 65 Gy. Preoperative radiotherapy is usually not advocated mainly to avoid a deleterious effect on the anastomotic healing.

The overall survival after surgery with or without additional postoperative radiotherapy varies between 52 and 91 % at 5 years and between 29 and 76 % at 10 years (Table 2) [9, 12, 20, 30, 29, 32]. The two largest series including 101 and 65 patients achieved 5-year survival rates of 52 and 73% [12, 32]. In those series, most patients received a course of postoperative radiotherapy and were recruited over a long time period.

Table 2 – Selected surgical series.

	Maziak [29]	Regnard [32]	Kanematsu [20]	Clough [9]	Molina [30]	Gaissert [12]
Study period	1963-95	1970-93	1972-98	1984-2003	1972-2002	1962-2002
Number	32	65	11	13	24	101
Surg+RT	78%	43%	83%	100%	54%	70%
Survival						
5 Y	79%	73%	91%	52%	57%	52%
10 Y	51%	57%	76%		45%	29%

Radiotherapy for unresectable disease

There are two goals: to restore a patent airway and to try to control the disease locally. Different methods are used to destroy the tumour locally and to restore the airway before radiotherapy: argon laser, cryosurgery, brachytherapy, argon beam coagulation; mechanical removal through the rigid bronchoscope [37].

In case a tumour cannot be resected, radiotherapy is usually proposed to a dose of 60 Gy or more, either after an endobronchial treatment or with an additional boost by brachytherapy [23]. Nevertheless, the data are scarce and most series are very heterogeneous including not only ACC but all types of tracheal tumours. Most reports were case reports or included only a few patients treated exclusively by radiotherapy, sometimes with concurrent chemotherapy. Usually, ACC appears to be a radiosensitive tumour with long term survival but with a high rate of local relapse even occurring after many years. In the large surgical series of Maziak *et al.*, six patients were judged to have unresectable disease [29]. Radiation doses ranged between 50 and 75 Gy. The mean survival was 74 months (range 1 to 172 months) but 5 out of the 6 patients had a local relapse. Subsequently, two patients were operated 7 and 8 years after the initial radiation. Similarly, Cheung reported two cases: one patient died from distant metastases without a local relapse and another had a local recurrence 8 years after the treatment [7]. Manninen reported 2 cases: one patient had a local relapse 98 months after a complete response [27]. Kanematsu reported 5 cases treated with radiation doses between 50 and 70 Gy. The 5-year survival rate reached 40% but all 5 patients developed a local recurrence [20]. Albers reported 14 cases of ACC treated by radiation after laser treatment: 8 patients developed a local relapse, 7 patients lived for 5 years [1].

The place of neutron therapy for tracheal ACC is unknown. Nevertheless, it was used with some success mainly for salivary gland tumours: in a series of 151 patients, the 5 year survival rate without local progressive disease reached 57% and the overall survival 72% [10].

Many reports dealing with radiotherapy for tracheal tumours have outlined better results, local response or survival, with higher radiation doses but in most series the number of patients with an ACC was too small to allow a multivariate analysis for this histology [6, 8, 11, 26, 31]. Concurrent chemoradiotherapy is now an appealing approach for many tumours including head and neck and lung cancers. Several case reports of ACC have showed good response using a platinum-based chemotherapy, given concurrently with radiation as observed in our case (Fig. 1) [2, 35]. By analogy, interesting results have been observed for head and neck localisations using carboplatin and paclitaxel: 5 patients with an unresectable lesion were controlled locally [16].

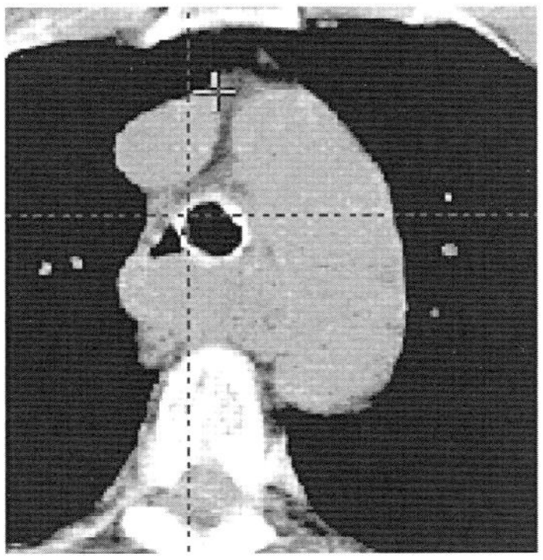

Fig. 1. This woman presented with severe dyspnoea. An endobronchial prosthesis was inserted before radiotherapy. The tumour extended posteriorly through the bronchial wall with an oesophageal compression. 66 Gy was delivered with weekly cisplatin and the prosthesis could be removed at the end of the radiation. She is in complete remission 2 years later.

High-dose rate brachytherapy is interesting either for palliation but also as a boost after external radiotherapy. Carvalho reported 3 cases treated with endobronchial brachytherapy for a local relapse after external radiation treatment: in the only case of ACC, the local relapse occurred after 9 years [5]. A complete response was observed after 3 fractions of 7.5 Gy prescribed at one cm; the patient was alive at 5 years with a tracheal stenosis. One main concern with this technique is our ability to obtain a good position of the catheter within the lumen, ideally centrally located to avoid delivering too high a dose to the mucosa. This explains the complications reported by different authors. Schraube reported two cases of necrotizing tracheitis after 3 to 4 fractions of 5 Gy each following an external beam dose of 46 to 50 Gy [34]. Harms reported 7 cases including 2 ACC treated by 50 Gy external radiation followed by a boost with HDR brachytherapy: 3 to 5 fractions of 5 Gy were delivered [17]. For the two cases of ACC, a complete and a partial response were observed but one patient developed a tracheal stenosis and a chondronecrosis. A special tracheal applicator is available: the outer cover can be expanded to move the radiation source away from the tracheal mucosa [31].

Case report

A 64-year-old man developed dyspnoea. The work-up showed a tumour obstructing 80% of the trachea. The tumour was 6 cm in length and started just above the carina (Fig. 2). The FDG-PET was negative. An endoscopic resection was performed for palliation followed by a course of external irradiation delivering 66 Gy. Two weeks later, a fiberbronchoscopy showed a good response with a small nodule remaining at the junction of the trachea and the main bronchus. A boost with HDR brachytherapy delivered an additional 8 Gy. The patient is still in complete remission 3 years later.

To conclude, complete response and long term survival can be achieved with radiotherapy for inoperable tracheal ACC. Radiation should deliver doses in the range of 60 to 70 Gy with a careful and precise technique to avoid excessive toxicity to surrounding tissue (the lungs and spinal cord). If a boost by HDR brachytherapy is planned, then the dose of external radiation needs to be adapted. Due to the possible extension into the submucosa, Kaminski *et al.* recommended margins of 4 to 5 cm above and below the gross disease [19] (Fig. 3). Combining radiation with chemotherapy is an interesting approach using a platinum-based schedule.

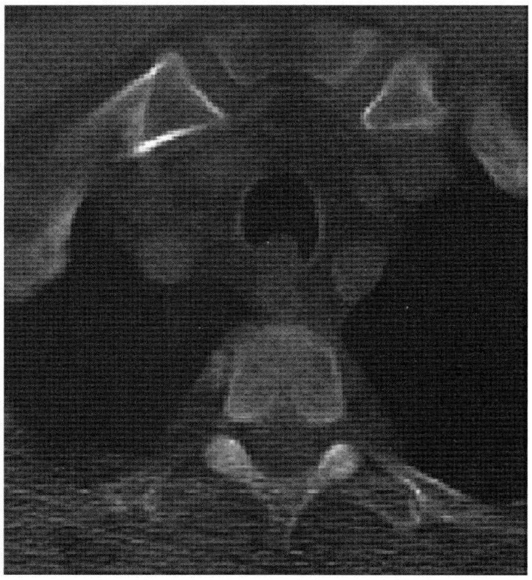

Fig. 2. This CT was performed after a laser resection. Notice the tumour extent through the bronchial wall.

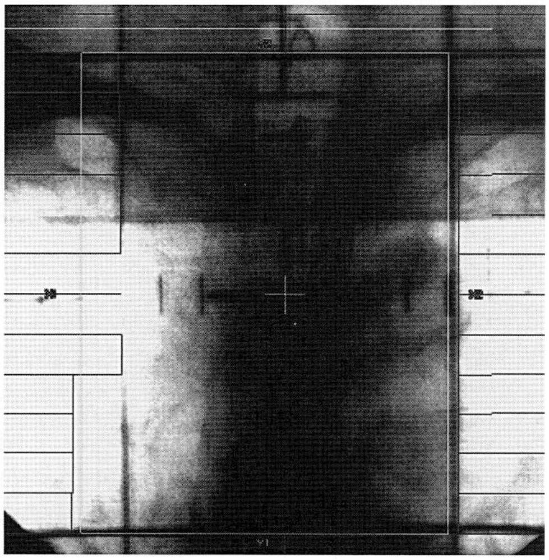

Fig. 3. Anterior radiation field for a tumour extending from the carina to the sternal notch.

Chemotherapy

Chemotherapy experience is mainly from the treatment of salivary gland tumours where it is reserved for the palliative management of advanced disease: objective responses are infrequent but stabilization of disease is observed [22]. Cisplatin-anthracycline combinations have showed some activity: the rate of objective response was 28%. The new targeted therapies may be of interest. Amongst the different molecular targets, the overexpression of EGFR is quite variable amongst ACC. A phase II trial of gefinitib did not report any objective response, only a stabilization of the disease.

Conclusions

ACC is a rare tumour of the trachea. Surgery is the primary treatment and should be performed by experienced thoracic surgeons. Postoperative radiotherapy is recommended especially in case of positive margins. For unresectable disease, radiotherapy should aim to deliver a dose in excess of 60 Gy with a careful technique and a boost by HDR brachytherapy may be considered. This is a slow growing tumour and late relapses are seen, requiring a long follow-up.

References

1. Albers E, Lawry T, Harrell J. *et al.* (2004) Tracheobronchial adenoid cystic carcinoma. A clinicopathologic study of 14 cases. Chest 125: 1160-65
2. **Allen AM, Rabin MS, Reilly JJ *et al.* (2007) Unresectable adenoid cystic carcinoma of the trachea treated with chemoradiation. J Clin Oncol 25: 5521-3**
3. Bhattacharyya N (2004) Contemporary staging and prognosis for primary tracheal malignancies: a population-based analysis. Otolaryngol Head Neck Surg 131: 639-42
4. Campistron M, Rouquette I, Courbon F *et al.* (2007) Adenoid cystic carcinoma of the lung : interest of 18 FDG PET/CT in the management of an atypical presentation. Lung Cancer 59: 133-6
5. Carvalho H, Figueiredo V, Pedreira WL *et al.* (2005) High dose-rate brachytherapy as a treatment option in primary tracheal tumors. Clinics 60: 299-304
6. Chao MW, Smith JG Laidlaw C *et al.* (1998) Results of treating primary tumors of the trachea with radiotherapy. Int J Radiat Oncol Biol Phys 41: 779-85
7. Cheung AY (1989) Radiotherapy for primary carcinoma of the trachea. Radiother Oncol 14: 279-85
8. Chow DC, Komaki R, Libshitz HI *et al.* (1993) Treatment of primary neoplasms of the trachea. The role of radiation therapy. Cancer 71: 2946-52
9. Clough A, Clarke P (2006) Adenoid cystic carcinoma of the trachea: a long-term problem. ANZ J Surg 76: 751-3
10. Douglas JG, Laramore GE, Austin-Seymour M *et al.* (2000) Treatment of locally advanced adenoid cystic carcinoma of the head and neck with neutron radiotherapy. Int J Radiat Oncol Biol Phys 46: 551-7
11. Fields J, Rigaud G, Emami B (1989) Primary tumors of the trachea. Results of radiation therapy. Cancer 63: 2429-33
12. **Gaissert HA, Grillo HC, Shadmehr MB *et al.* (2004) Long-term survival after resection of primary adenoid cystic and squamous cell carcinoma of the trachea and carina. Ann Thorac Surg 78: 1889-97**
13. Gaissert HA, Mark EJ (2006) Tracheobronchial gland tumors. Cancer Control 13: 286-94
14. Gelder CM, Hetzel MR (1993) Primary tracheal tumours: a national survey. Thorax 48: 688-92

7

15. Grillo HC, Mathisen DJ, Wain JC (1992) Management of tumors of the trachea. Oncology 6: 61-8
16. Haddad RI, Posner MR, Busse PM *et al.* (2006) Chemoradiotherapy for adenoid cystic carcinoma: preliminary results of an organ sparing approach. Am J Clin Oncol 29: 153-7
17. Harms W, Latz D, Becker H *et al.* (1999) HDR-brachytherapy boost for residual tumour after external beam radiotherapy in patients with tracheal malignancies. Radiother Oncol 52: 251-5
18. **Honings J, van Dijck J, Verhagen A *et al.* (2007) Incidence and treatment of tracheal cancer: a nationwide study in the Netherlands. Ann Surg Oncol 14: 968-76**
19. Kaminski JM, Langer CJ, Movsas B (2003) The role of radiation therapy and chemotherapy in the management of airway tumors other than small-cell carcinoma and non-small-cell carcinoma. Chest Surg Clin N Am 13: 149-67
20. Kanematsu T, Yohena T, Uehara T *et al.* (2002) Treatment outcome of resected and nonresected primary adenoide cystic carcinoma of the lung. Ann Thorac Cardiovasc Surg 8: 74-7
21. Kurien G, Cole I (1981) Primary carcinoma of the trachea. Clin Otolaryngol 6: 197-204
22. Laurie SA, Licitra L (2006) Systemic therapy in the palliative management of advanced salivary gland cancers. J Clin Oncol 24: 2673-8
23. Le Péchoux C, Baldeyrou P, Ferreira I, Maheé M (2005) Cylindromes thoraciques. Cancer Radiothérapie 9: 358-61
24. Licht PB, Friis S, Pettersson G (2001) Tracheal cancer in Denmark: a nationwide study. Europ J Cardio-Thorac Surg 19: 339-45
25. **Macchiarini P (2006) Primary tracheal tumours. Lancet Oncol 7: 83-91**
26. Makarewicz R, Mross M (1998) Radiation therapy alone in the treatment of tumours of the trachea. Lung Ca 20: 169-74
27. Manninen M, Pukander J, Flander M *et al.* (1993) Treatment of primary tracheal carcinoma in Finland in 1967-1985. Acta Oncol 32: 277-82
28. **Mathisen DJ (1999) Primary tracheal tumor management. Thorac Surg Oncol 8: 307-26**
29. Maziak DE, Todd TR, Keshavjee SH *et al.* (1996) Adenoid cystic carcinoma of the airway: thirty-two-year experience. J Thorac Cardiovasc Surg 112: 1522-32
30. Molina JR, Aubry MC, Lewis JE *et al.* (2007) Primary salivary gland-type lung cancer : spectrum of clinical presentation, histopathologic and prognostic factors. Cancer 15: 2253-9
31. Mornex F, Coquard R, Danhier S *et al.* (1998) Role of radiation therapy in the treatment of primary tracheal carcinoma. Int J Radiat Oncol Biol Phys 41: 299-305
32. Regnard JF, Fourquier P, Levasseur P *et al.* (1996) Results and prognostic factors in resections of primary tracheal tumors: a multicenter retrospective study. J Thorac Cardiovasc Surg 111: 808-14
33. Rousseau H, Dahan M, Lauque D *et al.* (1993) Self-expandable prostheses in the tracheobronchial tree. Radiology 188: 199-203
34. Schraube P, Latz D, Wannenmacher M (1994) Treatment of primary squamous cell carcinoma of the trachea: the role of radiation therapy. Radiat Oncol 33: 254-8
35. Videtic GM, Campbell C, Vincent MD (2003) Primary chemoradiation as definitive treatment for unresectable cancer of the trachea. Can Respir J 10: 143-4
36. Webb BD, Walsh G, Roberts DB *et al.* (2006) Primary tracheal malignant neoplasms: the Universisty of Texas MF Anderson Cancer Center experience. J Am Coll Surg 202: 237-246
37. Wood DE (2002) Management of malignant tracheobronchial obstruction. Surg Clin N Am 82: 621-42
38. Yang KY, Huang MH, Perng RP (1997) Revisit of primary malignant neoplasms of the trachea : clinical characteristics and survival analysis. Jpn J Clin Oncol 27: 305-9

Tracheal cancers

8

E. Touboul and F. Huguet

Five Essential Points

1. *Squamous cell carcinoma is the most common primary tracheal malignancy, followed by adenoid cystic carcinoma.*
2. *Bronchoscopy with tumour biopsies and CT scan are the most useful methods to assess diagnosis, size, tracheal site of the tumour, and extent.*
3. *Surgery with curative intent is considered to be the treatment of choice for resectable lesions.*
4. *The contraindications to surgery are the presence of multiple positive lymph nodes, involvement of more than 50% of the trachea in adults and 30% in children, mediastinal invasion of unresectable organs, and distant metastases.*
5. *Radiotherapy (with or without concurrent chemotherapy depending on histology) is proposed either as adjuvant therapy after resection, definitive treatment for unresectable and medically inoperable tumours, or palliative treatment for severe symptoms.*

Introduction

Primary malignant tumours of the trachea are rare and account for only 0.1-0.4% of all malignant disease [2, 13, 24]. In adults, 90% of primary tumours are malignant [13], compared with 10-30% in children [8]. Although the definitive diagnosis of these malignant tumours is often delayed, surgery should still be considered in most patients. However, radiotherapy with curative intent has been proposed for early-stage lesions or as an adjuvant after surgery, and for unresectable and medically inoperable lesions, or palliation of severe symptoms. Selection criteria and treatment indications have not been clearly defined due to the rarity of tracheal cancers. We report the evidence currently available to guide clinicians in the treatment of primary malignant tumours of the trachea.

Anatomy and pathology

The adult trachea is about 10-13 cm long and 1.5-2.5 cm wide. The trachea extends from the larynx to the carina, two-thirds being located in the thorax. The trachea is composed of 12-22 C-shaped cartilage rings (2 cartilage rings/cm), a posterior membrane, and fibrous tissue spanned by the trachealis muscle. The tracheal mucosa consists of ciliated pseudostratified columnar epithelium, lymphoid tissue, elastic fibres, nerves, blood vessels and mucous glands. The trachea is supplied by fine branches of the inferior thyroid artery and superior thyroid artery, while branches of the bronchial arteries supply the lowest part of the trachea. The draining lymph nodes are similar to those of bronchial carcinomas.

Primary malignant tumours can arise from the respiratory epithelium, salivary glands, and mesenchymal structures of the trachea (Table 1). According to various series, approximately 50% of malignant tracheal tumours are squamous cell carcinomas and 15-40% are adenoid cystic carcinomas [11, 13, 18]. The remaining malignant tumours form a heterogeneous histological group with little information available on their natural history and management [18]. Squamous cell carcinoma is mainly associated with cigarette smoking, and effects men 2 to 4 times more frequently than women in their sixth or seventh decade. Squamous cell carcinoma can be either ulcerative or exophytic and can arise most anywhere in the trachea. Synchronous mediastinal or pulmonary metastases are observed in about 30% of cases. Carcinomas of the oropharynx, larynx, or lung can also occur before, concurrently, or after tracheal squamous cell carcinoma in 40% of patients [11, 18]. On the other hand, adenoid cystic carcinoma is equally distributed between the sexes, is not associated with cigarette smoking and generally occurs during the fourth and fifth decade. Adenoid cystic carcinoma is often exophytic and progresses slowly over several years. The propensity to spread along both submucosal and perineural planes can explain the late local recurrences sometimes observed after resection. Only 10% of patients have regional lymph node or distant metastases.

Table 1 – Classification of primary malignant tracheal tumours.

Surface epithelium	Squamous carcinoma in situ Squamous cell carcinoma Adenocarcinoma Large-cell undifferentiated carcinoma Neuroendocrine tumours: - Typical or atypical carcinoids - Large-cell neuroendocrine tumour - Small-cell carcinoma
Salivary glands	Mucoepidermoid carcinoma Adenoid cystic carcinoma Carcinoma ex pleiomorphic adenoma
Mesenchyma	Soft-tissue type carcinoma Chondrosarcoma Malignant lymphomas Other…

Clinical presentation and diagnosis

The diagnosis is frequently delayed due to the nonspecific symptoms or absence of symptoms until the tumour occludes 50-70% of the tracheal luminal diameter. The symptoms can be explained by upper airway obstruction (dyspnoea, wheezing, and stridor), mucosal involvement and inflammation (haemoptysis and cough), and involvement of contiguous structures (dysphagia and hoarseness corresponding to recurrent laryngeal nerve palsy). Clinical symptoms vary according to the type of tumour [11]. Haemoptysis is usually an early symptom in patients with squamous cell carcinoma. Hoarseness and dysphagia mainly occur in patients with advanced disease but do not preclude operability. In contrast, wheezing and stridor are commonly present in patients with adenoid cystic carcinoma. Less than 25% of patients experience haemoptysis early in the course of the disease, which explains why many patients present at a stage of locally advanced disease [2, 12]. CT scan is the most useful method for diagnosis and to assess the size, extent, tracheal site of the tumour, and involvement of mediastinal lymph nodes and adjacent structures. CT imaging can allow multiplanar and three-dimensional reconstruction (virtual bronchoscopy) to accurately locate the tumour and delineate the relative position of the tumour with adjacent structures [10]. Magnetic resonance imaging (MRI) provides no advantages over CT, except for adenoid cystic lesions [1]. Bronchoscopy may be useful to obtain proximal and distal tumour biopsies and can assess the site and relative location of the tumour and the trachea [38]. Endoscopic ultrasound is also useful to assess the extent of tracheal invasion [23]. Thoracic and abdominal CT, brain CT or brain MRI are useful for distant staging of the disease. However, 18F-labelled fluorodeoxyglucose positron emission tomography (FDG-PET) is now used to detect mediastinal lymph node metastases and visceral metastases from carcinomas [37]. FDG-PET is also used to improve target definition and tumour coverage for treatment with CT-based three-dimensional conformal radiotherapy [7]. Pulmonary function tests can detect upper airway obstruction and a flow-volume loop presenting characteristic flattening of both inspiratory and expiratory phases is usually observed in fixed upper airway obstruction. Pulmonary function tests can be useful in assessing the response after local treatment.

Treatment modalities

Primary malignant tumours of the trachea are usually treated by surgery, endoscopic resection and radiotherapy.

Surgery with curative intent

Anaesthesia must be carefully managed. Various surgical techniques, depending on the site of the tumour, can be used to treat primary malignant tumours of the trachea: laryngectomy with resection of the upper trachea, resection of the trachea, carina or carina and lungs [16, 17]. A collar incision with manubriotomy is used for tumours of the cervical and most cranial portion of the intrathoracic trachea. Median sternotomy or right posterolateral thoracotomy is used for tumours of the lower part of the trachea. Anatomical mobilisation can allow about half of the trachea to be resected in adults and about one third of trachea in children, allowing resection followed by primary reconstruction, but the extent of cancer resection is limited by the amount of tension on anastomoses. The blood supply to the lateral segment must be preserved. Lymph nodes should not be extensively dissected to avoid severely compromising the blood supply to the remaining trachea. Anastomoses must be performed meticulously. Tracheal replacement with allogeneic aorta is an experimental treatment for extensive lesions involving more than 50% of the length of the trachea, but requires further prospective studies [40].

Endotracheal resection

Endotracheal tumours can be removed by biopsy forceps and section, electrocoagulation, photodynamic therapy, laser, or argon coagulation [18, 21, 27, 29]. However, these treatment modalities are more often palliative and can be used in patients with life-threatening airway obstruction until subsequent curative local treatment.

Radiotherapy

External radiation therapy with CT-based three-dimensional conformal radiotherapy (3D-CRT) with FDG-PET image fusion [7, 15] is recommended. New RT techniques with respiration-controlled treatment procedures [36] and intensity-modulated radiotherapy [6, 19] improve the conformity of the plan facilitating normal-tissue sparing and dose escalation. In patients with incomplete resection, administration of 60 Gy photon radiotherapy postoperatively given as five 2 Gy fractions per week can destroy residual microscopic carcinoma in tracheal margins and regional lymph nodes. In locally advanced disease, the total dose needs to be increased to 68-70 Gy given as five 2 Gy fractions per week over 6.8 - 7 weeks. Some data suggest that a total dose higher than 60 Gy increases local control and improves overall survival [4, 5, 9, 14, 22, 26, 30, 31]. A boost with endotracheal high-dose-rate brachytherapy could allow dose escalation at the target volume. Endotracheal high-dose-rate brachytherapy seems to improve local tumour control when used after 46-60 Gy external-beam radiotherapy at a dose of 3 x 5 to 4 x 5 Gy [20, 35]. However, the place of endotracheal brachytherapy boost irradiation has not yet been established and further studies are necessary.

Endobronchial stents

Silicone or expandable stents can be used to achieve durable palliation in carefully selected patients with unresectable or medically inoperable lesions [39].

Chemotherapy

Cisplatin-based chemotherapy can be used in combination with radiotherapy in patients with unresectable malignant epithelial tumours. Concurrent chemo-radiotherapy has not yet been assessed prospectively in primary malignant tracheal tumours.

Management guidelines

Surgery with curative intent is the primary and most curative treatment. Surgery also provides histological confirmation of complete tumour removal and permanently relieves airway obstruction [18]. Resectability should be established before any other treatment. The absolute contraindications to surgery are the presence of multiple positive lymph nodes, involvement of more than 50% of the trachea in adults and 30% in children, mediastinal invasion of unresectable organs, and distant metastases [11, 18]. Operative mortality ranges between 5 and 10% [3, 12, 28, 32-34]. Some authors recommend systematic postoperative radiotherapy to a total dose of 45 Gy over 4.5 weeks in patients with negative margins or complete resection and 65 Gy over 6.5 weeks in those with positive airway margins or incomplete resection [18]. Other authors propose adjuvant radiotherapy only in patients with positive airway margins or with incomplete resection [33]. Five-year survival ranges from 36 to 47% in patients with squamous cell carcinoma compared with 66 to 79% in patients with adenoid cystic carcinoma, depending on the series (Table 2). In patients with operable tumour, prognostic factors for increased survival are: complete resection, negative airway margins, and adenoid cystic histology [12, 24]. The impact of tumour depth or length and lymph node involvement on survival is not well known due to lack of data to formulate a precise pathological staging [25].

Table 2 – Survival rate after resection for primary malignant tumours of the trachea.

Histological type	Authors	n pts	Follow-up (years)	Survival (%)	
				5-year	10-year
Squamous cell carcinoma	Regnard [33] 1996	94	23	47	36
	Perelman [32] 1996	45	29	36	27
	Gaissert [12] 2004	90	41	39	18
Adenoid cystic carcinoma	Regnard [33] 1996	65	23	73	51
	Perelman [32] 1996	21	29	66	56
	Maziak [28] 1996	38	32	79	51

pts: patients.

For unresectable and medically inoperable lesions, definitive high-dose external radiotherapy is indicated at doses of more than 60 Gy over six weeks. The 5-year survival rate ranges between 12 and 30% (Table 3). However, published series are heterogeneous and do not present the results according to histological type and do not compare results between radiotherapy with curative intent and with palliative intent. Concurrent cisplatin-based chemotherapy can be used in tracheal carcinomas.

Other local treatments such as endobronchial stents or endotracheal debridement are considered to be local palliative measures to relieve airway obstruction.

Table 3 – Treatment results following definitive irradiation.

Authors	n pts	Radiation dose (Gy)	Median survival (months)	5-year survival (%)	Local control (%)
Cheung [4] 1989	19	40-60	5	–	5 at 15 months
Fields [9] 1989	18	40-65	10*	25*	86 if > 60 Gy 9 if < 60 Gy
Chow [5] 1993	12	50-66	26	–	75 if > 60 Gy 12 if < 60 Gy
Schraub [35] 1994	11	40-60 ± brachytherapy	31	30	45 at 6 months
Jeremic [22] 1996	22	56-70	24	25	–
Chao [3] 1998	42	40-60	12.5	–	44 if ≥ 50 Gy 3 if < 50 Gy at 2 years
Makarewicz [26] 1998	23	20-60 ± brachytherapy	26 if ≥ 60 Gy 7.2 if < 60 Gy	–	–
Mornex [30] 1998	84	30-70	16 if ≥ 56 Gy 6 if < 56 Gy	12 if ≥ 56 Gy 5 if < 56 Gy	69 if ≥ 56 Gy 34 if < 56 Gy

pts: patients.
* median survival: 6.5 months for squamous cell carcinoma, and 5-year survival rate: 0% for squamous cell carcinoma.

Conclusion

Primary malignant tumours of the trachea are rare. Squamous cell carcinoma is the most common malignant tumour, followed by adenoid cystic carcinoma. Nonspecific symptoms often lead to delayed diagnosis. Resection with primary reconstruction is considered to be the treatment of choice for resectable lesions. Radiotherapy (with or without concomitant chemotherapy in carcinomas) is proposed as adjuvant therapy after tracheal resection, and as curative treatment or palliative treatment for unresectable and medically inoperable lesions. All other local treatments such as debridement or endobronchial stents can be used as palliative treatment in patients with inoperable tumour and/or life-threatening airway obstruction.

References

1. Akala S, Okhubo Y, Park J *et al.* (2001) Multiplanar reconstruction MR image of primary adenoid cystic carcinoma of the central airway. Clin Imaging 25: 332-6
2. Bhattacharyya N (2004) Contemporary staging and prognosis for primary tracheal malignancies: a population-based analysis. Otolaryngol Head Neck Surg 131: 639-42
3. Chao MWT, Smith JG, Laidlaw C *et al.* (1998) Results of treating primary tumors of the trachea with radiotherapy. Int J Radiat Oncol Biol Phys 41: 779-85
4. Cheung AY (1989) Radiotherapy for primary carcinoma of the trachea. Radiother Oncol 14: 279-85
5. Chow DC, Komaki R, Libshitz HI *et al.* (1993) Treatment of primary neoplasms of the trachea. The role of radiation therapy. Cancer 71: 2946-52
6. Christian JA, Bedford JL, Webb S *et al.* (2007) Comparison of inverse-planned three-dimensional radiotherapy and intensity-modulated radiotherapy for non-small-cell lung cancer. Int J Radiat Oncol Biol Phys 67: 735-41
7. Deniaud-Alexandre E, Touboul E, Lerouge D *et al.* (2005) Impact of computed tomography and 18F-deoxyglucose coincidence detection emission tomography image fusion for optimization of conformal radiotherapy in non-small-cell lung cancer. Int J Radiat Oncol Biol Phys 63: 1432-41
8. Desai DP, Holinger LD, Gonzales-Crussi F (1998) Tracheal neoplasm in children. Ann Otol Rhinol Laryngol 107: 790-806
9. Fields JN, Rigaud G, Emami BN (1989) Primary tumors of the trachea. Results of radiation therapy. Cancer 63: 2429-33
10. Finkelstein SE, Summers RM, Nguyen DM *et al.* (2004) Virtual bronchoscopy for evaluation of airway disease. Thoracic Surg Clin 14: 79-86
11. Gaissert HA (2003) Primary tracheal tumors. Chest Surg Clin N Am 13: 247-56
12. **Gaissert HA, Grillo HC, Shadmehr MB (2004) Long-term survival of resection of primary adenoid cystic and squamous cell carcinoma of the trachea and carina. Ann Thorac Surg 78: 1889-96**
13. Gelder CM, Hetzel MR (1993) Primary tracheal tumours: a national survey. Thorax 48: 688-92
14. Green N, Kulber H, Landman M *et al.* (1985) The experience with definitive irradiation of clinically limited squamous cell cancer of the trachea. Int J Radiat Oncol Biol Phys 11: 1401-5
15. Greenberger JS, Kalend A, Sciurba F *et al.* (1996) Development if multifield three-dimensional conformal radiotherapy of lung cancer using a total lung dose/volume histogram. Radiat Oncol Invest 3: 243-55
16. Grillo HC (2003) Development of tracheal surgery: a historical review. Part 2: treatment of tracheal disease. Ann Thorac Surg 75: 1039-47
17. Grillo HC (2003) Development of tracheal surgery: a historical review. Part 1: techniques of tracheal surgery. Ann Thorac Surg 75: 610-9
18. Grillo HC, Primary tracheal tumours. In: Grillo HC (2004) Surgery of the trachea and bronchi. Hamilton, London: BC Decker, 208-47

19. Grills IS, Yan D, Martinez AA *et al.* (2003) Potential for reduced toxicity and dose escalation in the treatment of inoperable non-small cell lung cancer: a comparison of intensity-modulated radiation therapy (IMRT), 3D conformal radiation, and elective nodal irradiation. Int J Radiat Oncol Biol Phys 57: 875-90
20. Harms W, Latz D, Becker H *et al.* (1999) HDR-brachytherapy boost for residual tumour after external beam radiotherapy in patients with tracheal malignancies. Radiother Oncol 52: 251-5
21. Hooper RG, Jackson FN (1985) Endobronchial electrocautery. Chest 87: 712-4
22. Jeremic B, Shibamoto Y, Acimovic L *et al.* (1996) Radiotherapy for primary squamous cell carcinoma of the trachea. Radiother Oncol 41: 135-8
23. Kurimoto N, Murayama M, Yoshiota S *et al.* (1999) Assessment of usefulness of endobronchial ultrasonography in determination of depth of tracheobronchial tumor invasion. Chest 115: 1500-6
24. Licht PB, Früs S, Pettersson G (2001) Tracheal cancer in Denmark: a nationwide study. Eur J Cardiothorac Surg 19: 339-45
25. Macchiarini P (2006) Primary tracheal tumours. Lancet Oncol 7: 83-91
26. Makarewicz R, Mross M (1998) Radiation therapy alone in the treatment of tumours of the trachea. Lung Cancer 20: 169-74
27. Mathisen DJ, Grillo HC (1989) Endoscopic relief of malignant/airway obstruction. Ann Thorac Surg 48: 469-75
28. Maziak DE, Todd TR, Keshavjee SH *et al.* (1996) Adenoid cystic carcinoma of the airway: thirty-two-year experience. J Thorac Cardiovasc Surg 112: 1522-31
29. Mc Caughan Jr JS, Williams TE (1997) Photodynamic therapy for endobronchial malignant disease: a prospective fourteen-year study. J Thorac Cardiovasc Surg 114: 940-6
30. Mornex F, Coquard R, Danhier S *et al.* (1998) Role of radiation therapy in the treatment of primary tracheal carcinoma. Int J Radiat Oncol Biol Phys 41: 299-305
31. Muller A, Stockamp B, Schnabel T (2000) Successful primary radiation therapy of adenoid cystic carcinoma of the lung. Oncology 58: 15-7
32. Perelman MI, Koroleva N, Kirjukov J *et al.* (1996) Primary tracheal tumours. Semin Thorac Cardiovasc Surg 8: 400-2
33. Regnard JF, Fourquier P, Levasseur P (1996) Results and prognostic factors in resections of primary tracheal tumours: a multicenter retrospective study. J Thorac Cardiovasc Surg 111: 808-13
34. Schneider P, Schirren J, Muley T *et al.* (2001) Primary tracheal tumours: experience with 14 resected patients. Eur J Cardiothorac Surg 20: 12-8
35. Schraube P, Latz D, Wannenmacher M (1994) Treatment of primary squamous cell carcinoma of the trachea: the role of radiation therapy. Radiother Oncol 33: 254-8
36. Simon L, Giraud P, Dumas JL *et al.* (2007) [Pratical recommendations for breathing-adapted radiotherapy]. Cancer/Radiother 11: 214-24
37. Toloza EM, Harpole L, Mc Crory DC (2003) Noninvasive staging of non-small cell lung cancer: a review of the current evidence. Chest 123: 137s-46s
38. Wood D (2001) Bronchoscopic preparation for airway resection. Ches Surg Clin N Am 11: 735-48
39. Wood DJ (2002) Management of malignant tracheobronchial obstruction. Surg Clin North Am 82: 621-42
40. Wurtz A, Porte H, Conti M *et al.* (2006) Tracheal replacement with aortic allografts. N Engl J Med 355: 1938-40

Section 8

Malignancies of the skin

Unusual cutaneous malignancies: cutaneous adnexal tumours

1

B. Guillot

Five Essential Points

1. *Some cutaneous adnexal tumours may have a primary visceral conterpart and complete examination and tomodensitometry or PET scan are mandatory in these cases :*
   a. *Adenoid cystic carcinoma and primary tumour of salivary glands*
   b. *Apocrine carcinoma and metastasis of breast carcinoma*
   c. *Sebaceous carcinoma and primary breast or gastro-intestinal tract tumours*
   d. *Mucinous carcinoma and primary breast or gastro-intestinal tract tumours.*
2. *Local recurrences are frequent despite extensive surgery. Nodal and distant metastases are not uncommon.*
3. *Surgery is the treatment of choice of these tumours.*
4. *The surgical margins are debated: 1 to 3 cm-wide margins, and even more are recommended according to prognosis of the tumour.*
5. *Radiotherapy may be helpful in some selected situations; there is no curative treatment for metastatic lesions that are usually fatal.*

Introduction

Cutaneous carcinomas are frequent neoplasms arising from epidermal cells and are classically divided into basal cell carcinoma (BCC), squamous cell carcinoma (SCC) and skin adnexal carcinoma. Basal cell carcinoma and squamous cell carcinoma are currently reported with an increasing incidence (approximatively 85/100,000 per year for BCC and 25/100,000 per year for SCC in Europe). In contrast to these frequent tumours, skin adnexal carcinomas are very rare tumours even though their overall incidence is unknown. Many different histological subtypes have been reported but usually in short series or individual clinical reports. Although a classification based on the type of cell primitively involved in proliferation is largely accepted, the current terminology is often heterogenous, increasing the confusion regarding description and proposed management. This paper will briefly review clinical and histological characteristics of the main skin adnexal tumours and principles of treatment according to updated information from the literature.

Classification

The classification of adnexal skin tumours is based on the cellular origin of the malignancy: sudoral (eccrine or apocrine glands), hair follicle and sebaceous origin [1-16]. The main entities described are listed in Table 1.

1

Table 1 – Classification of cutaneous adnexal tumours.

Malignant tumours of cutaneous sweat glands	Eccrine origin	Porocarcinoma Hidradenocarcinoma Spiradenocarcinoma Malignant cylindroma Syringoid carcinoma Microcystic adenoid carcinoma Adenoid cystic carcinoma Mucinous carcinoma
	Apocrine origin	Syringocystadenocarcinoma Apocrine carcinoma Paget's disease
	Eccrine and apocrine origin	Malignant mixed tumours of the skin
Malignant tumours of pilosebaceous origin	Hair and hair follicle	Trichilemmal carcinoma Trichoblastic carcinoma Malignant proliferating trichilemmal cyst Pilomatrix carcinoma
	Sebaceous glands	Sebaceous carcinoma Basal cell carcinoma with sebaceous differentiation

Main anatomo-clinical entities

Tumours of sudoral origin [16, 21]

Eccrine tumours

Porocarcinoma: porocarcinoma is the more frequent adnexal tumour arising from the intra-epidermal ductal portion of the eccrine sweat gland. In about 30 to 50% of cases, porocarcinoma occurs on a preexistent benign poroma. Porocarcinoma generally appears after 50 years but is sometimes described in younger patients. Two main clinical subsets have been described: superficial porocarcinoma appears as a flat erythemateous or slighty pigmented lesion with polycyclic borders that slowly increase in size. The second type is trabecular porocarcinoma and features an exophytic, often ulcerated, nodule mainly located on the limbs or the feet. Histological examination of the superficial subtype displays acanthosis, with malignant cells, appearing as isolated nests in the epidermis. The lesion is well demarcated but isolated tumoral cells in the lymphatic vessels can be observed. In the trabecular form, the tumour is irregular with anastomotic trabecular walls. As in the superficial type, isolated cells may be observed in lymphatics. Porocarcinoma malignant cells show a characteristic porome-like differentiation and cytologic atypia and express carcinoembryonic antigen (CEA) and epithelial membrane antigen (EMA). Tumoral evolution may be local, regional and general. Tumour cells can swiftly invade lymphatic vessels, a process resulting in frequent *in transit* cutaneous or subcutaneous metastasis and lymph node invasion [11]. Visceral metastases mainly involve lungs, retroperitoneum, bones, or liver. Local, lymph node and visceral metastases occur in 17%, 19% and 11% of patients respectively. All reported patients with visceral metastasis died from their disease [19]. The main prognostic factors include high mitotic rate (more than 14 mitosis per high power field), lymphatic invasion and thickness of the primary tumour (more than 7 millimeters).

Hidradenocarcinoma [21]: this tumour is very rare and may occur during all ages of life. A slight male predominance is observed. The main locations are scalp, face and extremities. A previous chronic lesion is sometimes observed: radiation dermatitis, scars or benign hidradenoma. Clinical appearance is usually non-specific: erythematous plaque or nodule with telangiectasia or ulceration.

Some histological criteria may help to differentiate a malignant from benign sudoral tumour: poorly limited tumour, deep invasion of tumoral lobules and high frequency of mitosis. The tumour is located in the dermis and is composed of two cell types: clear cells and spindle cells. Clear cells are round and rich in glycogen and express PAS whereas spindle cells are present at the periphery of the lobules. As in other eccrine tumours, hidradenocarcinoma cells express cytokeratins, EMA, CEA and S100 protein.

The risk of local recurrence is high, probably about 50%. Nodal involvement usually precedes visceral metastasis that occur in 39% and 28% of patients respectively.

Adenoid cystic carcinoma: this rare tumour usually affects the scalp of elderly patients. The lesion appears as a plaque or a nodule, often resulting in local alopecia. Trunk and extremities may be involved but more rarely [15]. Histologically, this tumour cannot be distinguished from its salivary gland counterpart and salivary glands must be thoroughly investigated to eliminate a metastatis of a primary salivary neoplasm. Adenoid cystic carcinoma is a dermal tumour with monomorphous basaloid cells arranged in a cribriform or trabecular growth pattern. Tumour cells express pankeratin, EMA, CEA and in some case CD117, the two latter markers being used to rule out the diagnosis of adenoid basal cell carcinoma. The risk of local recurrence is high and metastases have been reported particularly in the lung.

Microcystic adnexal carcinoma: this tumour seems to be more frequent in female patients and may be observed during all ages of life even though it is more common after 50 years of age. The lesion appears as a flesh-colored or yellowisch plaque or nodule, with poorly limited borders. The tumour is indurated and often follows a protracted local evolution. The occurrence of the tumour is usually difficult to date with accuracy but local dysesthesias are frequently described by patients. Differential diagnosis includes morpheiform basal cell carcinoma or scar. The main location of the lesion is upper lip but other locations have also been described: axilla, scalp, buttocks). Among risk factors, previous radiation therapy and immunosuppression are often identified. Histologically, the tumour appears as a poorly delimited proliferation of epithelial cells infiltrating dermis and subcutaneous tissue. Perineural invasion may be observed. Tumoral cells are small, basaloid, with minimal atypia. A single layer of tumour cells are arranged as tubular or ductal structures in the dermis. The stroma is clearly sclerotic. Malignant cells express EMA, CEA and in most cases CD5.

This tumour is locally aggressive with frequent local relapses. Conversely, the occurrence of nodal or visceral metastases have been very rarely described [8].

Mucinous carcinoma: this tumour is mainly located on the head, especially eyelids and scalp, and on the trunk (axilla) in elderly people. Clinical appearence features a large erythemateous or flesh-colored nodule which can evolve toward ulceration over time. Histologically, the lesion appears as a well-delineated mass involving the dermis with no connection with the epidermis. The tumour cells are polygonal with a pale eosinophilic PAS positive cytoplasm. These cells express EMA, CEA and CK7. Cutaneous metastasis of adenocarcinoma [23], especially of breast or gastrointestinal tract origin, represent the main differential diagnosis. Accordingly, a comprehensive clinical examination is mandatory, along with PET-scan and conventional radiological imaging. Evolution of this tumour is frequently marked with local recurrences but distant metastases are rarely observed.

Other eccrine tumours [16]: among the other rare eccrine tumours, malignant cylindroma, spiradenocarcinoma or syringoid carcinoma are rarely described. These tumours have high recurrence rates and may display metastatic evolution.

Apocrine tumours

Apocrine carcinoma: less frequent than eccrine carcinoma, apocrine carcinoma exhibits an aggressive behaviour. These tumours are mainly located on the trunk and especially on axillary or genital areas and appear as an erythemateous nodule slowly increasing in size and sometimes ulcerated [20]. Histologically, the tumour is a poorly demarcated nodule located in the dermis and composed of tubular or ductal structures. Tumour necrosis, cytological pleiomorphism and high mitotic activity are sometimes observed. Tumour cells are PAS positive and express EMA, CEA, and sometimes S100 protein. The presence of androgen receptors and the lack of oestrogen or progesterone receptors is helpful to distinguish between apocrine carcinoma and metastatic breast carcinoma. Recurrences are frequently observed owing to deep extension of the tumour in the dermis. Distant metastases have been described in rare cases.

Tumour of pilosebaceous origin [1]

Hair and hair follicle

Trichilemmal carcinoma: this rare tumour usually affects elderly people and appears as an exophytic nodule quickly increasing in size and often ulcerated. The main locations are the face, the scalp and the neck [18]. Histological examination discloses a well-delineated proliferation connected to the epidermis and the pilosebaceous structures, a pattern highly reminiscent of the outer root sheath of the hair follicle. Tumour cells are PAS positive.

The rapid local extension sharply contrasts with an indolent general evolution. Indeed, recurrences are rare and no cases of metastasis have ever been described.

Pilomatrix carcinoma: this tumour occurs more frequently *de novo* than by malignant evolution of a benign pilomatrixoma but such an event has already been described, although unfrequently [22]. This malignancy can be observed in middle-aged people and in children. The most frequent location is the head and especially pre- and retro-auricular areas but scalp, back or limbs may also be affected. Local recurrences are often observed and distant metastasis can occur, especially in the lung [25]. Histologically, the tumour appears as a dermal proliferation of shadowed cells without visible nucleus, associated with basophilic cells. It differs from benign pilomatricoma by its poor limitation, asymetrical growth pattern, infiltration of adjacent tissues and numerous cytonuclear atypia. Differential expression of some epithelial keratins and of beta-catenin may help to distinguish between benign and malignant forms of the tumour [4].

Sebaceous glands

Sebaceous carcinoma: two types of sebaceous carcinoma have been described: eyelid sebaceous carcinoma derived from modified sebaceous glands such as Mebomius or Zeis glands, and carcinoma arising in other parts of the body, mainly face, scalp, trunk or genitalia. A large retrospective study of 1,349 cases [5] showed that the tumour was more frequent in men and that the median age at diagnosis was 73 years. Prognosis of eyelid location and other subsets seems to be identical, contrasting with previous reports showing a worst prognosis of eyelid-located lesions. The malignancy appears as a large polylobulated erythemateous or yellowish nodule, sometimes ulcerated. Local recurrences are frequently observed. Nodal or distant visceral metastasis is possible. Overall 5-year and 10-year survival rates have been estimated at 71% and 46% respectively. This carcinoma is responsible for 147 of 473 deaths observed in the series of 1,349 reported cases.

This tumour may be associated with Muir and Torre syndrome, a disease associating skin sebaceous tumours, multiple keratoacanthomas and colonic or genitourinary malignancies [14]. This syndrome is a rare genodermatosis related to mutation of hMSH2 and hMLT1 genes. In this syndrome, the prognosis of sebaceous carcinoma seems to be more favourable than in isolated forms.

Histological examination reveals a proliferation of basaloid cells with frequent mitosis and atypias. These cells are arranged as solid sheets displaying asymetry and poor circumscription. Peripheral palissading is usually absent. In immunohistochemistry, sebaceous carcinoma expresses cytokeratin (AE1 and AE3), EMA, CA 15-3 and androgen receptors but not CEA.

Treatment of skin adnexal carcinomas

Treatment of primary tumours

Surgery is the treatment of choice of all subtypes of cutaneous adnexal carcinoma. Classical carcinoma surgery may be used but two-step surgery may enhance the quality of the margin control and Mohs micrographic surgery has also been used in some studies, with an excellent control of the disease, especially in carcinoma of eccrine origin [7, 24, 26].

However, optimal lateral margins remain to be defined but should be tailored according to the risk of local recurrences and of life-threatening distant metastasis. In this perspective, three prognostic subsets can be defined:

- Tumours with good prognosis: those with low risk of local recurrence and with no significant risk of distant metastasis.
- Tumours with poor prognosis: those with high risk of recurrence including a high risk of distant metastasis.
- Tumours of intermediate prognosis: those with high risk of local recurrence but low risk of distant metastasis.

The first subset essentially includes trichilemmal carcinoma that has a relatively good prognosis with possible local recurrences but exceptional distant metastasis. Tumours with intermediate prognosis are represented by microcystic adnexal carcinoma, adenoid cystic carcinoma and mucinous carcinoma whereas tumours with poor prognosis include porocarcinoma, hidradenocarcinoma, apocrine carcinoma, sebaceous carcinoma and pilomatrix carcinoma.

In the good prognosis group, a 1 cm-wide margin is proposed followed by clinical survey every six months. For the intermediate prognosis group, a larger, 2 to 3 cm-wide margin is recommended followed by clinical survey every three months. In some cases, especially for microcystic adnexal carcinoma, a 5 cm margin is proposed but recurences can still occur despite these very large margins. Regarding the poor prognosis group, a wide excisison with margins of at least 3 cm are recommended. If these large margins cannot be respected due to anatomical or functional conditions, a strict histological examination of lateral margins by the pathologist is mandatory. In these cases, a two-step surgery or Mohs micrographic surgery can be very helpful in local control of the disease.

Radiotherapy is usually not proposed as a first-intention therapy for cutaneous adnexal carcinomas. Indeed, adnexal cutaneous tumours are usually considered to be radioresistant. However, radiotherapy may be proposed when surgery is impossible, either because the tumour is unresectable or when a second surgical step, theoretically mandatory in case of incomplete primary surgery, is impossible or results in major local defects. When radiotherapy is used, high doses ranging from 50 to 70 Gy are usually necessary [10]. Eventually, the use of radiotherapy as adjuvant therapy in some selected cases of cutaneous adnexal tumours has been proposed [6, 8].

Medical treatment cannot be proposed in these overly aggressive tumours. A case of trichilemmal carcinoma, a tumour with a good prognosis, has been treated with imiquimod with a good result [12] but this therapeutic option should be used only when surgery is impossible.

Lymph nodes

Systematic histological analysis of regional lymph nodes is not usually proposed when clinical examination or node echography do not reveal macroscopic disease. However, the sentinel lymph node biopsy procedure may be proposed and can result in earlier identification of micrometastasis [2]. However, the impact of this procedure on overall survival remains unknown. In case of definite nodal involvement, the main treatment remains surgery: a full lymphadenectomy in first intention, often associated with adjuvant radiotherapy despite the lack of strong evidence for this approach.

Distant metastasis

In case of unique metastasis, surgery can be proposed but this possibility remains very rare. In other cases, chemotherapy is possible but the response rate is low. The main drugs are selected by analogy with squamous cell carcinoma or adenocarcinoma and include cyclophosphamide, vincristine, platinum, 5 fluoro-uracile, bleomycin or anthracycline. More recently, docetaxel alone [17] or a combination of paclitaxel with interferon alpha [9] have been proposed in cases of porocarcinoma with promising results. Recently, capecitabine has been succesfully used in a case of metastatic hidradenocarcinoma [13] but was ineffective in an apocrine carcinoma even in association with trastuzumab [3]. Immunotherapy, alone or in combination with isotretinoin or chemotherapy has been used in porocarcinoma with transient positive results [11]. However, chemo or immunotherapy currently remain palliative treatments in these rare tumours. Targeted therapies are under investigation in some cutaneous carcinomas and their use in cutaneous adnexal tumours will perhaps represent a new hope for these rare but aggressive skin tumours.

References

1. **Alsaad KO, Obaidat NA, Ghazarian D (2006) Skin adnexal neoplasms – part 1: an approach to tumours of the pilosebaceous unit. J Clin Pathol , 60: 129-44**
2. Bogner PN, Fullen DR, Lowe L *et al.* (2003) Lymphatic mapping and sentinel lymph node biopsy in the detection of early metastasis from sweat gland carcinoma. Cancer 97: 2285-9

3. Cham PMH, Niehans GA, Foman N, Suwaytee P (2008) Primary cutaneous apocrine carcinoma presenting as carcinoma erysipeloides. Br J Dermatol, 158: 194-5
4. Cribier B, Worret WI, Braun-Falco M *et al.* (2006) Expression of hair and epithelial keratins and transcription factors HOXC13, LEF1, and beta-catenin in a malignant pilomatricoma: a histological and immunohistochemical study. J Cutan Pathol 33: 1-9
5. **Dasgupta T, Wilson LD, Yu JB (2009) A retrospective review of 1,349 cases of sebaceous carcinoma. Cancer 115: 158-65**
6. Dowd MB, Kumar RJ, Sharma R, Murali R. (2008) Diagnosis and management of sebaceous carcinoma: an australian experience. ANZ J Surg 78: 158-63
7. Friedman PM, Friedman RH, Jiang SB *et al.* (1999) Microcystic adnexal carcinoma: collaborative series review and update. J Am Acad Dermatol 41: 225-31
8. Gabillot-Carré M, Weill F, Mamelle G *et al.* (2006) Microcystic adnexal carcinoma: report of seven cases including one with lung metastasis. Dermatology, 212: 221-8
9. Gutermuth J, Audring H, Voit C *et al.* (2004) Antitumour activity of paclitaxel and interferon-alpha in a case of metastatic eccrine porocarcinoma. J Eur Acad Dermatol Venereol 18: 477-9
10. Harari PM, Shimm DS, Bangert JL, Cassady JR (1999). The role of radiotherapy in the treatment of malignant sweat gland neoplasms. Cancer 65: 1737-40
11. Huet P, Dandurand M, Pignodel C, Guillot B (1996). Metastazing eccrine porocarcinoma: report of a case and review of the literature. J Am Acad Dermatol 35: 860-4
12. Jo JH, Ko HC, Jang HS *et al.* (2005) Infiltrative trichilemmal carcinoma treated with 5% imiquimod cream. Dermatol Surg 31: 973-6
13. Jouary T, Kaiafa A, Lipinski P *et al.* (2006) Metastatic hidradenocarcinoma: efficacy of capecitabine. Arch Dermatol 142: 1366-7
14. Lazar AJF, Lyle S, Calonje E (2007) Sebaceous neoplasia and Torre-Muir Syndrome. Curr Diagn Pathol 13: 301-19
15. Naylor E, Sarkar P, Perlis CS *et al.* (2008) Primary cutaneous adenoid cystic carcinoma. J Am Acad Dermatol 58: 636-41
16. **Obaidat NA, Alsaad KO, Ghazarian D (2007) Skin adnexal tumours – part 2: an approach to tumours of cutaneous sweat glands. J Clin Pathol 60: 145-59**
17. Plunkett TA, Hanby AM, Miles DW, Rubens RD (2001) Metastatic eccrine porocarcinoma: response to docetaxel (Taxotere) chemotherapy. Ann Oncol 12: 411-4
18. Reis JP, Tellechea O, Cunha MF, Baptista AP (1993) Trichilemmal carcinoma: review of 8 cases. J Cutan Pathol 20: 44-9
19. Robson A, Greene J, Ansari N *et al.* (2002) Eccrine porocarcinoma (malignant eccrine poroma): a clinicopathologic study of 69 cases. Am J Surg Pathol 26: 272-4
20. Robson A, Lazar AJ, Ben Nagi J *et al.* (2008) Primary cutaneous apocrine carcinoma: a clinico-pathologic analysis of 24 cases. Am J Surg Pathol 32: 682-90
21. **Rutten A, Requena L (2008) Sweat gland carcinoma of the skin. Hautarzt 59: 151-60**
22. Sassmannshausen J, Chaffins M. (2001) Pilomatrix carcinoma: report of a case arising from a previously excised pilomatrixoma and a review of the literature. J Am Acad Dermatol 44: 358-61
23. Terada T, Sato Y, Furukawa K, Sugiura M (2004) Primary cutaneous carcinoma initially diagnosed as a metastatic adenocarcinoma. Tohoku J Exp Med 203: 345-8
24. **Thomas CJ, Wood GC, Marks VJ (2007) Mohs micrographic surgery in the treatment of rare agressive cutaneous tumors: the Geisinger experience. Dermatol Surg 33: 333-9**
25. Tselis N, Heyd R, Vogt HG, Zamboglou N (2006) Pilomatrix carcinoma with lymph node and pulmonary metastasis. Stralenther Onkol 182: 727-32
26. Wildemore JK, Lee JB, Humphreys TR (2004). Mohs micrographic surgery for malignant eccrine neoplasms. Dermatol Surg 30: 1574-9

Kaposi's sarcoma

2

Y.M. Kirova

Five Essential Points

1. *The survival of patients with HIV-related Kaposi's sarcoma is usually dictated by the degree of severity of the underlying immuno-suppression and survival cannot therefore be a particularly useful endpoint for evaluating therapy for Kaposi's sarcoma.*
2. *The viral origin provides opportunities for both prevention and treatment.*
3. *New drugs aimed at inhibiting angiogenesis and older ones, such as Thalidomide, which have anti-angiogenic properties, may be worth exploring.*
4. *Their effectiveness will be in the earlier stages of disease – by the time a patient has widespread disease, particularly if there is visceral involvement, it is unlikely that treatment strategies based on preventing angiogenesis will have any meaningful clinical benefit.*
5. *Radiotherapy provides a good palliation of symptoms.*

History

Moriz Kaposi in 1872 was the first author who described patients presenting with "sarcoma idiopaticum multiple hemorrhagicum" [14]. In 1912 Sternberg termed this pathology "Kaposi's sarcoma" – now referred to as classical Kaposi's sarcoma – an indolent tumour seen typically in patients of Mediterranean or East European Jewish origin. Since then various forms of Kaposi's sarcoma have been observed and described [15]. In 1914, Hallenberg described the first cases of African or endemic Kaposi's sarcoma. In the 1960s the first reports discussing Kaposi's sarcoma following organ transplantation and immune-suppressive therapy were published [25]. In 1981, the epidemic Kaposi's sarcoma associated to AIDS was described by Hymes [9].

Pathogenesis and epidemiology

Kaposi's sarcoma (KS) is associated with the herpes virus or human herpes virus 8 designated HHV-8 (KSHV). The virus has been identified using PCR-based techniques in all forms of Kaposi's sarcoma: classical Mediterranean; endemic African; paediatric, epidemic (HIV-related). HHV-8 is closely related to Epstein-Barr virus (EBV). HHV-8 like EBV may be transmitted in saliva. Although the rate of HHV-8 infection in homosexual men is related to the number of sexual partners, there is no evidence to suggest that transmission is exclusively through sexual contact. The evidence from Africa on HHV-8 prevalence in children suggests that the infection is acquired through normal social contacts in the family. In the developed world, the sero-prevalence of HHV-8 in the general population is estimated to be 5-10%; for HIV positive homosexual men 30%. In Africa, the general prevalence is much higher, over 15% and increases with age: <2% under the age of 5; 15% between 15 and 40 years; >27% in population older than 40 [10, 23].

The development and progression of Kaposi's sarcoma is, particularly in the earlier stages, heavily dependent upon cytokines. The KS-associated herpes virus/human herpes virus 8 open reading frame 74 encodes a constitutively active G protein-coupled receptor known as vGPCR that binds CXC chemokines with high affinity. Recently Jensen *et al.* showed that conditional transgenic expression of vGPCR by cells of endothelial origin triggers an angiogenic program *in vivo*, leading to development of an angioproliferative disease that resembles KS. This angiogenic program consists partly in the expression of the angiogenic factors placental growth factor, platelet-derived growth factor B, and inducible NO synthase by the vGPCR-expressing cells. The continued vGPCR expression is essential for progression of the KS-like phenotype and that down-regulation of vGPCR expression results in reduced expression of angiogenic factors and regression of the lesions [13].

Kaposi's sarcoma was the most frequent neoplasm occurring in AIDS patients and the first one to be described in AIDS [9, 15, 16, 21]. By the end of 1998, nearly 57,000 people in USA had developed Kaposi's sarcoma as a result of HIV related immunosuppression. The incidence of Kaposi's sarcoma as an AIDS defining illness in the USA has declined since 1993, the year in which the definition of AIDS was changed to allow a low (< 200) CD count to be considered an AIDS defining criterion. Part of this decrease is likely to be artefactual: patients with HIV infection are diagnosed as having AIDS earlier in the natural history of the infection before they have time to develop Kaposi's sarcoma. Some of the decrease is related to the highly active retroviral therapy (HAART) [19, 20]. In the early days of the HIV epidemic, the majority of patients died from opportunistic infections. With the development of treatment and prophylaxis of Pneumocystis carinii pneumonia (PCP), there was a change in the mortality pattern, an increasing proportion of patients dying from malignancies such as Kaposi's sarcoma and non- Hodgkin's lymphomas (NHL). With the development of HAART, one might anticipate a relative decline in Kaposi's sarcoma as a cause of death in HIV-positive individuals. In 2000 in USA about 1 000 HIV positive men and 100 HIV-positive women were diagnosed with AIDS because they had developed Kaposi's sarcoma. Cohort data suggested that the risk of developing Kaposi's sarcoma is 35% at ten years after the acquisition of infection with HIV plus HHV-8. It is much more difficult to unravel the epidemiology of HIV-related Kaposi's sarcoma in the developing world. Under-reporting of HIV-related Kaposi's sarcoma, together with higher background rates of Kaposi's sarcoma not related to HIV, results in difficulty in obtaining accurate estimates [10].

Clinical features

The classic lesion of Kaposi's sarcoma is a raised macula which is purplish in colour and which may be surrounded, because of extravagated red cells, by a yellowish halo. Individual lesions are, at first inconspicuous particularly in those with dark skin, but will increase in both size and number. Lesions may also coalesce into plaques and they may ulcerate and bleed [3, 10, 15]. Kaposi's sarcoma may develop preferentially at sites of previous trauma. Oedema is almost always a feature of Kaposi's sarcoma and its severity may appear out of all proportion to the visible skin lesions. This is because Kaposi's sarcoma will involve and obstruct dermal and sub-dermal lymhatics as well as spreading directly to lymph nodes. Facial and periorbital oedema, genital oedema and oedema of the legs are the main clinical manifestations of this phenomenon [15, 16]. The lesion is moist, while in protected sites, such as perineum, the glans penis and axilla, may become exuberant and polypoid. Surface ulceration and bleeding may occur. Secondary infection of Kaposi's sarcoma is common, particularly in the oral cavity, and will exacerbate any associated pain or swelling [28].

Endemic (African) Kaposi's sarcoma

In the 1950's Kaposi's sarcoma was recognized as a relatively common neoplasm endemic in native populations in Equatorial Africa, comprising approximately 9% of all cancers diagnosed in Ugandan males. African Kaposi's sarcoma follows two main clinical patterns: an indolent neoplasm identical to the classic disease seen in Europe and North America, or an aggressive form presented with exophytic tumours possibly invading the subcutaneous and surrounding tissue including the underlying bone. Oedema and ulceration of coalescing skin nodules often develop, particularly in the lower limbs. In Africa, both the indolent and locally aggressive forms of Kaposi's sarcoma occur with a male and female ratio of 1.5 to 1, comparable to that observed with the classic Kaposi's sarcoma, but in most cases patients in Africa are significantly younger than their European counterparts [7, 10, 15].

Classical (Mediterranean) Kaposi's sarcoma

This is the original disease described by M. Kaposi in 1872 [14]. The patient is typically an elderly male and in some cases female, presenting with gross oedema of both legs and multiple Kaposi's sarcoma lesions, particularly in the upper thighs and groin. The natural course of disease is indolent; the main symptoms are swelling and stiffening of the legs. Visceral involvement is uncommon.

Paediatric (lymphadenopathic) Kaposi's sarcoma

This variant of Kaposi's sarcoma is also seen in Africa, primarily in children. In these cases, the generalized lymphadenopathy is frequently associated with organ involvement. The prognosis is very poor with 100% fatality within 3 years [7, 10].

Epidemic (HIV-related) Kaposi's sarcoma

The clinical features of HIV-related Kaposi's sarcoma are characterized by extreme variability [1, 2, 9, 10, 8, 15, 16, 17, 28, 29]. The clinical patterns vary from small cutaneous Kaposi's sarcoma lesions to patients presenting aggressive disease involving multiple cutaneous sites, with extensive oedema and involvement of major organs, especially the lung and GI tract [7, 10]. The psychological burden of HIV-related Kaposi's sarcoma should not be underestimated. Kaposi's sarcoma can be used as a barometer of underlying immunosuppression: each new lesion reminds patients that their immune system is failing. Kaposi's sarcoma is highly visible disease. This can cause patients to feel outcast from their community or social group. The classic clinical presentation of cutaneous epidemic Kaposi's sarcoma is given in Figure 1.

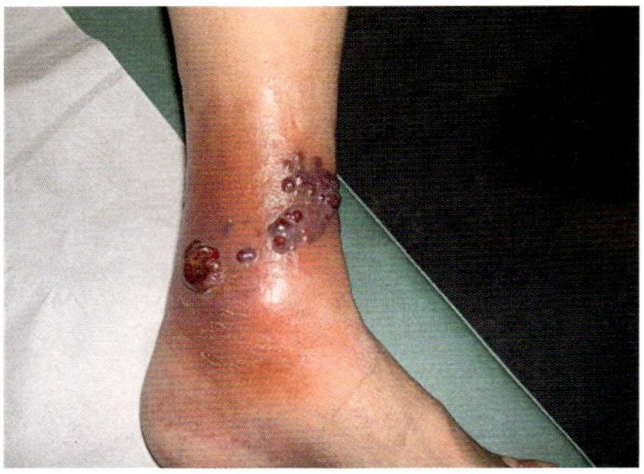

Fig. 1. Clinical presentation of epidemic Kaposi's sarcoma.

Diagnosis and staging

Diagnosis can only be made when histological proof of Kaposi's sarcoma is obtained. The most useful classification is that of the AIDS Clinical Trials Group (ACTG) staging system for AIDS related malignancies (Table 1) [17]. This classification is also applicable to classical, endemic, and paediatric Kaposi's sarcoma with involvement of cutaneous and muco-cutaneous structures, lymph nodes and visceral organs.

Table 1 – ACTG Staging System for Kaposi's sarcoma (KS).

	Good risk (0) All of the following	Poor risk Any of the following
Tumour (T)	Confined to skin and/or lymph nodes and/or minimal oral disease (non-nodular KS confined to the palate)	T-associated oedema or ulceration Extensive oral KS GI KS KS in other non-nodal viscera
Immune system (I) **Systemic illness (S)**	CD4 cells =/> 200 microL No history of OI or thrush No "B" symptoms (fever, night sweats, > 10% weight loss, diarrhea more than 2 weeks) PS > 70 Karnofsky	CD4 cells =/< 200 microL History of OI or thrush "B" symptoms (fever, night sweats, >10% weight loss, diarrhea more than 2 weeks) PS =/< 70 Karnofsky Other HIV-related illness (neurological disease, LNH)

Management

The management of Kaposi's sarcoma must be tailored to the clinical and social circumstances of the individual patient [7, 10, 19, and 20]. Watchful waiting strategy is a perfectly legitimate strategy. Given the heterogeneity of the disease itself, and the heterogeneity of the circumstances in which it is encountered, there is no universal imperative dictating immediate intervention. The normal rules of palliative treatment apply: in particular, the concept that the treatment should not be worse than the disease itself [10]. The management of Kaposi's sarcoma depends also on the clinical type and the stage of disease. For AIDS patients the treatment must take into account not only tumour regression but also the potential effects of any treatment on the patient's immune and haematological status [7].

Systemic treatment

The antiviral treatment is currently a part of the life of HIV+ patients.

Kaposi's sarcoma may be amenable to immunotherapy because of its clear association with immunodeficiency status.

Cytotoxic chemotherapy is the treatment used for patients with widespread cutaneous or visceral Kaposi's sarcoma or progressive disease. In some cases of non-HIV related tumours new anti-angiogenic treatments could be used [24]. The growing knowledge of Kaposi's sarcoma biology provides multiple opportunities for rational targeted therapies. Further research is needed to better understand the mechanisms by which Kaposi's sarcoma develops and to develop therapeutic strategies that prevent resistance to treatment [8].

Radiotherapy

Radiotherapy is the mainstay of local treatment for Kaposi's sarcoma [1-6, 10, 15, 16, 18, 22, 26-28]. Orthovoltage is suitable for the treatment of solitary lesions. The use of bolus is required when using megavoltage machines and electrons [10, 16]. The ICRU recommendations must be respected [11, 12]. Small localized lesions of Kaposi's sarcoma may be treated by local field irradiation and excellent response rates were obtained with doses as low as 20 Gy. Various doses and schedules have been reported for the treatment of endemic Kaposi's sarcoma, varying from a single dose of 8 Gy to fractionated regimens of 40-45 Gy [5, 6, 16]. Stelzer [27] randomized skin lesions to one of 3 regimens: single fraction of 8 Gy; 20 Gy in 10 fractions and 40 Gy in 20 fractions. Complete response (CR) rates (CR 79% and 83%) and duration of control was superior in the 20 and 40 Gy arms to the single fraction arm (CR 50%). Acute and late toxicities did not exceed RTOG grade I and were more pronounced with higher doses. In the series of Creteil, France [16] a 92% objective response (CR 66%; PR 26%) was reported for 6,464 skin lesions treated by two split-course protocols of 10 Gy in 4 fractions (low dose) or 20 Gy in 8 fractions (high dose) followed by a rest, then a boost of 10 Gy in 4 fractions. The high dose regimen delivered a total dose of 30 Gy in 12 fractions over 5 weeks.

Oral lesions of Kaposi's sarcoma treated by radiotherapy have been associated with severe mucositis following conventional doses in HIV-positive patients [4, 16, 26]. Chak *et al.* [4] in their 9 patients progressively reduced doses to the oral cavity using 2 Gy fractions from a total of 18 Gy eventually down to 12 Gy. The experience of Creteil showed good response rates and well tolerated treatment with a total dose of 15.2 Gy and 1.6-1.9 Gy/fraction, 7.6-8Gy/week) [16, 28].

Kaposi's sarcoma of genitals (penis, scrotum) has been treated with radiotherapy [1, 14, 16] in doses ranging from single fractions of 6 Gy to 20 Gy in 4 or more fractions. No specific problems have been noted regarding treatment responses or reactions at the site [10].

Small lesions of eyelids and conjunctiva can be irradiated effectively with orthovoltage therapy or electron beams using internal and external eye shields for lens protection with varying doses [10, 16]. Local reactions at doses of 20 Gy in 10 fractions are acceptable.

Radiotherapy can be used also for nodal and visceral lesions as palliative treatment with rapid relief of symptoms [10].

References

1. Belembaogo E, Kirova Y, Le Bourgeois JP (1997) Localisations génitales du sarcome de Kaposi épidémique: étude sur 71 patients. Cahiers d'Oncologie 6: 271-2

2

2. Belembaogo E, Kirova Y *et al.* (1998) Radiothérapie du sarcome de Kaposi épidémique: Expérience de l'hôpital Henri Mondor. Cancer/Radiother 2: 49-52
3. **Calitchi E, Kirova Y, Le Bourgeois JP (1998) Radiothérapie et tumeurs cutanées. Cancer/Radiother 2: 556-65**
4. Chak LY *et al.* (1988) Radiation therapy for AIDS-related Kaposi's sarcoma. J Clin Oncol 6: 863-7
5. Cohen L (1962) Dose, time and volume parameters in radiation therapy of Kaposi's sarcoma. Br J Radiol 35: 485-8
6. Cooper JS (1988) The influence of dose on the long term control of the classic Kaposi's sarcoma by radiotherapy. Int J Radiat Oncol Biol Phys 15: 1141-6
7. De Vita VT (1997) In: De Vita VT, Hellman S, Rosenberg SA (eds) Cancer: Principles and Practice of Oncology, Fifth Edition, Lippincott-Raven Publishers, Philadelphia, 1997, p. 2445-67
8. Dittmer DP, Krown SE (2007) Targeted therapy for Kaposi's sarcoma and Kaposi's sarcoma-associated herpesvirus. Curr Opin Oncol 19: 452-7
9. Hymes KB, Cheng T *et al.* (1981) Kaposi's Sarcoma in homosexual men; a report of 8 cases. Lancet 8247: 598-600
10. **IAEA-TECDOC-1224: The role of radiotherapy in the management of cancer patients infected by HIV 2001; Munro A, Kirova Y: Kaposi's sarcoma: 15-24**
11. ICRU. Report 50 (1993) Prescribing, recording, and reporting photon beam therapy. Washington DC: International Commission on Radiation Units and Measurements.
12. ICRU. Report 62: (supplement to ICRU Report 50) (1999) Prescribing, recording, and reporting photon beam therapy. Bethesda, MD: International Commission on Radiation Units and Measurements
13. Jensen KK, Manfra DJ *et al.* (2005) The human herpes virus 8-encoded chemokine receptor is required for angioproliferation in a murine model of Kaposi's sarcoma. J Immunol 174: 3686-94
14. **Kaposi M (1872) Idiopathisches multiple pigmentsarcom der haut. Arch Dermatol Syphiol 4: 256**
15. Kirova Y, Belembaogo E *et al.* (1997) Sarcome de Kaposi. Cancer/Radiother 1: 277-82
16. **Kirova Y, Belembaogo E *et al.* (1998) Radiotherapy in the Management of Epidemic Kaposi's Sarcoma. A Retrospective Study of 643 Cases. Radiother Oncol 46: 19-22**
17. Krown SE, Testa MA *et al.* (1997) AIDS-related Kaposi's sarcoma: prospective validation of the AIDS Clinical Trials Group staging classification. AIDS Clinical Trials Group Oncology Committee. J Clin Oncol 15: 3085-92
18. Le Bourgeois JP, Chavaudra J *et al.* (1992) In: Breast cancer in Radiothérapie oncologique. 2nd ed. Paris Hermann p. 237-253
19. Ledergerber B, Telenti A *et al.* (1999) Risk of HIV related Kaposi's sarcoma and non-Hodgkin's lymphoma with potent antiretroviral therapy: prospective cohort study. Swiss HIV Cohort Study. Br Med J 319: 23-4
20. Martinez V, Caumes E *et al.* (2006) Remission from Kaposi's sarcoma on HAART is associated with suppression of HIV replication and is independent of protease inhibitor therapy. Br J Cancer 94: 1000-6
21. **Mitsuyasu RT (1987) Clinical variants and staging of Kaposi's sarcoma. Semin Oncol 14 (2 Suppl 3): 13-8**
22. Perez CA, Brady LW (1992) In: Principles and practice of radiation oncology. 2nd ed. Philadelphia: J.B. Lippincott Company, p. 877-969
23. Plancoulaine S, Abel L *et al.* (2000) Human herpesvirus B transmission from mother to child and between siblings in an endemic population. Lancet 356: 1062-5
24. Rubegni P, Sbano P *et al.* (2007) Thalidomide in the treatment of Kaposi's sarcoma. Dermatology 215: 240-4
25. Siegel JH, Janis R *et al.* (1969) Disseminated visceral Kaposi's sarcoma. Appearance after human renal homograft operations. JAMA 207: 1493-6
26. Stein ME, Lakier R *et al.* (1993) Radiation therapy in endemic (African) Kaposi's sarcoma. Int J Radiat Oncol Biol Phys 27: 1181-4
27. Stelzer KJ, Griffin TW (1993) A randomized prospective trial of radiation therapy for AIDS-associated Kaposi's sarcoma. Int J Radiat Oncol Biol Phys 27: 1057-61
28. Yu SJ, Kirova Y *et al.* (1997) Oral Epidemic Kaposi's Sarcoma and Radiotherapy. Chinese Journal of Radiation Oncology 6: 179-82
29. Zoufaly A, Schmiedel S *et al.* (2007) Intestinal Kaposi's sarcoma may mimic gastrointestinal stromal tumor in HIV infection. World J Gastroenterol 13: 4514-6

Dermatofibrosarcoma protuberans (DFSP)

R.G. Panizzon

3

Five Essential Points

1. *Dermatofibrosarcoma protuberans (DFSP) is a fibrohistiocytic tumour of intermediate malignancy with a tendency to recur locally.*
2. *Young males and females are equally affected; Africans more than Caucasians. DFSP presents mostly on the trunk, as a multinodular protuberant firm tumour of blue-red colour.*
3. *The diagnosis is often made late because of the difficulty to distinguish DFSP from other mesenchymal tumours. CD34 stain is of help as stromelysin-3. DFSP is characterized by an infiltrative growth of the subcutaneous or muscular tissue.*
4. *Wide excision with a margin of 3 to 5 cm is the treatment of choice with Moh's or micrographic surgery, especially for local recurrences.*
5. *Local recurrences or metastases may be treated by radiotherapy or the tyrosine kinase antagonist Imatinib mesylate.*

Definition

Dermatofibrosarcoma protuberans (DFSP) is a malignant fibrohistiocytic tumour of intermediate malignancy of the skin which grows locally with infiltration and rarely metastasizes [27]. The tumour is mainly localized on the trunk and proximal extremities and tends to recur locally [10, 21]. The tumour is encountered in 1 per 100.000 inhabitants/year. The mean age of these patients is around 40 years [3, 14]. Tumours may occur already in childhood and there are also descriptions of congenital tumours [25]. Often the juvenile precursor lesion of DFSP is called giant cell fibroblastoma [17]. The tumour is equally frequent in men and women and the mortality rate is low.

Pathogenesis

The pathogenesis of DFSP is not clearly understood. New genetic research has found some chromosome translocations which show a fusion in chromosome regions of 17q22 and 22q13. This gene location is exactly the same as the codons of alpha-helix of type 1 collagen (COL 1A 19) and the beta chain of the platelet-derived growth factor (PDGF beta). These ring chromosomes express COL1A 1-PDGF beta-fusion protein which is the continuous stimulator of DFSP cells in the way PDGF receptor is bound [20]. This new finding could point the way towards a pathogenetically-based therapy.

Table 1 – Distribution of Dermatofibrosarcoma protuberans (AFIP).

Trunk	47.4 %
Lower extremity	19.9 %
Upper extremity	18.2 %
Head and neck	14.5 %

Diagnosis

Clinical findings

DFSP is mostly a skin coloured sometimes brown-yellow or reddish non-characteristic, elevated, firm and irregularly shaped and sometimes multinodular tumour of several years development (Fig. 1). An exact clinical diagnosis is often impossible. The extension of the tumour is often seen at the dermal-subcutaneous border but is also seen in the deeper subcutaneous or in the muscular tissue [2]. Very often the diagnosis is made by incisional biopsies, more rarely in excisional biopsies.

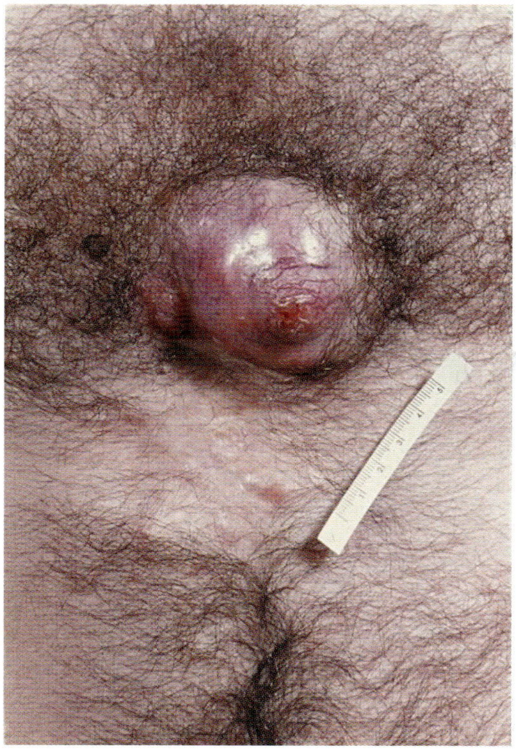

Fig. 1. Clinical appearance of Dermatofibrosarcoma protuberans in a 28-years-old man.

Histopathology

The histopathological findings show densely arranged atypical spindel and pleomorphic cells with a characteristic cartwheel or woven pattern (Fig. 2). Differentiation from dermatofibroma or dermatomyofibroma is mostly made by immunohistochemistry with CD34 or factor XIIIa staining [8, 26, 28]. DFSP shows regular positivity with CD34 whereas the antifactor XIIIa is often negative. Recently it was shown that with the help of Stromelysin-3 expression a differen-

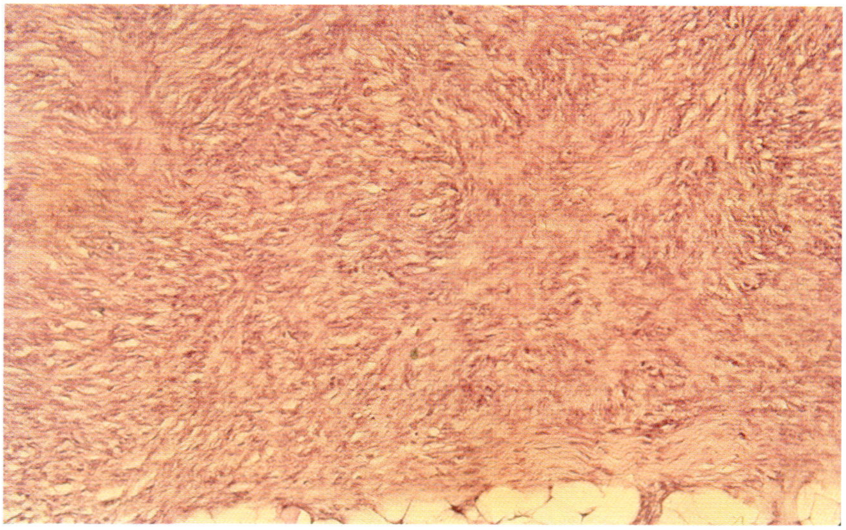

Fig. 2. Histological picture of Dermatofibrosarcoma protuberans HE, objective × 10.

tiation of dermatofibroma from dermatofibrosarcoma protuberans is possible [6]. Sometimes DFSP cells may contain melanin and then are called Bednar tumour. Sometimes less differentiated fibrosarcomatous areas can be found in DFSP which are less clearly stained with CD34 [10, 13]. These areas could be responsible for recurrence or even metastasis [5]. Furthermore one may distinguish myxoid types of DSFP [29]. The tumour regularly infiltrates in the deeper dermis and the subcutaneous structures, while a perineural growth is also described. DFSP is specified as a fibrohistiocytic tumour with intermediate malignancy.

Diagnosis of tumour spread

In case of recurrences or doubt of metastatic spread, an ultrasound of lymph nodes or a thorax X-Ray is recommended. Tumour extension can also be estimated by CT or MRI imaging [24]. However, the fine subclinical extension of this tumour should be kept in mind.

Prognosis and staging

DFSP is a locally infiltrating tumour and therefore local recurrence is quite frequent, and is strongly related to the treatment applied. In the literature, local recurrences are described in up to 80% of patients, while on the other hand, lymph node metastases are seldom described. Lung metastases occur rarely – in about 5% of the cases, especially in locally recurrent tumours or those with a fibrosarcomatous pattern [9, 13].

A simple staging with 3 levels is proposed:

- Stage 1: sole primary tumour
- Stage 2: loco-regional recurrence
- Stage 3: distant metastases.

It has also been proposed to differentiate stage 1a without, and 1b with a sarcomatous pattern.

Treatment modalities

Surgical treatment

Surgical treatment is the treatment of choice of DSFP. Since we have to consider a locally aggressive and infiltrating pattern with subclinical extension, particularly in horizontal direction, microscopically controlled surgery is of major importance and is characterized by a low recurrence rate. Depending on excision margins the reported recurrence rates were for 1 cm 70.7%, with 2 cm 39.7%, with 3 cm 15.5% and with 5 cm 5.2 % [19].

Microscopically controlled surgery (MCS)/Moh's surgery

The MCS or Moh's surgery should be done with paraffin sections, since cryosections are insufficiently sensitive [11]. With the Moh's technique, a topographically exact analysis of the dermal-subcutaneous extension and characterization contributes to and guarantees tumour free excision margins. In addition, immunohistochemical staining with CD34 may be necessary. The excision margin in primary excision should be at least between 3 cm and 5 cm. In very extensive tumours or in difficult localizations the site of the excision should be left open until there is evidence of complete excision. This is not only important for safety reasons but also considering the cosmetic result.

With this method the local recurrence rate is between 0 and 3%. Nouri *et al.* reported that in a review of 221 patients with DFSP treated by MCS only 5 (2.3%) had a recurrence [15].

Conventional surgery

All non microscopically-controlled surgical procedures can give rise to high recurrence rates since DFSP is characterized by local and deep infiltration and the recurrence rate is higher. Kimmel *et al.* showed though, on an investigation of 98 patients, that if a standard width of excision margin of 4 cm is respected, the clearance rate will be 95% [7].

Table 2 – Recurrence rate (RR) metastases in DFSP.

Author	RR %	Meta %	Meta/wide exc.
Diaz-Cascajo [4]	–	–	1/3
Goldblum [5]	22	0	0/18
Mentzel [12]	58	14.7	0/6
O'Connell [16]	–	–	0/2
Pizarro [18]	42	33	–

Radiotherapy

DFSP is considered a relatively radiosensitive tumour since with postoperative radiation, the risk of local recurrence can be markedly reduced although there are several reports of high recurrence rates [22]. Primary inoperable tumours are an indication for radiotherapy, or if there is a postoperative situation with insufficient margin clearance. Radiotherapy may also be considered after multiple recurrences. The irradiation field comprises the primary tumour site, the postoperative scar and a safety margin of 3 to 5 cm. The total dose is in the range of 46 to 60 Gy with conventional fractionation [23].

Ballo *et al.* investigated 16 patients who received radiation therapy for DFSP and whose resection margins were either positive or negative [1]. The only patient who showed recurrence six years after treatment was one with gross disease, *i.e.* a control of 95%.

Systemic therapy

Up to now an efficient chemotherapy has not been identified. Recently, there have been reports of DFSP cases where the expression of synthesis of COLIAI-PDGF/3 is present and where the stimulation of the DFSP cells through a PDGF beta-receptor could be inhibited with a tyrosine kinase-inhibitor [20, 22]. Treatment with Imatinib/ST-S71 (Glivec) is possible. Studies are ongoing with this treatment modality.

Follow-up

Guidelines for follow-up of DFSP have not been specified. In order to detect local recurrences as early as possible, clinical check-ups are necessary. We recommend three-monthly check-ups during the first year, then every 6 months for another two years, and then once yearly thereafter. During follow-up, the patient should be checked for lymph node and possibly distant metastases.

References

1. Ballo MT, Zagars GK, Pisters P *et al.* (1998) The role of radiation therapy in the management of dermatofibrosarcoma protuberans. Int J Radiat Oncol Biol Phys 40: 823-7
2. Brabant B, Revol M, Vergote T *et al.* (1993) Dermatofibrosarcoma protuberans of the chest and the shoulder. Plast Reconstr Surg 92: 459-62
3. Criscione VD, Weinstock MA (2007) Descriptive epidemiology of dermatofibrosarcoma protuberans in the US, 1973 to 2002. J Am Acad Dermatol 56: 968-73
4. Diaz-Cascajo C, Weyers W, Borrego L *et al.* (1997) Dermatofibrosarcoma protuberans with fibrosarcomatous areas. Am J Dermatopathol 19: 562
5. Goldblum JR, Reith JD, Weiss SW (2000) Sarcomas arising in dermatofibrosarcoma protuberans. Am J Surg Pathol 24: 1125-30
6. Kim HJ, Lee JY, Seo YJ *et al.* (2007) Stromelysin-3 expression in the differential diagnosis of dermatofibroma and dermatofibrosarcoma protuberans. Br J Dermatol 157: 319-24
7. **Kimmel Z, Ratner D, Kim JY *et al.* (2007) Peripheral excision margins for dermatofibrosarcoma protuberans. Ann Surg Oncol 14: 2113-20**
8. Kutzner H (1993) Expression of the human progenitor cell antigen CD 34 (HPCA-1) distinguishes dermatofibrosarcoma protuberans from fibrous histiocytoma in formalin-fixed paraffin-embedded tissue. J Am Acad Dermatol 28: 613-7
9. Lal P, Sharma R, Mohan H *et al.* (1999) Dermatofibrosarcoma protuberans metastasizing to lymph nodes. J Surg Oncol 72: 178-80
10. Lopes JM, Paiva ME (1991) Dermatofibrosarcoma protuberans. A histological and ultrastructural study of 11 cases with emphasis on the study of recurrences and histogenesis. Pathol Res Pract 187: 806-13
11. Massey RA, Tok J, Strippoli BA *et al.* (1998) A comparison of frozen and paraffin sections in dermatofibrosarcoma protuberans. Dermatol Surg 24: 995-8
12. Mentzel T, Beham A, Katemkamp D *et al.* (1998) Fibrosarcomatous ("high grade") dermatofibrosarcoma protuberans. Am J Surg Pathol 22: 576
13. Minter RM, Reith JD, Hochwald SN (2003) Metastatic potential of dermatofibrosarcoma protuberans with fibrosarcomatous change. J Surg Oncol 82: 201-8

3

14. **Monnier D, Vidal C, Martin L *et al.* (2006) Dermatofibrosarcoma protuberans: a population based cancer registry. J Eur Acad Dermatol Venereol 20: 1237-42**
15. Nouri K, Lodha R, Jimenez G *et al.*. (2002) Mohs micrographic surgery for dermatofibrosarcoma protuberans. Derm Surg 28: 1060-4
16. O'Connel JX, Trotter MJ (1996) Fibrosarcomatous dermatofibrosarcoma protuberans: a variant. Mod Pathol 9: 273
17. Perry D, Schultz L, Dehner L (1993) Giant cell fibroblastoma with dermatofibrosarcoma protuberans-like transformation. J Cut Pathol 20: 451-4
18. Pizarro GB, Fanburg JC, Miettinen M (1997) Dermatofibrosarcoma protuberans with fibrosarcomatous transformation: re-explored. Mod Pathol 10: 13A
19. Ratner D, Thomas CO, Johnson TM *et al.* (1997) Mohs micrographic surgery for the treatment of dermatofibrosarcoma protuberans. J Am Acad Dermatol 37: 600-13
20. Rubin BP, Schnetze SM, Eary JF *et al.* (2002) Molecular targeting of platelet derived growth factor B by imatinib mesylate in a patient with metastatic dermatofibrosarcoma protuberans. J Clin Oncol 20: 3586-91
21. Smola MG, Soyer HP, Scharnagl E (1991) Surgical treatment of dermatofibrosarcoma protuberans. A retrospective study of 20 cases with review of the literature. Eur J Surg Oncol 17: 447-53
22. **Sirvent N, Maire G, Pedeutour F (2003) Genetics of dermatofibrosarcoma protuberans family of tumors. From ring chromosomes to tyrosine kinase inhibitor treatment. Gens Chromosomes Cancer 37: 1-19**
23. **Sun LM, Wang CJ, Huang CC *et al.* (2000) Dermatofibrosarcoma protuberans: treatment results of 35 cases. Radiother Oncol 57: 157-81**
24. Torregiani WC, Al-Ismail K, Munk PL *et al.* (2002) Dermatofibrosarcoma protuberans:MR imaging features. Am J Roentgenol 178: 989-93
25. Weinstein JM, Drolet BA, Esterly BN *et al.* (2003) Congenital dermatofibrosarcoma protuberans. Arch Dermatol 139: 207-11
26. Weiss SW, Nickoloff BJ (1993) CD34 is expressed by a distinctive cell population in peripheral nerve, nerve sheath tumors and related lesions. Am J Surg Pathol 17: 1039-45
27. **Weiss SW (2008) Fibrohistiocytic tumors of intermediate malignancy. In: Enzinger-Weiss (eds) Soft tissue tumors. Mosby, pp 371-402**
28. Wick MR, Ritter JH, Lind AC *et al.* (1999) The pathological distinction between deep penetrating dermatofibroma and dermatofibrosarcoma protuberans. Semin Cutan Med Surg 18: 91-8
29. Zamecnik M, Michal M, Mukensnabl P (1998) Composite tumor consisting of dermatofibrosarcoma protuberans and myxofibrosarcoma. J Cut Pathol 25: 445-9

Merkel cell carcinoma: A challenge in cancer management

4

K.T. Beer

Five Essential Points

1. *MCC is an aggressive skin tumour which varies widely in clinical presentation.*
2. *An interdisciplinary approach is needed to provide optimal therapy.*
3. *The mainstay of curative treatments are radical surgery for primary tumour and lymph nodes and postoperative radiotherapy.*
4. *Lymphatic skip lesions are common and present a challenge for the definition of radiotherapy volumes.*
5. *The role of chemotherapy in locoregional disease is not yet defined and chemotherapy should be used within protocols.*

Introduction

Merkel cell carcinoma (MCC) is a rare tumour entity that has recently attracted the interest of oncologists. Often various specialists are involved in the treatment of MCC, such as general practitioners, plastic surgeons, dermatologists, medical oncologists, and radiation oncologists, each with a different approach to treatment options. In such rare tumour entities, this type of non-standardised management complicates the establishment and improvement of definitive treatment concepts [4, 27]. This chapter gives an overview of the pertinent diagnostic and therapeutic questions with regard to MCC.

MC was described for the first time by Toker in 1972 as a "trabecular carcinoma of the skin" [43, 44]. The cellular origin of this tumour was unclear at that time and, for this reason, the condition was given numerous other names, such as primary small cell carcinoma of the skin, primary neuroendocrine carcinoma of the skin, cutaneous apudoma, extrapulmonary carcinoid of the skin. Finally, Merkel cell carcinoma was adopted after a malignant transformation of Merkel cells, located in the basal layer of the epidermis became the supposed cause of this tumour [28, 40].

Epidemiology

MCC accounts for less than 1% of cutaneous malignancies. In a study of 1,124 cases of MCC identified in the Surveillance, Epidemiology, and End Results (SEER) database, the incidence increased over a 15-year period, from 0.15 cases per 100,000 in 1986 to 0.44 cases per 100,000 in 2001. Overall, the 2-year survival rate is 50-70%, depending on the stage (see below). Interestingly, survival is higher in women than in men. Caucasians have a 20-fold increased age-adjusted relative risk of developing MCC compared to Africans. The gender incidence reported in most studies is approximately equal for males and females, although some authors report an elevated female-to-male ratio of up to 4:1. The mean patient age at diagnosis is about 75 years, only 5% of cases occurring before 50 years [1, 36].

Clinical appearance and etiology

MCC usually appears as firm, painless, shiny lumps on the skin, red, pink, or blue in color and varying in size [3, 13, 15, 21, 22, 34]. Figures 1 and 2 are two exam-

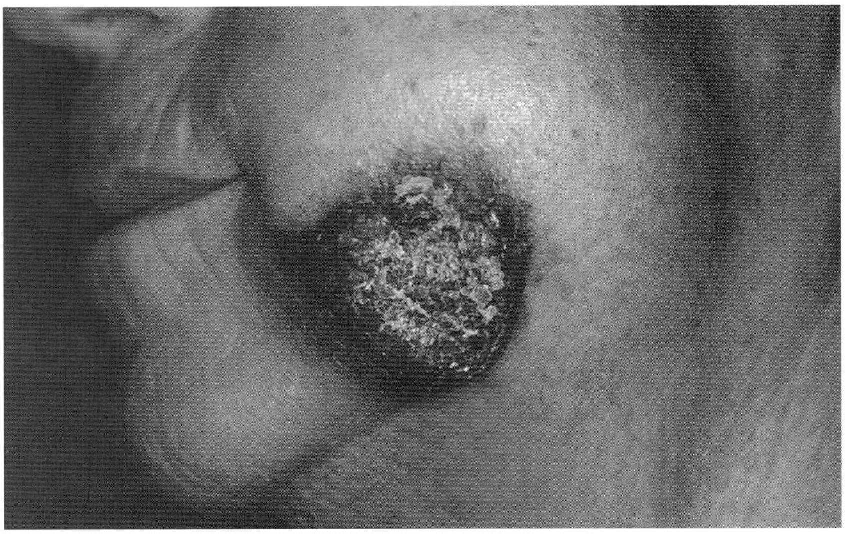

Fig. 1. Locally advanced Merkel cell carcinoma.

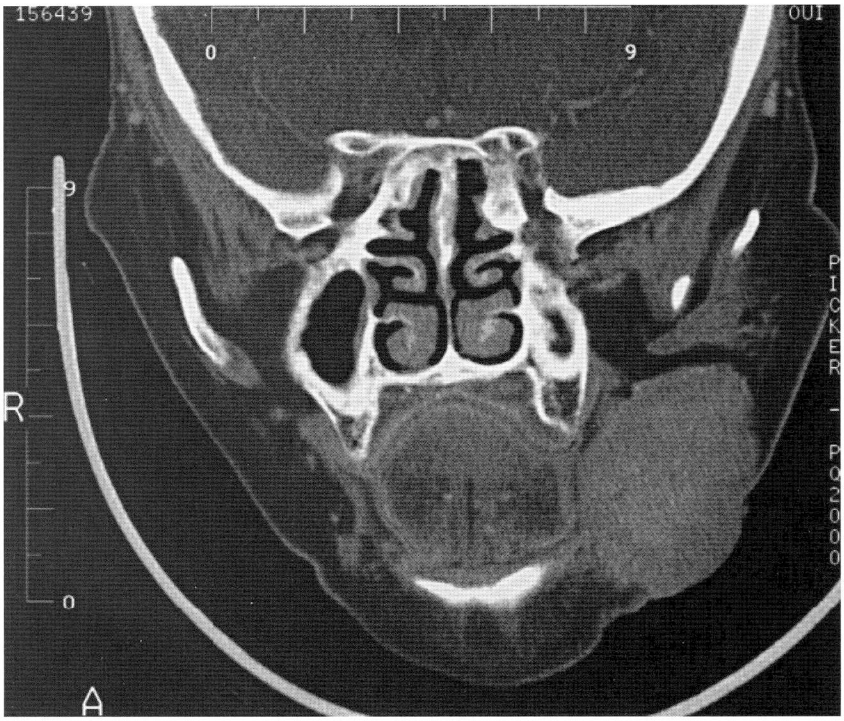

Fig. 2. Sagittal CAT reconstruction of the tumour in Figure 1.

ples of the possible clinical and radiological presentation of Merkel cell carcinoma. MCC is usually found on sun-exposed areas of the head, neck, arms, and legs. It grows rapidly and metastasizes often, even if the primary tumour is relatively small, to regional lymph nodes with haematogenous spread to bone, liver, lungs, and brain. The rate of distant metastases is in a range of 20 to 50% after initial treatment [34, 36]. Despite the typical presentation as a small primary tumour, occult or overt metastases are detected in 10 to 30% of cases at the time of the diagnosis. In addition, there is a high rate of nodal relapse (50 to 75%) and systemic relapse (30 to 50%) after local treatment. MCC can mimic other malignant skin lesions such as melanoma, adnexal tumours or lymphoma by clinical appearance [3], so an initial diagnosis has frequently to be revised. An etiologic role for chronic exposure to solar ultraviolet radiation (UVR) is suggested, mainly due to the markedly increased risk for Caucasian patients as opposed to African patients and the predominant location of MCC on sites of maximal cumulative UVR exposure, such as the head and neck region. Both the frequency and the aggressiveness of MCC increase after immunosuppression, organ transplantation, and B-cell neoplasia. MCC is not associated with Epstein-Barr virus or human papilloma-virus infection. Recently, a novel polyomavirus has been described in a series of MCC patients, suggesting that such tumours may be caused by a virus, such as others that occur with increased frequency in immunosuppressed patients [10, 18].

Histology

Merkel cell carcinoma is usually found within the dermis but may extend into the subcutaneous tissue. The combination of vesicular nuclei with small nucleoli, abundant mitoses, and apoptosis is characteristic of this tumour. Morphologically several differential diagnoses are considered, such as melanoma, lymphoma or extraskeletal Ewing sarcoma [40, 41]. With electron microscopy the presence of dense granula, associated with the neuro-secretory membrane points to its neuroendocrine origin [13, 44]. Nowadays, the diagnosis of MCC is based on immunohistochemical assessment. MCC often shows a specific immuno-histochemical expression of neuron-specific enolase (NSE), cytokeratin 20, neurofilament, synaptophysin, CD 57, and chromogranin A [26, 28]. Histologically, MCC has been classified into three distinct subtypes [17, 20, 37]: trabecular (the least frequent), intermediate (the most frequent, aggressive), and small cell.

Stage

No widely accepted or standardised staging classification according to prognosis is available. A commonly used staging system is based on clinical presentation:

- *Stage IA:* Primary tumour smaller than 2 cm with no evidence of spread to lymph nodes or distant sites.
- *Stage IB:* Primary tumour 2 cm or larger with no evidence of spread to lymph nodes or distant sites.
- *Stage II:* Regional node involvement but no evidence of distant metastases.
- *Stage III:* Presence of systemic metastases beyond the regional lymph nodes.

Diagnostic work up

Suspect lesions should be biopsied and an immuno-histological work up is mandatory to exclude other, more common skin tumours. According to the clinical presentation, a staging procedure including CT scan of the head and neck, thorax, abdomen and pelvis is advised [16]. Indium octreotide scintigraphy can be used to stage primary and metastatic disease [19].

Currently, the role of PET/PET-CT is under evaluation for staging [24, 39].

Treatment options

In general, surgery is the first therapeutic measure. Generous margins of 3 cm are recommended, although compromises have to be made for radicality according to the localisation of the tumour. The regional lymph nodes are resected simultaneously with the primary tumour, often with a sentinel lymphadenectomy [2, 48]. To evaluate locoregional lymph node metastases a sentinel node biopsy is frequently performed [30]. Radiotherapy is used to improve local and regional control as MCC is extremely radiosensitive [25]. However, despite radical locoregional treatment, local recurrences are frequent with concomitant lymphatic and hematogeneous metastases. Although the true value of cytostatic treatment is still unknown, various chemotherapeutic schemes are reported to be effective.

Management by stage

Stage I Merkel Cell Carcinoma

Wide local excision has been recommended whenever possible for patients with stage I MCC [2, 6, 48]. Frozen section control has also been recommended, especially when the tumour is in an anatomical site not amenable to wide margins. Some authors have advocated the use of Mohs micrographic surgery as a tissue-sparing technique [6]. The reported relapse rate is similar to or better than that of wide excision, but comparatively few cases have been treated in this manner and definitive clinical studies have yet to be conducted. The role of elective lymph node dissection (ELND) in the absence of clinically positive nodes is unclear. ELND has been recommended for larger tumours, tumours with more than 10 mitoses per high-power field, lymphatic or vascular invasion, and the small-cell histologic subtypes. Sentinel lymph node (SLN) biopsy has been suggested as an alternative to complete ELND for the proper staging of MCC. SLN biopsy has a lower morbidity than complete nodal dissection. Furthermore, for MCC sites with uncertain lymphatic drainage, such as those on the back, SLN biopsy techniques can be used to identify the pertinent lymph node beds. Several authors have found the use of SLN biopsy techniques in patients with MCC to be reliable and reproducible while a meta-analysis showed that SLN positivity is strongly predictive of a high short-term risk of recurrence and that subsequent therapeutic lymph node dissection was effective in preventing short-term regional nodal recurrence [31,47]. Because of the aggressive nature of MCC and the high incidence of locoregional recurrence after surgery alone, many authors advocate adjuvant radiation therapy to the primary site and to the regional lymph node bed [29]. Data from prospective, randomised trials are not available. Retrospective studies have reported that radiation therapy was used in patients with larger tumours, tumours with lymphatic invasion, tumours approaching the surgical margins and locally unresectable tumours. Improved locoregional control has been achieved with resection followed by radiation therapy as compared to surgery alone in these retrospective non-randomized reports [9, 23]. Studies suggest that the appropriate total dose is about 50 Gy to the surgical bed and the draining regional lymphatics, delivered in 2 Gy fractions [5, 9, 33]. For patients with unresected tumours or tumours with microscopic evidence of spread beyond the resected margins, higher doses of 56 Gy to 65 Gy have been recommended [8, 30, 32, 33]. A study by Müller *et al.* [34] gives a locoregional recurrence rate of 65% in stage I patients after surgery alone. With additional RT, the rate decreased to 43%. There are hints that recurrences develop predominently outside the radiotherapy volume in non-metastasizing disease, indicating the need to choose the appropriate treatment volumes judiciously [38].

Stage II Merkel Cell Carcinoma

In the literature, lymphatic recurrence rates of more than 50% are found after surgery alone [34]. As discussed previously, one difficulty is the erratic lymphatic spread of MCC and consequently, the definition of the extent of the lymphatic resection or, in the case of radiotherapy, of the treatment volume since so-called skip lesions do not follow a regular pattern of spread. Therefore, there is no standard in the literature with regard to lymphatic irradiation. Wide local excision of the primary tumour, whenever possible, and regional lymph node dissection have been recommended for patients with stage II MCC [23, 29]. Many authors advocate adjuvant radiation therapy to the primary site and to the regional lymph node bed [5, 33]. Again, and similar to Stage I, data from prospective, randomised trials are not available. Based on available retrospective reviews, radiation therapy has also been used.

Postoperative radiation therapy can improve locoregional control in stage II patients compared to surgery alone and can also improve survival [32]. Recommended doses are the same as those used in Stage I tumours. The role of adjuvant chemotherapy remains unproven but is advocated by some authors because of similarities between small cell lung cancer and MCC [42]. Studies have shown response rates of around 60% in the setting of locally advanced or metastatic disease using the same chemotherapy regimens as those used in patients with small cell lung cancer [11, 35]. The benefit of adjuvant chemotherapy has yet to be determined. Recently, it has been suggested that gene-expression profiling could establish distinct patterns for MCC subgroups and distinguish MCC from small cell lung cancer [45].

Stage III Merkel Cell Carcinoma

Chemotherapy is the most often used treatment for patients with stage III MCC [42]. The regimens employed are similar to those used for patients with small cell lung cancer. Cyclophosphamide, doxorubicin, vincristine and etoposide plus cisplatin are the most commonly used combinations. MCC often responds to chemotherapy initially, but this is usually short-lived and the impact on survival is uncertain. A recent phase II study has demonstrated the tolerability of chemotherapy in MCC [35]. However, its value in terms of improved survival, local control, and decreased distant metastases, remains to be defined [12, 46].

4

Recurrent Merkel Cell Carcinoma

Treatment options for patients with local recurrence include regional lymph node dissection and adjuvant radiation therapy if the regional nodes have not been previously treated. An alternative approach for patients who have not had a complete regional lymph node dissection would be a sentinel lymph node biopsy and complete nodal dissection if positive nodes are identified. When possible, adjuvant radiation therapy to the site of recurrence as well as to the regional lymph nodes is recommended after surgery. Chemotherapy may be an option for patients with unresectable recurrent tumours or for patients who have received their maximum tolerated radiation dose. Current research emphasises gene expression profiles to customise future treatment options [7].

References

1. Agelli M, Clegg LX (2003) Epidemiology of primary Merkel cell carcinoma in the United States. J Am Acad Dermatol 49: 832-41
2. Allen PJ, Zhang ZF, Coit DG (1999) Surgical management of Merkel cell carcinoma. Ann Surg;229: 97-105
3. Aydin A, Kocer NE, Bekerecioglu M *et al.* (2003) Cutaneous undifferentiated small (Merkel) cell carcinoma, that developed synchronously with multiple actinic keratoses, squamous cell carcinomas and basal cell carcinoma. J Dermatol 30: 241-4
4. **Bichakjian CK, Lowe L, Lao CD *et al.* (2007) Merkel cell carcinoma: critical review with guidelines for multidisciplinary management. Cancer 110: 1-12**
5. Bischof M, van Kampen M, Huber P *et al.* (1999) Merkel cell carcinoma: the role of radiation therapy in general management. Strahlenther Onkol 175: 611-5
6. Boyer JD, Zitelli JA, Brodland DG *et al.* (2002) Local control of primary Merkel cell carcinoma: review of 45 cases treated with Mohs micrographic surgery with and without adjuvant radiation. J Am Acad Dermatol 47: 885-92
7. Brunner M, Thurnher D, Pammer J *et al.* (2008) Expression of VEGF-A/C, VEGF-R2, PDGF-alpha/beta, c-kit, EGFR, Her-2/Neu, Mcl-1 and Bmi-1 in Merkel cell carcinoma. Mod Pathol 21: 876-84
8. Decker RH, Wilson LD (2006) Role of radiotherapy in the management of merkel cell carcinoma of the skin. J Natl Compr Canc Netw 4: 713-8
9. Eich HT, Eich D, Staar S *et al.* (2002) Role of postoperative RT in the management of Merkel cell carcinoma. Am J Clin Oncol 25: 50-6
10. **Feng H, Shuda M, Chang Y *et al.* (2008) Clonal integration of a polyomavirus in human Merkel cell carcinoma. Science 319: 1096-100**
11. Feun LG, Savaraj N, Legha SS *et al.* (1988) Chemotherapy for metastatic Merkel cell carcinoma. Review of the M.D. Anderson Hospital's experience. Cancer 62: 683-5
12. Garneski KM, Nghiem P (2007) Merkel cell carcinoma adjuvant therapy: current data support radiation but not chemotherapy. J Am Acad Dermatol 57: 166-9
13. Gloor F, Heitz PU, Hofmann E *et al.* (1982) The neuroendocrine Merkel cell carcinoma of the skin. Switzerland Med Wochenschr 112: 141-8
14. Goessling W, McKee PH, Mayer RJ (2002) Merkel cell carcinoma. J Clin Oncol 20: 588-98
15. Gollard R, Weber R, Kosty MP *et al.* (2000) Merkel cell carcinoma: review of 22 cases with surgical, pathologic, and therapeutic considerations. Cancer 88: 1842-51
16. Gollub MJ, Gruen DR, Dershaw DD (1996) Merkel cell carcinoma: CT findings in 12 patients. Am J Roentgenol 167: 617-20
17. Gould VE, Moll R, Moll I *et al.* (1985) Neuroendocrine (Merkel) cells of the skin: hyperplasias, dysplasias, and neoplasms. Lab Invest 52: 334-53
18. Guillot B, Foulongne V, Dereure O *et al.* (2008) Merkel cell carcinoma: A new virus linked to a rare form of cancer. Ann Dermatol Venereol 135: 637-8

19. Guitera-Rovel P, Lumbroso J, Gautier-Gougis MS *et al.* (2001) Indium-111 octreotide scintigraphy of Merkel cell carcinomas and their metastases. Ann Oncol 12: 807-11
20. Haag ML, Glass LF, Fenske NA (1995) Merkel cell carcinoma. Diagnosis and treatment. Dermatol Surg 2: 669-83
21. **Heath M, Jaimes N, Lemos B *et al.* (2008) Clinical characteristics of Merkel cell carcinoma at diagnosis in 195 patients: the AEIOU features. J Am Acad Dermatol 58: 375-81**
22. Helmbold P, Schroter S, Holzhausen HJ *et al.* (2001) Merkel cell carcinoma: a diagnostic and therapeutic challenge. Chirurg 72: 396-401
23. Herbst A, Haynes HA, Nghiem P (2002) The standard of care for Merkel cell carcinoma should include adjuvant radiation and lymph node surgery. J Am Acad Dermatol 46: 640-2
24. Iagaru A, Quon A, McDougall IR *et al.* (2006) Merkel cell carcinoma: Is there a role for 2-deoxy-2-[f-18]fluoro-D-glucose-positron emission tomography/computed tomography? Mol Imaging Biol 8: 212-7
25. **Jabbour J, Cumming R, Scolyer RA *et al.* (2007) Merkel cell carcinoma: assessing the effect of wide local excision, lymph node dissection, and radiotherapy on recurrence and survival in early-stage disease – results from a review of 82 consecutive cases diagnosed between 1992 and 2004. Ann Surg Oncol 14: 1943-52**
26. Kurokawa M, Nabeshima K, Akiyama Y *et al.* (2003) CD56: a useful marker for diagnosing Merkel cell carcinoma. Dermatol Sci 31: 219-24
27. Longo MI, Nghiem P (2003) Merkel cell carcinoma treatment with radiation: a good case despite no prospective studies. Arch Dermatol 139: 1641-3
28. Mackintosh J, Willis EJ, Friedlander M (1988) Merkel Cell Tumours. In: Williams CJ, Krikorian JG, Green MR, Raghavan D, eds. Textbook of uncommon cancer. John Wiley & Sons, Chichester New York Brisbane Toronto Singapore, pp. 913-923
29. Marks ME, Kim RY, Salter MM (1990) Radiotherapy as an adjunct in the management of Merkel cell carcinoma. Cancer 65: 60-4
30. **McAfee WJ, Morris CG, Mendenhall CM *et al.* (2005) Merkel cell carcinoma: treatment and outcomes Cancer 104: 1761-4**
31. Mehrany K, Otley CC, Weenig RH *et al.* (2002) A Metaanalysis of the Prognostic Significance of Sentinel Lymph Node Status in Merkel cell Carcinoma. Dermatol Surg 28: 113-7
32. Mojica P, Smith D, Ellenhorn JDI (2007) Adjuvant radiation therapy is associated with improved survival in Merkel cell carcinoma of the skin. J Clin Oncol 25: 1043-7
33. Morrison WH, Peters LJ, Silva EG *et al.* (1990) The Essential role of radiation therapy in securing locoregional control of Merkel cell carcinoma. Int J Radiat Oncol Biol Phys 19: 583-91
34. Müller A, Keus R, Neumann N *et al.* (2003) Management of Merkel cell carcinoma: case series of 36 patients. Oncol Rep 10: 577-85
35. Poulsen M, Rischin D, Walpole E *et al.* (2003) Trans-Tasman Radiation Oncology Group. High-risk Merkel cell carcinoma of the skin treated with synchronous carboplatin/etoposide and radiation: a Trans-Tasman Radiation Oncology Group Study – TROG 96:07. J Clin Oncol 21: 4371-6
36. Poulsen MG, Rischin D, Porter I *et al.* (2006) Does chemotherapy improve survival in high-risk stage I and II Merkel cell carcinoma of the skin? Int J Radiat Oncol Biol Phys 64: 114-9
37. Ratner D, Nelson BR, Brown MD et al. (1993) Merkel cell carcinoma. J Am Acad Dermatol 29: 143-56
38. Salvador Alonso R, Lahbabi I, Ben Hassel M *et al.* (2008) Recurrences of Non Metastatic Merkel Cell Carcinoma after Surgery and Radiotherapy Occur More Frequently Outside the Irradiated Fields Int J Radiat Oncol Biol Phys 72: S508
39. Shintani SA, Foote RL, Lowe VJ *et al.* (2008) Utility of PET/CT Imaging Performed Early After Surgical Resection in the Adjuvant Treatment Planning for Head and Neck Cancer Int J Radiat Oncol Biol Phys 70: 322-9
40. Smith PD, Patterson JW (2001) Merkel cell carcinoma (neuroendocrine carcinoma of the skin). Am J Clin Pathol 115: S68-78
41. Su LD, Lowe L, Bradford CR *et al.* (2002) Immuno-staining for cytokeratin 20 improves detection of micrometastatic Merkel cell carcinoma in sentinel lymph nodes. J Am Acad Dermatol 46: 661-6

42. Tai PT, Yu E, Winquist E *et al.* (2000) Chemotherapy in neuroendocrine/Merkel cell carcinoma of the skin: case series and review of 204 cases. J Clin Oncol 18: 2493-9
43. Tang CK, Toker C (1978) Trabecular carcinoma of the skin: an ultrastructural study. Cancer 42: 2311-21
44. Toker C (1972) Trabecular carcinoma of the skin. Arch Dermatol 105: 107-10
45. Van Gele M, Boyle GM, Cook AL *et al.* (2004) Gene-expression profiling reveals distinct expression patterns for Classic versus Variant Merkel cell phenotypes and new classifier genes to distinguish Merkel cell from small-cell lung carcinoma. Oncogene 23: 2732-42
46. Voog E, Biron P, Martin JP *et al.* (1999) Chemotherapy for patients with locally advanced or metastatic Merkel cell carcinoma. Cancer 85: 2589-95
47. Wagner JD, Evdokimow DZ, Weisberger E *et al.* (2004) Sentinel node biopsy for high-risk nonmelanoma cutaneous malignancy. Arch Dermatol 140: 75-9
48. Yiengpruksawan A, Coit DG, Thaler HT *et al.* (1991) Merkel cell carcinoma. Prognosis and management. Arch Surg 126: 1514-9

Langerhans cell histiocytosis (LCH)

M.H. Seegenschmiedt

5

Five Essential Points

1. *LCH is a rare disease, in which uncontrolled proliferation of Langerhans cells involves one or more body systems or tissues, which leads to different clinical manifestations. Children are mostly affected, but also adults develop LCH, and differential diagnosis should include LCH.*
2. *Single-system disease is the predominant clinical presentation and accounts for more than 60% of patients. The skeleton is the mostly affected organ system.*
3. *An important prognostic parameter is single- (only one organ/organ system or tissue involved) versus multi-system (more than one organ/organ-system or tissue involved) disease.*
4. *Radiotherapy is an important and effective tool for local lesions in both single- and multi-system disease. Usually low doses in the range of 8-20 Gy are applied leading to high local reponse rates, but open questions remain.*
5. *Chemotherapy is a very important and effective tool in multi-system disease, nevertheless there remain open questions. Outcome to initial systemic therapy has been found to be a prognostic factor in disease.*

Introduction

Langerhans cell histiocytosis (LCH) is a rare semimalignant disease involving uncontrolled clonal proliferation of Langerhans cells, *i.e.* abnormal cells deriving from bone marrow and capable of migrating from skin to lymphnodes. LCH can involve one or more body systems or tissues, leading to different clinical manifestations. The disease is part of a group of clinical syndromes called histiocytoses characterized by pathologic proliferation of histiocytes (a former term for dendritic cells and macrophages). These diseases are related to other forms of abnormal proliferation of white blood cells, such as leukemias and lymphomas.

LCH used to be called histiocytosis X, but was renamed in 1985 by the Histiocyte society and nowadays includes other diseases previously designated as eosinophilic granuloma, Hand-Schüller-Christian syndrome or Abt-Letterer-Siwe disease.

Although LCH is considered to be a typical pediatric disease, more and more adults are newly diagnosed and disease diagnosed in childhood can continue during adult life. In contrast, primary isolated pulmonary LCH (mostly in adults) represents a special entity, requiring (non-radiotherapeutic) treatment, and is not addressed in this chapter [42].

General

Epidemiology & etiology

LCH is a very rare disorder with an incidence of 0,2-1 per 100,000 children under the age of 15 years with a slight preponderance for the male gender [28, 41]. More than two thirds of LCH are diagnosed in childhood, but adults can also be affected. The incidence in adults may be underestimated due to wrong or incomplete differential diagnosis in this age group, reliable epidemiological data only exist for children [20, 22, 30].

The etiology of LCH is unknown [21, 25]. Langerhans cells belong to the normal human cellular environment, especially the mononuclear-phagocytic system, however their transformation to pathologic cell clones via bone marrow precursor cells remains unclear. Clonal proliferation is found in isolated and disseminated LCH, but clonality itself is not a prognostic factor. Harms and Müller as well as Liebermann *et al*. considered LCH to be a benign, possibly reactive process according to their clinical and pathologic findings, and found no evidence of a hereditary cause [20, 30]. An immune dysregulation and viral infection are further discussed but, as yet, not confirmed. In contrast, smoking has been identified as an essential risk factor especially in LCH of adults and in primary isolated pulmonary LCH [42].

Pathohistology and pathophysiology

Langerhans histiocytes are antigene-presenting dendritic cells of the mononuclear-macrophage system derived from pluripotential stem cells. Maturation extends from proliferating monoblasts and promonocytes (in bone marrow) to nonproliferating monocytes in the blood and various peripheral tissues. The more immature the L cells are, the more acute are the clinical manifestations: promonocytes and monocytes are found in monocytic leukemia, mature macrophages often occur in uni- or multifocal osseous LCH.

Using electron microscopy Birbeck granules can be identified, which is the most reliable diagnostic criterion for LCH. Langerhans cells display an intense CD 1a surface antigen-reaction and a strong staining for S-100 [15, 20,]. Cell proliferation ranges from 3% to 48%, and parallel, clinical manifestations range from small, slowly developing lesions to rapidly progressive lesions with a highly proliferating growth pattern [30]. Three different stages can be found:

1. The *proliferative stage* which is defined by proliferative Langerhans histiocytes with clinical lesions situated in cutaneous manifestations and due to a large proliferation index- in superficial lymph nodes.
2. The granulomatous stage which is characterized by various cell types: Langerhans histiocytes, eosinophilic, macrophages, giant-cells, lymphocytes and neutrophilic cells can be found; lesions occur in uni- or multifocal bony disease (previously eosinophilic granuloma) and represent a longer disease history.
3. The *xanthomathous or scaring stage*, in which Langerhans cells absorb lipids, obscuring their correct identification; this stage was previously seen in Hand-Schüller-Christian-disease.

The final result of a spontaneously healing lesion is an unspecific scar.

Radiotherapeutic rationale

The exact target mechanisms or cells affected by radiotherapy in LCH remain unclear. Even low doses of ionizing radiation which do not reach a normal cell-killing level have been shown to induce partial or even complete remission of disease; thus, either radiotherapy suppresses an inflammatory process with cascades of enzymes as in other benign diseases and so reduces *de novo*-Langerhans cells, or Langerhans cells are very sensitive to irradiation [18, 38].

Clinical course of disease

Single-system LCH is the predominant clinical presentation responsible for more than 60% of all patients In almost two-thirds of all cases, the most frequent presentation is single- and multi-system disease of the bone. The frequency of isolated involvement of skin, hypothalamic-pituitary area, or lymph nodes is much lower. Single-system LCH usually has a "benign course" even with possible spontaneous remission [22, 30, 41]. The percentage of reactivation in osseous single-system disease is reported to be as low as 18% in a larger series [41]. Howarth *et al.* found a large difference in osseous recurrences between patients with unifocal (11%) and multifocal lesions (60%) [22]. In both series, disease reactivation was defined as either local recurrence of the initial lesion or development of other lesions in the skeleton. They also observed 5% local recurrences [22].

The frequency of reactivated non-osseous single-system LCH, apart from pulmonary disease, cannot be evaluated reliably due to lack of large clinical series. The definition of disease reactivation in involvement of the hypothalamic-pituitary area is difficult, because most patients need hormone replacement therapy [37]. The course of solitary cutaneous or lymph node involvement is unpredictable and can vary from spontaneous complete remissions to a rare generalization of disease [41]. It is unknown, how often single-system advances to multi-system disease, but it seems to be a rare event [41]. Multi-system disease is more aggressive than single-system disease, requiring a systemic therapy. Spontaneous remissions may also occur in multi-system disease, but this less frequent than in single-system disease.

Diagnostic work-up

Diagnostic staging is most important, as the patient´s history and physical examination are difficult to interpret due to the possibility of other unspecific disease. Histological biopsy and clinical examination can ensure the definitive diagnosis, whereas the other diagnostic procedures including imaging and laboratory testing have to define, in each case, the extent of disease on which to base further therapeutic decisions.

Clinical work-up

Bony manifestations of LCH may lead to local pain and/or swelling. In osseous single-system LCH, symptoms can develop over many years. Other symptoms – depending on anatomical site – may involve exophthalmus, otitis media, tooth loss or hearing impairment; neurologic deficits (dysesthesia or paraplegia) are found in patients with extensive disease of the spine. Dermal LCH is associated with unclear pruritus, generalized rash, mucosal changes, unclear soft tissue swelling or symptoms lasting over months or years with changing degrees of extent and possible spontaneous remissions. Polydypsia and polyuria point to a hypothalamic-pituitary LCH involvement. Lymphadenopathy without infection may present as a first symptom of the disease. Dyspnoea, tachypnoea or cough can occur in the pulmonary type of LCH.

Careful examination of the whole skeleton is necessary paying attention to the skull, spine, pelvis, long bones, ribs, and mandible, as these sites account for over 50% of all LCH cases [24]. Lymph nodes have to be evaluated, especially the cervical chain. Despite low incidence, a baseline neurological examination is recommended, so as not to overlook advanced bony lesions in the skull, base of skull or spine being associated with neurological and endocronological deficits.

The whole skin requires careful examination, especially scalp, external ears and intertriginous areas. Careful examination of the oral mucosa and gingiva can reveal isolated mucosal lesions or mucosal lesions combined with underlying bony manifestations. Percussion and auscultation of the lung is a basic requirement to identify possibly advanced stages of lung disease, as pulmonary LCH occurs in up to 42% of cases. Abdominal palpation can reveal possible hepatomegaly and/or splenomegaly in multi-system disease.

Diagnostic imaging

Plain radiography reveals lytic bony lesions with poorly to well-defined margins with or without sclerosis. Larger and more aggressive cases appear with moth-eaten bony destruction and poorly defined margins. Skull lesions are lytic with sharp borders and a "punched out" appearance. Oral LCH displays "floating teeth" resulting from complete destruction of the underlying bone leaving the teeth without any bony contact. Advanced lesions of the spine present a collapse of vertebral bodies, known as "vertebra plana". Lesions in long bones are typically of oval shape. Healing bony lesions display trabeculation and recalcification of lytic areas, development of sclerosis in nonsclerotic lesions, and loss of distinct margins.

Plain radiography is also useful to detect interstitial lung disease or superimposed infections and pneumothorax. In advanced stages, nodular, reticular, and reticonodular pulmonary opacities and diffuse cysts can be detected ("honeycomb" appearance). Even today, radiographic skeletal survey remains the first recommended diagnostic tool for evaluation of bony involvement in LCH.

Computed tomography (CT) and magnetic resonance imaging (MRI) provide detailed information about soft tissue involvement with or without bony disease, or about bony lesions in anatomically complex areas [31]. MRI determines lesion extent, marrow edema, and soft tissue involvement. Ultrasonography identifies intra-abdominal lymphadenopathy, hepatomegaly, splenomegaly and lymphadenopathy or soft tissue involvement in other regions of the body accessable to the examination. Bone scintigraphy is a complementary imaging technique to detect skeletal lesions with increased uptake of radionuclide activity even before radiographic defects are visible. Scintigraphy determines the activity of bony lesion and differentiates quiescent and active lesions with impact on treatment decision or monitoring the response to treatment (follow-up). Positron emission tomography (PET) is a very innovative diagnostic imaging method useful for staging or evaluating early response [3].

Laboratory testing

The following tests should be carried out:

- Urinary status may identify patients with diabetes insipidus caused by an hypothalamic-pituitary LCH involvement.

- Liver function tests provide information about possible hepatic infiltration and successive dysfunction in multi-system disease.
- Endocrine evaluation can reveal abnormal growth hormone levels, abnormal FSH/LH levels with hypogonadism, abnormal prolactin levels with galactorrhoea, or abnormal TSH levels with hypothyroidism.
- Immunologic parameters (*e.g.*, immunoglobulin levels, T and B cell number and function) can identify combined immunodeficiency cases presenting as LCH.

Histological examination

Histological examination of suspicious lesions is the only definitive diagnostic test. Material can be obtained by ultrasonography-, CT- or MR-guided biopsies, by open biopsies of bones or other involved tissues (*e.g.* skin, gum, lymph node), by curettage of bony structure, or by resection of parts of the bone or other involved tissues. The material for histological examination has to be sufficient, and preserved carefully to allow a definitive diagnosis.

Staging systems

The most important classification is the definition of two categories of disease extent by The Histiocyte Society, differentiating between "Single-system disease" (only one organ/organ system or tissue involved) and "Multi-system disease" (more than one organ/organ system or tissue involved at the same time) [26]. Other advanced classifications are shown on Tables 1A-C [11, 16, 19].

Treatment

Most patients receive multiple treatments – simultaneously or sequentially with a short gap between different therapies. Thus, interpretation of treatment results according to treatment modality is difficult and complicated by variations in age

Table 1A – Staging system according to Egeler and D´Angio [11].

Restricted LCH - Biopsy proven skin rash, no other site of involvement. - Monostotic lesion, with or without diabetes insipidus, adjacent lymph node involvement or skin rash. - Polyostotic lesions, consisting of several bones or more than two lesions in one bone, with or without diabetes insipidus, adjacent lymph node involvement or skin rash.
Extensive LCH - Visceral organ involvement with or without bone involvement, diabetes insipidus, adjacent lymph node involvement and skin rash but without signs of organ dysfunction. - Visceral involvement, with or without bone lesions, diabetes insipidus, adjacent lymph node involvement and skin rash with signs of organ involvement of lung, liver or haemopoeitic system.

Table 1B – Staging system according to Gadner *et al.* [16].

Stage 1	Isolated uni- or bifocal bone involvement.
Stage 2	Multifocal bone involvement.
Stage 3	Involvement of all soft tissues, with or without bone involvement, with no organ dysfunction.
Stage 4	All patients with liver, lung, or bone marrow dysfunction.

5

Table 1C – Staging system according to JCRT [19].

Stage	Description
IA	Single, monostotic bone lesion.
IB	Multiple lesions in one or more bones.
II	> 24 months of age at diagnosis, plus one or more of the following: diabetes insipidus, involvement of teeth or gingiva, lymph node involvement, skin involvement or seborrhoea, mild lung involvement, or focally positive bone marrow.
IIIA	< 24 months of age with involvement of any system listed in stage II.
IIIB	> 24 months of age with liver or spleen involvement, massive nodal involvement; advanced lung involvement; diffuse bone marrow involvement.
IV	Spleen > 6 cm below costal margin and fever for over 1 month with or without any or all of the above systems involved.
V	"Special" monocytosis in peripheral blood in addition to stage III or stage IV findings.

and other prognostic factors such as clinical stage. Usually there is a lack of differentiation between therapy results in adolescents and children, variations in radiotherapy, chemotherapy, and chemotherapeutic agents.

Surgery

Surgical intervention can range from open biopsies of suspicious lesions – to allow a definitive diagnosis of disease – to complex reconstructive bone surgery in spine lesions. The aim is the complete removal of lesions to reach a persistent local control.

No clinical studies have been reported with regard to surgery in adult patients, while various pediatric reports (not detailed here) show relatively good results after surgery alone or with adjuvant radiation therapy.

Chemotherapy

Systemic treatment of multi-system disease aims at reducing or even eradicating the pathologic cell clones in the involved organ system and tissue in order to reach a complete or partial systemic disease control [7]. Single-agent chemotherapy as first-line treatment minimizes treatment-related morbidity [17]; poor responders may still have the possibility to benefit from salvage chemotherapy [10, 16, 33]. Chemotherapy is also applied for (progressive) single-system disease to obtain durable local control in patients with multifocal osseous single-system disease [41].

The AIEOP-CNR-HX 83 study prospectively tested the outcome of patients stratified into good and poor prognostic groups according to the absence or presence of organ dysfunction at time of diagnosis [8]. The treatment of the good prognosis group consisted of the sequential use of vinblastine (for 3 months), followed by doxorubicin (for 3 months), and finally etoposide (equally for 3 months). The poor risk group received 9 courses of combination therapy including vincristine, cyclophosphamide, doxorubicin and prednisolone. After an observation time of 4 years, 92% of 84 evaluable patients were alive. The complete response rate after the different monotherapy periods was 63% with vinblastine, 43% with doxorubicin and 88% with etoposide. In the poor risk group, only 2 out of 11 patients (18%) had a complete remission. 6 patients died and 7 had chronic disease.

Another multi-agent regimen for multi-system disease was published by Egeler *et al.* including cytosine arabinoside, vincristine and prednisolone [10]. Eight of 10 patients without organ dysfunction and 5 of 8 patients with organ dysfunction at diagnosis reached complete remission of disease after an observation period between 3 and 12 years.

The two DAL-HX 83 and DAL-HX 90 studies prospectively registered newly diagnosed patients to follow their courses and tested the hypothesis that in disseminated LCH intensified chemotherapy initiated soon after diagnosis would decrease disease activity and mortality and prevent recurrences and chronic disease [16]. 275 patients under the age of 18 years were entered in both studies. Minkov *et al.* reported the findings of both studies in patients with multi-system disease and found an overall response to applied therapy in 56 of 63 patients (89%) at any time during the disease course [33]. Thirteen of these patients had complete remissions, 37 patients continuous regression of disease. In 9 patients, progressive disease was seen and the last 4 patients had stable disease (no change). Nearly 90% of responders achieved response within the 6 weeks of initial treatment and 92% of responders were disease free at last evaluation. In contrast, 8 of the 9 non-responders died within a median time of 6 months.

The first international randomized LCH-I trial of The Histiocyte Society prospectively assessed the effectiveness and toxicity of a 6-month treatment with vinblastine *versus* etoposide in previously untreated patients [17]. 148 patients (of whom 143 were evaluable) under the age of 18 years were entered in the study. Vinblastine and etoposide were equally effective. An overall response occurred in 88 of 143 patients (62%) at varying times during the course of the disease. Twenty-nine patients (20%) died within a median time of 6 months from diagnosis. The second international randomized LCH-II study of The Histiocyte Society is still ongoing. Multiagent chemotherapy is used in all patients and inclusion of etoposide is randomly assigned. The aim is the assessment of the effectiveness of etoposide [29].

Bisphosphonates

Bisphosphonates have been prospectively proven to be of use in the treatment of bony metastases of breast cancer, prostate cancer, and multiple myeloma. They can be used in (multiple) bony lesions in osseous single-system disease or in bony lesions in multi-system disease of LCH. The role of bisphosphonates in unifocal bony lesions (in osseous single-system disease) sofar remains unclear. The aim is the reduction of pathologic bone arrosions and support of bony remodeling. A possible problem in children is the lack of data on possible long-term effects on growing bone [23]. In addition, bisphosponates seem to affect pulmonary LCH due to antimacrophage activity [5].

Elooma *et al.* reported on the use of pamidronate in two adults with multifocal osseous single-system disease to achieve pain relief, regression of lesions, and biochemical evidence of decreased bone resorption [13]. Arzoo *et al.* reported that pamidronate in a 23-year-old woman with multifocal bony involvement in multi-system disease resulted in complete pain relief and in stabilization of lesions [1].

Immune therapy

Corticosteroids are used as local or systemic therapy. Bony, cutaneous, subcutaneous, and mucosal lesions in both single-system and multi-system disease are treated by intralesional or perilesional infiltrations often combined with the transcutaneous biopsy. Systemic corticosteroids are applied in multi-system disease parallel to chemotherapy to reach systemic disease control. In the LCH-I study all

5

patients received one initial dose of high-dose methylprednisolone to relieve general symptoms (swelling, pain, fever). Immune modulation with cyclosporine A was reported as an adjuvant treatment option in high-risk patients with progressive multi-system disease. Thalidomide and Psoralen ultraviolet A (PUVA) therapy are treatment options in cutaneous LCH.

Minkov *et al.* reported a series of 26 patients receiving cyclosporine A [32]. Regression was observed in 15% of the patients. Culic *et al.* reported on 3 patients, who received interferon-α (IFN-α) as consolidation therapy after induction chemotherapy with etoposide [9]. All patients remained disease-free.

Bone marrow transplantation was reported from Stoll *et al.* in one patient with progressive multi-system disease, who remained disease-free for more than 41 months after transplantation [39].

As reported in a meta-analysis comprising 53 patients, Bertram *et al.* confirmed immobilization as an adequate therapy in bony lesions in the cervical spine [2].

Radiotherapy

Radiotherapy is applied for symptoms and anticipation of possible clinical complications and problems. Radiotherapy should be considered only when it is clearly warranted by the presence of disease progression or when location and extent of disease are a threat to the functioning of critical organs [6].

For radiotherapy the optimal dose and a dose-effect relationship has still not been established. So far, the recommended total doses are 6 to 10 Gy in children and 15 to 20 Gy in adults, but these recommendations have to be carefully reviewed [6].

Management and clinical outcome after radiotherapy can be divided into outcome results in osseous single-system disease, non-osseous single-system disease, and multi-system disease.

Table 2 summarizes the possible radiotherapeutic indications which have been applied in the past.

Table 2 – Indications for radiation therapy in LCH.

- Functionally inoperable bony lesions.
- Difficulty to operate on bony lesions.
- Bony lesions that recur despite other therapies.
- Recurrent bony lesions after surgical removal (?).
- Wide bony lesions after surgical removal (?).
- Incompletely resected bony lesions (?).
- Progressive bony lesions under other therapies.
- Otologic involvement.
- Ulcers of skin, vulva, oral cavity and digestive tract.
- Large lymph nodes causing dyspnea or atelectasis.
- Partial diabetes insipidus.
- Lesions associated with severe pain and other symptoms.

Radiotherapy for osseous single-system disease

Literature data concerning radiotherapy in LCH deal with uni- or multifocal osseous single-system disease. Series with more than seven patients are presented in a textbook for non-malignant disorders [36, 38]. Kilpatrick *et al.* summarize 106 patients

with predominance of unifocal bony disease [25]. The age of these patients ranged from 0 to 71 years with a clear majority of children. More than two thirds of the patients were treated by radiotherapy alone. If adjuvant treatment modalities were used, mostly surgery was applied. Total dose of radiotherapy, if mentioned at all, usually ranged from 3 to 43 Gy.

As in cancer treatment, local control in Langerhans cell histiocytosis is defined as either complete remission, partial remission, no change, or as progressive disease. A complete remission requires a radiographically-proven complete disappearance of the respective lesion. Progressive disease is present, if signs of a further local progression are documented within the region treated by radiotherapy. Local control rates range from 79-100% with less than 100%-local control rate only in some of the cited clinical series. Complete remission rates also range from 79 to100% with a 100% complete remission rate in some series.

Figure 3 demonstrates a complete remission of an unifocal bony lesion in osseous single-system disease following radiotherapy alone up to a dose of 16 Gy.

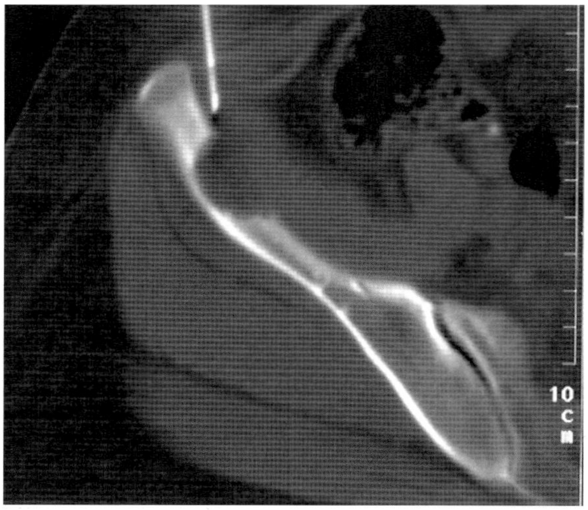

Fig. 1. 42 year old female with unifocal lesion in the right os ilium (single-system disease).

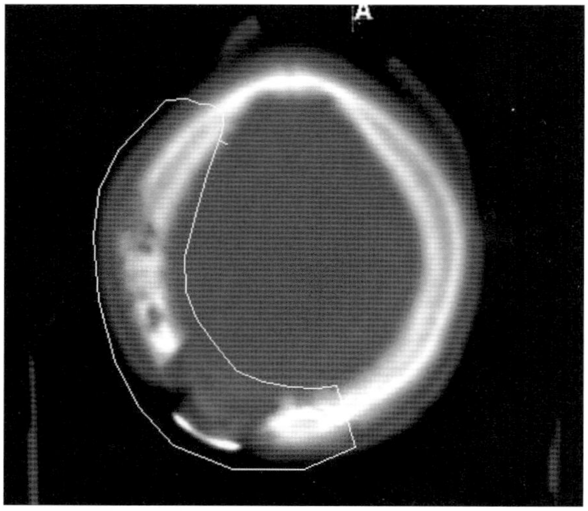

Fig. 2. 24 year old male with parietal and parieto-occipital skull lesion as part of a multifocal single-system osseous LCH: planning-CT with outlined planning target volume.

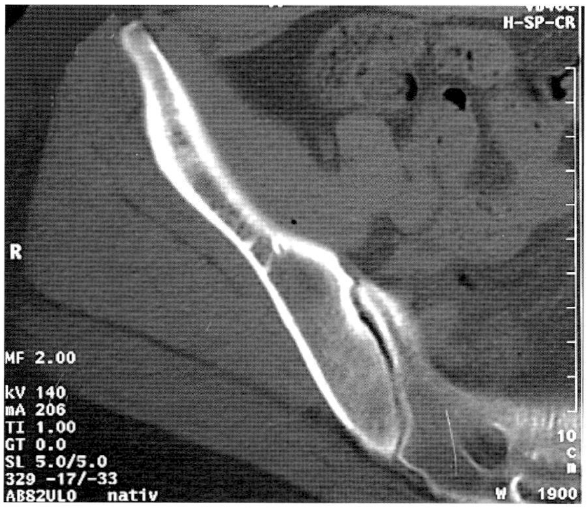

Fig. 3. Patient in Figure 1 with unifocal lesion in the right side of the pelvis (os ilium) in osseous single-system disease: post-radiotherapy CT 25 months after radiotherapy alone (16 Gy) showing complete recalcification.

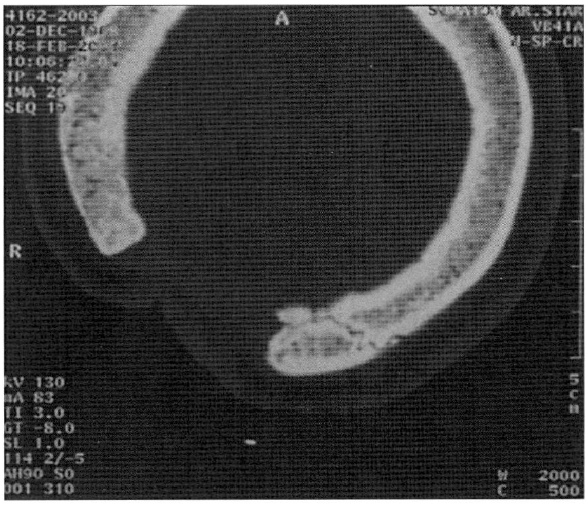

Fig. 4. Patient in Figure 2 with bony lesions in the parietal and parieto-occipital skull in multifocal osseous single-system disease: post-radiotherapy CT 3 months after radiotherapy showing mostly recalcification in addition to the bony resection.

The bony structure in the right pelvis has been restored completely without further signs of a disease activity.

Figure 4 reveals an early response of multifocal bony lesions in osseous single-system disease following radiotherapy alone up to a dose of 20 Gy. The bony structure has been restored mostly with small remaining lytic parts of the initial lesion.

Radiotherapy for non-osseous single-system disease

Few data exist concerning radiotherapy in non-osseous single-system disease, and is mostly presented as single case reports. The organ system which is most often irradiated in non-osseous single-system disease is the hypothalamic pituitary area associated with diabetes insipidus. In such cases, treatment outcome has to be divided into radiographic and laboratory response. Laboratory response is defined by the need for antidiuretic hormone (ADH) replacement therapy. In most cases, irradiation with doses of approximately 6 Gy (in children) to 18 Gy (in adults) leads to a complete normalization of the initially thickened tissue in the pituitary area, but not to a normalization of laboratory parameters. Nevertheless, Rosenzweig *et al.* saw two complete remissions (radiographic and laboratory) with the best prognosis for those patients, in whom radiotherapy started immediately after diagnosis [37].

Circumscribed dermal and mucosal lesions can resolve with radiotherapy alone, but more extensive lesions can also recur.

LCH of the brain is usually treated with a combination of surgery and postoperative irradiation often leading to complete remissions.

Results of radiotherapy in non-osseous series with more than five patients since 1970 are presented in a recent textbook on radiotherapy for non-malignant disorders [38]. The largest series are the ones from Greenberger *et al.* with 83 patients, and from Kilpatrick *et al.* with 66 patients [19, 25]. The age of the patients ranged from 0 to 71 years with a clear majority of children. The usual adjuvant treatment was chemotherapy due to its effect in multi-system disease. Total dose of radiotherapy, if mentioned, ranged from 1,4 to 45 Gy. Local control rates range from 75% to 100%, complete remission rates from 0-85%.

Radiotherapy for multisystem disease

In a German multicentre patterns-of-care study the current clinical experience with radiotherapy of Langerhans' cell histiocytosis in adults was evaluated in 123 institutions by use of a questionnaire. Only 23 of the 123 institutions (18.7%) reported

clinical experience with radiotherapy of Langerhans' cell histiocytosis of adults. Eighteen institutions with 98 patients were evaluable. The majority of patients (72 of 98) was treated on a linear accelerator. The median single dose of radiotherapy was 2 Gy, while the median total dose was 24 Gy. Eighty-one of 89 evaluable patients (91%) reached a local control of the treated lesion(s), 69 of those had a complete remission. Eight of 89 patients (9%) developed an in-field recurrence, 87.8% of patients while experienced no acute and 97% of patients no late side effects of radiotherapy. In conclusion, clinical experience with radiotherapy of Langerhans' cell histiocytosis in adults in Germany is still very limited. Nevertheless, the clinical result, high remission and local control rates, confirm the effectiveness of radiotherapy in the multidisciplinary treatment of this disease. Future patients should be systematically included into a prospective radiotherapy registry [35, 38].

Discussion

Treatment Indications

Decisions regarding treatment should be well balanced between expected morbidity from the disease and expected morbidity of the treatments given. It should be considered that there is a high chance of spontaneous resolution and favourable outcome in patients who have single-system disease, and the risk of a secondary progression to multi-system disease is rare.

Surgery, radiotherapy or their combination are the mostly used treatments. Intralesional injection of corticosteroids can lead to local healing. While chemotherapy usually is not indicated in solitary osseous lesions, it can be an excellent option for recurrent lesions. The role of bisphosphonates in unifocal osseous single-system disease has not yet been defined.

Radiotherapy indications are:

1) recurrent lesions following resection or other treatments,
2) functional inoperable (or difficult to operate) lesions in certain body sites, or
3) lesions, where surgery would lead to functional loss [6, 12].

Radiotherapy may be indicated after resection of wide and/or recurrent lesions, or as an adjuvant form of therapy after incomplete resection of lesions. Radiotherapy can be used as first-line therapy and as an alternative to other forms of treatment in all parts of the skeleton.

Multifocal bony lesions in osseous single-system disease often require local treatment of one or more lesions due to pain and/or imminent fractures or neurological complications caused by osseous involvement of the spine [4, 6, 19, 25, 43]. Bisphosphonates induce remission and prevent osseous progression [13, 14, 23]. Chemotherapy reduces the incidence of reactivation and disease morbidity. Thus, Titgemeyer *et al.* suggests an early start of systemic therapy, even in cases of rapid osseous progression [41].

Isolated LCH-lesions of skin, mucosa may be allowed to resolve without treatment, but in case of associated complications such as pain, swelling, or ulceration with bleeding, excisions, psoralen ultraviolet A-therapy, radiotherapy or injection of corticosteroids may be necessary. A special entity is the isolated involvement of the hypothalamic-pituitary area, in which rapidly given radiotherapy can lead to complete remissions [37].

Treatment of disseminated LCH is difficult due to a very high mortality rate, and probability of spontaneous remission in multi-system disease is low. It seems

to be important to reach an early response using multi-agent chemotherapy to discriminate between responders and non-responders. Progression under effective chemotherapy is a poor prognostic factor; adjuvant immune modulation or bone marrow transplantation can be salvage strategies [17, 34].

Sequelae of treatment

Late effects of surgery can be persisting osseous defects or loss of function following extensive resections of bony lesions, especially the possibility of development of a scoliosis in the pretreated spine. The risk of secondary leukemia, as an important possible late effect of chemotherapy, is reported as being about 1% in patients treated with etoposide [17].

As the total dose of radiotherapy rarely exceeds 20 Gy, acute and sub-acute side effects are very rare. Most literature data do not provide any information about acute side effects of radiotherapy. We recommend a systematic registration of such effects and the use of the Common Toxicity Criteria (CTC) score.

Radiotherapy also bears a small risk of secondary malignancies. Greenberger *et al.* report a rate of 3.9% for induction of malignant tumours [18]. Due to higher life expectancy, cured children have a higher probability of developing malignant tumours than adults. In addition, the use of older radiotherapy techniques may play a role. As there is a known tendency of patients with LCH to develop second malignancies, it is difficult to relate these to any form of treatment [26, 29].

Prognostic factors

Prognostic factors in patients with Langerhans cell histiocytosis have been established many years ago and were confirmed by Gadner *et al.* (2001) [17]. Age under 2 years, involvement of more than 4 organs with dysfunction, are important negative prognostic factors in this disease.

The French Langerhans' Cell Histiocytosis Study Group found male sex, involvement of lymph nodes, bone marrow and liver, partial response and failure to treatment to be significant variables for a poor prognosis in multivariate prognostic analysis [40].

Howarth *et al.* found, that important factors for predicting recurrent disease included both bone and mucocutaneous involvement, both osseous and extra-osseous involvement, relapse after treatment of patients with osseous and multisystem disease, more than 2 bones involved, the presence of mucous membrane LCH, and the presence of hepatosplenomegaly in patients less than 3 years of age at presentation [22].

Involvement of more than 2 bones also was associated with a poor prognosis in the series of Kilpatrick *et al.* [25].

In patients with poor prognostic factors, Gadner *et al.* found a positive impact of the response to the initial 6 weeks of treatment [17]. This new prognostic factor had a more significant effect on outcome than did the factor of age at diagnosis and an effect equal to that of the extent of organ involvement at diagnosis. The importance of response to initial therapy as a prognostic factor was confirmed by Minkov *et al.* [33].

References

1. Arzoo K, Sadeghi S, Pullarkat V (2001) Pamidronate for bone pain from osteolytic lesions in Langerhans´-cell histiocytosis. N Engl J Med 345: 225
2. Bertram C, Madert J, Eggers C (2002) Eosinophilic granuloma of the cervical spine. Spine 27: 1408-13

3. Blum R, Seymour JF, Hicks RJ (2002) Role of 18FDG-positron emission tomography scanning in the management of histiocytosis. Leukemia Lymphoma 43: 2155-7
4. Boutsen Y, Esselinckx W, Delos M, Nisolle JF (1999) Adult onset of multifocal eosinophilic granuloma of bone: A long-term follow-up with evaluation of various treatment options and spontaneous healing. Clin Rheumatol 18: 69-73
5. Brown RE (2001) Bisphosphonates as alveolar macrophage therapy in pulmonary Langerhans cell histiocytosis? Med Pediatr Oncol 36: 641-3
6. Cassady JR (1987) Current role of radiation therapy in the management of histiocytosis X. Hematol Oncol Clin N Am 1: 123-9
7. Ceci A, Terlizzi MD, Colella R *et al.* (1988) Etoposide in recurrent childhood Langerhans cell histiocytosis: An italian coopoerative study. Cancer 62: 2528-31
8. Ceci A, Terlizzi MD, Colella R *et al.* (1993) Langerhans´cell histiocytosis in childhood: Results from an Italian Cooperative AIEOP-CNR-HX 83 study. Med Pediatr Oncol 21: 259-64
9. Culic S, Jakobson A, Culic V *et al.* (2001) Etoposide as the basic and interferon-alpha as the maintenance therapy for Langerhans cell histiocytosis: A RTC. Pediatr Hematol Oncol 18: 291-4
10. Egeler RM, De Kraker J, Voute PA (1993a) Cytosine-arabinoside, vincristine, and prednisolone in the treatment of children with disseminated Langerhans cell histiocytosis with organ dysfunction: Experience at a single institution. Med Pediatr Oncol 21: 265-70
11. Egeler RM, D'Angio GJ (1995) Langerhans cell histiocytosis. J Pediatr 127: 1-11
12. El-Sayed S, Brewin TB (1992) Histiocytosis X: does radiotherapy still have a role? Clin Oncol 4: 27-31
13. Elooma I, Blomqvist C, Porkka L *et al.* (1989) Experiences of clodronate treatment of multifocal eosinophilic granuloma of bone. J Intern Med 1: 59-61
14. Farran RP, Zaretski E, Egeler RM (2001) Treatment of Langerhans cell histiocytosis with pamidronate. J Pediatr Hematol Oncol 23: 54-6
15. Favara BE, Feller AC, Pauli M *et al.* (1997) Contemporary classification of histiocytic disorders. Med Pediatr Oncol 29: 157-66
16. Gadner H, Heitger A, Grois N *et al.* (1994) A treatment strategy for disseminated Langerhans cell histiocytosis. Med Pediatr Oncol 23: 72-80
17. **Gadner H, Grois N, Arico M *et al.* (2001) A randomized trial of treatment for multisystem Langerhans´cell histiocytosis. J Pediatr 138: 728-34**
18. Greenberger JS, Cassady JR, Jaffe N *et al.* (1979) Radiation therapy in patients with histiocytosis: Management of diabetes insipidus and bone lesions. Int J Radiat Oncol Biol Phys 5: 1749-55
19. Greenberger JS, Crocker AC, Vawter G *et al.*. (1981) Results of treatment of 127 patients with systemic histiocytosis (Letterer-Siwe Syndrome, Schuller-Christian Syndrome and Multifocal Eosinophilic Granuloma). Medicine 60: 311-38
20. Harms D, Müller KM (2001) Pathologische Aspekte der Langerhans-Zell-Histiozytose. Mit besonderer Berücksichtigung auch der pulmonalen LCH. Pathologe 22: 175-83
21. Herzog KM, Tubbs RR (1998) Langerhans cell histiocytosis. Adv Anat Pathol 5: 347-58
22. Howarth DM, Gilchrist GS, Mullan BP *et al.* (1999) Langerhans cell histiocytosis. Diagnosis, natural history, management, and outcome. Cancer 85: 2278-90
23. Kamizono J, Okada Y, Shirahata A, Tanaka Y (2002) Bisphosphonate induces remission of refractory osteolysis in Langerhans cell histiocytosis. J Bone Miner Res 17: 1926-8
24. Kilborn TN, Teh J, Goodman TR (2003) Paediatric manifestatios of Langerhans cell histiocytosis: A review of the clinical and radiological findings. Clin Radiol 58: 269-78
25. **Kilpatrick SE, Wenger DE, Gilchrist GS *et al.* (1995) Langerhans´cell histiocytosis (histiocytosis X) of bone. A clinicopathologic analysis of 263 pediatric and adult cases. Cancer 76: 2471-84**
26. Ladisch S, Gadner H (1994) Treatment of Langerhans cell histiocytosis – Evolution and current approaches. Br J Cancer 70(Suppl 13): 541-6
27. **Ladisch S, Gadner H, Arico M *et al.* (1994) A randomized trial of etoposide *vs* vinblastine in disseminated Langerhans cell histiocytosis. The Histiocyte Society. Med Pediatr Oncol 23: 107-10**
28. Ladisch S, Jaffe ES (1995) The histiocytoses. In: Pizzo PA, Poplack DG (eds) Principles and practice of pediatric oncology. Lippincott, Philadelphia, pp 617-30

29. Ladisch S (1998) Langerhans cell histiocytosis. Curr Opin Hematol 5: 54-8
30. Lieberman PH, Jones CR, Steinman RM *et al.* (1996) Langerhans cell (eosinophilic) granulomatosis. A clinicopathologic study encompassing 50 years. Am J Surg Pathol 20: 519-52
31. Meyer JS, De Camargo B (1998) The role of radiology in the diagnosis and follow-up of Langerhans cell histiocytosis. Hematol Oncol Clin North Am 12: 307-26
32. Minkov M, Grois N, Broadbent V *et al.* (1999) Cyclosporine – a therapy for multisystem Langerhans cell histiocytosis. Med Pediatr Oncol 33: 482-5
33. Minkov M, Grois N, Heitger A *et al.* (2002) Response to initial treatment of multisystem Langerhans cell histiocytosis: An important prognostic indicator. Med Pediatr Oncol 39: 581-5
34. Minkov M, Grois N, Braier J *et al.* (2003) Immunosuppressive treatment for chemotherapy-resistant multisystem Langerhans cell histiocytosis. Med Pediatr Oncol 40: 253-6
35. **Olschewski T, Seegenschmiedt MH and the German Cooperative Group on "Radiotherapy for Benign Diseases" (2006) Strahlentherapie der Langerhans-Zell-Histiozytose. Ergebnisse und Schlussfolgerungen einer nationalen Patterns-of-Care-Studie. Strahlentherapie und Onkologie 182: 629-34**
36. Olschewski T, O Micke, MH Seegenschmiedt (2008) Langerhans Cell Histiocytosis. In: Seegenschmiedt MH, HB Makoski, KR Trott, LW Brady (eds) Radiotherapy for Non-Malignant Disorders-Contemporary Concepts and Clinical Results. Springer-Verlag, Berlin, Heidelberg, New York, ISBN10: 354062550X; 397-424
37. Rosenzweig KE, Arceci RJ, Tarbell NJ (1997) Diabetes insipidus secondary to Langerhans cell histiocytosis: Is radiation therapy indicated? Med Pediatr Oncol 29: 36-40.
38. **Seegenschmiedt MH *et al.* (2008) Radiotherapy for Non-Malignant Disorders, 1st Edition, Springer Publishers, Heidelberg New York, ISBN10: 354062550X**
39. Stoll M, Freund M, Schmid H *et al.* (1990) Allogeneic bone marrow transplantation for Langerhans´cell histiocytosis. Cancer 66: 284-8
40. The French Langerhans´Cell Histiocytosis Study Group (1996) A multicenter retrospective survey of Langerhans´cell histiocytosis: 348 cases observed between 1983 and 1993. Arch Child Dis 75: 17-24
41. Titgemeyer C, Grois N, Minkov M *et al.* (2001) Pattern and course of single-system disease in Langerhans cell histiocytosis. Data from the DAL-HX 83- and 90-Study. Med Pediatr Oncol 37: 108-14
42. Vassallo R, Ryu JH, Colby TV *et al.* (2000) Pulmonary Langerhans´-cell histiocytosis. N Engl J Med 342: 1969-78
43. Willis B, Ablin A, Weinberg V *et al.* (1996) Disease course and late sequelae of Langerhans´cell histiocytosis: 25-year experience at the University of California, San Francisco. J Clin Oncol 14: 2073-82

Section 9
Other malignancies

Primary bone lymphoma (Osteolymphoma)

1

D. Christie

Five Essential Points

1. *Primary bone lymphoma is a rare tumour and there is a lack of prospective studies. The term Osteolymphoma is proposed to avoid literature-searching problems.*
2. *The distribution of tumours reflects the location of bone marrow and there is a tendency for homing to occur.*
3. *Standard treatment for a Stage IA lesion would include CHOP-R chemotherapy and radiotherapy to a dose of 45 Gy. CNS prophylaxis would be considered for parameningeal tumours.*
4. *Five-year survival and local control rates are commonly around 75 %.*
5. *If the risk of fracture is high, orthopaedic fixation should be considered prior to treatment. There are also ways of giving the treatment that limit the risk afterwards.*

Introduction

Primary bone lymphoma (or Osteolymphoma) is a rare form of non-Hodgkin's lymphoma occurring primarily in bone. Although pathologically similar to the more common form of the disease that occurs in lymph nodes, it has some special features including patterns of presentation, the need for orthopaedic stabilisation, and a tendency to both occur and then reoccur in multiple bony sites. There are some special problems with the staging of the disease, the assessment of response to treatment and subsequent pathological fractures. The term Osteolymphoma has been proposed to overcome difficulties in literature searching.

Epidemiology

Primary bone lymphoma or Osteolymphoma (OL) is a rare form of non-Hodgkin's lymphoma (NHL) arising primarily in bone. The term Osteolymphoma was proposed [3,4] in studies from Australasia in order to overcome difficulties in literature searching, although it is yet to gain acceptance. If the terms "bone" and "lymphoma" are used in a computer search, thousands of scientific articles are identified, as nearly all articles about lymphoma of any type will mention bone marrow. If the terms "primary bone lymphoma" are used, many articles that use any one of many alternative terms, such as "primary lymphoma of bone" will be missed.

Most studies of OL are small, but there are a few large, retrospective reports [5, 18, 20]. The largest modern series is from the IELSG, which recently collected data on 499 cases in their IELSG-14 retrospective study. The Trans-Tasman Radiation Oncology Group has been conducting one of the first prospective studies, details of which are available from their website.

It is likely that early reports included cases of Ewing's sarcoma, which would later be excluded by immunohistochemistry. While the exact incidence is difficult to define, the relative incidence of OL has been described in a variety of ways, but is usually reported as either the proportion of all malignant primary bone tumours or as a proportion of all extranodal lymphomas, both usually around 5%. OL can occur in children [15], but most reports describe adults with a mean age of 45-60 years [7, 18] and a wide age range (15-99 years) and there is usually a slight predominance of males (55-60%).

OL has been noted in association with other conditions including the HIV virus [22, 28], sarcoidosis [11], Gaucher disease [2, 14], hereditary exostoses [17], Paget's disease [18, 23], osteomyelitis [18] and following some specific treatments including hip replacements [10, 27], CLL after cladarabine chemotherapy [21] and renal transplants [15]. However, because of their inconsistency, these indicate neither aetiology nor any predisposition towards the condition.

The distribution of OL at various sites around the skeleton reflects the distribution of bone marrow and thus concentrates in the axial skeleton and proximal parts of the long bones. It is possible that a homing mechanism may be active as the initial presentation of OL may involve multiple bony sites in the absence of any soft tissue disease [3]. Similarly, recurrences also tend to occur in bone. However the mechanism remains unknown and there are difficulties in distinguishing true OL from secondary involvement of bone by soft tissue lymphoma masses.

Pathology

To classify OL, a surgical biopsy is required. The maximum size of the biopsy should be limited to two millimetres as there is a risk of pathological fracture. Most reported series predate modern lymphoma classification systems, but most recent reports classify the majority of cases as diffuse large B-cell NHL. Various other types have been noted, but no other type predominates. There are case reports of T-cell OL [12] and most other histological types of lymphoma. Additional detail about pathological findings and other diagnostic issues will soon be available [6].

In early disease the most commonly affected bone is the femur [18] but every bone in the body is a potential site for OL and many case reports describe cases in specific bones, such as bones of the thumb, the feet, the jaws, etc. The commonest presenting features are pain (90%), swelling (30%), and pathological fracture (15%). Spinal cord compression and B-symptoms are both relatively uncommon at 10%. LDH levels are elevated in around 30% of patients. Most patients present with unifocal disease. Multifocal disease can present either within a single bone (monostotic disease) or in different bones (polyostotic disease). It can be difficult to determine whether a tumour has permeated a bone extensively, or whether separate tumours are present. Soft tissue disease may also be present (20%), most commonly regional nodes, although other nodes and other soft tissues can be affected. Median tumour sizes are 5 – 10 cm, but can vary widely between 1 and 30 cm. Extraosseous extension appears in around 50% of cases and can make it difficult to distinguish disease that has arisen in bone from that which has arisen in adjacent lymph nodes and involved bone secondarily.

Imaging

The typical plain film appearance of an OL tumour is lytic, around half are also blastic. The cortex can show permeative, moth-eaten or destructive patterns. Occasionally there is onion skin layering, breach of the periosteum or a sunburst appearance, although these latter features more typically occur in sarcomatous bone lesions rather than OL. CT scanning may contribute by demonstrating cortical breakthrough and extraosseous extension [16, 19]. MRI scanning may reveal the extent of disease in more detail including the replacement of trabecular bone and bone marrow by tumour [9, 24]. Bone lesions show up well on isotope bone scanning (Tc-99). PET scanning has tended to take over the role of functional imaging from gallium scanning, but often does not fully cover the limbs [26]. An example of a patient who presented with a lytic lesion in the lower femur that required fixation is shown in Figures 1-2. The patient was found on isotope bone scanning (Fig. 3) to have multiple bony sites of disease and was successfully treated using the treatments described below.

A

B

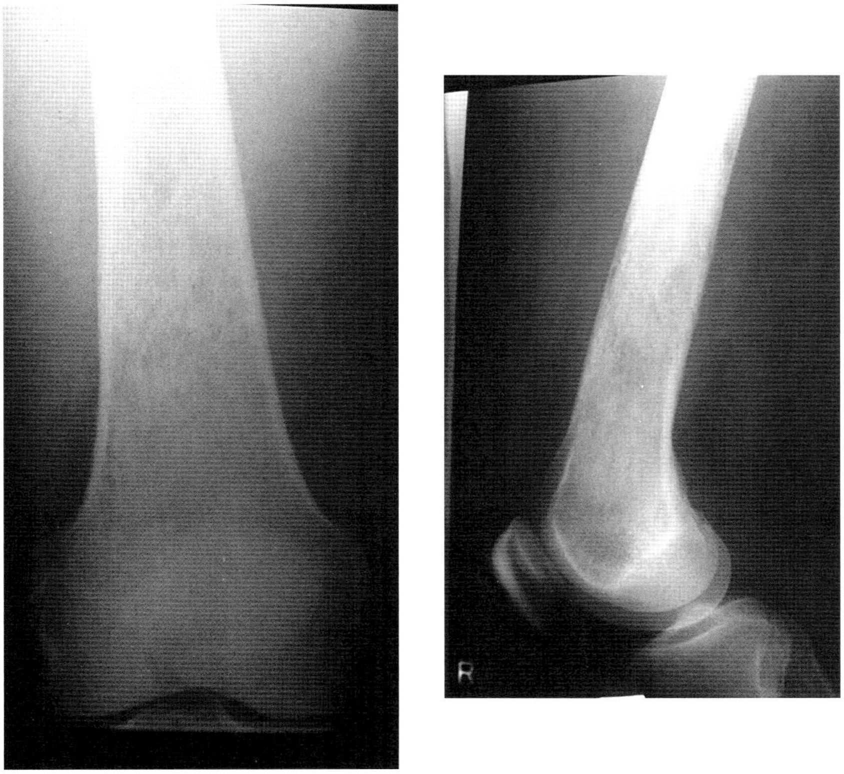

Fig. 1A and 1B. Plain films (AP and lateral views) of a patient showing a permeative OL lesion in the distal femur.

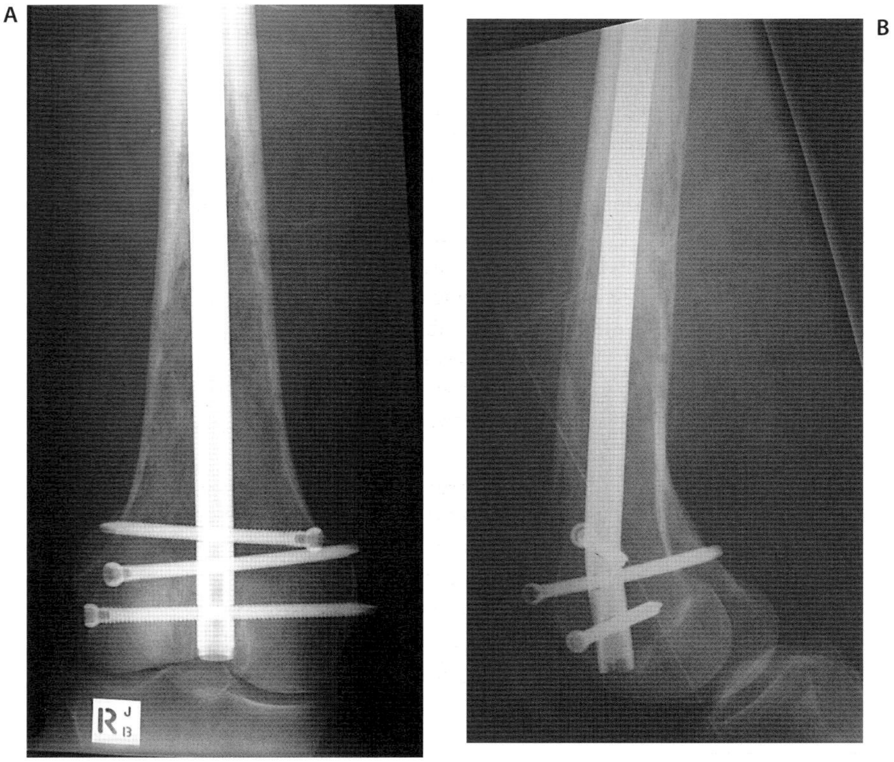

Fig. 2A and 2B. Plain films of the same patient following internal fixation.

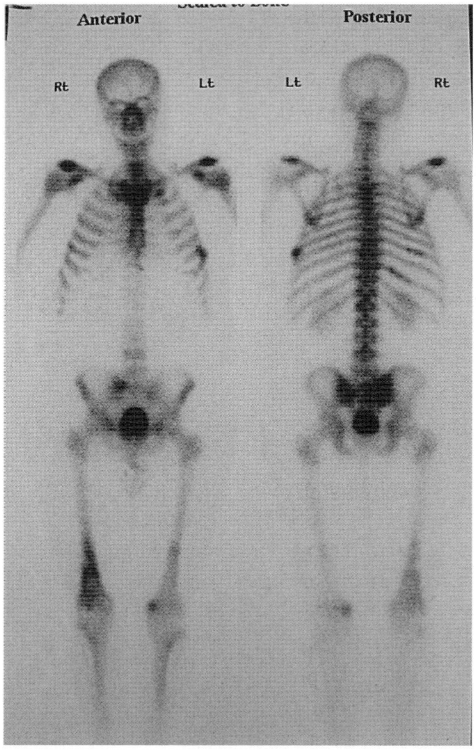

Fig. 3. Bone scan of the same patient showing additional lesions in the pelvis and rib cage.

Prognostic factors

Prognostic factors have been noted, but inconsistently. In the study by Ostrowski [18], there were significantly worse survival rates on univariate analysis for patients with multifocal disease, advanced disease, disease site (mandible and maxilla worst), presentation prior to 1960, and age over 50 years. Nineteen patients who received chemotherapy had worse survival although the difference was not statistically significant and perhaps indicated advanced disease. Others have reported multivariate analyses showing better outcomes with younger age [1, 7, 30], IPI score [20], the dose of radiotherapy [7], the use of multimodality therapy [1] and the use of rituximab [20]. The IELSG 14 study, reported in abstract, showed significantly better results with age under 60 years, ECOG performance status less than 2, normal LDH, combined modality therapy, higher radiation dose and more than three cycles of chemotherapy [5].

No established criteria for the diagnosis of OL exist, and there is disagreement over the inclusion of cases with multifocal or soft tissue disease. It would seem reasonable to include patients if they present with either a single focus of bony disease, multiple foci of bony disease, or predominantly bony disease that exceeds in volume any associated soft tissue disease. Tumours arising in parameningeal locations should be examined further with a CSF specimen and MRI scanning of the overlying dura. CNS involvement by OL is rare.

Staging

Staging is usually performed using the Ann Arbor system, but rarely identifies any patients with stage III disease. Care is required to limit the diagnosis of stage IV to those with diffuse involvement of bone marrow beyond any focus of bony disease detectable as a tumour by imaging. An International Prognostic Index (IPI) score can be assigned, such that the primary tumour does not contribute any points to the score for extranodal disease, but any other extranodal sites would do so.

Orthopaedic stabilisation and treatment

After diagnosis, orthopaedic involvement may be required to ensure stability and should be expedited so that other treatments are not delayed [8]. Staging investigations can be completed while recovering from surgery, when required.

The role of surgery is otherwise limited. Many of the first reports of OL reported treatment by radiotherapy alone, and local control rates were high (80%). However, long-term survival was limited by distant failure and no recent series has advised treatment by radiotherapy alone. Most patients reported in the last 20 years have received combined treatment with chemotherapy and radiotherapy [1, 5, 20], although wide variations in specific details of the treatments were reported when a case of OL was circulated for expert comment [29].

Chemotherapy has usually preceded radiotherapy. The most commonly used type of chemotherapy has been six cycles of conventional CHOP chemotherapy (cyclophosphamide, adriamycin, vincristine and prednisone). The chemotherapy can vary: for example the substitution of mitozanthrone to limit cardiac exposure to anthracyclines and accelerating the treatment by using a 14-day cycle with colony stimulating factors. Rituximab should be routinely added (R-CHOP) [20] for those with CD-20 positive immunohistochemistry. Intrathecal methotrexate treatment should be included for patients that have a high risk of CNS involvement.

Radiotherapy doses of 36-45 Gy in 1.8-2.0 Gy fractions are usually prescribed. The volume to be treated should consider adjacent sensitive organs such as the lung or kidney. It is usually possible to treat the whole of an affected bone while minimising the risk of late effects. Whole bone treatment overcomes the difficulty in locating the border of a permeative lesion. When whole bone treatment appears risky due to exposure of adjacent organs, wide margins (3-5 cm) around pre-chemotherapy tumour margins within bone is a reasonable alternative. Margins around the soft tissue or extraosseous borders can be further reduced to 1-2 cm around post-chemotherapy volumes where the distinction between normal and abnormal tissue is easier. For patients with multifocal disease, it is reasonable to add a lower radiation dose, say 30 Gy to areas of initially bulky tumour, providing the number and size of affected sites is limited to 2 or 3.

Responses to treatment are difficult to assess as uptake can be seen for many years on isotope bone scans and architectural effects on plain films. Rather than the traditional criteria for nodal disease, the designation of response is usually made when pain and swelling have resolved, and any abnormal soft tissue disease has resolved on imaging with CT, MRI or PET scanning. Complete response would be considered to have occurred if there is evidence of bone healing on plain films and if there are no other signs of progressive disease during the follow-up period. The description of response rates in reports of this condition should be regarded with caution. Rates of 5-year overall survival around 75% are often reported.

Toxicity

With the treatment of OL there is a special form of toxicity, which is pathological fracture. These can occur despite the absence of local recurrence. They can lead to persisting non-union of bone and disability can result if they occur in the lower limb. The risk of a fracture following treatment is likely to be higher if various features are present. These include architectural disturbance of bone due to the previous tumour, pathological fractures that were present prior to treatment, osteonecrosis due to radiotherapy, the use of higher doses of steroids in association with CHOP chemotherapy and other medical conditions such as osteomyelitis, Paget's disease and osteoporosis, particularly for older, female patients. Pathological fractures were reported in detail in two studies [13, 25] describing eleven patients with pathological fractures. These patients had relatively high radiation doses (over 50 Gy), large fraction sizes and local recurrences were present in some cases. Other reports have had much lower rates of pathological fracture than these two. To prevent fractures developing after treatment, regimens should include orthopaedic fixation of fractures before treatment where indicated, limited use of corticosteroids with chemotherapy, limited radiation doses and fraction sizes. Pain or disability after treatment should be investigated. Osteoporosis and osteomyelitis should be treated appropriately.

References

1. **Beal K, Alen L, Yahalom J (2006) Primary bone lymphoma: treatment results and prognostic factors with long term follow-up in 82 patients. Cancer 106(12): 2652-6**
2. Bohm P, Kunz W, Horny HP, Einsele H (2001) Adult Gaucher disease in association with primary malignant bone tumors. Cancer 91(3): 457-62
3. Christie D, Barton MB, Bryant G *et al.* (1999) Osteolymphoma (primary bone lymphoma): an Australian review of 70 cases. Aust NZ J Med 29: 214-9
4. Christie D, Cahill SP, Barton M (1996) Primary bone lymphoma (Osteolymphoma). Australas. Radiol. 40: 319-23
5. **Christie D, Gracias E, Mary Gospodarowicz M *et al.* (2007) Patterns of Outcome and Prognostic Factors in Primary Bone Lymphoma (Osteolymphoma): A survey of 499 cases by the International Extranodal Lymphoma Study Group. Abstract 0717 presented to the European Haematology Association 12th Congress 2007, Hematologica 92(s1): 267**
6. Christie D, Vose J (2008) Bone Lymphoma. In Cavalli F, Stein H, Zucca E. Extranodal Lymphomas: Pathology and Management. Publ. by Informa Healthcare, London, UK
7. **Fairbanks RK, Bonner JA Inwards CY *et al.* (1993) Treatement of stage IE primary lymphoma of bone. Int J Radiat Oncol Biol Phys 28: 363-72**
8. Gabel GT, Sim FH, Beabout JW *et al.* (1989) Non-Hodgkin's Lymphoma of Bone. Mayo Clinic Tumor Rounds 12(8): 1139-42
9. Hicks DG, Gokan T, O'Keefe *et al.* (1995) Primary lymphoma of bone. Correlation of magnetic resonance imaging features with cytokine production by tumour cells. Cancer 75: 973-80
10. Ito H, Shimzu A. (1999) Malignant lymphoma at the site of a total hip replacement. Orthopaedics 22(1): 82-4
11. Kobayashi H, Kato Y, Hakamada M *et al.* (2001) Malignant lymphoma of the bone associated with systemic sarcoidosis. Intern Med 40(5): 425-38
12. Lones MA, Sanger W, Perkins SL, Mediros LJ (2000) Anaplastic large cell lymphoma arising in bone: Report of a case of monomorphic variant with the t(2;5)(p23;q35) translocation. Arch Pathol Lab Med 124(9): 1339-43
13. Lucraft HH (1991) Primary lymphoma of bone: A review of 13 cases emphasising orthopaedic problems. Clin Oncol 3: 265-9
14. Manz M, Riessen R Poll L *et al.* (2001) High grade lymphoma mimicking bone crisis in Gaucher's disease. Brr J Haematol 113(1) 191-3
15. Maxymiw WG, Wood RE, Lee L (1991) Primary mulitfocal Non-Hodgkin's Lymphoma of the jaws presenting as periodontal disease in a renal transplant patient. Int J Oral Maxillofac Surg 20: 69-70
16. Mulligan ME, Kransdorf MJ (1993) Sequestra in primary lymphoma of bone: Prevalence and radiologic features. AJR 160: 1245-8
17. Neben K, Werner M, Bernd L *et al.* (2001) A man with hereditary exostoses and high grade non-Hodgkin's lymphoma of the bone. Ann Hematol 80(11): 682-4
18. **Ostrowski M, Unni KK, Banks P *et al.* (1986) Malignant lymphoma of bone. Cancer 58: 2646-55**
19. Phillips WC, Kattapuram SV, Dosoretz DE *et al.* (1982) Primary lymphoma of bone: relationship of radiographic appearance and prognosis. Diagnostic Radiol 144(2): 285-90
20. **Ramadan KM, Shenkier T, Sehn LH *et al.* (2007) A clinicopathological study of 131 patients with primary bone lymphoma: a population-based study of successively treated cohorts from the British Columbia cancer agency. Ann Oncol 18: 129-35**
21. Robak T, Kasznicki M, Bartkowiak J *et al.* (2001) Richter's syndrome following cladirabine therapy for chronic lymphocytic leukemia first manifested as pathological fracture of the femur. Leuk Lymphoma 42(4): 789-96
22. Sipsas NV, Kontas A, Panayiotkopoulos *et al.* (2002) Extranodal non-Hodgkin lymphoma presenting as a soft tissue mass in the proximal femur in a HIV+ patient. Leuk Lymphoma 43(12): 2405-7
23. Stephens GC, Lennington WJ, Schwartz HS (1994) Primary lymphoma and Paget's disease of the femur. AJCP 101(6): 783-6

24. Stiglbauer R, Augustin I, Kramer J *et al.* (1992) MRI in the diagnosis of primary lymphoma of bone: Correlation with histopathology. J Comput Assist Tomogr 16(2): 248-53
25. Stokes SH, Walz BJ (1983) Pathological fracture after radiation therapy for primary non-Hodgkin's malignant lymphoma of bone. Int J Radiat Oncol Biol Phys 9: 1153-9
26. Sweet DL, Mass D, Simon MA, Shapiro CM (1981) Histiocytic lymphoma (Reticulum cell sarcoma) of bone. JBJS 63(1): 79-84
27. Syed AA, Agarwal M, Fenelon G, Toner M (2002) Osseous malignant non-Hodgkin's B-cell Lymphoma associated with total hip replacement. Leuk Lymphoma 43(11): 2213-6
28. Thurner MM, Rieger A, Kleibl-Popov C, Schindler E (2001) Malignant lymphoma of the cranial vault in an HIV-positive patient: imaging findings. Eur Radiol 11(8): 1506-9
29. Tsang RW, Gospodarowicz MK, O'Sullivan B (2002) Staging and management of localised non-Hodgkin's lymphomas: Variation among experts in radiation oncology. Int J Radiat Oncol Biol Phys 52(4): 747-56
30. Zinzani PL, Carillo G, Ascani S *et al.* (2003) Primary bone lymphoma: Experience with 52 patients. Haematologica 88: 280-5

Erdheim-Chester disease

R.C. Miller

2

Five Essential Points

1. *ECD is a member of the Juvenile Xanthogranuloma family of non-Langerhans cell histiocytoses. Immunohistochemical staining demonstrates cells that are CD68+, CD1a-, S100weakly+ or SD100-, and Langerin- in ECD.*
2. *The clinical presentation of ECD typically consists of symmetric long bone involvement with lipid-laden macrophages. Fifty percent of patients present with visceral involvement, additionally.*
3. *Prognosis in ECD is poor in comparison to other histiocytic disorders, with a 57% rate of mortality in the largest series in the literature.*
4. *No recognized curative therapy exists. Cladribine and Interferon alpha-2a are recently recognized treatment options with systemic activity against ECD.*
5. *External beam radiotherapy can provide palliation of local symptoms, but the effect may be temporary.*

Introduction and Purpose

This chapter reviews diagnostic criteria and treatment options for Erdheim-Chester disease, a rare non-Langerhans cell histiocytosis. The rarity of this disease process has prevented the performance of clinical trials to prospectively determine treatment options. Treatment recommendations are based on individual case reports and small case series.

Classification of histiocytic disorders

Erdheim-Chester disease (ECD) belongs to a collection of disease entities involving abnormal proliferation of histiocytes. The definition of a histiocyte has expanded over time from its original conception as a macrophage to now include both macrophagic and monocytic cells involved in phagocytosis, antigen presentation, and other functions in the immune response. Histiocytic disorders form a continuum of illnesses which reflect the underlying function and extent of dedifferentiation of the type of histiocyte involved. Dendritic cells, which are involved in the presentation of foreign antigens to lymphocytic cell, were first described in the skin by Langerhans in 1868. Their presence, in immature form, or absence differentiates the histiocytic disorders into two broad categories, Langerhans cell histiocytosis (LCH) and Non-Langerhans cell histiocytosis. LCH, formerly known as Histiocytosis X, is an illness with a variable clinical course, typically affecting the bones, skin, liver, the lymphatic system, and other organs. It is a rare disorder,

2

typically affecting pediatric patients. Non-Langerhans cell histiocytic disorders fall into two categories, the Juvenile Xanthogranuloma (JXA) family and the non-JXA family. Erdheim-Chester Disease is a systemic variant of the JXA family [36, 37].

Diagnostic criteria of Non-Langerhans cell histiocytosis

Non-Langerhans cell histiocytoses are characterized by an accumulation of histiocytes that do not include a population of Langerhans cells. Langerhans cells can be recognized histopathologically by phenotype as well as through immunohistochemical staining (CD1a+/Langerin+/S100+). Within the Non-Langerhans Cell histiocytoses, JXA and non-JXA cells can be differentiated by immunostains. JXA family cells, and those of Erdheim-Chester disease, are typically positive for factor XIIIa+, CD68, CD 163, fascin, and CD14. Expression of CD1a, S100, and Langerin is typically negative or equivocal. Birbeck granules are absent [36].

In the setting of Erdheim-Chester disease, biopsies of bone tissue demonstrate lipid-laden macrophages in a fibrotic substrate. Whether the disease represents a polyclonal response induced by cytokines or whether it represents monoclonal process has yet to be defined, although monoclonal cell populations in ECD have been reported, with some investigators arguing that ECD represents a neoplastic process [11, 34]. Immunohistochemical staining demonstrates cells that are CD68+, CD1a-, S100weakly+/SD100-, and Langerin- in ECD. However, these findings must be interpreted within the clinical picture to confirm the diagnosis of Erdheim-Chester disease [2, 27].

Clinical features of Erdheim-Chester disease

Following the confirmation of the presence of a Non-Langerhans Cell histiocytosis by histopathological and immunostaining, a specific clinical diagnosis can be accomplished using two broad criteria as outlined in Figure 1: the presence or absence of cells characteristic of the JXA family and the presence or absence of cutaneous and systemic involvement of disease process.

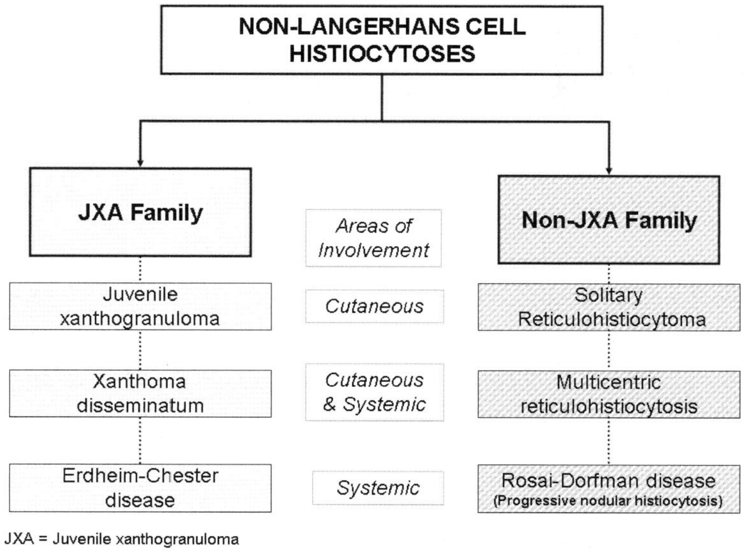

Fig. 1. The Non-Langerhans Cell histiocytoses [37].

The clinical presentation of Erdheim-Chester disease was initially noted by Chester in 1930 [10]. Patients are typically middle-aged, with a range of 7 to 84 years of age (mean 53 years) at diagnosis having been reported. Clinically, Erdheim-Chester disease is characterized by systemic involvement of lipid containing macrophages, typically presenting with involvement of the diaphyses and metaphyses of long bones, with or without involvement of other organs. The lesions appear as symmetric osteosclerosis on plain film radiographs. Figure 2 demonstrates typical symmetric uptake in bilateral tibias by radionuclide scan in the setting of Erdheim-Chester disease. In comparison to LCH, Erdheim-Chester has a greater propensity for involvement of the long bones and appendicular skeleton in contrast to the relatively greater involvement of small and flat bones in LCH. In Erdheim-Chester disease, the lower extremities are more frequently involved than the upper extremities. The later age at diagnosis, as well as typical pattern of bone involvement, differentiates ECD from xanthoma disseminatum in young children, whose histiocytes show a similar immunohistochemical staining pattern. Cutaneous lesions are less common than in most other diseases of the JXA family. Extra-osseous involvement is present in approximately 50% of cases. Retroperitoneal fibrosis, central nervous system involvement, exophthalmos, and xanthomas are common systemic manifestations. Figure 3 illustrates involvement of the brainstem as depicted by magnetic resonance imaging. Interstitial lung disease may be present

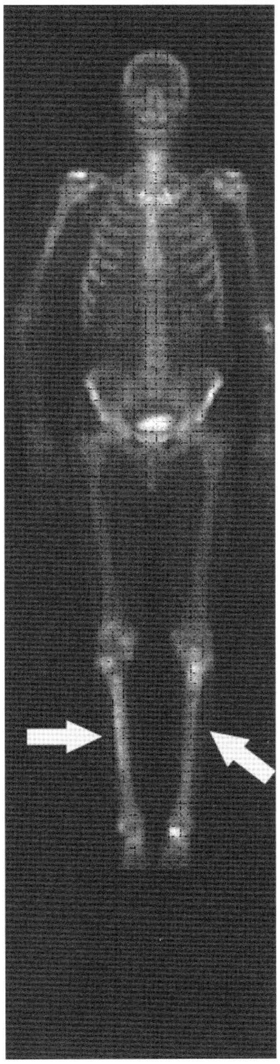

Fig. 2. Radionuclide bone scan of an ECD patient showing characteristic bilateral uptake of radionuclide in the long bones of the lower extremities.

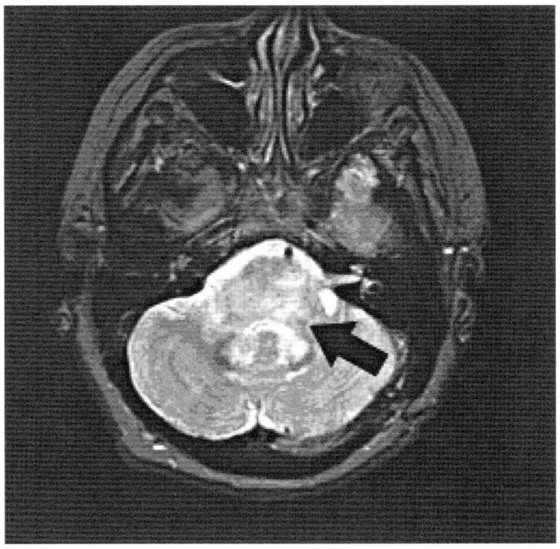

Fig. 3. Axial T2 magnetic resonance imaging scan of progressive cerebral involvement of ECD. Note involvement of brainstem, primarily on left.

in approximately one in three cases. Death from ECD typically occurs from pulmonary, either pulmonary fibrosis or respiratory failure, or cardiac failure. Prognosis in Erdheim-Chester disease is variable, with involvement of visceral organs carrying with it a more negative prognosis. Given the rarity of this disease, there are few large series in the medical literature allowing for comparison of the effects of treatment and outcomes. In the largest series reported to date, that of Veyssier-Belot *et al.*, 22 of 37 (57%) patients succumbed to the disease [8, 24, 27, 31, 35].

Systemic Therapy

No definitive treatment options yet exist for ECD. The very rare nature of the illness has prevented any systematic investigation into treatment options or the conduct of prospective research in this area. Reports of the efficacy of systemic therapy, as well as local therapy, consist of case reports and retrospective case series reviewing prior published case reports. Additionally, some patients appear in the literature in multiple manuscripts, having first been described as a case reports and then later in collected cases series, making the very limited number patients with specific treatment and outcomes data reported in the medical literature appear slightly larger than may be the case.

By analogy with Langerhans cell histiocytosis, steroids are often used for symptom palliation, although ECD can be resistant to such therapy. Cytotoxic chemotherapy such as vinca alkaloids and doxorubicin, have been employed on a case by case basis, without a definitive benefit being show. Stem cell transplantation has also been attempted. Immunosuppression has also been evaluated, also with inconclusive results [5, 6, 35]. Cladribine has been employed given its effect on monocytic cells [9, 24, 30]. Interferon alpha-2a has also been reported to have been used with success in controlling systemic ECD [7, 12, 13, 17, 23].

Local therapy

Given the diffuse nature of the underlying disease process, surgery has less of a role in the treatment of ECD in comparison to the LCH. Radiotherapy has historically been used in the treatment of LCH, both definitively as well as for palliative purposes. Additionally, its use has been explored in the treatment of non-Langerhans Cell Histocytoses, both for members of the JXA family such as such as primary orbital xanthogranulomas, and for diseases of the non-JXA family, such Rosai-Dorfman disease [15, 25, 26, 28]. By analogy, as well as given the known radiosensitivity of histiocytes, radiotherapy has also been employed for palliative treatment of lesions of ECD. No large series of ECD patients treated with palliative radiotherapy have been reported. Sporadic case reports have appeared in the literature documenting a pain response in patients receiving external beam radiotherapy for palliation of bone involvement with ECD. A reduction of pain is reported following therapy, although the long term efficacy of such treatment is difficult to ascertain based on the very limited nature published. Radiation doses employed typically range from 10 to 20 Gy, once again analogous to the treatment techniques employed for radiotherapeutic treatment of LCH [16, 20, 22]. A review of the effect of palliative radiotherapy on bone pain in six patients from the Rare Cancer

Solitary plasmacytoma

R.W. Tsang

3

Five Essential Points

1. *The median age for patients with solitary plasmacytoma is 55 – 65 years, on average about 10 years younger than those with multiple myeloma.*
2. *Radiation therapy is the standard treatment for solitary plasmacytoma, expecting local control in over 90% of cases.*
3. *Over 60% of patients with solitary plasmacytoma of bone will progress to myeloma.*
4. *Extramedullary plasmacytoma has a lower rate of progression to myeloma, approximately 25-30%.*
5. *Persistence of an elevated M-protein following radiation therapy predicts for progression to myeloma.*

Introduction

Plasma cell neoplasms comprised 22% of the mature B-cell neoplasms in the Surveillance, Epidemiology, and End Results program (SEER) of the United States [26]. The majority of these are multiple myeloma, a generalized malignancy of terminally differentiated B-cells, with localized solitary plasmacytoma accounting for less than 6% of cases. This chapter will chiefly address the management of solitary plasmacytomas, as the treatment of multiple myeloma is mainly with systemic chemotherapy and the role of local therapy is restricted for palliation of symptoms. The recommended tests for the work up of plasmacytoma are to rule out the presence of systemic myeloma, as outlined in Table 1. A diagnosis of solitary plasmacytoma is made when all the following criteria are satisfied [10]: a histologically confirmed single lesion with negative skeletal imaging outside the primary site, normal bone marrow biopsy (less than 10% monoclonal plasma cells), and no myeloma-related organ dysfunction. The median age at diagnosis of solitary plasmacytoma is 55-65 years, on average about 10 years younger than patients with multiple myeloma [28, 32, 35]. Males are affected more often (male:female ratio 2:1) [28]. A monoclonal protein (M-protein) is present in 30-75% of cases (especially for a bone presentation), usually minimally elevated (IgG < 35 g/L, IgA < 20 g/L, and urine monoclonal kappa or lambda < 1.0 g/24 h) [10, 37]. Some patients with suspected solitary plasmacytoma of bone will be upstaged following magnetic resonance imaging (MRI) detection of multiple vertebral lesions or bone marrow disease [21, 23, 36], or positivity on ^{18}F-fluorodeoxyglucose positron emission tomography (FDG-PET) [29].

Solitary plasmacytoma (SP) most commonly presents in bone (80%). Such cases are considered Stage I multiple myeloma according to the Durie Salmon staging

3

Table 1 – Diagnostic Workup for Solitary Plasmacytoma.

General • History and Physical examination • Complete blood count, and blood smear, chemistry panel including calcium and creatinine
Standard laboratory tests • Bone marrow aspirate and trephine biopsy • Serum $\beta_2$microglobulin, albumin, C-reactive protein, and lactate dehydrogenase • M-protein measurement: ➢ Serum protein electrophoresis (SPEP), and immunofixation for quantification of immunoglobulins ➢ Urine protein electrophoresis ➢ Free light chain measurements in serum and urine (if conventional M-protein is negative or equivocal)
Imaging studies • Skeletal survey • Computed tomography (CT) and magnetic resonance imaging (MRI) where indicated: ➢ To visualize soft tissue tumour, detailed assessment of local disease extent and bulk ➢ To assess vertebral column osteopenia and compression fractures, and spinal cord • Optional: ^{18}F-FDG-PET to detect local extension, or search for occult disease

system [11]. The most frequent location is the vertebra [28]. Symptoms consist of pain, neurologic compromise, and occasionally pathologic fracture. A lytic lesion is typical, sometimes with contiguous soft tissue involvement. Less commonly SP presents in an extramedullary site (20%), usually in the upper respiratory passages [1, 28, 32, 34]. The histologic diagnosis of extramedullary plasmacytoma (EMP) can be difficult, and the main differential diagnosis is extranodal marginal zone lymphoma [1, 16].

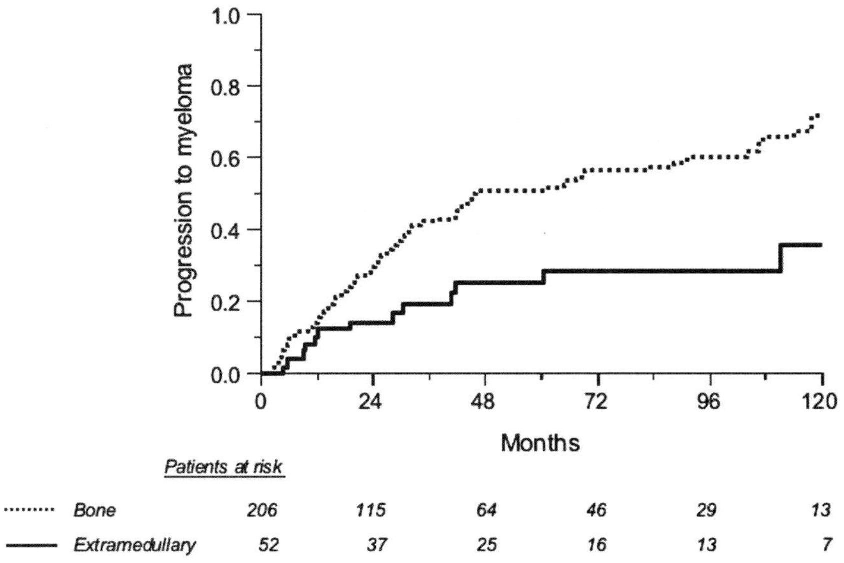

Fig. 1. Solitary plasmacytoma treated with radiation therapy (n = 258): the probability of progression to multiple myeloma according to bone (dotted line) *vs* extramedullary (solid line) localization (p = 0.0009), used with Permission from Elsevier Inc.

Management of solitary plasmacytoma

Radiation therapy (RT) is the standard treatment for solitary plasmacytoma. Surgery is considered for bone instability or fracture, or when there is rapidly progressive neurologic deterioration such as spinal cord compression [10, 31]. For patients treated with surgical excision, RT is still indicated for microscopic residual disease. Surgery alone without RT leads to an unacceptably high local recurrence rate [28]. A review of the recent literature for solitary bone plasmacytoma (Table 2) indicated a high local control rate with RT (79-91%), but a modest overall survival of approximately 50% at 10 years. This is because of a high progression rate to multiple myeloma, a finding consistently reported by many investigators (Table 2) [19, 28, 35, 37]. Over 60% of patients with solitary bone tumour will progress to myeloma (Table 2), usually within two to four years after treatment. Therefore, solitary plasmacytoma of bone appears to be an early form of multiple myeloma. The presence of low level M-protein pre-radiation is very common, and by itself is not associated with a higher risk of progression to multiple myeloma.

Table 2 – Solitary plasmacytoma: Representative treatment results in the last 15 years, 1993-2007.

First author, year	Institution	No. of patients (median f/u)	Local control	Progression to myeloma (10-year rate)	Overall survival (10-year rate)
Solitary Plasmacytoma of Bone (series including more than 30 patients):					
Galieni, 1995[13]	Siena, Italy**	32** (69 months)	91%*	~ 68%	49%
Tsang, 2001[35]	Princess Margaret Hospital	32 (95 months)	87%	64% (8-year rate)	65% (8-year rate)
Wilder, 2002[37]	MD Anderson Cancer Center	60 (94 months)	90%	62%	59%
Ozsahin, 2006[28]	RARE Cancer Network**	206** (56 months)	79% (10-year rate)	72%	52%
Extramedullary Plasmacytomas (series including more than 15 patients):					
Susnerwala, 1997[33]	Christie Hospital	25 (73 months)	79%	8%*	59% (5-year rate)
Liebross, 1999[21]	MD Anderson Cancer Center	22	95%	44% (5-year rate)	50%
Galieni, 2000[14]	Siena, Italy**	46** (118 months)	92%	15%*	78% (15 years)
Strojan, 2002[32]	Slovenia Cancer Registry	26 (61 months)	87%	8%	61%
Chao, 2005[8]	Australia**	16 (66 months)	100%	31%	54%
Ozsahin, 2006[28]	RARE Cancer Network**	52** (56 months)	74% (10-year rate)	36%	72%
Tournier-Rangeard, 2006[34]	Centre Alexis Vautrin, France	17 (80.5 months)	73% (10-year rate)	36%	63%

* Crude rate, **Multiple Institutions.

The addition of adjuvant chemotherapy to RT is theoretically attractive in an attempt to eradicate subclinical disease to prevent the disease relapsing as myeloma. One randomized trial suggested a benefit with adjuvant melphalan and prednisone given for 3 years after RT [2]. However this was a small study and the concerns regarding prolonged use of alkylating agents on the bone marrow does not justify its routine use.

For extramedullary plasmacytomas (EMP), complete surgical excision may be curative for small lesions. However most patients with larger lesions or with tumour location not amenable to complete excision should receive local RT. Postoperative RT is indicated for incompletely excised lesions. In contrast to bone localization, EMPs are well-controlled with local radiation (Table 2), with a much lower rate of progression to myeloma, ranging from 8-44% [8, 14, 22, 28, 32-34]. Therefore a substantial proportion of patients are cured of their disease. Although the 10-year survival varied widely in the recent literature (range 50%-78%), the two largest series reported 10-year survival rates of 72% [28] and 78% [14].

Radiation therapy techniques

The accurate evaluation of tumour extent is paramount to the success of RT management. MRI is extremely useful to delineate the gross tumour volume (GTV) both within and beyond bone. This is especially important for the head and neck areas (*e.g.* paranasal sinuses), where inflammatory changes may be difficult to distinguish from tumour based on CT scans. Currently, the role of FDG-PET in defining tumour extent to assist with radiation therapy planning requires further investigation.

Clinical target volumes (CTV) should encompass probable routes of microscopic spread, recognizing that barriers to the extension of local disease will vary according to anatomic location, as will the morbidity of treating adjacent normal tissues (Fig. 1). While coverage of the entire involved bone have been recommended by some authors, a study of palliative RT to only the symptomatic area for multiple myeloma found that recurrence in the untreated portion of the bone was rare [5]. Similarly, among 30 patients with solitary plasmacytoma treated with RT that encompassed only the tumour with a margin, no marginal recurrences were seen [18]. Prophylactic regional lymph node coverage is not necessary in solitary plasmacytoma of bone as the regional nodal failure rate was low after local radiation without intentional coverage of adjacent nodes (*i.e.* 0%-4%) [18, 22, 33, 35]. For EMP, nodal involvement at presentation is observed in 10-20%, and occasional nodal failure in the literature led to a common practice of extending the RT coverage to the draining lymph node region. After reviewing a series of 26 patients with EMP and contrasting the results with the literature, Strojan *et al.* concluded that prophylactic nodal radiation is probably unnecessary [32]. Therefore the need for prophylactic nodal coverage is controversial.

Planning target volumes (PTV) should account for setup variation from day to day and organ motion issues, typically adding 5-10 mm to the CTV depending on the immobilization technique employed. Overall, RT field edges are typically 2-3 cm from gross tumour seen on imaging (Fig. 2). Although parallel-opposed fields are commonly adequate to encompass disease, CT based planning and the use of conformal or intensity-modulated radiation therapy (IMRT) techniques should be used when needed to treat the PTV adjacent to critical structures. This is especially important in extramedullary disease involving the head and neck areas where avoidance of the eyes, optic pathways, and salivary glands is desirable to minimize

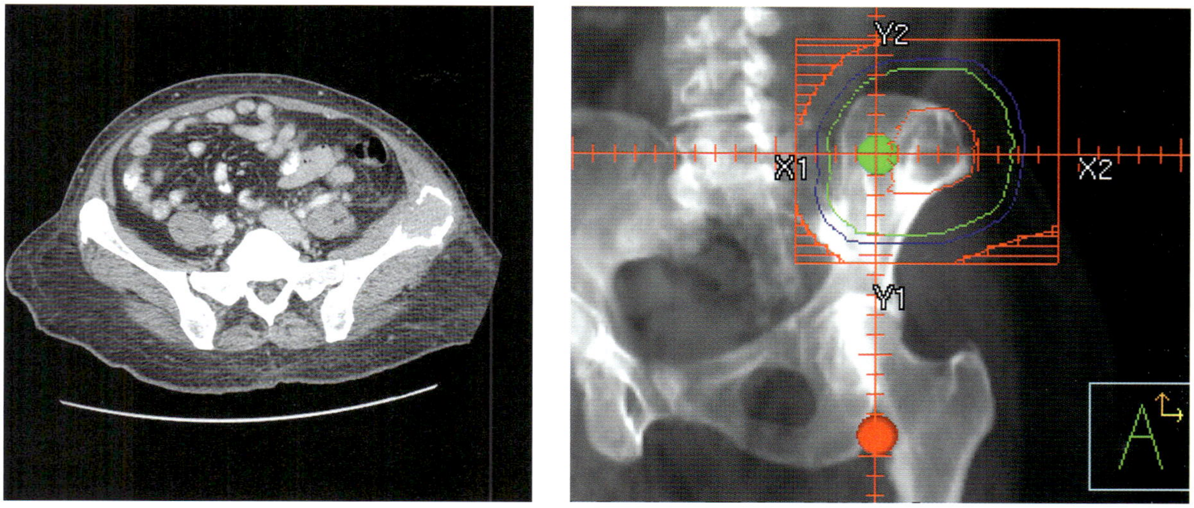

A B

Fig. 2. A solitary plasmacytoma of the left iliac bone in a 54 year old woman.

A. Axial CT scan showing 5 cm lytic bone lesion involving the superior and anterior aspect of the ilium, with a soft tissue component.

B. Radiation treatment with oblique parallel opposed fields (angled 20 degrees from the vertical), with combination of 6 MV and 18 MV beams, 4,000 cGy in 20 fractions. The contours represent the GTV (inside red line), CTV (green line), and PTV (blue line). See text for further details.

morbidity. With proper planning and treatment procedures, the RT management of plasmacytomas may produce transient local morbidity but severe late toxicity is not expected.

Radiation Therapy Dose

Reports examining RT dose-response in plasmacytoma have produced varying results. Plasmacytomas are radiation-sensitive tumours, as most studies documented response rates > 85% for patients treated with ≥ 35 Gy. Some investigators reported better local control following doses ≥ 45 Gy [12, 34], while others have found no indication of improved outcome with higher doses [18, 28]. A dose-response analysis of 81 patients by Mendenhall *et al.* led to a recommendation of a minimum dose of 40 Gy, for both bone and extramedullary lesions [25]. In that study, a total dose of ≥ 40 Gy gave a local failure rate of 6%, compared with a suboptimal 31% for lower doses [25]. Therefore the standard practice is to administer a dose of 40-45 Gy, or even higher for bulky tumours. However, in the largest of these studies (n = 258), there was no evidence of improved local control with RT doses ranging from 30-50 Gy, even for the subset of patients with tumours > 4 cm [28]. In fact there was a worse local control rate for the group receiving total dose ≥ 50 Gy, although not statistically significant [28]. Care must be exercised in interpreting these data as retrospective studies of dose-response are typically confounded by selection bias, as higher doses tend to be prescribed to larger tumours with a worse prognosis. What is known is that durable local control is obtained in > 85% of small tumours (< 5 cm) with 35 Gy-40 Gy, and there is little evidence that higher doses are necessary, regardless of bone or EMP locations. However, plasmacytomas of ≥ 5 cm have worse local control [28, 35], and doses of

45-50 Gy are recommended in these larger tumours. Despite this, one should be aware that the quality of evidence supporting the use of higher RT doses is limited, and local recurrences are still infrequently seen even after doses exceeding 50 Gy [28, 35].

Prognostic factors affecting outcome

Older age was reported to be associated with a higher risk of progression to myeloma in some studies [3, 6, 35] but not others [4, 15, 24, 28, 30]. A bony presentation was consistently demonstrated to have a higher risk of recurrence as myeloma with 10-year rate 76%, compared with an extramedullary presentation where the 10-year rate was 36% [28] (Fig. 1). Subclinical osteopenia [13] or abnormal MRI scan of the spine [23, 27, 36] reflect presence of occult disease and predicts for rapid progression to symptomatic myeloma. A suppression of the normal immunoglobulin classes, also known as immunoparesis, correlates with a higher risk of progressing to myeloma [13, 17]. Additionally, for those with an elevated M-protein pre-treatment, its persistence following RT predicts for progression to myeloma [9, 21, 37], as well as an abnormal serum immunoglobulin free light chain ratio at diagnosis [9]. Anaplastic plasmacytomas (those with a higher histologic grade) [33], and tumours with a high level of angiogenesis [20] are also associated with a poor outcome.

With respect to local control, initial tumour size is an important factor. Tumours smaller than 5 cm achieved a high level of local control with 35 Gy, whereas those 5 cm or larger had a local failure rate of 58% (7 out of 12 patients, total dose range 25-50 Gy) [35]. The importance of tumour bulk is also supported by additional studies [15, 24, 28].

Assessment of response and follow-up

Following treatment, it is common for a residual bone or soft-tissue abnormality to persist on follow-up imaging, and periodic re-imaging may be required every 4-6 months until any residual mass disappears or remains stable on consecutive scans. Following a period of stability, it is generally not beneficial to continue routine imaging of the treated site.

Since there is a significant risk of recurrence of disease as multiple myeloma, repeat measurement of the M-protein may detect the onset of systemic disease prior to the development of symptoms [7, 37]. Complete blood counts should be taken periodically to evaluate bone marrow function. The occurrence of new bone pain requires further investigations, including imaging as appropriate.

References

1. Alexiou C, Kau RJ, Dietzfelbinger H *et al.* (1999) Extramedullary plasmacytoma: tumor occurrence and therapeutic concepts. Cancer 85(11): 2305-14
2. Aviles A, Huerta-Guzman J, Delgado S *et al.* (1996) Improved outcome in solitary bone plasmacytomata with combined therapy. Hematol Oncol 14(3): 111-7
3. Bataille R, Sany J (1981) Solitary myeloma: clinical and prognostic features of a review of 114 cases. Cancer 48(3): 845-51
4. Bolek TW, Marcus RB, Mendenhall NP (1996) Solitary plasmacytoma of bone and soft tissue. Int J Radiat Oncol Biol Phys 36(2): 329-33

5. Catell D, Kogen Z, Donahue B, Steinfeld A (1998) Multiple myeloma of an extremity: must the entire bone be treated? Int J Radiat Oncol Biol Phys 40(1): 117-9
6. Chak LY, Cox RS, Bostwick DG, Hoppe RT (1987) Solitary plasmacytoma of bone: treatment, progression, and survival. J Clin Oncol 5(11): 1811-5
7. Chang MY, Shih LY, Dunn P *et al.* (1994) Solitary plasmacytoma of bone. J Formos Med Assoc 93(5): 397-402
8. Chao M., Gibbs P, Wirth A *et al.* (2005) Radiotherapy in the management of solitary extramedullary plasmacytoma. Intern Med J 35(4): 211-5
9. Dingli D, Kyle RA, Rajkumar SV *et al.* (2006) Immunoglobulin free light chains and solitary plasmacytoma of bone. Blood 108(6): 1979-83
10. **Durie BG, Kyle RA, Belch A *et al.* (2003) Myeloma management guidelines: a consensus report from the Scientific Advisors of the International Myeloma Foundation. Hematol J 4(6): 379-98**
11. Durie BG, Salmon SE (1975) A clinical staging system for multiple myeloma. Correlation of measured myeloma cell mass with presenting clinical features, response to treatment, and survival. Cancer 36(3): 842-54
12. Frassica DA, Frassica FJ, Schray MF *et al.* (1989) Solitary plasmacytoma of bone: Mayo Clinic experience. Int J Radiat Oncol Biol Phys 16(1): 43-8
13. Galieni P, Cavo M, Avvisati G *et al.* (1995) Solitary plasmacytoma of bone and extramedullary plasmacytoma: two different entities? Ann Oncol 6(7): 687-91
14. Galieni P, Cavo M, Pulsoni A *et al.* (2000) Clinical outcome of extramedullary plasmacytoma. Haematologica 85(1): 47-51
15. Holland J, Trenkner DA, Wasserman TH, Fineberg B (1992) Plasmacytoma. Treatment results and conversion to myeloma. Cancer 69(6): 1513-7
16. Hussong JW, Perkins SL, Schnitzer B *et al.* (1999) Extramedullary plasmacytoma. A form of marginal zone cell lymphoma? Am J Clin Pathol 111(1): 111-6
17. Jackson A, Scarffe JH (1990) Prognostic significance of osteopenia and immunoparesis at presentation in patients with solitary myeloma of bone. Eur J Cancer 26(3): 363-71
18. Jyothirmayi R, Gangadharan VP, Nair MK, Rajan B (1997) Radiotherapy in the treatment of solitary plasmacytoma. Br J Radiol 70(833): 511-6
19. **Knobel D, Zouhair A, Tsang RW *et al.* (2006) Prognostic factors in solitary plasmacytoma of the bone: a multicenter Rare Cancer Network study. BMC Cancer 6(1): 118**
20. Kumar S, Fonseca R, Dispenzieri A *et al.* (2003) Prognostic value of angiogenesis in solitary bone plasmacytoma. Blood 101(5): 1715-7
21. Liebross RH, Ha CS, Cox JD *et al.* (1998) Solitary bone plasmacytoma: outcome and prognostic factors following radiotherapy. Int J Radiat Oncol Biol Phys 41(5): 1063-7
22. Liebross RH, Ha CS, Cox JD *et al.* (1999) Clinical course of solitary extramedullary plasmacytoma. Radiother Oncol 52(3): 245-9
23. Mariette X, Zagdanski AM, Guermazi A *et al.* (1999) Prognostic value of vertebral lesions detected by magnetic resonance imaging in patients with stage I multiple myeloma. Br J Haematol 104(4): 723-9
24. Mayr NA, Wen BC, Hussey DH *et al.* (1990) The role of radiation therapy in the treatment of solitary plasmacytomas. Radiother Oncol 17(4): 293-303
25. **Mendenhall CM, Thar TL, Million RR (1980) Solitary plasmacytoma of bone and soft tissue. Int J Radiat Oncol Biol Phys 6(11): 1497-501**
26. Morton LM, Wang SS Devesa SS *et al.* (2006) Lymphoma incidence patterns by WHO subtype in the United States, 1992-2001. Blood 107(1): 265-76
27. **Moulopoulos LA, Dimopoulos MA, Smith TL *et al.* (1995) Prognostic significance of magnetic resonance imaging in patients with asymptomatic multiple myeloma. J Clin Oncol 13(1): 251-6**
28. **Ozsahin M, Tsang RW, Poortmans P *et al.* (2006) Outcomes and patterns of failure in solitary plasmacytoma: A multicenter Rare Cancer Network study of 258 patients. Int J Radiat Oncol Biol Phys 64(1): 210-7**
29. Schirrmeister H, Buck AK, Bergmann L *et al.* (2003) Positron emission tomography (PET) for staging of solitary plasmacytoma. Cancer Biother Radiopharm 18(5): 841-5
30. Shih L., Dunn P, Leung WM *et al.* (1995) Localised plasmacytomas in Taiwan: comparison between extramedullary plasmacytoma and solitary plasmacytoma of bone. Br J Cancer 71(1): 128-33

3

31. Soutar R, Lucraft H, Jackson G *et al.* (2004) Guidelines on the diagnosis and management of solitary plasmacytoma of bone and solitary extramedullary plasmacytoma. Clin Oncol (R Coll Radiol) 16(6): 405-13
32. Strojan P, Soba E, Lamovec J, Munda A (2002) Extramedullary plasmacytoma: clinical and histopathologic study. Int J Radiat Oncol Biol Phys 53(3): 692-701
33. Susnerwala SS, Shanks JH, Banerjee SS *et al.* (1997) Extramedullary plasmacytoma of the head and neck region: clinicopathological correlation in 25 cases. Br J Cancer 75(6): 921-7
34. Tournier-Rangeard L, Lapeyre M, Graff-Caillaud P A. *et al.* (2006) Radiotherapy for solitary extramedullary plasmacytoma in the head-and-neck region: A dose greater than 45 Gy to the target volume improves the local control. Int J Radiat Oncol Biol Phys 64(4): 1013-7
35. Tsang RW, Gospodarowicz MK, Pintilie M *et al.* (2001) Solitary plasmacytoma treated with radiotherapy: impact of tumor size on outcome. Int J Radiat Oncol Biol Phys 50(1): 113-20
36. Van de Berg BC, Lecouvet FE, Michaux L *et al.* (1996) Stage I multiple myeloma: value of MR imaging of the bone marrow in the determination of prognosis. Radiology 201(1): 243-6
37. Wilder RB, Ha CS, Cox JD *et al.* (2002) Persistence of myeloma protein for more than one year after radiotherapy is an adverse prognostic factor in solitary plasmacytoma of bone. Cancer 94(5): 1532-7

Neuroendocrine tumours

4

K. Öberg

Five Essential Points

1. *Neuroendocrine tumours are a heterogeneous group of neoplasms.*
2. *The WHO classification system with TNM staging and grading might improve future therapy.*
3. *Surgery is still a cornerstone in the management of NETs.*
4. *Somatostatin analogs are the gold standard in the treatment of functioning NETs but new data also indicate a role in non-functioning NETs.*
5. *Management of NET patients should be concentrated in centres with a specific and clinical interest.*

Introduction

Neuroendocrine tumours (NETs) constitute a heterogenous group of malignancies that are considered to be rare. However, recent data indicate that this group of tumours has significantly increased in incidence and prevalence during the last decades (Fig. 1). The current incidence and prevalence is considered to be 5.25 and 35/100,000 people respectively [58]. The tumours derive from the diffuse neuroendocrine cell-system, spread throughout the gastrointestinal tract and the bronchopulmonary system. The increase in incidence is largely due to the introduction of more sensitive diagnostic tools as well as an overall increased awareness among physicians. NETs occur most frequently in the gastrointestinal tract (60%) with the second most common localization in the bronchopulmonary system (30%) [35, 58]. NETs can be both sporadic and part of familial syndrome, such as multiple endocrine neoplasia type 1, von Hippel-Lindau syndrome and neurofibromatosis. The genetic background is not fully elucidated but the inherited forms, such as multiple endocrine neoplasia type 1, depends on loss of a tumour suppressor gene encoding for the menin protein and localized on chromosome 11q13. The disease includes tumour formation in the pituitary, parathyroids, endocrine pancreas as well as in the adrenals. Von Hippel-Lindau disease develops many different types of tumours including endocrine pancreatic tumours and pheochromocytomas. The disease develops through loss of heterozygosity at 3p25.5 gene locus. Patients with neurofibromatosis, or Von Recklinghausen's disease (NF1), have loss of the NF1-gene, which is a tumour suppressor gene that is located on 17q11.2 and encodes a protein called neurofibromin. This gene is also involved in tuberous sclerosis [43].

Classification of NETs has been previously based on embryology and is divided into foregut, midgut and hindgut tumours. This old type of classification has now been abandoned and the 2000 WHO classification of endocrine tumours attempts to divide these into:

- well-differentiated endocrine tumours (benign or uncertain behaviour),
- well-differentiated endocrine carcinomas (low-grade malignant behaviour) and
- poorly differentiated endocrine carcinomas (high-grade malignant behaviour) [51].

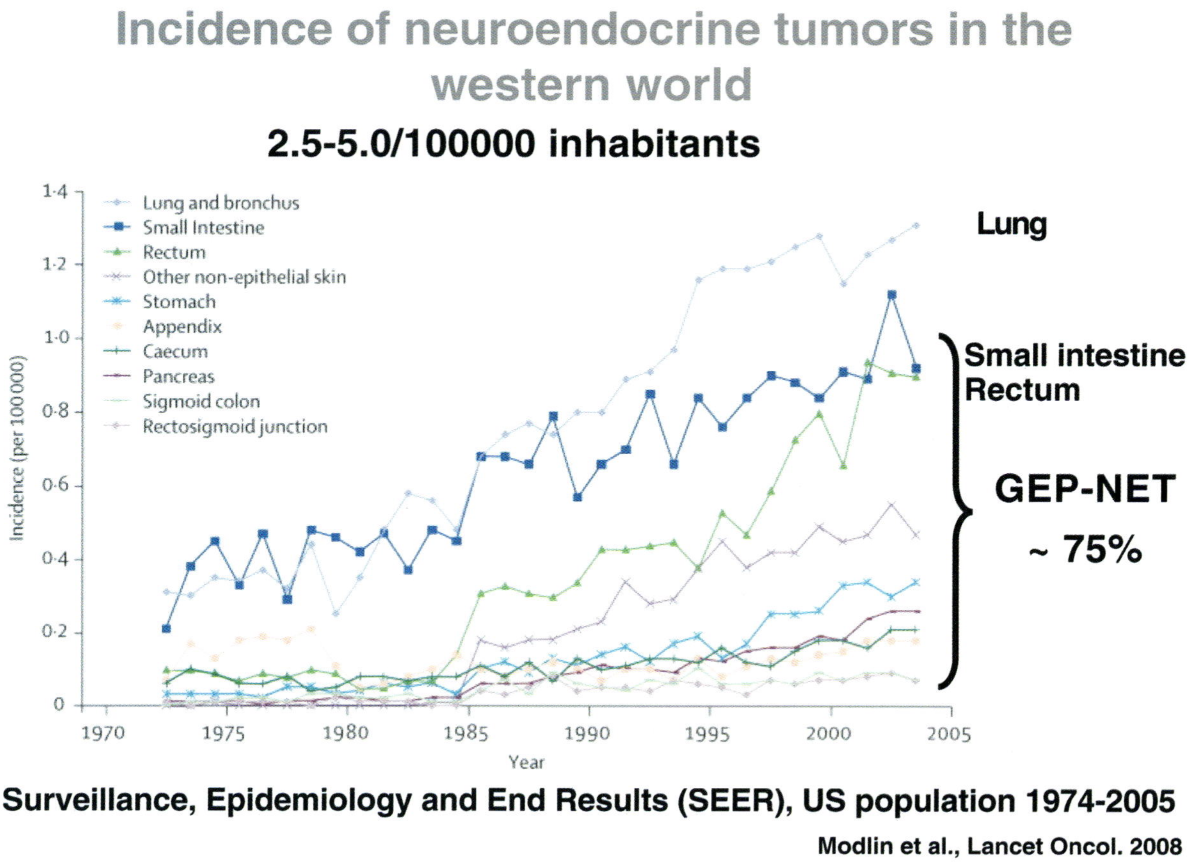

Fig. 1. Increasing incidence in NETS in the US population between 1973-2005. NETs, in all sites (appendix 250%; cecum 350%; bronchopulmonary and small intestine 420-460%; sigmoid 700%; rectum 900%, and stomach 1130%) have increased in incidence in the past 3 decades (NCI SEER database).

This classification has further been refined by the European Neuroendocrine Tumour Society (ENETS) with a TNM-classification and grading system [48]. The molecular genetic mechanism of NET development is complex and remains largely unknown. However, the new classification will give new insights into specific, genetic and molecular changes related to tumour subtypes.

The tumours tend to be slow growing (although aggressive variants exist) and often present a considerable diagnostic and therapeutic challenge. The primary tumour is usually small and clinical symptoms are often absent until the tumour has already metastasized. The majority of tumours are thus diagnosed at the stage at which the only curative treatment, radical surgery, is no longer an option.

Treatment

The treatment rationale is based on the following observations; a majority of the patients present with metastatic disease; there is a delay in diagnosis both from the side of the patient and the doctor, due to sometimes vague symptoms; a wide spectrum of clinical cause, indolent to very rapid progression; sometimes life-threatening clinical symptoms due to excessive hormone production; unique expression of peptide receptors, which can be targets for treatment; slow tumour progression makes it possible to test different therapies and finally good performance status despite extensive disease. The therapeutic objectives include amelioration of clinical symptoms, abrogation of tumour growth, improvement and maintenance of quality of life and hopefully prolongation of survival. Despite improved diagnosis and increased awareness of the disease with several therapeutic options, no significant increase in survival in metastatic disease has been obtained during the last decades in US [35, 58].

The following therapeutic options exist:

– *Surgery*
  - Resection
  - Debulking; cytoreductive
  - By-passing
  - Radiofrequency ablation
  - Liver transplantation
– *Embolization/Chemoembolization (TACE)*
  - Liver targeted
– *Radiotherapy*
  - External
  - Tumour targeted (I^{131}MIBG, Ind^{111}DTPA-Octreotide, Y^{90}-DOTATOC, Lu^{177} DOTA Octreotide)
– *Medical therapy*
  - Chemotherapy
  - Alpha interferon
  - Somatostatin analogs
  - Other biological therapies (VEGF, EGF inhibitors, RAD001).

Surgical Treatment

A majority of patients present with metastatic disease and therefore curative surgery is not an option in many cases. However, surgical interventions in combination with other treatment options, must always be considered even in individuals with incompletely resectable disease. The aim is to decrease tumour burden to facilitate symptom control and prevent complications. A more advanced surgery has evolved during the last decade and usually NETs are more easily resectable than adenocarinomas [2]. Small solitary non-invasive lesions in the stomach, duodenum and rectum can be treated with endoscopic local resection [21, 33]. For centrally localized bronchopulmonary typical carcinoids, conservative resection consisting of sleeve resection, wedge or segmental resection is the preferred treatment [10]. In atypical lung carcinoids more extensive surgical procedures such lobectomy or pneumonectomy to ensure minimum risk of recurrence is commonly advocated. Radiofrequency ablation, alcohol or cryotherapy are other debulking procedures and can be done from outside or during open surgery [2, 20]. Liver transplantation is an option in selected patients, who should be young with disease limited to the liver and not having undergone a Whipple procedure. Longterm progression-free survival is limited in patients with pancreatic endocrine tumours, whereas this somewhat better for carcinoid tumours of the small intestine [1].

Embolization and Chemoembolization

Embolization and chemoembolization is an option to reduce tumour mass and can be done at any time during the course of the disease. It has not been demonstrated whether an early embolization or a late procedure is preferable. It is also an open question whether plain embolization using microparticles (poly-vinyl alcohol or gel-foam powder) is as effective as chemoembolization with particles and cytotoxic agents. The overall results in terms of objective responses have been 25-50% for plain embolization and 35-75% for chemoembolization using microparticles together with streptozotocin or doxorubicin[19]. Most recently, embolization with radioactive beads (Y^{90}-labeled) has been introduced with encouraging results (SIR-Spheres or Spherex particles) [47]. The treatment is rather expensive and there is always the risk of leakage of the radioactive beads into the systemic circulation, in particular into the lungs. The precise role of this type of embolization has to be evaluated.

Radiotherapy (PRRT)

External beam irradiation has been used in the past with limited effect in these usually slow-growing tumours. Nowadays, therefore, external beam irradiation is only indicated for brain and bone metastases. Another type of radiotherapy that has emerged over the last decade is tumour targeted radioactive treatment or peptide receptor radiotherapy (PRRT). Radioactive MIBG (J^{131}, J^{125}) has been used in the treatment of malignant pheochromocytomas and also classical midgut carcinoid tumours with objective responses in about 20-30 % of the patients[40]. During the development of somatostatin receptor scintigraphy for detection of NETs, treatment with ^{111}Indium-DTPA-Octreotide was started with limited efficacy, with 10-15 % objective response. Today PRRT is based on ^{90}Yttrium-DOTA-Octreotide, ^{90}Yttrium-DOTATOC (emits ß-particles) and ^{177}Lutetium-DOTA-octreotate (emits ß-particles and γ-rays) [18]. The largest compilation of data on ^{177}Lutetium-DOTA-octreotate comes from the Rotterdam group indicating objective responses in 40 % (28 % PR, 16 % MR, 2 % CR) of the patients with stabilization of the disease in another 35 % [31]. Overall survival was 46 months and median survival from diagnosis was 128 months. Recent data from our own centre in 100 patients supports these results (to be published).

Medical Treatment – Chemotherapy (Table 1)

Cytotoxic treatment has been applied for treatment of NETs for more than three decades. Several different regimens of single agent or multi-agent chemotherapy have been tried with little, short-lasting or no effect in NETs. Early studies from the 1980's indicated a significant role for cytotoxic treatment in pancreatic endocrine tumours, in particular streptozotocin in combination with doxorubicin or 5FU giving objective responses in up to 70% of patients with duration of up to three years. However, recent studies using streptozotocin plus 5FU and doxorubicin report on 39% partial remission with a median response duration of 9.3 months, using more modern evaluation methods [25]. For patients with intestinal NETs such as classical midgut carcinoids, cytotoxic treatment has been of little or no value with objective responses in less than 25% of the patients with short duration (< 10 months). A recent study by Sun and co-workers using doxorubicin + 5FU or streptozotocin + 5FU or dacarbazine for metastatic carcinoids, report on a overall response rate of 16% with progression-free survival of 4.8 months [52]. Today, cytotoxic treatment is not recommended as first-line therapy for low-proliferating, well-differentiated

Table 1 – Chemotherapy.

Reference	Type of Tumour	Regimen	No. of Patients	Objective Response (%)	Response duration (months)	Median survival (months)
Moertel [37] *et al.*	Pancreatic	STZ STZ + 5-FU	42 42	36 63	17 17	16.5 26
Eriksson *et al.* [15]	Pancreatic	STZ + 5-FU or DOX	44	45	27.5	–
Moertel *et al.* [39]	Pancreatic	STZ + DOX STZ + 5-FU	36 33	69 45	18 14	26 18
Cheng and Saltz [9]	Pancreatic	STZ + DOX	16	6	18	–
McCollum *et al.* [32]	Pancreatic	STZ + DOX	16	6	3.9	20.2
Kouvaraki *et al.* [25]	Pancreatic	STZ + DOX + 5-FU	84	39	9.3	40
Moertel and Hanley [36]	Carcinoids	5-FU + cyclophosphamide STZ + 5-FU	47 42	33 33	– –	– –
Engstrom *et al.* [13]	Carcinoids	STZ + 5-FU DOX	80 81	22 21	8 6.5	16 12
Bukowski *et al.* [7]	Carcinoids	STZ + DOX + 5-FU + cyclophosphamide STZ + 5-FU + cyclophosphamide	56 9	31 22	– –	– 10.8
Sun *et al.* [52]	Carcinoids	DOX + 5-FU STZ + 5-FU	25 27	15.9 16	4.5 5.3	15.7 24.3
Moertel *et al.* [38]	Poorly differentiated	Cisplatin + etoposide	18	67	8	19
Mitry *et al.* [34]	Poorly differentiated	Cisplatin + etoposide	41	42	9	15
Fjallskog *et al.* [17]	Poorly differentiated	Cisplatin + etoposide	36	47	9	–
Kulke *et al.* [27]	Pancreatic carcinoid	Temozolomide + thalidomide	11 15	45 7	14 –	– –
Ekeblad *et al.* [12]	Foregut (pancreatic bronchial, thymus)	Temozolomide	35	14 (40% low 0^6-MGMT)	7	–
Kulke *et al.* [26]	Pancreatic carcinoid	Temozolomide + bevacizumab	18 16	24 0	9 –	– –

NETs. Poorly-differentiated NETs have demonstrated significant responses to a combination of cisplatinum (carboplatin) and etoposide with 40-60% objective responses. The same combination has not been of any benefit in well-differentiated slow-growing tumours. Temozolomide alone or in combination with thalidomide, bevacizumab or capecitabine has generated response rates of 14-60%. Patients with low expression of the enzyme O6-MGMT had a higher response rate, 40 % *versus* overall response rate of 14% [12]. Most recently, the combination of temozolomide with capecitabine and bevacizumab has generated significant antitumour responses in high proliferating tumours with Ki-67 values above 50%. This combination is now being evaluated in a larger cohort of poorly differentiated NETs.

4

Alpha Interferon

Alpha interferon was introduced in 1983 for treatment of well-differentiated low-proliferating NETs such as classical midgut carcinoids and is now registered in most European countries for treatment of low proliferating carcinoid tumours. Today more that 600 patients have been reported in the literature. Alpha interferon has an anti-proliferative effect through the blocking of the cell cycle transition from S to G_2 phase through activation of the Jak/Stat pathway. It also has an anti-angiogenic effect by inhibition of VEGF and b-FGF and it stimulates the immune system through increased natural killer cell activity. The dose has to be titrated individually, looking at the effect on bone marrow by reducing the leucocyte count to a lower normal level ($3x10^9$/Liter). Today recombinant alpha interferon, interferon-α2b (IntronA®) and interferon-α2a (Roceron®), are used at doses of 3-5MU, 3-5/week. Most recently, pegylated alpha interferons, Peg-IntronA® and Pegasys®, 50-150 µg/week have been introduced in the treatment. In 27 papers, comprising 679 patients, the median symptomatic response rate was 62%, biochemical response 50%, tumour response regression 10% and stabilisation 65%. The side-effects of alpha interferon are significant and therefore individually titrated doses are important. The most severe side-effects are chronic fatigue syndrome in up to 60% of the patients, and autoimmune reactions in 10-15% of the patients [5,11,22,41,44,46,50].

Somatostatin Analogs (Table 2, 3)

Somatostatin analogs are generally well-tolerated and long-acting somatostatin analog therapy is currently the treatment of choice for patients with functioning NETs with clinical symptoms related to hormone overproduction. Several somatostatin analogs have been developed during the last two decades: e.g. octreotide, lanreotide and vapreotide. All these have been applied in clinical trials, but today only octreotide and lanreotide are used in clinical pratice. Octreotide has an immediate release formulation (Sandostatin®) and long-acting formulation (Sandostatin LAR®) whereas lanreotide is only available as a long-acting formulation –

Table 2 – Neuroendocrine tumours. Somatostatin analogue therapy, summary of several trials.

Response		Standard dose	High dose	Slow release
		(100-1500 µg/d)	(> 3,000 µg/d)	(20-30 mg/d/2-4w)
Symptomatic n (%)		146/228 (64)	11/26 (42)	76/119 (63)
Biochemical n (%)	CR	6/54 (11)	1/33 (3)	3/119 (3)
	PR	116/211 (55)	24/83 (72)	76/119 (64)
	SD	72/211 (34)	7/33 (21)	21/119 (18)
	PD	11/211 (11)	1/33 (3)	19/119 (15)
Tumor n (%)	CR	–	1/53 (2)	–
	PR	7/131 (5)	6/53 (11)	4/119 (3)
	SD	50/131 (38)	25/53 (47)	94/119 (79)
	PD	74/131 (56)	21/51 (39)	21/119 (18)

CR, complete remission; PR, partial remission; SD, stable disease; PD, progressive disease.

Table 3 – Antiproliferative effect of somatostatin analogues in patients with progressive disease [39].

SSA	Dosage	n	CR	PR	SD	PD
Lanreotide	3000 µg/day	22	0	1	7	14
Lanreotide	30 mg/2 weeks	35	0	1	20	14
Octreotide	600-1500 µg/day	52	0	0	19	33
Octreotide	1500-3000 µg/day	58	0	2	27	29
Octreotide	600 µg/day	10	0	0	5	5
Lanreotide	15000 µg/day	24	1	1	11	11
		201	1 (0.5%)	5 (3%)	89 (44%)	106 (53%)

CR, complete remission; PR, partial remission; SD, stable disease; PD, progressive disease.

Somatuline Autogel®. Most recently, a new somatostatin analog – SOM230 or Pasireotide® – has come into clinical trials. The previous analogs, octreotide and lanreotide are octapeptides, binding preferentially to somatostatin receptor type 2 and receptor type 5 with high affinity and somewhat lower affinity for receptor type 3 [45]. However, SOM230 which is a cyclic hexapeptide binds with high affinity to somatostatin receptor 1, 2, 3 and 5 but not to 4 [6]. A majority of NETs express somatostatin receptor type 2, but more recent data have also indicated that these tumours might express receptor type 1, 3, 4 and 5 [23]. In future it will be possible to determine the specific profile of somatostatin receptor expression in each tumour using specific antibodies. New analogs that can bind to other receptors than receptor type 2 and 5 might be of benefit in the treatment. Most data on the clinical efficacy of somatostatin analogs has been generated from octreotide which has been in clinical use since the mid 1980's. The objective response rate in terms of significant tumour shrinkage is rather low, only about 5 %, but stabilization of the disease is seen in up to 40% of the patients. Biochemical responses are obtained in 40-60% of the patients and symptomatic response in 40-50% [14, 30, 42, 46, 49, 55, 56]. A very recent study (Promid-study) in metastatic carcinoid tumours evaluated in a randomized fashion, the treatment with Sandostatin LAR® 30 mg *versus* placebo [4]. A significant increase in time to progression was noted for octreotide, median 14 mo *versus* 6.0 mo, $p = 0.000072$. There was no difference between functioning or non-functioning tumours. The debate whether non-functioning tumours without hormone-related syndromes should be treated with somatostatin analogs seems to be settled by this study, indicating a role for somatostatin analogs also for this group of patients. High-dose treatment seems to be of benefit in patients resistant to standard dose of octreotide, giving significant antitumour responses [57]. A recent study with Pasireotide given in 40 patients resistant to standard octreotide LAR treatment, reported symptomatic improvement in 27% of the patients [29]. There are currently ongoing studies to compare Sandostatin LAR® with Pasireotide LAR® in patients with classical midgut carcinoid tumours. The antitumor effect of somatostatin analogs is not only inhibition of growth factor and growth factor receptor expression; there is also an effect on the immune system and an anti-angiogenic effect, also slowing down the transition from G1 to S-phase in the cell cycle [42]. A problem during longterm treatment is the development of resistance (tachyphylaxis), necessitating dose increase or withdrawal of the drug. The precise molecular mechanism has not been elucidated. The side-effects of somatostatin analog treatment are low, mainly some gastrointestinal problems such as borborygmia, diarrhea and sometimes also gallstone formation.

Combination Treatment – Alpha Interferon – Somatostatin Analog

Non-randomized trials have indicated a role of the combination of alpha interferon with somatostatin analog [54]. The theoretical background is based on data from pre-clinical studies on BON-cells and also the demonstration that alpha interferon can upregulate somatostatin type 2 receptor content. However, three randomized trials have not been able to clearly demonstrate an advantage in survival for the combination compared with single drug treatment [3, 16, 24]. However, these studies have inherited some important problems with low accrual rate of patients and the mixing of different subtypes of NETs. Ongoing randomized trials will hopefully sort out the role of the combination therapy.

Other Biological Treatments or Molecular Targeted Treatment

NETs express a large number of growth factors and growth factor receptors on the cell-surface and also in the tumour stroma [8, 53]. High expression of these molecules has stimulated the interest in using new molecular targeted treatments for NETs. The tumours are usually highly vascularised with expression of VEGF and other pro-angiogenic molecules. Therefore, treatment with VEGF inhibitors, such bevacizumab (Avastin®) and sunitinib, has been applied with responses in 10-20% of the patients [28, 61]. The PI3K-AKT mTOR pathway is also activated in NETs, which has led to treatment with inhibitors of the mTOR pathway, such as rapamycin (RAD001, Everolimus). Initial data indicate responses in up to 20% of the patients with a stabilization of the disease in 73% [60]. A recent study on RAD001 (Everolimus) (Radiant 1) in patients with cytotoxic refractory pancreatic endocrine tumours who were randomized to receive either RAD001 as single-drug or in combination with octreotide, gave partial remission in 8 % and 4% of patients respectively with progression-free survival of 9.3 and 12.9 months respectively [59].

Conclusion

Neuroendocrine tumours are a heterogenous group of tumours with varying malignant behaviour. A new WHO-classification refined with TNM-staging and a grading system might form a platform for more individualized and targeted treatment in the future. Figure 2 summarizes a treatment algorithm for neuroendocrine tumours as it stands today. New treatments have to be developed based on the unique features of neuroendocrine tumours such as peptide hormone receptor expression, APUD, characteristics and high vascularity. In centres dedicated to diagnosis and treatment of NETs, a significant improved overall survival has been obtained during the last decades (Fig. 3) but the standards of care have to be improved in general as indicated by figures from the large US database SEER [58]. The treatment of these patients should be concentrated in centres with scientific and clinical interest in these tumours.

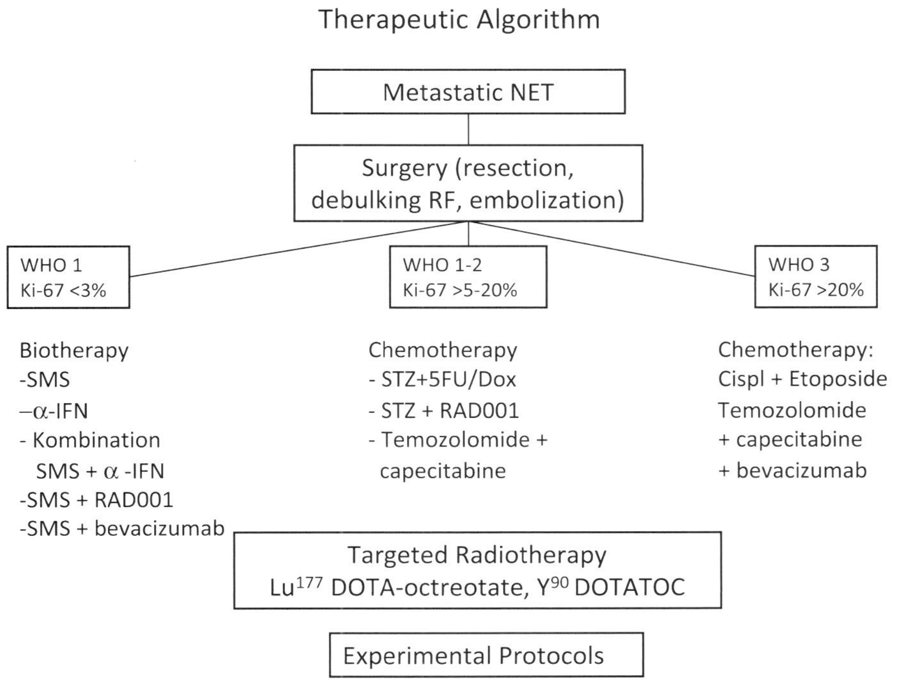

Fig. 2. Therapeutic algorithm for metastatic neuroendocrine tumours. The treatment is based on the WHO-classification for different types of NETs.

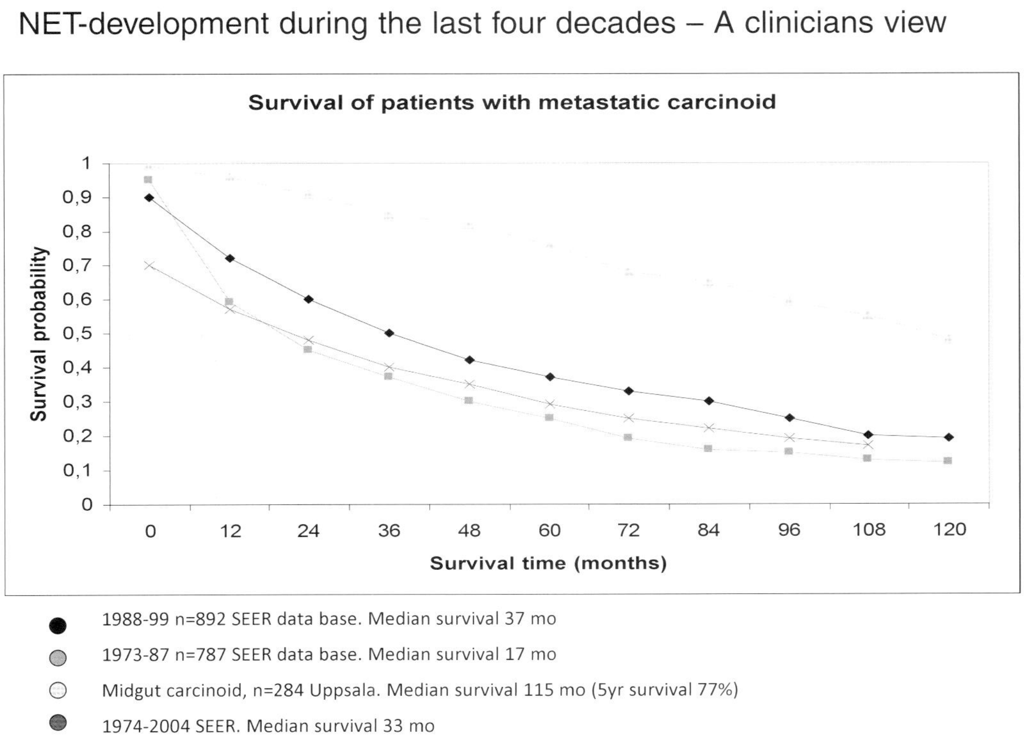

Fig. 3. Survival curves for metastatic carcinoid tumours. Note the difference in survival between a specialized centre (Uppsala) compared with standard of care in US from different time periods. The survival curve for 1973-87 is before the introduction of somatostatin analogs in the treatment.

References

1. Ahlman H, Friman S, Cahlin C *et al.* (2004) Liver transplantation for treatment of metastatic neuroendocrine tumors. Ann N Y Acad Sci 1014: 265-9
2. Akerstrom G, Hellman P (2007) Surgery on neuroendocrine tumours. Best Pract Res Clin Endocrinol Metab 21: 87-109
3. Arnold R, Rinke A, Klose KJ *et al.* (2005) Octreotide versus octreotide plus interferon-alpha in endocrine gastroenteropancreatic tumors: a randomized trial. Clin Gastroenterol Hepatol 3: 761-71
4. Arnold R *et al.* (2009) Placebo-controlled, double-blind, prospective randomized study of the effect of octreotide LAR in the control of tumor growth in patients with metastatic neuroendocrine midgut tumors: A report from the PROMID Study Group. ASCO GI Cancers Symposium. Abs.# 121. 2009
5. Biesma B, Willemse PH, Mulder NH *et al.* (1992) Recombinant interferon alpha-2b in patients with metastatic apudomas: effect on tumours and tumour markers. Br J Cancer 66: 850-5
6. Bruns C, Lewis I, Briner U *et al.* (2002) SOM230: a novel somatostatin peptidomimetic with broad somatotropin release inhibiting factor (SRIF) receptor binding and a unique antisecretory profile. Eur J Endocrinol 146: 707-16
7. Bukowski RM, Johnson KG, Peterson RF *et al.* (1987) A phase II trial of combination chemotherapy in patients with metastatic carcinoid tumors. A Southwest Oncology Group Study. Cancer 60: 2891-5
8. Chaudhry A, Funa K, Oberg K (1993) Expression of growth factor peptides and their receptors in neuroendocrine tumors of the digestive system. Acta Oncol 32: 107-14
9. Cheng PN, Saltz LB (1999) Failure to confirm major objective antitumor activity for streptozocin and doxorubicin in the treatment of patients with advanced islet cell carcinoma. Cancer 86: 944-8
10. Cooper WA, Thourani VH, Gal AA *et al.* (2001) The surgical spectrum of pulmonary neuroendocrine neoplasms. Chest 119: 14-8
11. Detjen KM, Welzel M, Farwig K *et al.* (2000) Molecular mechanism of interferon alfa-mediated growth inhibition in human neuroendocrine tumor cells. Gastroenterology 118: 735-48
12. Ekeblad S, Sundin A, Janson ET *et al.* (2007) Temozolomide as monotherapy is effective in treatment of advanced malignant neuroendocrine tumors. Clin Cancer Res 13: 2986-991
13. Engstrom PF, Lavin PT, Moertel CG *et al.* (1984) Streptozocin plus fluorouracil versus doxorubicin therapy for metastatic carcinoid tumor. J Clin Oncol 2: 1255-9
14. Eriksson B, Oberg K (1999) Summing up 15 years of somatostatin analog therapy in neuroendocrine tumors: future outlook. Ann Oncol 10 Suppl 2: S31-8
15. Eriksson B, Skogseid B, Lundqvist G *et al.* (1990) Medical treatment and long-term survival in a prospective study of 84 patients with endocrine pancreatic tumors. Cancer 65: 1883-90
16. Faiss S, Pape UF, Bohmig M *et al.* (2003) Prospective, randomized, multicenter trial on the antiproliferative effect of lanreotide, interferon alfa, and their combination for therapy of metastatic neuroendocrine gastroenteropancreatic tumors–the International Lanreotide and Interferon Alfa Study Group. J Clin Oncol 21: 2689-269655
17. Fjallskog ML, Granberg DP, Welin SL *et al.* (2001) Treatment with cisplatin and etoposide in patients with neuroendocrine tumors. Cancer 92: 1101-7
18. Forrer F, Valkema R, Kwekkeboom DJ *et al.* (2007) Neuroendocrine tumors. Peptide receptor radionuclide therapy. Best Pract Res Clin Endocrinol Metab 21: 111-29
19. Gupta S, Johnson MM, Murthy R *et al.* (2005) Hepatic arterial embolization and chemoembolization for the treatment of patients with metastatic neuroendocrine tumors: variables affecting response rates and survival. Cancer 104: 1590-602
20. Hellman P, Ladjevardi S, Skogseid B *et al.* (2006) Radiofrequency tissue ablation using cooled tip for liver metastases of endocrine tumors. World J Surg 26: 1052-6
21. Itoi T, Sofuni A, Itokawa F *et al.* (2007) Endoscopic resection of carcinoid of the minor duodenal papilla. World J Gastroenterol 13: 3763-4
22. Jacobsen MB, Hanssen LE, Kolmannskog F *et al.* (1995) Interferon-alpha 2b, with or without prior hepatic artery embolization: clinical response and survival in mid-

gut carcinoid patients. The Norwegian carcinoid study. Scand J Gastroenterol 30: 789-96
23. Kimura N, Pilichowska M, Date F *et al.* (1999) Immunohistochemical expression of somatostatin type 2A receptor in neuroendocrine tumors. Clin Cancer Res 5: 3483-7
24. Kolby L, Persson G, Franzen S, Ahren B (2003) Randomized clinical trial of the effect of interferon alpha on survival in patients with disseminated midgut carcinoid tumours. Br J Surg 90: 687-93
25. Kouvaraki MA, Ajani JA, Hoff P *et al.* (2004) Fluorouracil, doxorubicin, and streptozocin in the treatment of patients with locally advanced and metastatic pancreatic endocrine carcinomas. J Clin Oncol 22: 4762-71
26. Kulke MH (2006) A phase II study of temozolomide and bevacizumab in patients with advanced neuroendocrine tumors. ASCO annual Meeting. Abstract No. 4044 2006
27. Kulke MH, Stuart K, Enzinger PC *et al.* (2006) Phase II study of temozolomide and thalidomide in patients with metastatic neuroendocrine tumors. J Clin Oncol 24: 401-6
28. Kulke MH, Lenz HJ, Meropol NJ *et al.* (2008) Activity of sunitinib in patients with advanced neuroendocrine tumors. J Clin Oncol 26: 3403-10
29. Kvolls L (2006) Safety and efficacy of pasireotide (SOM230) in patients with metastatic carcinoid tumors refractory or resistant to octreotide LAR. Results of a phase II study. ASCO annual Meeting. Abstract No. 4082. 2006
30. Kvols LK, Moertel CG, O'Connell MJ *et al.* (1986) Treatment of the malignant carcinoid syndrome. Evaluation of a long-acting somatostatin analogue. N Engl J Med 315: 663-6
31. Kwekkeboom DJ, de Herder WW, Kam BL *et al.* (2008) Treatment with the radiolabeled somatostatin analog [177 Lu-DOTA 0,Tyr3]octreotate: toxicity, efficacy, and survival. J Clin Oncol 26: 2124-30
32. McCollum AD, Kulke MH, Ryan DP *et al.* (2004) Lack of efficacy of streptozocin and doxorubicin in patients with advanced pancreatic endocrine tumors. Am J Clin Oncol 27: 485-8
33. Merg A, Wirtzfeld D, Wang J *et al.* (2007) Viability of endoscopic and excisional treatment of early rectal carcinoids. J Gastrointest Surg 11: 893-7
34. Mitry E, Baudin E, Ducreux M *et al.* (1999) Treatment of poorly differentiated neuroendocrine tumours with etoposide and cisplatin. Br J Cancer 81: 1351-5
35. Modlin IM, Oberg K, Chung DC *et al.* (2008) Gastroenteropancreatic neuroendocrine tumours. Lancet Oncol 9: 61-72
36. Moertel CG, Hanley JA (1979) Combination chemotherapy trials in metastatic carcinoid tumor and the malignant carcinoid syndrome. Cancer Clin Trials 2: 327-34
37. Moertel CG, Hanley JA, Johnson LA (1980) Streptozocin alone compared with streptozocin plus fluorouracil in the treatment of advanced islet-cell carcinoma. N Engl J Med 303: 1189-94
38. Moertel CG, Kvols LK, O'Connell MJ, Rubin J (1991) Treatment of neuroendocrine carcinomas with combined etoposide and cisplatin. Evidence of major therapeutic activity in the anaplastic variants of these neoplasms. Cancer 68: 227-32
39. Moertel CG, Lefkopoulo M, Lipsitz S *et al.* (1992) Streptozocin-doxorubicin, streptozocin-fluorouracil or chlorozotocin in the treatment of advanced islet-cell carcinoma. N Engl J Med 326: 519-23
40. Mukherjee JJ, Kaltsas GA, Islam N *et al.* (2001) Treatment of metastatic carcinoid tumours, phaeochromocytoma, paraganglioma and medullary carcinoma of the thyroid with (131)I-meta-iodobenzylguanidine [(131)I-mIBG]. Clin Endocrinol (Oxf) 55: 47-60
41. Oberg K. (2001) Chemotherapy and biotherapy in the treatment of neuroendocrine tumours. Ann Oncol 12 Suppl 2: S111-14
42. Oberg K (2009) Somatostatin analogues. In: Howl J, Jones S (eds): Bioactive Peptides. CRC Press, Edition 2009; pp 169-187
43. Oberg K (2009) Genetics and molecular pathology of neuroendocrine gastrointestinal and pancreatic tumors (gastroenteropancreatic neuroendocrine tumors). Curr Opin Endocrinol Diabetes Obes 16: 72-8
44. Oberg K, Eriksson B (1991) The role of interferons in the management of carcinoid tumours. Br J Haematol 79 Suppl 1: 74-7

45. Patel YC (1999) Somatostatin and its receptor family. Front Neuroendocrinol 20: 157-98
46. Plockinger U, Wiedenmann B (2007) Neuroendocrine tumors. Biotherapy. Best Pract Res Clin Endocrinol Metab 21: 145-62
47. **Popperl G, Helmberger T, Munzing W *et al.* (2005) Selective internal radiation therapy with SIR-Spheres in patients with nonresectable liver tumors. Cancer Biother Radiopharm 20: 200-8**
48. Rindi G, D'Adda T, Froio E *et al.* (2007) Prognostic factors in gastrointestinal endocrine tumors. Endocr Pathol 18: 145-9
49. Ruszniewski P, Ducreux M, Chayvialle JA *et al.* (1996) Treatment of the carcinoid syndrome with the longacting somatostatin analogue lanreotide: a prospective study in 39 patients. Gut 39: 279-83
50. Shah T, Caplin M (2005) Endocrine tumours of the gastrointestinal tract. Biotherapy for metastatic endocrine tumours. Best Pract Res Clin Gastroenterol 19: 617-36
51. Solcia E, Kloppel G, Sobin L (2000) Histological Typing of Endocrine Tumours. In: Verlag S (ed) World Health Organization Histological Classification of Tumours, 2nd Edition, Springer, Berlin, Heidelberg, New York, Geneva, pp. 38-74
52. Sun W, Lipsitz S, Catalano P *et al.* (2005) Phase II/III study of doxorubicin with fluorouracil compared with streptozocin with fluorouracil or dacarbazine in the treatment of advanced carcinoid tumors: Eastern Cooperative Oncology Group Study E1281. J Clin Oncol 23: 4897-904
53. Terris B, Scoazec JY, Rubbia L *et al.* (1998) Expression of vascular endothelial growth factor in digestive neuroendocrine tumours. Histopathology 32: 133-8
54. Tiensuu Janson EM, Ahlstrom H, Andersson T, Oberg KE (1992) Octreotide and interferon alfa: a new combination for the treatment of malignant carcinoid tumours. Eur J Cancer 28A: 1647-50
55. Tomassetti P, Migliori M, Gullo L (1998) Slow-release lanreotide treatment in endocrine gastrointestinal tumors. Am J Gastroenterol 93: 1468-71
56. Tomassetti P, Migliori M, Corinaldesi R, Gullo L (2000) Treatment of gastroenteropancreatic neuroendocrine tumours with octreotide LAR. Aliment Pharmacol Ther 14: 557-60
57. Welin SV, Janson ET, Sundin A *et al.* (2004) High-dose treatment with a long-acting somatostatin analogue in patients with advanced midgut carcinoid tumours. Eur J Endocrinol 151: 107-12
58. **Yao JC, Hassan M, Phan A *et al.* (2008) One hundred years after "carcinoid": epidemiology of and prognostic factors for neuroendocrine tumors in 35,825 cases in the United States. J Clin Oncol 26: 3063-72**
59. Yao JC, Lombard-Bohas E, Baudin E *et al.* (2008) A Phase II trial of daily oral RAD001 (Everolimus) in patients with metastatic pancreatic neuroendocrine tumours (NET) after failure of cytotoxic chemotherapy. ESMO Congress Stockholm. Abs.#508PD 2008
60. Yao JC, Phan AT, Chang DZ *et al.* (2008) Efficacy of RAD001 (everolimus) and octreotide LAR in advanced low- to intermediate-grade neuroendocrine tumors: results of a phase II study. J Clin Oncol 26: 4311-8
61. Yao JC, Phan A, Hoff PM *et al.* (2008) Targeting vascular endothelial growth factor in advanced carcinoid tumor: a random assignment phase II study of depot octreotide with bevacizumab and pegylated interferon alpha-2b. J Clin Oncol 26: 1316-23